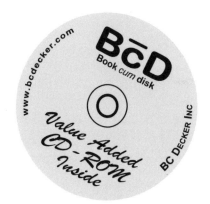

# PREFACE

It has been only nine years since the publication of the first edition of the *Atlas of Gastrointestinal Motility*. That book appeared 40 years after the publication of the first motility atlas (*Atlas of Esophageal Motility*), which was limited to the esophagus, consisted of five chapters, and was produced by a single institution (Mayo Clinic), with Dr. Charles Code as editor. By the time the first edition of the *Atlas of Gastrointestinal Motility* was published, the advances in our understanding of gastrointestinal motility and its disorders had expanded to the extent that our first edition comprised 17 chapters written by 25 contributors from a large number of centers. The fact that it took the field 40 years to reach this point and only nine years to warrant the present new edition demonstrates the rapid progress that has been made in our knowledge of gastrointestinal motility and its disorders. These advances have been made possible by new technology and by new and improved physiologic information that, in turn, has led to better comprehension, diagnosis, and treatment of disorders of gastrointestinal motility.

The present text, which consists of 33 chapters, updates the information contained in our first edition and expands its scope both in depth and breadth to include additional information in areas covered by our first *Atlas* as well as new discoveries in previously unexplored areas.

Motility disorders are disorders of neuromuscular function rather than structure. They may represent either primary disturbances of a gastrointestinal organ or part of an organ (eg, sphincters) or may result from systemic disorders (eg, sclerodema). Motility has entered a new era that transcends diagnostic boundaries and now extends to therapeutics. Today, more treatments are available for motility disorders. This step forward started with the introduction of biofeedback, initially to treat one disorder and subsequently other disorders. New treatment techniques are also being developed to electrically stimulate intestinal pacemakers and neuromuscular apparatus, and new drugs based on improved understanding of pathophysiology are being developed.

The first edition of this *Atlas* contained two major sections: one dealing with an overview of normal physiology and recording techniques, and the second dealing with application to clinical conditions. The present *Atlas* is organ centered, divided into two major parts, the second of which is composed of chapters within seven separate sections, each beginning with a description of normal physiology and recording techniques for a specific organ, followed by a clinical discussion of the pathophysiology and motility tests pertinent to that particular organ system. We feel that this organization provides a more compact and cohesive focus. (The first section deals with basic physiology of the gastrointestinal tract with an emphasis on neural and smooth muscle physiology.) In keeping with the traditional concept of an atlas, this text focuses on descriptions of techniques using graphic pictorial tracings to illustrate diagnostic and therapeutic applications of motility studies in clinical disorders.

The authors hope that this *Atlas* will help all health care providers (physicians, physician assistants, nurses, and students) and researchers interested in the neuromuscular function of the gut. We also hope that this *Atlas* will further appreciation and understanding of normal gastrointestinal motility and disorders of motility, enhance diagnostic accuracy, and thereby improve the treatment of patients with motility disorders of the digestive tract.

The field of gastrointestinal motility continues to evolve rapidly, and we look forward with anticipation to further exciting developments.

Kenneth L. Koch, MD
Michael D. Crowell, PhD
Marvin M. Schuster, MD

*Addendum*

To honor Marvin Schuster, our friend, colleague and mentor who has contributed so extensively to the field of gastrointestinal motility and whose vision led to the publication of the first edition of the *Atlas*, we and the publisher felt strongly that this book should be named the *Schuster Atlas of Gastrointestinal Motility*.

Kenneth L. Koch, MD
Michael D. Crowell, PhD

*Schuster*
*Atlas of*

# GASTROINTESTINAL
# MOTILITY

## *in Health and Disease*

### SECOND EDITION

*Schuster*
*Atlas of*
# GASTROINTESTINAL
# MOTILITY

*in Health and Disease*

## SECOND EDITION

Marvin M. Schuster, MD, FACP, FAPA, FACG

Michael D. Crowell, PhD, FACG

Kenneth L. Koch, MD

2002
BC Decker Inc
Hamilton • London

**BC Decker Inc**
P.O. Box 620, L.C.D. 1
Hamilton, Ontario L8N 3K7
Tel: 905-522-7017; 800-568-7281
Fax: 905-522-7839; 888-311-4987
E-mail: info@bcdecker.com
www.bcdecker.com

02 03 04 05 /PC/ 9 8 7 6 5 4 3 2

ISBN 1-55009-104-2

Printed in Canada

## Sales and Distribution

*United States*
**BC Decker Inc**
P.O. Box 785
Lewiston, NY 14092-0785
Tel: 905-522-7017; 800-568-7281
Fax: 905-522-7839; 888-311-4987
E-mail: info@bcdecker.com
www.bcdecker.com

*Canada*
**BC Decker Inc**
20 Hughson Street South
P.O. Box 620, LCD 1
Hamilton, Ontario L8N 3K7
Tel: 905-522-7017; 800-568-7281
Fax: 905-522-7839; 888-311-4987
E-mail: info@bcdecker.com
www.bcdecker.com

*Foreign Rights*
**John Scott & Company**
International Publishers' Agency
P.O. Box 878
Kimberton, PA 19442
Tel: 610-827-1640
Fax: 610-827-1671
E-mail: jsco@voicenet.com

*Japan*
**Igaku-Shoin Ltd.**
Foreign Publications Department
3-24-17 Hongo
Bunkyo-ku, Tokyo, Japan 113-8719
Tel: 3 3817 5680
Fax: 3 3815 6776
E-mail: fd@igaku-shoin.co.jp

*U.K., Europe, Scandinavia, Middle East*
**Elsevier Science**
Customer Service Department
Foots Cray High Street
Sidcup, Kent
DA14 5HP, UK
Tel: 44 (0) 208 308 5760
Fax: 44 (0) 181 308 5702
E-mail: cservice@harcourt.com

*Singapore, Malaysia,Thailand, Philippines, Indonesia, Vietnam, Pacific Rim, Korea*
**Elsevier Science Asia**
583 Orchard Road
#09/01, Forum
Singapore 238884
Tel: 65-737-3593
Fax: 65-753-2145

*Australia, New Zealand*
**Elsevier Science Australia**
Customer Service Department
STM Division
Locked Bag 16
St. Peters, New South Wales, 2044
Australia
Tel: 61 02 9517-8999
Fax: 61 02 9517-2249
E-mail: stmp@harcourt.com.au
Web site: www.harcourt.com.au

*Mexico and Central America*
**ETM SA de CV**
Calle de Tula 59
Colonia Condesa
06140 Mexico DF, Mexico
Tel: 52-5-5553-6657
Fax: 52-5-5211-8468
E-mail: editoresdetextosmex@prodigy.net.mx

*Argentina*
**CLM (Cuspide Libros Medicos)**
Av. Córdoba 2067 - (1120)
Buenos Aires, Argentina
Tel: (5411) 4961-0042/(5411) 4964-0848
Fax: (5411) 4963-7988
E-mail: clm@cuspide.com

*Brazil*
**Tecmedd**
Av. Maurílio Biagi,, 2850
City Ribeirão Preto – SP – CEP: 14021-000
Tel: 0800 992236
Fax: (16) 3993-9000
E-mail: tecmedd@tecmedd.com.br

# CONTRIBUTORS

**Sami R. Achem,** MD, FACP, FACG
Department of Internal Medicine
Mayo Graduate School of Medicine
Rochester, Minnesota

**Fernando Azpiroz,** MD, PhD
Section of Research
Vall d'Hebron University Hospital
Barcelona, Spain

**Nagammapudur S. Balaji,** MS, FRCS
Department of Surgery
University of Southern California
Los Angeles, California

**Gabrio Bassotti,** MD, PhD, FACG
Department of Clinical and Experimental Medicine
University of Perugia Medical School
Perugia, Italy

**Nancy N. Baxter,** PhD, MD
Department of Surgery
Mayo Graduate School of Medicine
Rochester, Minnesota

**Michael Camilleri,** MD
Department of Medicine
Mayo Graduate School of Medicine
Rochester, Minnesota

**Donald O. Castell,** MD
Department of Medicine
Medical University of South Carolina
Charleston, South Carolina

**June A. Castell,** MS
Department of Medicine
Medical University of South Carolina
Charleston, South Carolina

**Mohan Charan,** MD
Department of Gastroenterology
Graduate Hospital
Philadelphia, Pennsylvania

**Paola Ciamarra,** MD
Department of Pediatrics
University of Pittsburgh
Pittsburgh, Pennsylvania

**Michael D. Crowell,** PhD, FACG
Department of Gastrointestinal Physiology and Motility
The Johns Hopkins University School of Medicine
Baltimore, Maryland

**Michael M. Delvaux,** MD
Gastroenterology Unit
Toulouse Hospital
Toulouse, France

**Kenneth R. DeVault,** MD, FACG
Department of Internal Medicine
Mayo Graduate School of Medicine
Rochester, Minnesota

**Ghislain Devroede,** MD
Department of Surgery
University of Sherbrooke
Sherbrooke, Quebec

**Carlo Di Lorenzo, MD**
Department of Pediatrics
University of Pittsburgh
Pittsburgh, Pennsylvania

**Voeker F. Eckardt, MD**
Department of Gastroenterology
German Clinic for Diagnostics
Wiesbaden, Germany

**Paul Enck, PhD**
Department of General Surgery
University of Tübingen
Tübingen, Germany

**Robert S. Fisher, MD**
Department of Medicine
Temple University School of Medicine
Philadelphia, Pennsylvania

**James J. Galligan, PhD**
Department of Pharmacology and Toxicology
Michigan State University
East Lansing, Michigan

**R. Matthew Gideon**
Department of Medicine
Graduate Hospital
Philadelphia, Pennsylvania

**Steven Heymen, MA**
Department of Medicine
University of North Carolina
Chapel Hill, North Carolina

**Walter J. Hogan, MD**
Department of Medicine
Medical College of Wisconsin
Milwaukee, Wisconsin

**Philip O. Katz, MD**
Department of Medicine
Graduate Hospital
Philadelphia, Pennsylvania

**Gordon L. Kauffman, Jr, MD**
Department of Surgery
Pennsylvania State University
Hershey, Pennsylvania

**Howard S. Kaufman, MD**
Department of Surgery
The Johns Hopkins University School of Medicine
Baltimore, Maryland

**John E. Kellow, MD, FRACP**
Department of Medicine
University of Sydney
Sydney, Australia

**Ramesh K. Khurana, MD, FAAN**
Department of Neurology
The Johns Hopkins University School of Medicine
Baltimore, Maryland

**Doe-Young Kim, MD, PhD**
Gastroenterology Research Unit
Mayo Graduate School of Medicine
Rochester, Minnesota

**Linda C. Knight, PhD**
Department of Diagnostic Imaging
Temple University School of Medicine
Philadelphia, Pennsylvania

**Kenneth L. Koch, MD**
Department of Medicine
Pennsylvania State University
Hershey, Pennsylvania

**Moritz A. Konerding, MD**
Department of Anatomy
Johann-Guteuberg Mainz University
Mainz, Germany

**Brian E. Lacy, PhD, MD**
Department of Medicine
The Johns Hopkins University School of Medicine
Baltimore, Maryland

**Jianmin Liu, MD**
Department of Medicine
Veterans Medical Research Foundation
San Diego, California

**Alan H. Maurer, MD**
Department of Diagnostic Imaging
Temple University School of Medicine
Philadelphia, Pennsylvania

**Ravinder K. Mittal, MD**
Department of Medicine
University of California
San Diego, California

**William C. Orr, PhD**
Department of Psychiatry and Behavioral Sciences
University of Oklahoma Health Sciences Center
Oklahoma City, Oklahoma

**Henry P. Parkman, MD**
Department of Medicine
Temple University School of Medicine
Philadelphia, Pennsylvania

**John H. Pemberton, MD**
Department of Surgery
Mayo Graduate School of Medicine
Rochester, Minnesota

**Jeffrey H. Peters, MD, FACS**
Department of Surgery
University of Southern California
Los Angeles, California

**Charlene M. Prather, MD**
Division of Gastroenterology and Hematology
Saint Louis University
Saint Louis, Missouri

**William J. Ravich, MD**
Department of Medicine
The Johns Hopkins University School of Medicine
Baltimore, Maryland

**Beatrice Salvioli, MD**
Department of Internal Medicine
San Orsola Malpighi Academic Hospital
Bologna, Italy

**Sushil K. Sarna, PhD**
Departments of Medicine and Physiology
University of Texas Medical Branch
Galveston, Texas

**Marvin M. Schuster, MD, FACP, FAPA, FACG**
Department of Medicine
The Johns Hopkins University School of Medicine
Baltimore, Maryland

**Reza Shaker, MD**
Department of Medicine
Medical College of Wisconsin
Milwaukee, Wisconsin

**Arnold Wald, MD**
Department of Medicine
University of Pittsburgh Medical Center
Pittsburgh, Pennsylvania

**William E. Whitehead, PhD**
Department of Medicine
University of North Carolina
Chapel Hill, North Carolina

**Jackie D. Wood, MS, PhD**
Departments of Physiology and Internal Medicine
Ohio State University College of Medicine
Columbus, Ohio

*As before, we dedicate this work*
*to the scientists, teachers, students and patients*
*who have taught us much*
*and from whom we continue to learn.*

# CONTENTS

## Other Conditions Related to Motility Dysfunction

## Surgical Therapies

## Conclusion

# PART I

# Physiologic Basis of Gastrointestinal Motility

# CHAPTER 1

# Myoelectrical and Contractile Activities of the Gastrointestinal Tract

*Sushil K. Sarna*

## SUMMARY

The mixing and propulsive motor functions of the gut are regulated by three types of contractions: (a) rhythmic phasic contractions, (b) ultrapropulsive contractions, and (c) tone. The rhythmic phasic contractions cause mixing and slow net distal propulsion in the postprandial and interdigestive states. The efficacy of these contractions in mixing and propulsion depends on their spatial and temporal characteristics. Propagation of contractions is essential for propulsion of ingesta. These contractions are regulated by enteric neurons and slow waves generated by circular smooth muscle cells and interstitial cells of Cajal. The ultrapropulsive contractions are of two types: (a) giant migrating contractions (GMCs) that cause caudal mass movements and (b) retrograde giant contractions (RGCs) that cause oral mass movements. The GMCs, but not the phasic contractions, cause descending inhibition of contractions and relaxation of tone. Under certain conditions, they also produce the sensation of abdominal cramping. Retrograde giant contractions rapidly regurgitate the luminal contents of the upper half of the small intestine into the stomach in preparation for vomitus expulsion by somatomotor response. The precise role of a tonic contraction, which may last from a few minutes to a few hours, is not known, but it is thought that it may enhance the efficacy of phasic and ultrapropulsive contractions by reducing the lumen diameter. The intensity of mixing and the rate of propulsion differ widely in different organs of the gut. Accordingly, the presence of the three types of contractions and their spatial and temporal organizations also differ markedly among the gut organs.

The primary motor functions of the gastrointestinal tract are to (a) mix, agitate, and propel the ingesta at rates that allow efficient absorption of food components; (b) keep the upper gastrointestinal tract clean of residual food, secretions, and bacteria in the interdigestive state; and (c) rapidly propel luminal contents over long distances without regard to digestion or absorption in situations such as swallowing, vomiting, defecation, and mass movements. In addition, the junctions of major organs and the beginning and end of the gut have specialized features, the function of which is to minimize reflux of luminal contents but under appropriate conditions allow a regulated transfer of luminal contents in the caudad direction. The objectives of this chapter are to (a) illustrate the motor patterns that perform the above diverse motor functions in different organs of the gut and (b) discuss the cellular, electrophysiologic, and neurochemical mechanisms that regulate these motor patterns.

## REGULATION OF MIXING AND PROPULSION

The efficacy of mixing and propulsion depends on the frequency, amplitude, duration, and direction of propagating contractions and their frequency and distance of propagation.[1,2] The frequency of contractions determines how often the contractions attempt to mix and propel. Obviously, the greater the frequency, the greater the mixing and/or propulsion will be. The amplitude of contraction governs how much of the lumen

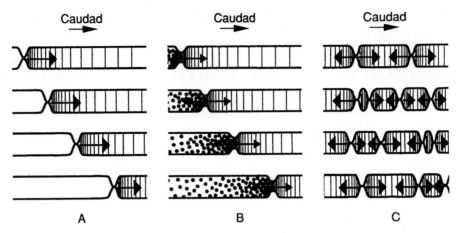

**FIGURE 1.1.** Relationship between the spatial and temporal parameters of contractions and mixing and propulsion. **A**, A strong lumen-occluding contraction that propagates effectively propels the luminal contents in the direction of its propagation. The contents will be propelled approximately to the distance of propagation of the contraction. **B**, A non-lumen-occluding contraction that propagates is less effective in propulsion than the lumen-occluding contraction because some of the contents will escape through the opening and left behind the contraction. These contents will be mixed and stirred during their escape through the partially open lumen. **C**, Spatially uncoordinated or nonpropagating contractions mostly mix and agitate luminal contents with very little propulsion. Reproduced with permission from Sarna SK, Otterson MF. Small intestinal physiology and pathophysiology. In: Owyang A, editor. Gastrointestinal clinics of North America. Philadelphia: WB Saunders; 1989. p. 375–405.

will be occluded by each contraction. Complete occlusion will be more effective in mixing and propulsion than partial occlusion (Fig. 1.1). The longer duration of contractions accentuates their mixing and propulsive abilities. Collectively, these parameters are referred to as the temporal parameters of contractions.

Propagation of contractions is essential for propulsion of ingesta. Unlike the cardiovascular system, where propulsion is achieved by increasing the pressure in a localized compartment (the heart), propulsion in the gut occurs when a circular muscle contraction propagates and pushes the contents ahead of it in the direction of its propagation. Three spatial parameters govern the efficacy of propulsion: (a) the direction of propagation of contractions, (b) the frequency of propagating contractions, and (c) the mean distance over which contractions propagate. A higher frequency of propagating contractions will produce more frequent propulsions in the direction of their propagation, and, finally, a longer mean distance of propagation of contractions means that the luminal contents are propelled over a greater distance with each propagated contraction.

## TYPES OF GUT CONTRACTIONS AND THEIR REGULATION

The above diverse motor functions of the gut are achieved by three distinct types of contractions generated in the muscle layers of the gut: (a) rhythmic phasic contractions (b) tone, and (c) ultrapropulsive contractions (Fig. 1.2).

### Rhythmic Phasic Contractions

These contractions occur in the fasting and postprandial states. They produce mixing, agitation, and slow net distal propulsion of ingesta. There is no fixed spatial and temporal organization of postprandial phasic contractions to achieve these functions in response to the ingestion of a given meal. For example, in response to the same meal given twice, the spatial and temporal patterns of contractions at a given time would be different, but their overall mean values may be the same. The spatial and temporal parameters of these contractions depend, however, on the nutritional make-up, volume, and consistency of the digesta. In the interdigestive state, the phasic contractions are organized as migrating motor complexes in the upper gut to cleanse it and to keep bacteria in the distal small intestine.

### Regulation of Phasic Contractions

The spatial and temporal characteristics of phasic contractions are regulated by slow waves generated in the muscle layers and the enteric neurons consisting of postsynaptic excitatory and inhibitory motoneurons, interneurons, and sensory neurons (Fig. 1.3). The activity of the enteric neurons may be modulated by input from the spinal cord, the central nervous system (CNS) via the parasympathetic and sympathetic neurons, and endocrine and paracrine hormones

The interior of smooth muscle cells is maintained at a negative potential (–50 to 60 mV) with respect to the extracellular medium by ionic transport mechanisms (Fig. 1.4). This potential is called the resting membrane potential. The membrane potential exhibits periodic depolarizations that govern the excitability of the smooth muscle cells to contract by triggering the inward movement of $Ca^{2+}$ ions, primarily through the long-lasting L-type $Ca^{2+}$ channels in the membrane and subsequent release of $Ca^{2+}$ from the intracellular stores. The slow wave consists of three components: upstroke, plateau, and repolarization. The ionic mechanisms of the upstroke are

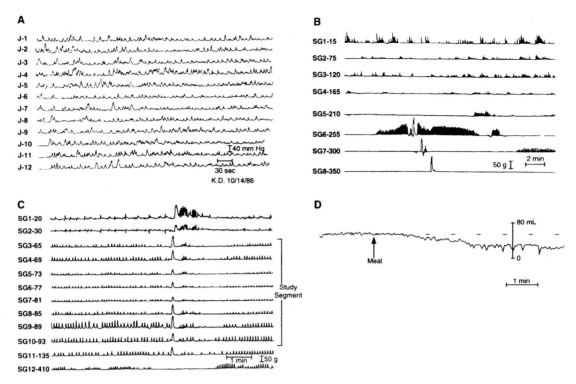

**FIGURE 1.2.** Three different types of contractions in the small intestine. **A,** Rhythmic phasic contractions recorded from human jejunum by a manometric tube with side holes 2 cm apart. **B,** Giant migrating contraction (GMC) recorded from canine small intestine with strain gauge transducers. The GMC originated at a distance of 255 cm from the pylorus and propagated to the end of the ileum in about 2 minutes. The GMC started during a phase 3 activity. Note the differences between the amplitudes and durations of phasic contractions in phase 3 activity and the GMC. SG1 to SG8 represent the strain gauge transducers and the numbers after them their distances from the pylorus. (Reprinted with permission from Sarna SK, Otterson MF. Small intestinal physiology and pathophysiology. Gastroenterol Clin North Am 1989;18:375–405. **C,** A retrograde giant contraction began 135 cm from the pylorus and propagated orad to the proximal duodenum. SG1 to SG12 represent the strain gauge transducers and the numbers after them their distances from the pylorus. Reproduced with permission from Cowles VE, Sarna SK. Effect of *Trichinella spiralis* infection on intestinal motor activity in the fasted state. Am J Physiol 1990;259:G693–701. **D,** Increase of tone recorded by a barostat from the human ileum after the ingestion of a meal. The barostat recorded a decrease in its volume owing to an increase in tone. Adapted from Coffin B, Léman M, Flourié B, et al. Ileal tone in humans: effects of locoregional distensions and eating. Am J Physiol 1994;267:G569–74.

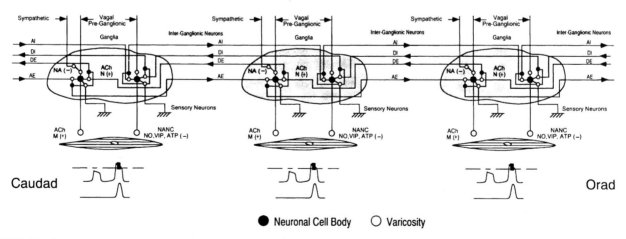

● Neuronal Cell Body    ○ Varicosity

**FIGURE 1.3.** Illustration of the myogenic and neurochemical regulation of gastrointestinal phasic contractions. The smooth muscle generates spontaneous slow waves and is innervated by excitatory and inhibitory postsynaptic enteric neurons. The physiologic neurotransmitter of the excitatory neurons is acetylcholine (ACh). The putative neurotransmitters of the inhibitory motor neurons are nitric oxide (NO), vasoactive intestinal peptide (VIP), and adenosine triphosphate (ATP). The slow wave is superimposed with spikes when the excitatory neurotransmitter is released. The sensory neurons provide feedback to the enteric ganglia regarding the mechanical and chemical stimuli from the luminal contents. The excitatory and inhibitory motoneurons with cell bodies in the enteric ganglia also receive descending and ascending inputs from the proximal and distal ganglia, respectively, as well as input from the extrinsic and sympathetic neurons that can modulate their output. NANC, nonadrenergic noncholinergic; NA, noradrenaline; N, nicotinic receptor; M, muscarinic receptor; AI, ascending inhibition; DI, descending inhibition; DE, descending excitation; AE, ascending excitation.

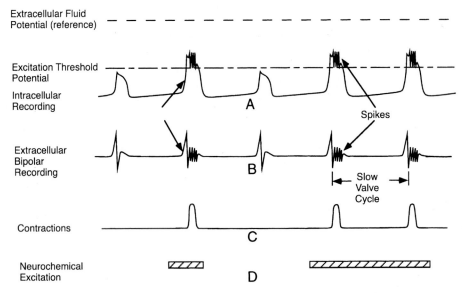

**FIGURE 1.4.** Illustration of regulation of rhythmic phasic contractions by slow waves and spikes. **A,** The resting membrane potential of smooth muscle cells is negative with respect to the extracellular fluid potential. The depolarization during spontaneous slow waves does not exceed the excitation threshold; therefore, no contractions occur. The release of acetylcholine by neurochemical excitation depolarizes the plateau phase of the slow waves beyond the excitation threshold; spikes are superimposed on the plateau phase and the cell contracts. **B,** This diagram illustrates the morphology of slow waves and spikes when they are recorded by extracellular bipolar electrodes. **C,** This illustration shows the contractions associated with spikes. Adapted from Sarna SK. In vivo myoelectric activity: methods, analysis and interpretation. In: Wood JD, editor. Handbook of physiology, gastrointestinal motility and circulation. Bethesda (MD): American Physiological Society; 1989. p. 817–63.

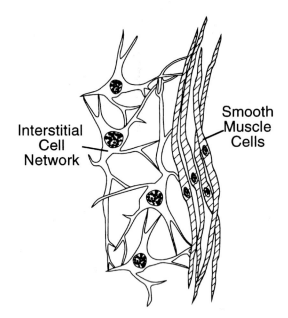

**FIGURE 1.5.** Illustration of interstitial cells of Cajal (ICC) and smooth muscle cells. The processes of ICC form gap junctions and with the adjacent circular smooth muscle and with other ICC. The driving of circular muscle slow wave by ICC is thought to occur via these gap junctions. Adapted from Sanders KM. A case for interstitial cells of Cajal pacemakers and mediators of neurotransmission in the gastrointestinal tract. Gastroenterology 1996;111:492–515.

not fully understood. It has been suggested, however, that the slow waves in circular muscle cells may be triggered by specialized cells called the interstitial cells of Cajal (Fig. 1.5). The plateau phase is caused by $Ca^{2+}$ influx through the L-type

channels. The repolarization of membrane potential may be attributable to the inactivation of the $Ca^{2+}$ channels, opening of $Ca^{2+}$-activated $K^+$ channels, or both. The membrane potential during the plateau of the slow wave is in the range of –40 to –50 mV. Patch clamp studies show that, at these potentials, the inward $Ca^{2+}$ current is minute. As a result, the muscle contraction associated directly with a slow wave alone is so tiny that it is not detected visually or by conventional transducers used to record in vivo contractions. These tiny contractions are, however, detectable in vitro muscle strips when they are stretched in a muscle bath environment.

However, if an excitatory neurotransmitter, such as acetylcholine (AChL), is released from the excitatory motoneurons in conjunction with slow-wave depolarization, the membrane potential depolarizes further, and when it exceeds an excitation threshold, spikes, superimposed on the plateau phase, occur. The spikes depolarize the membrane to the range of 0 to +30 mV, the range in which the inward $Ca^{2+}$ currents are maximal.[3] This $Ca^{2+}$ influx and the subsequent release of $Ca^{2+}$ from the intracellular stores ($Ca^{2+}$-induced $Ca^{2+}$ release) raise the cytosolic-free ($Ca^{2+}$) levels, which is one of the initial steps in triggering a cascade of signaling pathways in the cells to cause a phasic contraction. As shown later, during Phase 1 activity of the migrating motor complex (MMC) cycle, slow waves are present but spikes are absent, and there are no contractions. Spikes are superimposed on slow waves during Phases 2 and 3 of the MMC cycle and in the postprandial state and are accompanied by phasic contractions. Spikes are essential to cause meaningful phasic contractions in all major organs of the gut.

In summary, the occurrence of phasic contractions requires two conditions to be met: (a) there must be a slow-wave depolarization with spikes on the plateau phase and (b) an excitatory neurotransmitter must be present on the cell surface during the depolarization. The slow waves are omnipresent, but the release of neurotransmitters is intermittent. This means that the maximum frequency of phasic contractions at a given location cannot exceed the frequency of slow waves at that site. The actual frequency of contractions depends on how many slow waves had concurrent release of the excitatory neurotransmitter. Although both ACh and Substance P are known excitatory neurotransmitters, ACh is the established physiologic neurotransmitter of in vivo gut contractions. All spontaneous contractions in the stomach, small intestine, and colon in the intact conscious state are blocked by atropine, the nonspecific antagonist of muscarinic receptors. On the other hand, the in vivo blockade of neurolkinin ($NK_1$) receptors does not inhibit spontaneous contractions in the canine gut.

Since $Ca^{2+}$ influx during a contraction is caused by spikes, the total influx and its duration are governed by the number of spikes superimposed on a slow wave and their amplitude, which, in turn, determines the amplitude and duration of contractions.

The smooth muscle cells also are innervated directly by nonadrenergic noncholinergic (NANC) inhibitory neurons (see Fig. 1.3), the putative mediators of which are nitric oxide (NO), vasoactive intestinal polypeptide (VIP), and adenosine triphosphate (ATP). The understanding of the precise role of each of these neurotransmitters in different parts of the gut is still evolving. There is evidence, however, that NO plays a prominent role in regulating the inhibition of in vivo phasic contractions and relaxation of tone.

In addition to producing relaxation in sphincters, the inhibitory neurons play important roles in the motility functions of gut organs. For example, by competing with the excitatory input, they may fine-tune the spatiotemporal patterns of contractions that produce optimal mixing and propulsion. Systemic administration of NO synthase inhibitor delays gastric emptying, suggesting that in response to neuronal feedback from the proximal small intestine, NO released from the gastric NANC neurons may have optimized the gastropyloroduodenal contractions.[4] The inhibition of NO synthase alters the spatiotemporal characteristics of these contractions and hence delays gastric emptying. Similarly, the inhibitory neurons may fine-tune the spatiotemporal characteristics of contractions in the proximal small intestine in response to neurohormonal input from the ileum (ileal brake). The role of NANC inhibitors in descending inhibition is discussed in the section on GMCs.

As noted above, the slow waves and spikes regulate the timing, maximum frequency, amplitude, and duration of contractions. However, uncoordinated occurrence of contractions along the gut would primarily cause to and fro movements of the ingesta, resulting in mixing, agitation, and stirring but little or no propulsion (see Fig. 1.1C). The contractions must

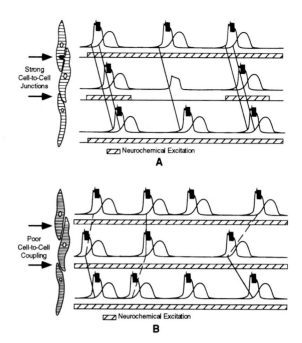

**FIGURE 1.6.** Propagation of contractions in a segment depends on the coordination (phase locking) of slow waves and concurrent neurochemical excitation of the segment. The left diagram shows the cell-to-cell junctions (gap junctions) between adjacent cells to produce electrical coupling. The intrinsic frequencies of the three cells decrease from the top to the bottom in **A** and **B**. In **A**, the electrical coupling among the three cells is strong because of gap junctions; therefore, the slow waves of the three cells become phase locked. When concurrent neurochemical excitation is present in all three cells, the contraction propagates from the top cell to the bottom cell. For the middle section of A, the slow waves were phase locked, but concurrent neurochemical excitation did not occur in all three cells; hence, the contraction did not propagate from the top to the bottom. Instead, it occurred locally in the first and the third cells. In **B**, because of poor coupling among the three cells, the slow waves were not phase locked. Under these circumstances, even though neurochemical excitation occurred in all three cells concurrently, the contractions did not propagate; they occurred randomly in the three cells. Reproduced with permission from Sarna SK, Otterson MF. Myoelectrical and contractile activities. In: Schuster MM, editor. Atlas of gastrointestinal motility in health and disease. Baltimore: Williams and Wilkins; 1993. p. 3–47.

propagate to propel. Propagation of phasic contractions is regulated, in part, by the coordination of slow waves along the circumference and length of the gut. The smooth muscle cells communicate with neighboring cells at specialized cell-to-cell junctions called gap junctions (Fig. 1.6). At these junctions, the cells approximate each other, or a projection from the membrane of one cell protrudes into a cavity of similar shape of an adjacent cell to facilitate communication. The degree of communication or electrical coupling depends on the distance between the membrane at the cell-to-cell junction. Shorter distances between the membranes and cylindrical protrusions assist in stronger coupling. This coupling allows the slow waves generated in adjacent cells to coordinate with each other in time and frequency.

The slow-wave oscillations of the gastrointestinal smooth muscle cells have the characteristics of relaxation oscillators; that is, if two cells are electrically coupled, one cell can alter the frequency and timing of oscillation of the other cell without altering its other intrinsic characteristics. If the coupling between two adjacent cells is strong and the difference between their intrinsic frequencies relatively small, the higher-frequency cell is able to entrain the frequency of the lower intrinsic frequency cell to that of its own. This means that both cells will begin to oscillate at the higher frequency, and the oscillation of the lower intrinsic frequency cell will begin with a short time lag (phase lag), after that of the higher-frequency cell (see Fig. 1.6A). This produces spatial coordination of slow waves. Because each cell can contract only once during its depolarization, the cell with the higher intrinsic frequency will contract first if spikes are present on its slow-wave plateau phase, followed a short while later by a contraction of the lower intrinsic frequency cell if spikes are present on that call's slow-wave plateau phase as well (see Fig. 1.6A). If the lower intrinsic frequency cell is located distal to the higher intrinsic frequency cell, as is the case throughout the stomach and the small intestine, the contractions will seem to propagate from the higher intrinsic frequency to the lower intrinsic frequency cells in the caudal direction (see Fig. 1.6A). If the lower intrinsic frequency cell, which has now acquired the higher frequency of the proximal cell, similarly drives the next distal cell, the contraction of these three cells will occur at the same frequency and seem to propagate from the most proximal to the most distal cell (eg, the first and third sets of contractions in Fig. 1.6A). Therefore, one of the factors that determine the distance of propagation of contractions in the gastrointestinal tract is the number of cells in which slow waves are entrained as above. The slow waves are usually strongly coupled in the circumferential direction so that, at a given point, the cells along the circumference almost contract together to give the appearance of a ring contraction.

If the coupling between the cells is weak, their slow waves do not become entrained. In this case, the depolarizations of adjacent cells occur without spatial coordination (see Fig. 1.6B). Even though all three cells in Figure 1.6B are concurrently excited by neurohormonal control, the contractions are discoordinated because of the lack of coordination of slow waves in the three cells. This type of spatial discoordination is commonly observed in the distal small intestine and the colon and is associated with slower propulsion than that in the proximal small intestine, where the slow waves are entrained.

Another factor that regulates the distance of propagation of contractions is the number of contiguous cells that concurrently receive excitatory neurotransmitter release in their vicinity (see Fig. 1.6). As stated earlier, the autonomous depolarizations of slow waves do not exceed the contractile-excitation threshold potential to produce a meaningful contraction. An excitatory neurotransmitter, such as ACh, must be present for the depolarization to exceed the contractile-excitation threshold potential. In Figure 1.6A, although the slow-wave depolarizations are coordinated in space (phase locked) in all three cells in every cycle, the contraction prop-

agates from the most proximal to the most distal cells only when all three cells are concurrently stimulated by an excitatory neurotransmitter (first and third contractions). At the time of the second slow wave in Figure 1.6A, only the proximal and the distal cells received neurochemical excitation; the middle cell did not. In this case, isolated contractions occurred in the proximal and the distal cells, but there was no propagation. This type of spatial coordination of slow waves occurs in the stomach and the proximal small intestine; these organs therefore exhibit propagating contractions over relatively long distances.

The gastrointestinal tract contains millions of smooth muscle cells. The contractions of each single cell, of approximate length of a few hundred micrometers, alone can hardly be sufficient to produce a contraction sufficient to cause mixing and propulsion. In practice, several thousand cells encompassing the entire circumference of a short segment (1–1.5 cm) have nearly the same intrinsic frequency, and the coupling along the circumference, at least in the stomach and the upper small intestine, is strong enough to fully entrain all of these circumferential cells with a minimal phase lag so that they seem to oscillate together. The projections of the enteric motoneurons are such that all cells in a circular band receive concurrent neurotransmitter release. The circumferential coordination of slow waves and neurotransmitter release produces bands or rings of contractions. However, the intrinsic frequency of bands of smooth muscle cells decreases in the distal direction in the stomach and the small intestine. The coupling and the propagation of contractions among single cells, as illustrated in Figure 1.6, therefore becomes the coupling and propagation of contractions between adjacent bands of smooth muscle cells.

The control of spatial and temporal organization of rhythmic phasic contractions to mix and propel luminal contents in the gastrointestinal tract can therefore be summarized as follows:

1. Neurotransmitter release from the postsynaptic excitatory motoneurons determines whether contractions will occur in a given segment. Acetylcholine is the physiologic neurotransmitter for most spontaneous in vivo phasic contractions. Nitric oxide, VIP, and ATP are putative inhibitory neurotransmitters in the gut. If both excitatory and inhibitory neurotransmitters are released concurrently in a segment, the occurrence of contractions will depend on the summation of these opposing effects.

2. When an excitatory neurotransmitter is present on the membrane of a smooth muscle cell, it will contract only when its membrane depolarizes. Therefore, the timing and frequency of contractions stimulated by neuronal input depend on the oscillations of slow waves. The maximum frequency of phasic contractions cannot exceed the frequency of slow waves. Only one phasic contraction occurs during each slow-wave depolarization, and its duration is less than or equal to that of the slow wave.

3. The spatial coordination of contractions, that is their direction and distance of propagation, is governed by the length of the segment that exhibits phase-locked slow waves and the length of the contiguous segment that receives concurrent excitatory neurotransmitter release.

## Integrated Control of Phasic Contractions

From the above, it is clear that several regulatory systems (neurons, neurotransmitters and hormones, slow waves, spikes, and signal transduction within cells) work together to produce the desired temporal and spatial organization of contractions to mix and propel the ingesta. The neural control is composed of the CNS, autonomic nerves (the vagus, pelvic, and sympathetic nerves), and enteric neurons. The sensory nerves detect the presence of food components in the lumen through mechano- and chemoreceptors and send the information to the enteric ganglia via the interneurons. Although balloon distention has been used extensively as a stimulus to study the effect of stretch on gut motor activity in vivo and in vitro, no significant distention of the gut occurs during normal digestion and absorption of a meal. The sensory neurons, however, detect the chemical nature of the ingesta and the stroking of the villi by the luminal contents. As discussed later, distention can occur distal to a GMC that causes a mass movement. The postsynaptic motoneurons release the appropriate neurotransmitter to stimulate or inhibit contractions of the smooth muscle cells. As explained above, the muscle cells contract only during slow-wave depolarization. The postsynaptic neurons also receive input from the other descending and ascending interneurons and extrinsic nerves that may modulate the neurotransmitter release at the neuroeffector junction The CNS and the extrinsic nerves provide voluntary control over swallowing and defecation.

It must be noted, however, that some enteric neurons also have internal clocks that make them fire spontaneously and periodically without necessarily any input from the lumen-sensing neurons. The periodic firing of presynaptic neurons generates the migrating motor complex in the fasting state when there is little or no nutritional load in the stomach and the small intestine to stimulate contractions. This periodic neuronal firing is inhibited by the presence of nutrients in the upper gut.

The chemicals that affect gut smooth cells are synthesized in the neurons and endocrine-paracrine cells. These substances may act on smooth muscle cells in the neurocrine mode (released from enteric postsynaptic neurons), paracrine mode (released from specialized cells in the immediate surroundings of the smooth muscle), endocrine mode (released from the endocrine cells or glands), or a combination of three modes. There are several categories of endogenous substances, such as cholinergics, amines, peptides, and fatty acid–derived compounds that have been shown to affect gut contractions. Basically, these can be divided into two classes: excitatory and inhibitory. In addition to contracting or inhibit-

ing contractions, these substances also produce chemical transmission at synapses in extrinsic and interneuronal pathways to mediate reflex actions. It must be noted that we know a lot more about the localization, production, and pharmacologic effects of these substances than their physiologic or pathologic roles. It is noteworthy that in the intact conscious state, there is some debate as to whether the circulating hormones or drugs act on neurons or smooth muscle cells to affect contractions. Recent findings show that in the intact conscious state, the prokinetic agents act on neurons to stimulate contractions. Although, in vitro, these same compounds exhibit a direct effect on smooth muscle cells, that may not be the way of their influence on gut motility in the intact state.

## Ultrapropulsive Contractions

The phasic contractions cause mixing and slow net distal propulsion of ingesta. However, there are situations when the luminal contents have to be propelled rapidly without regard for digestion or absorption. This motor function is achieved by two types of ultrapropulsive contractions: (a) GMCs that produce mass movements in the caudal direction and (b) RGCs that produce mass movements in the orad direction.

The GMCs are two to four times larger in amplitude and four to six times longer in duration than the maximum amplitude and duration of rhythmic phasic contractions, respectively (Fig. 1.7). In addition, unlike the phasic contractions, the GMCs propagate uninterruptedly over long distances at a velocity of $\geq 1$ cm/sec from the point of their origin in the small intestine or the colon. Because of the large amplitude, they completely occlude the lumen. Their uninterrupted rapid propagation over long distances propels the luminal contents trapped ahead of them rapidly over the entire distance of their propagation. Because of their long duration, GMCs simultaneously contract a 20- to 30-cm-long segment, which increases the efficacy for propulsion by reducing the chance of any luminal contents escaping through and being left behind. In health, the GMCs occur just a few times a day, normally in the terminal ileum and proximal colon only. In pathologic states, such as inflammation, the frequency of GMCs is increased dramatically, and they can begin in the duodenum and propagate all the way to the ileum in just a few minutes. Often, the small intestinal GMCs cross over to the colon from where they have the potential to propagate all the way to the rectum to cause defecation.

The phasic contractions cause to and fro movements of the ingesta and propulsion over small distances at a time. As such, there are no large volumes of luminal contents being propelled that may distend the distal receiving segment. In the case of propulsion by a GMC, however, whatever is trapped ahead of it is rapidly propelled over long distances without any to and fro movement. This means that luminal contents ahead of a GMC can accumulate into a large bolus, which may distend the receiving segment of the small intestine or the colon. Such rapid propulsion would be facilitated if the spontaneous phasic contractions in the distal receiving segment were inhibited to minimize resistance to rapid propulsion (see Fig. 1.7). In addition, the distal receiving segment should relax its tone to accommodate the large bolus ahead of a GMC. Both of these functions are achieved by descending interneurons that stimulate the postsynaptic inhibitory motoneurons to produce inhibition of phasic contractions and relaxation of tone.

The term "peristalsis" was originally described by Bayliss and Starling[5] as a contraction proximal to the bolus and relaxation distal to it, causing rapid propulsion. The GMCs fit this description rather than the phasic contractions (Fig. 1.8). No relaxation of tone or inhibition of phasic contraction is seen distal to phasic contractions (see Fig. 1.2A).

The occurrence of GMCs has also been associated with intermittent abdominal pain. This pain may be caused by (1) the strong force with which the GMCs contract the gut wall and stimulate the sensory receptors beyond their nociceptive threshold; (2) the bolus that is being propelled by the GMC, which distends the distal receiving segment beyond its nociceptive threshold (Fig. 1.9); (3) ischemia caused by reduced blood flow in the segment that is contracted for long periods of 20 to 30 seconds by the GMC; and (4) a signal from the sensory receptors in the mesentery caused by altered blood flow or distortion during a GMC. Not all GMCs are, however, perceived to be painful. Impairment in the descending inhibition and hyperalgesia may be the major factors for the sensation of pain caused by a GMC.

The mechanisms of generation of GMCs are not completely understood. It is known, however, that (1) the neurotransmitter for their generation is also ACh.[6] It seems that the release of ACh at the neuroeffector junction for a duration

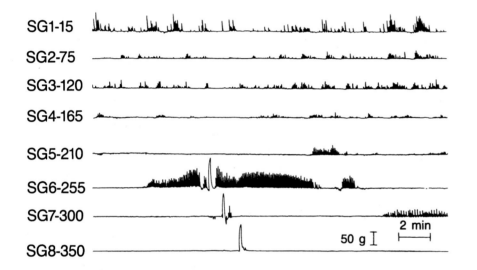

**FIGURE 1.7.** A giant migrating contraction (GMC) originating at a distance of about 255 cm distal to the pylorus. Note the occurrence of GMC during a Phase 3 activity at the same site. The GMC propagated rapidly to the end of the small intestine. The top five strain gauge (SG) transducers show rhythmic phasic contractions. Note the relatively large amplitude and duration of GMC when compared with those of the phasic contractions. Reproduced with permission from Sarna SK, Otterson MF. Small intestinal physiology and pathophysiology. Gastroenterol Clin North Am 1989;18:375–405.

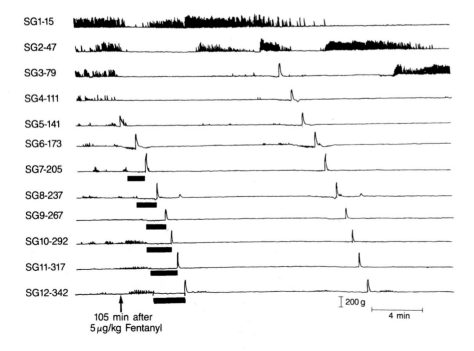

**FIGURE 1.8.** Giant migrating contractions are preceded by descending inhibition indicated by *dark horizontal bars*. The descending inhibition is typical of peristalsis as originally defined by Bayless and Starling.[7] In contrast, the phasic contractions shown in Figure 1.2A do not produce descending inhibition. SG, strain gauge transducers.

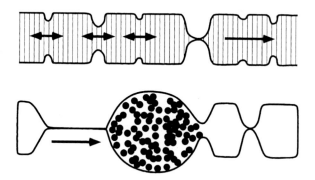

**FIGURE 1.9.** In the top diagram, the phasic contractions partially or completely occlude the lumen. These contractions mix, agitate, and slowly propel the luminal contents in the aboral direction without causing significant distention of the receiving segment. In the bottom diagram, the giant migrating contraction occludes the lumen of a long segment and traps the luminal contents ahead of it, and when it propagates rapidly, the build-up of the bolus causes distention of the distal receiving segment. If the ongoing contractions in the distal receiving segment are not inhibited and its tone is not relaxed, the bolus will meet resistance, causing more distention. This may be perceived as painful if the distention exceeds the nociceptive threshold.

longer than that required for a phasic contraction may be required to stimulate a GMC. Calcitonin gene–related peptide (CGRP), given close intra-arterially, is a reliable stimulus for the generation of the GMCs.[6] It acts on presynaptic neurons to release ACh at the neuroeffector junction to stimulate a GMC. Smaller doses of CGRP stimulate only phasic contractions, whereas larger doses stimulate both GMCs and phasic contractions; (2) GMCs require enteric descending interneurons for propagation; they do not propagate beyond a translocation and reanastomosis in the gut wall, which interrupts the enteric neuronal continuity[7]; (3) the cellular signal transection processes that generate GMCs are somewhat different than those that stimulate phasic contractions[6]; (4) the GMCs are not regulated by slow waves.[8] Their duration is several times longer than that of a slow-wave cycle.

Stimulation or inhibition of GMCs is an attractive target for drug development to treat specific motility disorders. As noted below, an increase in the frequency of GMCs causes motor diarrhea, and a decrease in their frequency causes constipation. Pharmacologic stimulation of GMCs can therefore produce frequent mass movements to overcome sluggish transit. Stimulation of GMCs in the distal colon may produce not only a mass movement but also descending relaxation to overcome outlet obstruction. On the other hand, pharmacologic inhibition of GMCs in gut inflammation or infection and diarrhea-predominant irritable bowel syndrome may reduce the number of mass movements, urgency of defecation, and abdominal cramping if hyperalgesia accompanies the motility disorder. Recent studies show that some of the cellular signaling pathways for the stimulation of GMCs differ from those for the stimulation of phasic contractions. It should therefore be possible to stimulate or inhibit GMCs selectively without concurrently affecting the phasic contractions and tone.

### Retrograde Giant Contractions

Retrograde giant contractions are ultrapropulsive contractions that propagate in the orad direction. They are 1.5 to 2 times larger in amplitude and 2 to 4 times longer in duration than the phasic contractions of Phase 3 activity. The RGCs begin in the mid-to-distal small intestine and propagate orad, up to the antrum, at a velocity of about 8 to 10 cm/sec (see Fig. 1.2C). They regurgitate the contents of the upper small intestine into the stomach in preparation for vomitus expulsion. It is noteworthy that vomitus expulsion itself is not caused by RGCs but is a somatomotor response caused by the contraction of the abdominal and diaphragmatic muscles.

The initiation of an RGC preceding vomiting is regulated by the CNS via the vagal nerves. Bilateral truncal vagotomy abolishes the RGCs stimulated by apomorphine but preserves retching and vomiting.[9] The CNS also regulates the orad propagation of RGCs and coordinates it with retching and vomiting. The enteric nervous system modulates the orad propagation of RGCs and determines the amplitude and duration of RGCs. The neurotransmitter for the stimulation of RGCs at the neuroeffector junction is also ACh.[9]

### Tonic Contraction

A tonic contraction is a sustained increase in tone that may last from several minutes to several hours (see Fig. 1.2D). The precise role of tone in gut motor function has not been established, but it is thought to enhance the efficacy of phasic contractions in mixing and propulsion by narrowing the lumen. The weaker phasic contractions that may not occlude the lumen on their own may do so if they are superimposed on a tonic contraction. As noted earlier, the tone is not regulated by slow waves.

## MOTOR PATTERNS OF MAJOR GUT ORGANS

The motor functions of the major gut organs differ widely. The motor function of the esophagus is primarily to transfer the swallowed bolus rapidly into the stomach without regard to mixing and propulsion (Fig. 1.10). The head of a bolus takes ~ 2 to 5 seconds to traverse a length of about 30 cm in the human esophagus. The motor function of the stomach is to mix the ingesta with gastric secretions, agitate the mixture to break down the food into small-sized particles, and empty them into the duodenum at a rate that allows efficient digestion and absorption of food components in the small intestine. The head of a typical meal begins to empty from the stomach in about 10 to 20 minutes, but the total gastric emptying time depends on the consistency, calories, and nutritional components in the meal. The motor function of the proximal small intestine is to mix and agitate the ingesta but propel it relatively quickly so that it does not act as an obstruction to further gastric emptying. However, when the digesta reaches the distal small intestine, mixing and agitation intensify, but propulsion slows down for efficient reabsorption of bile acids.

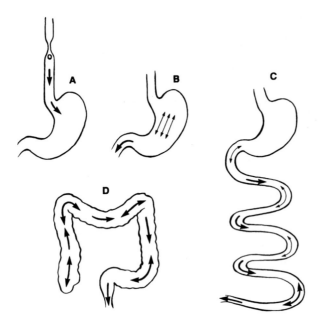

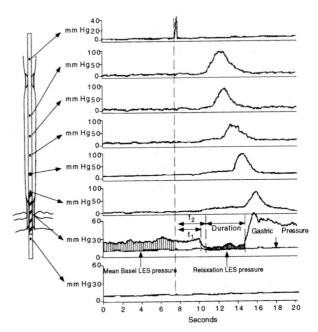

**FIGURE 1.10.** Mixing and motor functions of the major gut organs differ widely. **A**, The primary motor function of the esophagus is a mass movement to rapidly transfer the swallowed bolus to the stomach without regard for any mixing for digestion and absorption. **B**, Gastric motor function requires mixing, trituration, and regulated emptying in small volumes. **C**, The upper small intestine has relatively faster transit along with some mixing. The transit rate slows distally in the small intestine, and mixing and agitation intensify. **D**, Mixing and agitation are further intensified in the colon while the transit rate becomes even slower.

**FIGURE 1.11.** An esophageal contraction following a swallow that produces a mass movement in the esophagus without regard for digestion and absorption. This contraction has the characteristics of a giant migrating contraction (GMC). The esophagus does not normally show rhythmic phasic contractions. Descending inhibition, including relaxation of the lower esophageal sphincter (LES), precedes the esophageal GMC. Reproduced with permission from Shi G, Ergin GA, Mantie M, Kahrilas PJ. Lower esophageal sphincter relaxation characteristics using a sleeve sensor in clinical manometry. Am J Gastroenterol 1998;93:2373–9.

The head of a typical meal takes about 2 hours to traverse a length of 6 to 8 meters of small intestine in humans. The colon maintains homeostasis by reabsorbing water and electrolytes and serves as a temporary storage place so that defecation can occur in a socially acceptable manner in humans. A bolus may take 36 to 48 hours to traverse a length of about 1 meter in the human colon. Thus, the rate or propulsion slows down, and mixing and agitation are intensified distally in the gut. Accordingly, the type of contractions each organ generates, and their spatial and temporal organization, would also be different. The following sections illustrate the different patterns of contractions that correspond to the above functions in major gut organs.

### Esophagus

The motor function of the esophagus is essentially to produce a mass movement after each swallow. This is achieved by contractions that have the characteristics of GMCs, that is, large amplitude, long duration, and rapid uninterrupted propagation over the entire length of the esophagus (Fig. 1.11). As is typical of a GMC, the esophageal contractions are preceded by descending inhibition/relaxation that accommodates the bolus as it is propelled distally, and it also prevents another GMC from originating at a distal location while the present GMC is still propagating. The

descending inhibition also relaxes the lower esophageal sphincter to let the bolus pass through it.

### Stomach and Pylorus

The motor functions of the stomach are to (a) act as a reservoir for the ingested meal on its arrival in the fundus; (b) gradually transfer the ingesta to the body and the antrum of the stomach, mix it with gastric secretions, and agitate it for breakdown to smaller-sized particles; and (c) empty the ingesta at a rate that allows efficient digestion and absorption of food components in the small intestine.

Figure 1.12 shows the motor activity of the stomach during the entire period of emptying of a solid meal. The fundus does not exhibit the usual spontaneous phasic contractions in the postprandial state because it acts as a reservoir that does not require mixing movements. The fundus relaxes when a meal is ingested and then contracts gradually to transfer its contents to the body and the antrum of the stomach. The phasic contractions are coordinated (phase locked) throughout the corpus and antrum (Fig. 1.13). The contractions are smaller in amplitude in the corpus and do not occlude the lumen, thus causing mainly mixing movements. The contractions in the antrum are larger in amplitude, and, because of the smaller antral lumen size, they occlude it and are therefore effective in gastric emptying.

The pyloric phasic contractions play a major role in the regulation of gastric emptying. The pylorus is not a classic sphincter in the sense that it is not closed by a tonic contraction that relaxes to let the contents pass through. Instead, the pylorus is a narrow opening that is periodically constricted by phasic contractions generated in its circular muscle layer. As the distally propagating antral contraction approaches the pylorus, it attempts to push the contents through it. The pyloric contractions are phase locked with the antral contractions. Because of narrow pyloric size, they close the pylorus shortly after the onset of the antral contraction. The time lag between the onset of the antral contraction and the pyloric closing by its phasic contraction gives the window during which gastric emptying occurs in spurts. The size of the pyloric opening also determines the maximum size of the particle that can pass through it. Once the pylorus is closed by its phasic contraction, the gastric contents ahead of the distally propagating antral contraction face resistance and are retropropelled to cause aggressive mixing and agitation to break them down to small particle

sizes. In a complete antro-phylorioduodenal coordination, a propagated contraction begins in the duodenum soon after a bolus of chyme is emptied from the stomach to propel it and make space for additional gastric emptying.

The stomach does not generate GMCs. The RGCs that begin in the small intestine propagate only up to the antrum.

### Small Intestine

The motor functions of the small bowel (a) mix, agitate, and slowly propel its contents in the aborad direction; (b) keep the lumen clean in the interdigestive state: (c) rapidly retropropel the contents of the upper small intestine into the stomach in preparation for vomitus expulsion; and (d) occasionally produce aboral mass movements.

The postprandial motor functions of mixing and slow net distal propulsion are achieved primarily by phasic contractions. The rate or propulsion is faster in the upper small intestine. Accordingly, the phasic contractions are coordinated in space and are entrained at the same frequency

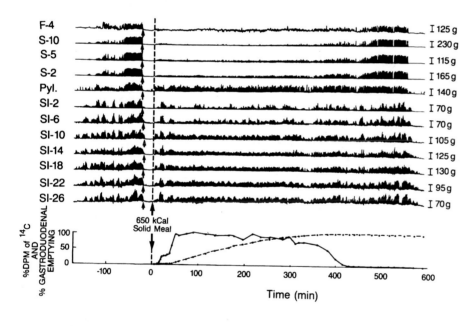

**FIGURE 1.12.** Recordings of canine fundus (F), gastric pyloric (Pyl), and duodenal motor activities during complete gastric emptying of a solid meal. The *arrows* show the cyclic motor activity in the stomach and migrating motor complex in the small intestine (SI) before the ingestion of the meal. These complexes were disrupted after ingestion of the meal and reappeared after the meal was completely emptied. The *bottom graph* shows the cumulative emptying of the meal (*broken line*). Reproduced with permission from Haba T, Sarna SK. Regulation of gastroduodenal emptying of solids by gastropyloroduodenal contractions. Am J Physiol 1993;264:G261–71.

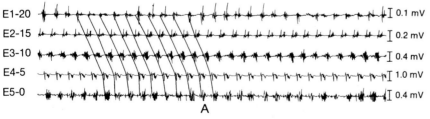
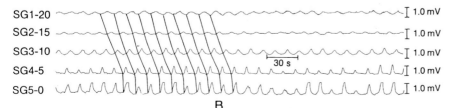

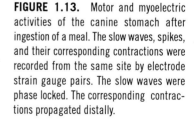

**FIGURE 1.13.** Motor and myoelectric activities of the canine stomach after ingestion of a meal. The slow waves, spikes, and their corresponding contractions were recorded from the same site by electrode strain gauge pairs. The slow waves were phase locked. The corresponding contractions propagated distally.

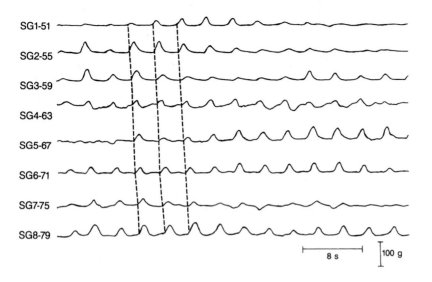

**FIGURE 1.14.** The phasic contractions propagate in the duodenum over relatively long distances and hence produce relatively rapid propulsion. SG, strain gauge transducers. The numbers after this symbol denote the distances of the transducers from the pylorus. Reproduced with permission from Sarna SK, Otterson MF. Small intestine physiology and pathophysiology. Gastroenterol Clin North Am 1989;18:375–405.

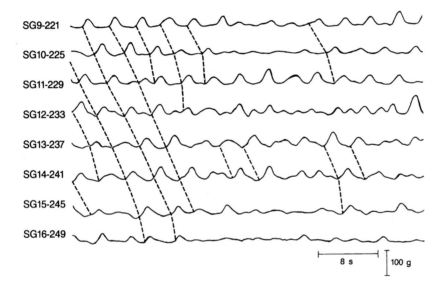

**FIGURE 1.15.** The propagation of contractions deteriorates in the mid to small intestine as compared with that shown in Figure 1.14. SG, strain gauge transducers. The numbers after SG indicate the distance of the transducers from the pylorus. Reproduced with permission from Sarna SK, Otterson MF. Small intestine physiology and pathophysiology. Gastroenterol Clin North Am 1989;18:375–405.

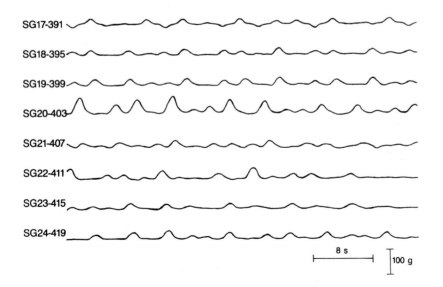

**FIGURE 1.16.** The distal ileum has mostly nonpropagating contractions (compare with Figs. 1.14 and 1.15), resulting in slower transit. SG, strain gauge transducers. The numbers after SG denote the distances of the transducers from the pylorus. Reproduced with permission from Sarna SK, Otterson MF. Small intestine physiology and pathophysiology. Gastroenterol Clin North Am 1989;18:375–405.

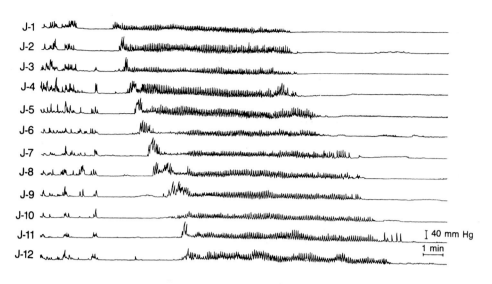

**FIGURE 1.17.** A migrating motor complex (Phase 3 activity) recorded from the human jejunum (J). The recording was made with a manometric tube with side holes 2 cm apart. Note the orderly distal propagation of the group of contractions as a whole. Reproduced with permission from Sarna SK, Soergel KH, Harog JM, et al. Spatial and temporal patterns of human jejunal contractions. Am J Physiol 1989;20: G423–32.

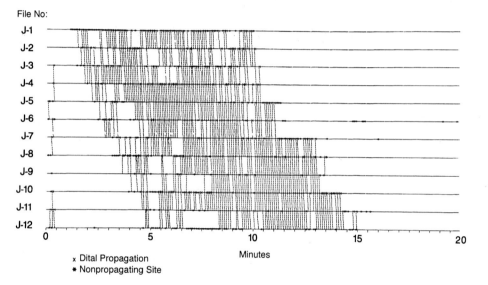

**FIGURE 1.18.** Computer-assisted analysis of propagation of phasic contractions within Phase 3 activity. The lines connect the start of phasic contractions shown in Figure 1.17. The propagation of individual phasic contractions brings the luminal contents to the forefront of Phase 3 activity. When Phase 3 activity migrates distally, as shown in Figure 1.17, the contents are propelled ahead of it. Reproduced with permission from Sarna SK, Soergel KH, Harog JM, et al. Spatial and temporal patterns of human jejunal contractions. Am J Physiol 1989;20:G423–32.

(Fig. 1.14). The spatial coordination of contractions deteriorates along the length of the small intestine (Figs. 1.15 and 1.16). Correspondingly, the rate of propulsion decreases, and mixing increases distally.

In the fasting state, phasic contractions become organized as migrating motor complexes consisting of Phase 1 activity that has little or no contractile activity, Phase 2 activity that shows intermittent single or groups of contractions, and Phase 3 activity that is a group of the largest-amplitude phasic contractions occurring at their maximum frequency, and the entire group of contractions migrates distally in an organized fashion (Fig. 1.17). The large amplitude and repetitive occurrence of these phasic contractions in a given segment are effective in propelling the residual food, debris, and secretions to the forefront of Phase 3 activity. As Phase 3 activity migrates to the terminal ileum, the luminal contents are emptied into the colon. It is noteworthy that the actual propulsion of debris is caused by the propagating phasic contractions within Phase 3 activity (Fig. 1.18).

The phasic contractions within Phases 2 and 3 are controlled by the myogenic and neurochemical controls discussed in the previous sections. However, there are no major luminal contents present in the interdigestive state to provide a sensory stimulus to initiate these contractions. It seems that, like several other neurons, some neurons in the gut can oscillate spontaneously and generate a series of action potentials to produce Phase 3 activity. It is noteworthy that the distal propagation of Phase 3 contractions as a group is also regulated by the enteric interneurons rather than the extrinsic neurons.[10]

The small intestine has built-in protective mechanisms against accidental ingestion of toxic substances by rapidly expelling them. The first step in this process is the initiation of an RGC (see Fig. 1.2C) that regurgitates the contents of the upper half of the small intestine into the stomach. Once there, the somatomotor response takes over and causes vomitus expulsion of gastric contents by a coordinated response of contraction of diaphragmatic and abdominal muscles and

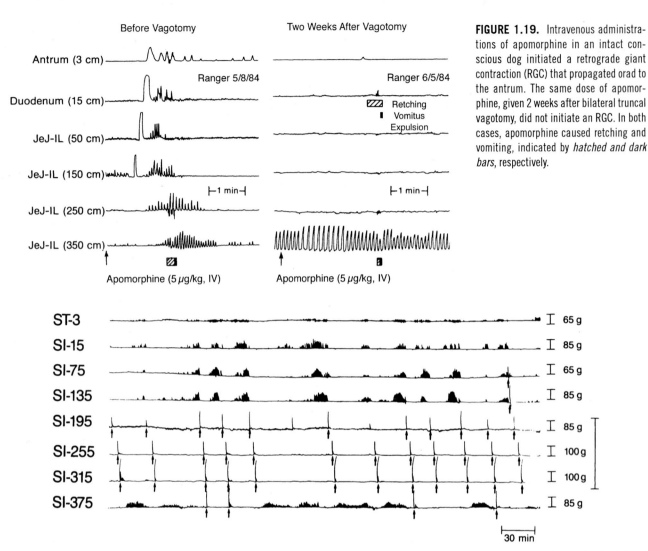

**FIGURE 1.19.** Intravenous administrations of apomorphine in an intact conscious dog initiated a retrograde giant contraction (RGC) that propagated orad to the antrum. The same dose of apomorphine, given 2 weeks after bilateral truncal vagotomy, did not initiate an RGC. In both cases, apomorphine caused retching and vomiting, indicated by *hatched and dark bars*, respectively.

**FIGURE 1.20.** Effect of inflammation on the motor activity of the canine small intestine (SI) recorded with strain gauge transducers. Inflammation was induced in the study segment by mucosal exposure to ethanol and acetic acid. The phasic contractions and migrating motor complexes were present in the upper small intestine and in the terminal ileum that were not inflamed, but they were suppressed in the inflamed segment. The frequency of giant migrating contractions (GMCs) (indicated by *arrows*) was significantly increased in the inflamed segment. The GMCs caused mass movements, resulting in diarrhea. Many of the ileal GMCs propagate into the colon to cause mass movements there as well. When one of these GMCs propagates all the way to the rectum, it causes uncontrollable defecation. ST, stomach. Reproduced with permission from Jouët P, Sarna SK, Singaram C, et al. Immunocytes and abnormal gastrointestinal motor activity during ileitis in dogs. Am J Physiol 1995;269:G913–24.

relaxation of the stomach and the lower and upper esophageal sphincters. The regurgitation by RGCs is an orad mass movement and is preceded by inhibition of contractions and relaxation of tone in the orad receiving segment. The RGCs occur only in the upper half of the small intestine. An RGC may or may not be followed by vomitus expulsion. The RGCs induced by apomorphine are blocked by intravenous atropine, indicating that ACh is the neurotransmitter at the neuro-effector junction. They are also blocked following bilateral truncal vagotomy, indicating CNS control of their initiation (Fig. 1.19). The retching and vomiting produced by apomorphine are present after atropine and after vagotomy.

The caudal mass movements in the small intestine are produced by GMCs (see Fig. 1.7). Under normal conditions, such mass movements occur in the fasting state only in the terminal ileum, once or twice a day. In small intestinal acute inflammation (Fig. 1.20), infections (Fig. 1.21), radiation enteritis, and Crohn's disease, the frequency of GMCs is increased dramatically. Under these conditions, they can begin anywhere in the small bowel and rapidly propagate, usually to the end of the terminal ileum. The GMCs can be stimulated pharmacologically by intravenous administration or morphine, erythromycin (Fig. 1.22), and loperamide and by mucosal irritation with substances, such as vinegar. Pharmacologically stimulated GMCs usually originate in the duodenum and propagate to the ileocolonic junction. It is possible that the abdominal discomfort felt by some subjects after erythromycin is attributable to the stimulation of GMCs that originate in the upper small intestine.

The occurrence of a GMC has been associated with abdominal cramping in patients with irritable bowel syndrome

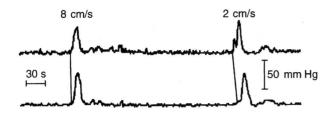

**FIGURE 1.21.** Manometric recording from the proximal small intestine of a patient with severe late radiation enteropathy and significant gram-negative overgrowth shows two giant migrating contractions propagating at 8 cm/sec and 2 cm/sec, respectively. Reproduced with permission from Husebye E, Skar V, Hoverstad T, et al. Abnormal intestinal motor patterns explain enteric colonization with gram-negative bacilli in late radiation enteropathy. Gastroenterology 1995;109:1078–89.

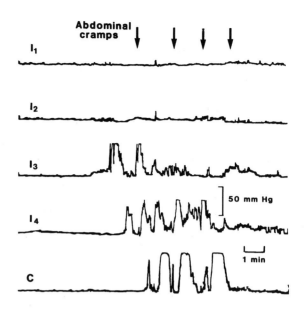

**FIGURE 1.23.** The occurrence of giant migrating contractions in patients with irritable bowel syndrome was associated with abdominal cramping, indicated by arrows. $I_1$ to $I_4$, ileal recording sites with a manometric tube; C, cecum. Reproduced with permission from Kellow JE, Phillips SF. Altered small bowel motility in irritable bowel syndrome is correlated with symptoms. Gastroenterology 1987;92:1885–93.

(Fig. 1.23) and in a patient with a functional bowel disorder (Fig. 1.24). It is important to understand that every GMC may not cause abdominal cramping as there are several factors that are involved in producing this sensation. However, the GMCs are more likely to be perceived as painful in conditions that cause hyperalgesia, such as gut inflammation, irritable bowel syndrome, and gut infection.

Figure 1.2D shows that ileal tone in humans is increased after ingestion of a meal. As discussed earlier, the increase in tone by itself may not have any direct effect on mixing or propulsive functions but it may enhance the efficacy of phasic and ultrapropulsive contractions.

### Colon

Because of the tight junctions in the colon villi, the rate of absorption is slow. Also, the colon has to temporarily store the feces and cause defecation under voluntary control for social reasons in humans and for self-protection in wild animal species. The slow rate of propulsion in the colon is achieved

by mostly discoordinated contractions (Fig. 1.25)[11,12]. In the canine colon, but not in the human colon, the phasic contractions are organized as migrating and nonmigrating motor complexes (Fig. 1.26), but the individual contractions within these complexes do not propagate or propagate over very short distances. The motor complexes in the colon may originate anywhere; they do not always migrate the entire length of the colon, and a small percentage of them may even migrate in the orad direction. Some groups of colonic contractions, constituting a motor complex, do not migrate at all

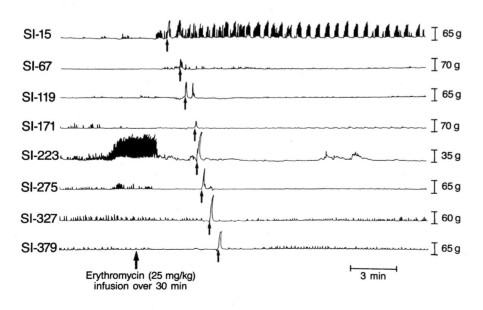

**FIGURE 1.22.** Intravenous administration of erythromycin stimulated a giant migrating contraction in the upper small intestine and it propagated all the way to the terminal ileum. SI, small intestinal strain gauge transducer. The numbers after the symbols indicate the distances of the transducers from the pylorus.

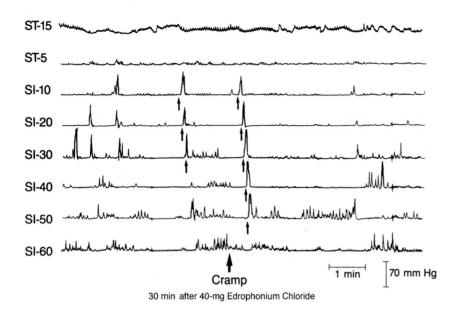

**FIGURE 1.24.** Manometric recording from a patient with symptoms of severe idiopathic abdominal cramping. The patient was administered edrophonium chloride that mimicked the sensation of abdominal cramping. Recording shows that the sensation of cramping was associated with giant migrating contractions (GMCs), which also occurred spontaneously in this patient prior to the administration of edrophonium chloride. Spontaneous GMCs are usually not recorded in the upper small intestine of normal subjects. ST, stomach; SI, small intestine.

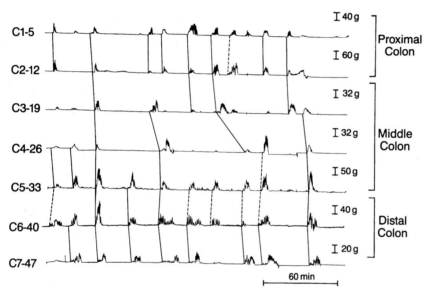

**FIGURE 1.25.** Canine colonic motor activity recorded with surgically implanted strain gauge transducers. The contractions are organized as migrating and nonmigrating motor complexes. The colonic motor complexes migrate mostly in the caudal direction, but their point of origin and distance of migration vary. Some complexes also seem to migrate in the oral direction; others do not migrate at all. C1 to C7, colonic strain gauge transducers. The numbers after these symbols denote their distances from the ileocolonic junction.

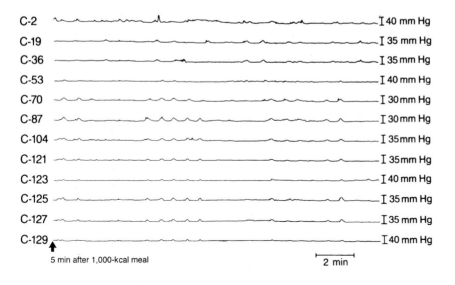

**FIGURE 1.26.** Manometric recording of human colonic motor activity showing random contractions 5 minutes after ingestion of a 1,000-kcal meal. C, colon. The numbers after C indicate the distances of the side holes from the leading tip of the tube. The tip of the tube was located in the ascending colon.

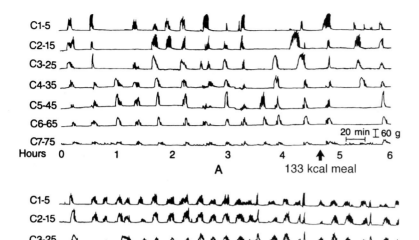

**FIGURE 1.27.** Colonic motor activity before and after a meal. The colonic motor complexes persist after a meal and their frequency is increased. C1 to C7 represent the strain gauge transducers. The numbers after these symbols denote their distances from the ileocolonic junction.

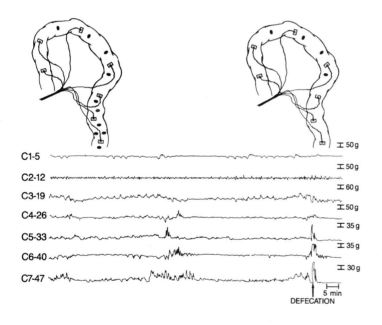

**FIGURE 1.28.** Colonic motor activity associated with defecation. The diagram (*upper left*) shows radiopaque markers distributed throughout the colon. Colonic motor activity consisted largely of uncoordinated contractions. Toward the end of the tracing, a giant migrating contraction (GMC) originated at strain gauge transducer C5 and propagated to the rectum, causing defecation. Immediately following defecation, all of the radiopaque markers distal to the origin of the GMC were expelled, indicating the rapid propulsive force of GMCs or mass movements. C1 to C7 represent strain gauge transducers. The numbers after these symbols indicate their distances from the ileocolonic junction. Reproduced with permission from Sethi AK, Sarna SK. Contractile mechanisms of colonic propulsion. Am J Physiol 1995; 268:G530–8.

or migrate over very short distances of a few centimeters. The colonic motor complexes are not disrupted by the ingestion of a meal (Fig. 1.27). In contrast to the colon, most migrating motor complexes in the small intestine originate in the proximal duodenum and migrate all the way to the terminal ileum. In particular, the small intestinal migrating motor complexes do not migrate in the orad direction and are disrupted by ingestion of a meal. The disorganization of motor complexes in the colon is consistent with the overall disorganization of its contractions that produce transit times of 36 to 48 hours in the normal human colon. In brief, the motor function of colonic motor complexes is different from that of small intestinal migrating motor complexes.

Colonic contractions in the human colon have not yet been reported to be organized as migrating and nonmigrating motor complexes. It is possible that they do not have this type of organization, but it is also possible that their absence is attributable to the conditions under which human colonic motor activity is usually recorded. Most manometric recordings require cleansing the colon, the effect of which on colonic motor activity is not known because the colon is seldom empty in the normal state. The effect of placing a manometric catheter in the colon on its motor activity is also not known. Finally, a manometric catheter does not record contractions that do not occlude the lumen. It is possible that one or more of these factors may contribute to the disruption of

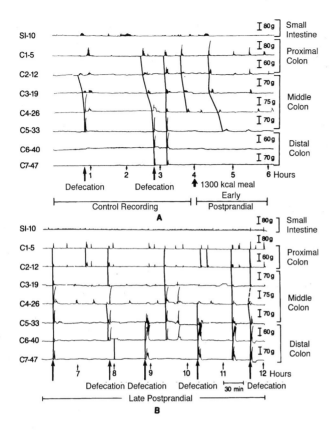

human colonic motor complexes if they are present normally.

Occasional mass movements seem to be essential for normal colonic motor function. In health, these mass movements occur just a few times in the proximal or the transverse colon and also precede defecation (Fig. 1.28). In both cases, the mass movements are caused by GMCs. The absence of mass movements indicated by a decrease in the frequency of GMCs or their total obliteration has been reported to be associated with constipation.[13] By contrast, the frequency of GMCs and mass movements are dramatically increased in experimental acute colonic inflammation[14] (Fig. 1.29) and in patients with ulcerative colitis.[15] The colonic GMCs are also perceived to be painful under certain conditions, particularly when the descending inhibition is impaired and the patients have hyperalgesia. The frequency of GMCs is increased, whereas the phasic contractions and tone are suppressed in colonic inflammation.

Figure 1.30 shows that colonic tone is also increased in ingestion of a meal.

## REFERENCES

1. Cowles VE, Sarna SK. Relation between small intestinal motor activity and transit in secretory diarrhea. Am J Physiol 1990;259:G420–9.
2. Schemann M, Ehrlein H-J. Postprandial patterns of canine jejunal motility and transit of luminal content. Gastroenterology 1986;90:991–1000.
3. Liu X, Rusch NJ, Striessnig J, Sarna SK. Down-regulation of L-type calcium channels in inflamed circular smooth muscle cells of the canine colon. Gastroenterology 2001;120:480–9.
4. Orihata M, Sarna SK. Inhibition of NO synthase delays gastric emptying of solid meals. J Pharmacol Exp Ther 1994;271:660–70.
5. Bayliss WM, Starling EH. The movements and innervation of the small intestine. J Physiol (Lond) 1899;24100–43.
6. Sarna SK. Molecular mechanisms of giant migrating contractions (GMCs) in normal and inflamed ileum [abstract]. Gastroenterology 1999;116:G4665.
7. Otterson MF, Sarna SK. Neural control of small intestinal giant migrating contractions. Am J Physiol 1994;266:G576–84.
8. Gonzalez A, Sarna SK. Different types of contractions in rat colon and their modulation by oxidative stress. Am J Physiol 2001;280:G546–54.
9. Lang IM, Sarna SK, Condon RE. Gastrointestinal motor correlates of vomiting in the dog: quantification and characterization as an independent phenomenon. Gastroenterology 1986;90:40–7.
10. Sarna SK. Cyclic motor activity; migrating motor complex: 1985. Gastroenterology 1985;89:894–913.
11. Sarna SK. Physiology and pathophysiology of colonic motor activity. Dig Dis Sci 1991;36:827–62.
12. Sarna SK. Physiology and pathophysiology of colonic motor activity. Dig Dis Sci 1991;36:998–1018.
13. Bassotti G, Gaburri M, Imbimbo BP, et al. Colonic mass movements in idiopathic chronic constipation. Gut 1988;29:1172–9.
14. Sethi AK, Sarna SK. Colonic motor activity in acute colitis in conscious dogs. Gastroenterology 1991;100:954–63.
15. Kern FJ, Almy TP, Abbot FK, Bogdonoff MD. The motility of the distal colon in nonspecific ulcerative colitis. Gastroenterology 1951;19:492–503.

**FIGURE 1.29.** Colonic motor activity in the fasting and postprandial states in a dog with acute colonic inflammation induced by mucosal exposure to ethanol and acetic acid. The colonic motor complexes are suppressed (compare with Fig. 1.27), whereas the frequency of giant migrating contractions (GMCs) is significantly increased. Several of the GMCs propagated to the rectum and caused defecation. C1 to C7 denote colonic strain gauge transducers. The numbers after these symbols indicate their distances from the ileocolonic junction. SI, small intestinal strain gauge transducer. Reproduced with permission from Seth AK, Sarna SK. Colonic motor response to a meal in colitis. Gastroenterology 1991;101:1537–46.

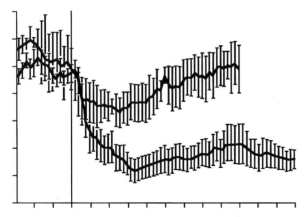

**FIGURE 1.30.** A barostat located in the colon showed a decrease in its volume on drinking water or ingesting a meal. The decrease of barostat volume indicates an increase in colonic tone. Reproduced with permission from Steadman CJ, Phillips SF, Camilleri M, et al. Variations of muscle tone in the human colon. Gastroenterology 1991;101:373–81.

# CHAPTER 2

# Neural and Humoral Regulation of Gastrointestinal Motility

*Jackie D. Wood*

The concept of the enteric nervous system (ENS) as a brain-in-the-gut has become firmly established during the 30 years since publication of the first article on the electrical behavior of single neurons in the myenteric plexus of the cat small intestine.[1] This work to record the neurophysiologic behavior of enteric neurons duplicated methods used for the brain and spinal cord. It was done with extracellular microelectrodes that detected spontaneous firing of single units, responses to electrical stimulation of synaptic inputs, and actions of putative neurotransmitters. Nishi and North[2] and Hirst and colleagues[3] were the first to apply intracellular microelectrode recording methods (ie, "sharp" microelectrodes) in studies of electrical and synaptic behavior of enteric neurons, followed by Wood and Mayer.[4] Since these early studies, a wealth of new information has accrued on the electrical and synaptic behavior and identification of neurotransmitters in the ENS. This, interpreted together with results from work on the neuronal control of gastrointestinal motility and secretion, has firmly established the conceptual perception of the ENS as an independent integrative system, as opposed to earlier views of relay distribution functions characteristic of other autonomic ganglia.

Abundant evidence now supports the concept of the ENS as a "second brain" with neural circuits organized for the local control and coordination of the activity of the musculature, secretory epithelium, and blood vascular system of the gut.[5] Organization of the activity of these effector systems, in turn, accounts for the moment-to-moment digestive behavior in the functioning bowel. Integrated circuits in the ENS account for programming of digestive and defense behaviors that include the digestive pattern of small intestinal motility, the migrating motor complex, power propulsion in defensive states, and reversed small intestinal propulsive motility during emesis.[6,7] Most evidence suggests that vertebrate evolution has positioned a minibrain in close proximity to the gut effector systems. Rather than crowding the $2 \times 10^8$ neurons required for automatic control of gut functions into the cranium as part of the "big brain" and relying on signal transmission over long unreliable pathways to the gut, natural selection placed the integrated microcircuits at the site of the effector systems. Like the central nervous system, the circuits at the effector sites have evolved as an organized array of different kinds of neurons interconnected by chemical synapses.

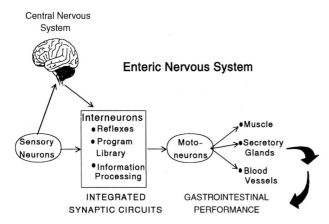

**FIGURE 2.1.** The neurophysiologic model for the enteric nervous system (ENS) is the same as for the central nervous system. Sensory neurons, interneurons, and motoneurons are connected synaptically for information transfer from sensory neurons, interneuronal integrative networks, motoneurons, and gastrointestinal effector systems. The ENS organizes and coordinates the activity of each effector system into the overall performance of the integrated organ. The bidirectional flow of neural signals is continuous between the central nervous system and the ENS.

Function in the circuits is determined by generation of action potentials within single neurons and chemical transmission of information at the points of contact between neurons. The same kinds of synaptic events as found in the central nervous system occur in the ENS and involve the same diverse array of excitatory and inhibitory neurotransmitter substances.

Organization of the connectivity of the neurons that form the ENS is the same as for all independent integrative nervous systems, whether it is the vertebrate brain or spinal cord or the simple nervous systems of invertebrate animals (Fig. 2.1). Like the brain and spinal cord, neurons of the enteric minibrain are synaptically connected for directional flow of neural traffic from sensory neurons to interneurons to motoneurons. Enteric sensory neurons are specialized for detection of the continuously changing conditions within the walls and luminal milieu of the digestive tract and transformation of the information into codes for processing by local area networks and the central nervous system. They code information on parameters such as contractile tension, muscle length, acidity, and osmolarity of luminal contents. Enteric interneurons are synaptically connected into local area networks that process the information generated by the sensory neurons. Networks of interneurons also hold a library of programs, any of which may be called up for generation of a particular pattern of organized digestive behavior. The interdigestive state of small intestinal behavior, or the coordinated secretory and powerful propulsive behavior in response to foreign antigens, is an example of a program in the enteric library.[6,7] Enteric motoneurons connect the interneuronal networks with the effector systems. They are the final common pathways for output from the nervous system to effectors that include the musculature, secretory epithelium, and blood vasculature. Communication from the interneuronal networks by way of the motoneurons directs each effector system to respond with appropriate strength and timing to ensure meaningful coordination with the responses of other effectors. This is the mechanism by which responses of the musculature, epithelium, and blood vasculature system are organized into a functional pattern of behavior at the level of the whole organ.

As with neuropathic changes in the central nervous system, insight into the neurophysiology of the ENS is basic to understanding of the normal and disordered functions of the digestive tract and to the development of strategies for rational therapy. Achalasia in sphincters, the neuropathic form of chronic intestinal pseudo-obstruction, gastroparesis, functional dyspepsia, and the irritable bowel syndrome (IBS) are among the disorders associated with disordered enteric nervous function.[6,7] The etiology of some of these disorders that are currently classified as "functional" also is expected to stem from subtle alterations in enteric neurophysiology. This is reminiscent of central neurologic disorders (eg, Parkinson's disease) that were initially categorized as functional diseases before electrical and synaptic behavior in the microcircuits of the specific brain nuclei and the identification of neurotransmitters and their synaptic actions were understood. The findings of the 1999 GlaxoWellcome landmark survey of IBS in women that nearly 1 in 12 American women has been diagnosed with IBS that seriously compromises quality of life contributes to current actions at national and international levels to raise awareness of this disease. The finding that IBS is two times more prevalent than cardiovascular disease (ie, hypertension) underscores the need for better understanding of enteric neuropathy in functional gastrointestinal disorders. To understand the pathophysiology, it goes without saying that normal neurophysiology of the ENS must be understood first.

## ENTERIC NEUROPHYSIOLOGIC METHODS

Progress in understanding the cellular neurophysiology of enteric neurons has followed advances in application of electrophysiologic and optical imaging methods of recording the electrical and synaptic behavior from single neurons in the ENS. Studies of this kind use modifications of the highly successful approaches to investigation of the brain and spinal cord and have progressed under the umbrella of the new subspecialty of neurogastroenterology.[8]

The guinea pig gastrointestinal tract continues to be the most studied model for electrophysiologic investigation of elements of the ENS. Published information on the electrical and synaptic behavior of guinea pig myenteric neurons exists for both the myenteric and submucous plexuses of the small and large intestine,[9–14] the gastric corpus and antrum,[15–18] gallbladder,[19–21] sphincter of Oddi,[22] and pancreas.[23,24] Fewer reports are available for other species; nevertheless, these are also expanding. Published reports are currently available for the cat,[25] mouse,[26] pig,[27,28] and human.[29]

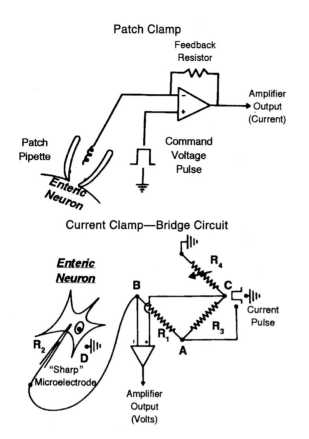

**Patch Clamp**

**Current Clamp—Bridge Circuit**

**FIGURE 2.2.** Current clamp and patch clamp are methods use in intracellular studies of electrical and synaptic behavior of enteric neurons. Patch clamp (*top*) recording is done with glass pipettes that are moved onto the surface of the neuron and the tip sealed to the surface membrane by application of slight suction. Ideally, the fire-polished pipette tip seals to the neuronal membrane with a resistance of more than 10 gigohms to isolate the patch of membrane under the pipette tip and to reduce current flow from the cell interior past the electrode seal when the patch is ruptured by added suction. Rupture of the patch by added suction or by permeabilizing the patch with nystatin or amphotericin B included in the pipette solution opens access to the neuronal interior for recording of whole-cell currents. The specialized amplifiers for patch clamp recording are essentially current-to-voltage converters with a high gain, owing to a large feedback resistor. Configuration of the amplifier is such that the potential inside the patch pipette may be either clamped at a steady level or clamped in command steps to membrane potentials dictated by experimental protocols. Whole-cell currents at the command potential are recorded at the amplifier output. Current clamp (*bottom*) uses "sharp" microelectrodes (tips <1 μm) and a Wheatstone bridge or equivalent circuit to pass electrical current across the neuronal membrane. A single microelectrode is used to inject current into the cell and to record the resulting change in electrotonic potential across the membrane. The current pulses are passed between points A and D (ground) The bridge circuit nulls the voltage drop that occurs across the resistance $R_2$ of the microelectrode so that only the potential across the membrane is recorded between points B and C. This is done by adjusting $R_4$ until the current between A and B equals the current between B and ground at D and the current between A and C equals the current between C and ground at D. When this adjustment is complete, the bridge is said to be balanced, and injection of the current pulse between A and ground does not change the potential between B and C.

## Electrophysiologic Methods

Properties and functions of enteric neurons can be investigated with extracellular and intracellular microelectrode methods of recording neuronal electrical behavior and with optical imaging of voltage-sensitive dyes. This, in conjunction with injection of intraneuronal markers from micropipette electrodes, provides insight into relations of electrophysiologic behavior, histoanatomy, and histochemistry.

## Extracellular Recording

Several different kinds of metal microelectrodes[1] and glass suction electrodes[30,31] may be used for extracellular recording. With extracellular recording, the uninsulated electrode tip may be designed to be small enough to detect the action potential discharge of cell bodies or fibers of single neurons (single-unit recording), or it may be sufficiently large to obtain "multiunit" recordings. Because the electrode tip is in the extraneuronal space, the most useful information obtained is on the occurrence of action potentials within a particular time frame. Extracellular recording has the advantage that discharge patterns of single units can be studied over prolonged time spans and multiple units can be recorded simultaneously for analysis of neuronal interactions. It has the disadvantage of being limited to recognition of relatively small numbers of units in the range of two to four units and is therefore of little value in attempts to study the spread of neural excitation over the spatial distribution

of an extended network of myenteric or submucous plexus. Multiple electrode arrays incorporated with microchip technology are one of the most promising approaches for this kind of research. Additional information can be derived from extracellular electrical recording by testing the effects of pharmacologic agents on the neural activity and by relating the neural activity to behavior of an effector system.

## Intracellular Recording

Intracellular recording is accomplished by impalement of the neurons with fine-tipped (< 0.5-μm diameter) glass pipettes filled with electrolyte solution (usually concentrated KCl).

These are referred to as "sharp electrodes," as opposed to "patch electrodes," which also accomplish intracellular recording but with much larger tip sizes sealed to the outside of the membrane. Intracellular recording with sharp microelectrodes or patch pipettes is technically more involved than extracellular recording; nevertheless, it provides a variety of information about the electrical and synaptic behavior of the neurons that is otherwise unobtainable.

Information on resting membrane potential, membrane resistance, ionic currents and channel behavior, and synaptic potentials is best obtained with intracellular recording. An advantage of intracellular recording with sharp microelectrodes is that the experimenter controls the membrane potential of a neuron by injecting electrical current into the cell through the recording microelectrode (Fig. 2.2). This is called "current clamp." Depolarizing current can be injected to excite the cell or hyperpolarizing current can be used to clamp the membrane potential away from action potential threshold and thereby reduce excitability. The amount of injected current and the corresponding change in transmembrane voltage are measurable parameters for which the ohmic equation $R = V/I$ is used to estimate the electrical resistance of the cell membrane. The resistance of the membrane is determined by its permeability to ions; consequently, changes in ionic conductance produced by synaptic transmitter substances, sensory stimuli, drugs, and so on are reflected by changes in membrane resistance. The resistance measured by intracellular current injection is referred to as input resistance because it is not a precise measure of the specific resistance of any given patch of cell membrane. The input resistance is determined not only by the specific membrane resistance but also by geometric variables such as the size of the cell body and the extent of branching of the processes—all of which are usually unmeasurable. Changes in the electrical characteristics of the microelectrodes during impalements can also distort measurements of input resistance in unpredictable ways. Consequently, most measurements are estimates, and only relative changes in input resistance produced by experimental manipulation are of consequence.

## Voltage Clamp Recording

Voltage clamp methods (see Fig. 2.2) provide information about the properties of ionic currents that pass across the cell membranes and the behavior of channels that account for changes in input resistance recorded in the current clamp mode. In general, voltage clamp permits ionic flow across a cell membrane to be measured as an electrical current while the membrane voltage is held constant with an electronic feedback circuit. This is advantageous because information about ion channel behavior is more easily obtained from an area of membrane with a uniform, controlled voltage than when the voltage is changing with time and in space between adjacent regions of membrane. Voltage control across the membrane is important in this kind of work because the opening and closing (gating) of many ionic channels of interest in enteric neuronal membranes are dependent on the transmembrane potential.

Single-electrode voltage clamp and patch clamp recording are two methods of voltage clamp that have been applied with success in work on enteric neurons. Single-electrode voltage clamp is accomplished with sharp microelectrodes that have the 0.2- to 0.5-μm tip sizes required for impalement of the small neurons. Specialized electronic circuitry is used to switch between current injection and sampling of the transmembrane voltage at switching frequencies in the order of 3 to 15 kHz. The amplifier switches between voltage measuring, usually about 70% voltage sampling and 30% current passing. In practice, the experimenter determines the set point (command voltage) at which the membrane potential is to be clamped by adjustment of the electronics. The amplifier then samples the transmembrane voltage at the determined frequency, and a sample and hold amplifier records that voltage while the system is switched to current injection of appropriate polarity and strength to clamp the membrane potential at the set point. Current required to clamp the membrane at the set point is the equivalent of the ionic current flowing across the membrane. The principal disadvantage of the single-electrode voltage clamp technique is the limitation imposed by the necessarily high resistance of the sharp electrode. The high resistance in combination with the capacitance inherent in the glass pipette limits the frequency at which switching between current injection and sampling can take place. Consequently, applications of single-electrode voltage clamp to enteric neurons have been limited to relatively slow electrical events occurring over several milliseconds or seconds. Action potential currents are too fast to be recorded effectively with a single-electrode voltage clamp and the high-resistance electrodes necessary for successful impalement. Nevertheless, useful information has been obtained with the method.[19,32–34]

Recording with patch pipettes (see Fig. 2.2) overcomes the inherent problems of voltage clamping with sharp electrodes. Patch pipettes have much larger tip diameters that are often heat polished to facilitate a seal with the surface of the neuron. Suction applied to the pipette establishes a tight, high-resistance seal (gigaohms) and is also used to destroy the membrane within the opening of the electrode. A second method used to preserve the intraneuronal milieu is called perforated patch recording. The presence of an antibiotic such as amphotericin B or nystatin in the patch pipettes permeabilizes the membrane following the formation of the seal between the pipette tip and membrane.[35] This prevents the diffusion of macromolecules from the cytoplasm into the pipette. Both the perforated patch and "broken" patch provide a low-resistance path to the neuronal interior that overcomes the inherent problems of a single-electrode clamp with sharp electrodes. The currents thus recorded are called whole-cell currents and represent the sum of the ion fluxes through many channels. Ion channels carrying the currents in whole-cell recording may be of different types and require appropriate methods to isolate individual currents by suppression of accompanying currents. For example, both $Na^+$ and $Ca^{2+}$ may carry current into the neuron when the clamp voltage is quickly stepped from the resting potential to zero potential. Treatment with the neurotoxin tetrodotoxin is a useful tool that selectively blocks $Na^+$ channels to permit study of $Ca^{2+}$ currents in isolation in this case.

Two general approaches are used to investigate the cellular neurophysiology of enteric neurons in the guinea pig. One is to record from the neurons in place in the gastrointestinal wall of dissected preparations; the other is to apply proteolytic enzymes to digest the ganglia free of the surrounding tissues. Ganglia dissociated in this manner may be studied acutely[36] or after a variable period in culture.[35,37] The enteric ganglia are imbedded within the gut wall, making microdissection necessary to expose the ganglia for electrical recording. Dissection is also a necessary step for enzymatic dissociation of the ganglia.[38]

## Optical Imaging

The myenteric and submucous plexuses are two-dimensional networks of neurons spread in a single layer around the circumference and in the longitudinal dimension of the bowel. Neuronal cell bodies in these networks are flat, with their neurites projecting from the edges of the soma in only the X-Y directions.[39] The ENS is one of the few, if not the only, integrative nervous systems that function with the neurons in a single plane rather than in clustered organization. Understanding of how excitation (ie, nerve impulses) spreads from neuron to neuron over extended distances of several centimeters in the two-dimensional networks is an absolute necessity for understanding how the brain-in-the-gut controls the musculature to generate the variety of motor patterns that are part of the physiology of the gastrointestinal tract. This kind of information cannot be obtained with microelectrode methods that are necessarily restricted to recording from no more than one or two neurons. Optical imaging with voltage-sensitive dyes is one of the primary methodologies on the horizon for application to the problems involved in studying the spread of excitation in the two-dimensional networks that make up the ENS.

Optical imaging of changes in neuronal electrical activity is based on the principle that compounds such as Di-8-ANEPPS incorporate in the neuronal membrane and change their spectral properties (ie, absorption or fluorescence) with changes in voltage across the membrane.[40,41] The changes in spectral emission during electrical events (eg, action and synaptic potentials) are detected by photodiode arrays, high-resolution video cameras, or laser scanning systems (Fig. 2.3). Application of this methodology to the ENS is in its infancy; nevertheless, the feasibility of recording action and synaptic potentials simultaneously from multiple neurons in the myenteric and submucous plexus in vitro has been demonstrated.[40,41] For example, Obaid and colleagues described the firing patterns of eight different neurons in the submucous plexus over a 3-minute period following application of nicotine.[40] Animation of the optical images of the eight neurons as they fired impulses over time can be accessed at the author's Website (<http://loco1.med.upenn.edu/~animation>).

## EXTRACELLULARLY RECORDED ELECTROPHYSIOLOGIC BEHAVIOR

Both spontaneous and stimulus-evoked patterns of action potential discharge are recorded extracellularly from neurons within myenteric and submucosal ganglia of intestinal segments in vitro[1,30,31,42-44] and in vivo.[45] Extracellular recording from the gastric myenteric plexus has not been reported. The neurons in the extracellular studies can be classified into three distinct groups on the basis of the pattern of action potential discharge. Neurons in the first group discharge periodic bursts of high-frequency spikes with silent interburst intervals and are called burst-type units. Neurons, some of which may be processes of spinal afferent neurons,

make up the second group. These are mechanosensitive units, which may be spontaneously active or silent and which can be induced by mechanical distortion of the ganglionic surround to discharge spikes at increased frequency. Neurons in the third group are called single-spike neurons because they continuously discharge spikes at irregular intervals and are unaffected by mechanical stimulation.

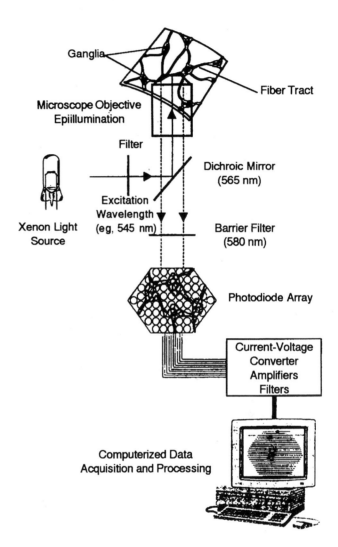

**FIGURE 2.3.** Imaging changes in neuronal membrane potentials with voltage-sensitive dyes in the ENS. Preparations of myenteric or submucous plexus are microdissected from the intestinal wall and placed in a chamber on the stage of an inverted epifluorescence microscope. The tissue is then exposed to the voltage-sensitive dye (eg, the styryl dye Di-8-ANEPPS) for 10 minutes in Krebs solution containing dimethyl sulfoxide followed by continuous superfusion with Krebs solution. Fluorescence of the dye is induced by a xenon light source. Excitation of the dye occurs at 530 nm with fluorescent emission selected at 565 nm with a diachronic mirror and a barrier filtration at 580 nm. The microscope image is projected onto an array of 464 photodiodes. Currents generated by the photodiodes are converted to voltage, amplified, filtered, and sent to the computer for storage and analysis. Optical recordings of action potentials and excitatory synaptic events with single-neuron resolution can be obtained with higher power objectives, and images from 100 to 150 ganglia may be recorded simultaneously with lower power objectives. Adapted from Neunlist et al.[41]

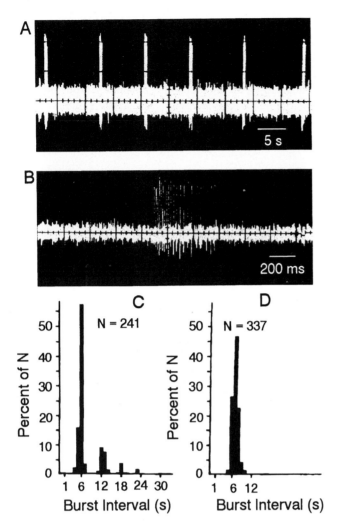

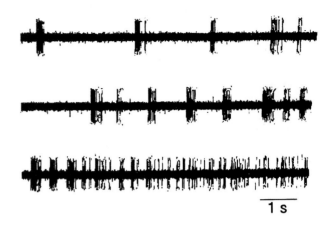

**FIGURE 2.5.** Discharge of an erratic burst-type neuron recorded extracellularly in the myenteric plexus of guinea pig small intestine. The discharge pattern shows conversion from a burst pattern to continuous spike discharge and reversion to a burst pattern. The record is continuous from top to bottom.

**FIGURE 2.4.** Discharge of a steady burst-type neuron recorded extracellularly in the myenteric plexus of cat small intestine. **A**, Burst pattern recorded with a slow time base. **B**, One burst of spikes shown with an expanded time base. **C**, Histogram of interburst interval distribution of consecutive bursts of spikes from a steady burster in the myenteric plexus of a cat small intestinal preparation. The ordinate is the proportion of the total number of intervals, and the abscissa represents the duration of the intervals. The neuron discharged either at intervals of 6 s or at multiples of the 6-s interval. **D**, Burst-interval histogram for a myenteric plexus neuron in the cat that discharged with only small variation around a mean interval of 6 s.

## Burst-Type Neurons

The steady, systematic discharge of burst-type units (Fig. 2.4) continues for several hours in segments of intestine in vitro. These and other enteric neurons are resistant to hypoxia, as reflected by the lack of effect on spike discharge of media with low oxygen partial pressure. This may reflect an adaptation for ischemic physiologic conditions known to occur periodically in the gut. The interburst intervals are temperature dependent. The duration of the interburst interval decreases at temperatures above 37°C and increases below this temperature. The temperature coefficient ($Q_{10}$) for this effect is 10 to 16 over a temperature range of 32 to 40°C. This

is the basis for suggestions that the neurons could be the deep body thermosensors known to be involved in nervous regulation of body temperature.[46]

Burst-type units are distinguished as either steady bursters or erratic bursters on the basis of the regularity of the interburst time intervals. Steady bursters discharge with relatively low statistical variance of interburst interval. Frequency distribution histograms for steady bursters are sometimes multimodal, and the secondary peaks on the histograms are distinct multiples of the time interval represented by the primary peak (see Fig. 2.4). This suggests that the timing of the bursts is determined by an oscillatory pacemaker mechanism and impulse generation fails during some cycles of the continuously running oscillator.

Firing patterns of erratic bursters are characterized by irregular interburst intervals and by periodic conversion to continuous discharge (Fig. 2.5). Variations in the duration of interburst intervals of some erratic bursters are repeated systematically in cyclical patterns. In these cases, each cycle of activity proceeds in a sequence of a silent period of relatively long duration followed by a series of bursts at regular intervals, progressive decrease in intervals separating successive bursts, and then continuous firing followed by the next silent period (see Fig. 2.5).

Elevated $Mg^{2+}$ blocks the ongoing activity of the erratic bursters but not that of the steady bursters.[47] It is known from intracellular studies that elevated $Mg^{2+}$ suppresses the release of neurotransmitters at synapses in the ENS. The effects of elevated $Mg^{2+}$ suggest that synaptic mechanisms are required for production of the erratic burst patterns, whereas burst pattern generation in the steady bursters involves an endogenous pacemaker mechanism. The results of intracellular recording suggest that the burst-type discharge does not originate in the cell bodies of the neurons but rather starts in the neuropil and propagates in dendrites to be recorded as they invade the soma.

Focal application of single electrical shocks either to the surface of a myenteric ganglion or to an interganglionic fiber tract evokes a burst of spikes that resembles the spontaneously discharged bursts of erratic bursters. These stimulus-evoked bursts appear to be synaptically mediated because they are reversibly blocked by elevated $Mg^{2+}$ and reduced $Ca^{2+}$ in the bathing medium. Nevertheless, the responses are unaffected by a variety of putative neurotransmitter substances and synaptic blocking drugs that include curare, hexamethonium, atropine, acetylcholine, norepinephrine, methysergide, 5-hydroxytryptamine (5-HT), naloxone, and morphine.[48] Several pharmacologic agents have been tested on the spontaneously occurring burst discharge.[1,31,49] In general, agents active at cholinergic synapses alter the ongoing discharge of the erratic bursters. Acetylcholine stimulates some of the units, and muscarinic or nicotinic blocking drugs sometimes halt the discharge of some. Burst-like discharge superimposed on oscillations of membrane potential is sometimes seen in intracellularly recorded responses to application of acetylcholine. No putative neurotransmitters or receptor-blocking drugs have been found to affect the discharge of the steady bursters. The available evidence suggests that the erratic bursters possess cholinergic receptors and that their discharge is driven by release of one or more unidentified transmitters from the long list known to be localized in the ENS (see the section on synaptic transmission below).

Steady bursters appear not to receive synaptic input. They may be continuously running oscillators that provide synaptic drive to the erratic bursters. Indications of driver-follower coupling have been observed on multiunit records as sequential temporal coupling by a constant time interval of the discharge of two different burst units.[50] This kind of activity is expected to continuously release neurotransmitters at neuromuscular junctions. Continuous release of inhibitory neurotransmitters is known to maintain states of ongoing inhibition of contractile activity in the autogenic intestinal musculature.[51]

Peptidergic neurotransmitters are colocalized with other neurotransmitters (eg, acetylcholine or 5-HT) in enteric neurons. Burst-type discharge is implicated as a mechanism for selective release of peptidergic neurotransmitters in these instances. The responses of several autonomic effector systems to neural stimulation are enhanced when the nerves are stimulated to discharge in high-frequency bursts.[52] Bursts of action potentials in the motor nerves to alimentary effectors are significantly more effective than sustained discharge in evoking responses. The frequencies of spike discharge within the bursts and the interburst intervals found to be most effective are within the range of discharge parameters of the burst-type units in the myenteric plexus. The pattern of discharge in the motor axon is undoubtedly an important determinant of the response of the effector system whether the effector is muscle or secretory cells.

Edwards and colleagues suggested that with colocalization of more than one neurotransmitter, one or the other transmitter could be released preferentially by modulating the pattern of spike discharge.[52] Enteric axons may function like some

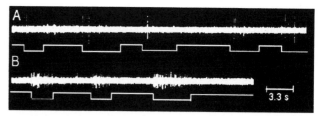

**FIGURE 2.6.** Mechanosensitive neurons in the ENS behave like slowly and rapidly adapting receptors elsewhere in the nervous system. **A,** Rapidly adapting mechanoreceptor in the myenteric plexus of cat small intestine. The unit discharged only at the onset of mechanical distortion of the ganglion, indicated by downward deflection of the bottom trace. **B,** Slowly adapting mechanoreceptor in the myenteric plexus of dog small intestine. The unit discharged at relatively constant frequency throughout each mechanical stimulus, indicated by downward deflections on the bottom trace.

sympathetic nerves in which norepinephrine, adenosine triphosphate (ATP), and neuropeptide Y are colocalized within the same release site. Low-frequency stimulation releases norepinephrine and ATP simultaneously from small granular vesicles while short, high-frequency bursts preferentially increase exocytosis of neuropeptide Y from large storage vesicles.[52, 53] A similar situation holds for enteric neurons that have formed synaptic contacts in culture. Neurons in these cultures synthesize acetylcholine and co-store it with the inhibitory neuromuscular transmitter vasoactive intestinal peptide.[54] Low-frequency electrical stimulation releases acetylcholine that acts at postsynaptic neurons to evoke nicotinic fast excitatory postsynaptic potentials (EPSPs). High-frequency stimulation (> 10 Hz) is required to release the peptide, which evokes slow synaptic excitation (slow EPSPs) in the same neurons.

## Mechanosensitive Neurons

Extracellular recording from single units within the myenteric plexus reveals three kinds of units that respond with an increased rate of discharge to mechanical stimulation. One kind of mechanosensitive unit behaves like a typical slowly adapting mechanoreceptor and another like a fast-adapting mechanoreceptor (Fig. 2.6). The third kind is activated by mechanical stimulation to discharge prolonged trains of spikes lasting up to 40 s (see Fig. 2.6). The discharge frequency of the third kind of unit is independent of the intensity of stimulation, and the discharge continues in a set pattern for many seconds after termination of the mechanical stimulus. The prolonged trains of spikes are the extracelullar correlates of the train-like discharge recorded intracellularly during slow EPSPs in afterhyperpolarization (AH)/Dogiel morphologic type II neurons. Enteric mechanosensitive units are activated by circular muscle contractions in preparations of small intestine in vitro.[1]

The units behaving like slowly adapting mechanoreceptors (see Fig. 2.6) show sustained discharge without signs of adaptation during a stimulus of constant intensity, and the frequency of discharge is directly related to the intensity of stimulation.[55] They may or may not show ongoing discharge prior to stimulation. The units that behave like fast-adapting mechanoreceptors (see Fig. 2.6) give an intensity-dependent discharge at the onset of the stimulus and quickly stop firing during a sustained stimulus.

Mechanosensitivity is a property of the three types of mechanosensitive units only and is not a general property of all myenteric ganglion cells. Other myenteric neurons may show low levels of ongoing discharge of action potentials that may be similar to those of the slowly adapting mechanosensitive neurons; nevertheless, these units are not excited by the same kind of mechanical stimulation that increases the firing rate of slowly adapting units.

The receptive fields of the slowly adapting mechanosensitive neurons are limited to the region of the ganglion and do not extend to the interganglionic fiber tracts.[42] The discharge patterns of both the fast- and slowly adapting mechanosensitive neurons, when recorded at the ganglia, are similar to patterns of discharge recorded in gastrointestinal vagal afferent fibers[56,57] and splanchnic nerves.[58,59] The mechanosensitive units recorded in the myenteric plexus apparently correspond to the "deep" tension receptors that discharge in vagal afferent fibers and that were shown by Iggo[57] to be localized within the muscularis externa. The probable location of the generator region of the "deep tension receptors" is within the periganglionic connective tissue or within the ganglia. Vagal afferents have been traced to their specialized terminations within the myenteric ganglia of the stomach and small intestine.[60,61] Binding of cholecystokinin to the A receptor subtype and serotonin to the 5-HT$_3$ receptor subtype on vagal afferents stimulates firing.[62,63] Histamine (H)$_1$ receptors, serotonergic 5-HT$_3$ receptors, and receptors for multiple kinds of cytokines stimulate firing of spinal afferents. Histamine and serotonin activate mechanosensory units at the level of myenteric ganglia.[55]

## Single-Spike Neurons

Single-spike neurons continuously discharge action potentials at relatively low frequencies with no consistent pattern to the activity. The ongoing discharge is sometimes altered but never blocked by elevated $Mg^{2+}$ and lowered $Ca^{2+}$ in the bathing solution, indicating that it is independent of synaptic input. Stimulation by acetylcholine and other nicotinic agonists is the most noteworthy characteristic of these units. Norepinephrine acts at alpha-adrenoceptors to reduce the discharge rate. This is consistent with nicotinic cholinergic synaptic input to these neurons because norepinephrine acts presynaptically to suppress the release of acetylcholine at nicotinic synapses in the enteric microcircuits.[64]

## INTRACELLULARLY RECORDED ELECTROPHYSIOLOGIC BEHAVIOR

With the exception of the gastric antrum and gallbladder, intracellular recording with "sharp" microelectrodes distinguishes two kinds of electrical behavior in enteric neurons.

These are referred to as AH type 2 and synaptic type I neurons. This arbitrary combination of terms recognizes Nishi and North[2] and Hirst and colleagues,[3] who published the first descriptions of the electrophysiology of the two types of neurons. These designations combine the alphabetical terms of Hirst and colleagues and the numeric designations of Nishi and North. Both terms are useful because AH type II neurons usually have Dogiel type II multipolar morphology, whereas S type I neurons are generally unipolar.

AH type 2 neurons are distinguished electrophysiologically by (1) higher resting membrane potentials and lower input resistances than S type I neurons; (2) no spike discharge to depolarizing current injection or discharge of one or two spikes only at the onset of intraneuronal injection of long-duration depolarizing current pulses (Fig. 2.7); (3) absence of anodal break excitation at the offset of hyperpolarizing current pulses; (4) prolonged postspike hyperpolarizing potentials; (5) $Ca^{2+}$ contribution to the inward current of the action potential; (6) tetrodotoxin-resistant action potentials; (7) exposure to multivalent cationic $Ca^{2+}$ entry blockers such as $Mn^{2+}$, $Mg^{2+}$, or $Cd^{2+}$, which depolarizes the neurons, increases input resistance, and augments excitability; and (8) activation of adenylate cyclase and elevation of intracellular cyclic adenosine monophosphate (cAMP), which depolarizes the cells, increases input resistance, and augments excitability. Aside from electrophysiologic properties, most AH neurons (ie, $\approx 80\%$), but not S neurons, contain the calcium-binding protein calbindin.[65] AH neurons comprise the largest proportion of neurons in the intestinal myenteric plexus (ie, $\approx 70\%$) and the smallest proportion of submucous plexus neurons (ie, <10%).

Most of the multipolar AH/Dogiel type II neurons in the intestinal myenteric plexus project one of their long processes out of the ganglion to pass through the circular muscle coat and into the mucosa. Because these terminals of AH-type neurons in the mucosa respond to release of serotonin from enterochromaffin cells in the mucosa and because mechanical stimulation of the mucosa activates enterochromaffin cells to release serotonin, there has been an inclination toward calling them "primary afferent neurons."[66,67] The behavior of AH neurons overall does not fit the classic neurophysiologic descriptions of primary sensory afferent neurons (ie, dorsal root and nodose ganglion cells) and is therefore a confusing misnomer. AH neurons are a unique population of neurons in the mammalian nervous system and would best be called simply "AH/Dogiel type II" to convey their functional significance in neural control of the bowel and to retain the term that has been used consistently since first being applied by Hirst and colleagues in 1974.[3]

S type I neurons are distinguished by (1) lower resting membrane potentials than AH neurons; (2) higher input resistance than AH neurons; (3) repetitive spike discharge throughout long-duration depolarizing current pulses (see Fig. 2.7); (4) frequency of repetitive discharge increases in direct proportion to the size of depolarizing pulses; (5) anodal break excitation at the offset of intraneuronally injected hyperpolarizing current pulses; (6) blockade of somal spikes

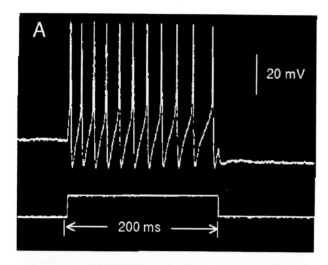

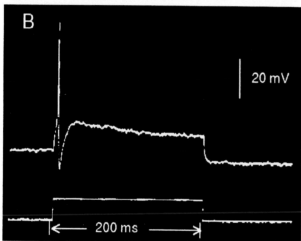

**FIGURE 2.7.** Responses evoked by intracellular injection of depolarizing current in AH- and S-type neurons in the myenteric plexus of guinea pig small intestine recorded with "sharp" intracellular microelectrodes. **A**, Injection of a 200-ms duration depolarizing pulse-evoked discharge of multiple spikes throughout the current pulse in an S-type neuron. **B**, Injection of a 200-ms duration depolarizing pulse in an AH-type neuron evoked a single spike only at the onset of the current pulse. The hyperpolarizing "sag" in voltage evident during the current pulse (*upper trace*) following the spike reflects activation of the ionic conductances responsible for the after-hyperpolarization in AH neurons. Upper traces are transmembrane voltage; bottom traces show timing of the injected current (see Fig. 2.2; current clamp method).

by tetrodotoxin; and (7) insensitivity to stimulation of adenylate cyclase by forskolin and elevation of cAMP.

Nicotinic fast EPSPs can be evoked experimentally in most all S-type neurons by electrical stimulation. Nevertheless, this cannot be used as the sole basis for classification because AH neurons have nicotinic receptors and may also receive fast synaptic input. S neurons are more likely to show spontaneously occurring fast EPSPs and spike discharge than AH neurons. Nevertheless, AH neurons discharge spontaneously when activated by excitatory neurotransmitters or paracrine signals.

## Membrane Electrophysiology: Resting Potentials

The resting membrane potential of enteric neurons is predicted by the Goldman-Hodgkin-Katz constant field equation.[68] Potassium conductance is the main determinant of the resting potential, which is usually less than the potassium equilibrium potential. In AH neurons, a component of the resting potassium conductance and consequently the resting potential are dependent on the concentration of free intracellular $Ca^{2+}$.[69–72] A steady influx of $C^{2+}$ is responsible for elevated intraneuronal levels that maintain $Ca^{2+}$-activated $K^+$ channels in an open state. This is reflected by high $K^+$ conductance, lowered input resistance, and hyperpolarized membrane potential in AH neurons in the absence of excitatory mediators.

Neurotransmitters and paracrine neuromodulators act to increase or decrease the $Ca^{2+}$-activated $K^+$ conductance, and this is the key mechanism for up and down modulation of excitability and input-output relations. The functional significance of resting potentials less than the $K^+$ equilibrium potential is provision of a mechanism whereby the membrane potential can be modulated in the hyperpolarizing or depolarizing direction, determined by whether the messenger substance acts to increase or decrease the $K^+$ conductance. In enteric neurons, inhibitory signal substances such as opioid peptides, galanin, and adenosine decrease neuronal excitability by increasing $K^+$ conductance and hyperpolarizing the membrane,[73–75] whereas excitatory messengers like substance P, serotonin, and histamine decrease resting potassium conductance, depolarize the membrane, and enhance excitability.[76,77]

The membrane of the cell body, the initial segments of neurites, and the neurites themselves (ie, axons and dendrites) are sites where action potentials are initiated in enteric neurons. Action potential generation in the cell bodies of AH neurons differs from spike-generating mechanisms in the cell bodies of S neurons and the neurites of the AH neurons.

## Membrane Electrophysiology: Action Potentials

The ionic mechanism of action potential generation in the cell bodies of AH neurons includes conductance changes for $Ca^{2+}$, $Cl^-$, $Na^+$, and $K^+$. Both $Na^+$ and $Ca^{2+}$ carry the inward current of the rising phase of the spike. A characteristic "shoulder," reminiscent of the plateau on cardiac action potentials, is present at the onset of the falling phase of the spike in AH neurons[13] that reflects activation of voltage-gated $Ca^{2+}$ conductance in N-type, high-voltage activated $Ca^{2+}$ channels[35] as the membrane is depolarized by inward $Na^+$ current. $\omega$-CgTx-MVIIC toxin from *Conus magus* is a selective blocker for the channel.[78] The $Na^+$ channels are typical of tetrodotoxin-sensitive channels found in neurons elsewhere.[79] Application of tetrodotoxin reduces the rate of rise, the amplitude, and the threshold but does not abolish the action potentials. The rate of rise of the spike in tetrodotoxin is increased by elevation of external $Ca^{2+}$, and the pure $Ca^{2+}$ spike in this case is abolished by multivalent ions that block $Ca^{2+}$ entry.[13,32,80–82] Dihydro-

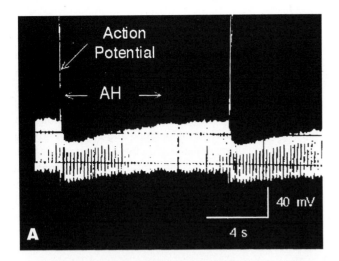

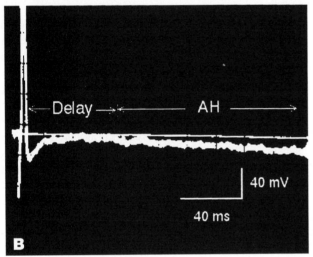

**FIGURE 2.8.** Postspike after-hyperpolarization in an AH myenteric neuron from guinea pig small bowel in vitro. **A,** Two action potentials were followed by the characteristic prolonged hyperpolarization of the cell membrane. Decreased amplitude of electrotonic potentials produced by intracellular injection of hyperpolarizing current pulses (see Fig. 2.2; current clamp method) reflects decreased input resistance during the hyperpolarization. **B,** One action potential and postspike hyperpolarization recorded with an expanded time base from the same neuron. The prolonged after-hyperpolarization was delayed in onset until about 40 ms after the hyperpolarizing undershoot of the action potential.

pyridines and other organic calcium entry blockers that suppress $Ca^{2+}$ conductance in gastrointestinal smooth muscles do not affect the $Ca^{2+}$ spikes in AH neurons.[4]

AH-type neurons possess the full complement of voltage-gated $K^+$ currents generally found in neurons elsewhere. These include A-type, delayed rectifier, and inwardly rectifying currents.[83,84] The falling phase of the spike is associated with time- and voltage-dependent activation of delayed rectifier $K^+$ channels. Shoulders on the falling phase of the spikes are prolonged by tetraethylammonium.[13] A prominent undershoot (ie, positive after-potential) of the repolarization phase in some of the neurons lasts for 10 to 15 ms (Fig. 2.8) and reflects delayed inactivation of the delayed rectifier.

Long-lasting hyperpolarizing after-potentials are the hallmark of the action potentials in AH neurons (see Fig. 2.8). The after-hyperpolarization activates slowly beginning from 45 to 80 ms after the positive after-potential (see Fig. 2.8) and lasts for up to 30 s. The amplitude of the after-potential summates when two or more spikes are fired in close sequence. An increase in membrane conductance reflected by a decrease in the input resistance occurs during the hyperpolarizing after-potentials (see Fig. 2.8). The amplitude of the after-potential is increased by elevation of extracellular $Ca^{2+}$ and is suppressed my multivalent ions that block $Ca^{2+}$ entry. Prolongation of the $Ca^{2+}$ spikes during suppression of the delayed rectifier $K^+$ channels by tetraethylammonium enhances the after-potentials.[13] The amplitude is reduced, and the duration of the hyperpolarizing after-potential is shortened in bathing media with reduced $Ca^{2+}$.[82] The polarity of the hyperpolarizing after-potential is reversed with current clamp of the membrane potentials to values greater than the $K^+$ equilibrium potential of $\approx -90$ mV. An inverse relation exists between the concentration of $K^+$ in the bathing solution and the amplitude of the after-potential, with a Nernstian decrease in the reversal potential for a 10-fold increase in extracellular $K^+$.[82–85] The outward current associated with the hyperpolarizing after-potential in single-electrode voltage clamp studies reverses at $\approx -82$ mV.[86] These findings were evidence that the hyperpolarizing after-potential is generated by an outward current carried by $K^+$ ions.

The outward $K^+$ current responsible for the hyperpolarizing after-potential appears to be carried by $Ca^{2+}$-activated $K^+$ channels. Evidence for this comes from voltage clamp results that suggest that the slow outward current is coupled temporally to inward $Ca^{2+}$ currents that are activated by depolarizing voltage steps.[86] The amplitude of the current of the hyperpolarizing after-potential is a direct function of the amount of $Ca^{2+}$ that enters the cell during depolarizing clamp steps or as the result of discharge of action potentials. A finite amount of $Ca^{2+}$ must enter before activation of the $K^+$ current takes place. Hirst and colleagues referred to this as "primer $Ca^{2+}$."[86] Total $Ca^{2+}$ entry determines only the amplitude of the $K^+$ current; it does not influence the time to peak current, the rate of activation of the current, or the rate of inactivation. Further evidence for the $Ca^{2+}$ dependence of $K^+$ current activation is the suppression of the current and the associated hyperpolarization by multivalent cations that block $Ca^{2+}$ entry.[69,81,82,85] This is consistent with the results obtained with optical imaging of intraneuronal $Ca^{2+}$ that show increased intraneuronal free $Ca^{2+}$ during the hyperpolarizing after-potential.[70] The after-hyperpolarization associated with the $Ca^{2+}$-activated $K^+$ current is reinforced by inwardly rectifying $K^+$ current as the membrane potential is hyperpolarized toward the $K^+$ equilibrium potential. Inwardly rectifying $K^+$ current in AH neurons activates at membrane potentials more negative than $-80$ mV.[83]

The details of the cellular physiology of the $Ca^{2+}$-activated current responsible for the after-hyperpolarization are not yet fully understood. Any postulated mechanism must account for the long 30- to 40-ms delay in activation of the current after the spike, the slow rates of activation, and inactivation and the fact that the entire event, which lasts for several seconds, is triggered by a very brief injection of $Ca^{2+}$ of shorter duration that the 3- to 4-ms action potential. The rates of development and decay of the hyperpolarizing after-potentials have temperature coefficients $(Q_{10})$ of 3,[85] which is suggestive of a metabolic process rather than passive diffusion of ions. The association of inactivation of the $Ca^{2+}$-activated $K^+$ channels and elevation of cytoplasmic cAMP[87] is consistent with involvement of biochemical mechanisms. Elevation of cAMP also closes the $Ca^{2+}$-activated $K^+$ channels that are open in AH neurons at rest. Whether the $Ca^{2+}$-dependent $K^+$ channels that are open at rest and the channels that are opened following the action potential are the same is unresolved.

The hyperpolarizing after-potentials function to lengthen the refractory period following the spike, and this automatically limits the frequency of spike discharge by the cell body. During slow synaptic excitation, discussed below, the neurotransmitter or paracrine modulator acts to reduce the hyperpolarizing after-potential, and this permits the somal membrane to fire repetitively at a higher frequency. Modulation of the after-potential by chemical messengers is part of the overall mechanisms by which the excitability and input-output relations of the neurons are governed.[13]

Somal action potentials in S-type neurons and spike generation by neurites of both AH- and S-type neurons are generated by classic mechanisms of activation and inactivation of time- and voltage-dependent $Na^+$ and $K^+$ conductance channels. The spikes are always abolished by sufficient concentrations of tetrodotoxin, and the rate of rise and amplitude are reduced in depleted $Na^+$. Unlike AH neurons, mechanisms for generation of repetitive spike discharge are always activated, and the cells will often discharge spontaneously, with the spikes preceded by ramp-like prepotentials. In contrast to AH neurons, S neurons fire continuously during long-lasting depolarizing current pulses (see Fig. 2.7), and the frequency of discharge is related directly to the size of the depolarizing pulse. Prominent positive after-potentials are associated with the spikes and are not followed by $Ca^{2+}$-dependent after-spike hyperpolarizing potentials like those in AH neurons. Unlike AH neurons, depletion of extracellular $Ca^{2+}$ or activation of adenylate cyclase by forskolin does not elevate excitability. Motoneurons to the musculature are S type.

### Enteric Neuronal Excitability: Plasticity

The patterns of electrophysiologic excitability in enteric neurons are not fixed and are often observed to change during the course of a 1- to 2-hour recording session in vitro. For example, the behavior of AH neurons can range from inexcitability to typical AH behavior to enhanced excitability with absence of the hyperpolarizing after-potentials and repetitive firing at elevated frequency. The neuron may not respond at all to the intraneuronal injection of depolarizing current and may later be found to have converted to a state of enhanced

excitability with behavior like that of an S-type neuron. Such neurons are identified as the AH type by excitatory response to forskolin, expression of calbindin, tetrodotoxin-insensitive spikes, and long-lasting hyperpolarizing after-potentials when in lesser states of excitability. Exposure of the neurons to adenosine or an adenosine $A_1$ receptor agonist converts the hyperexcitable state to inexcitability with transition through AH-type behavior and is a useful test for identification of neurons with elevated excitability as being the AH type.

Plasticity of electrophysiologic behavior appears to be a fundamental property of enteric neurons in most regions of the digestive tract and is probably an important determinant of the output functions of the circuits in which they reside. The behavioral states are probably determined by changes in concentrations of neurotransmitters, paracrine mediators, or hormones that may appear in the external milieu in the various digestive or pathophysiologic states of the bowel. For example, heightened neuronal excitability is found in the intestine after immune sensitization to a foreign antigen. This is due to mast cell degranulation and release of histamine, which is an excitatory mediator that acts like forskolin to elevate cAMP and enhance excitability.[88–90] In these cases, AH neurons are converted from their hypoexcitable state to superexcitability. In some experimental preparations, excitability is suppressed by elevated levels of endogenously released adenosine. In this situation, treatment with the degradative enzyme adenosine deaminase restores excitability.[91]

## SYNAPTIC TRANSMISSION

Fundamental mechanisms for chemically mediated synaptic transmission in the ENS are the same as elsewhere in the nervous system. Synaptic transmitters are released by $Ca^{2+}$-triggered exocytosis from stores localized in vesicles at axonal terminals or transaxonal varicosities. Release is triggered by the depolarizing action of action potentials when they arrive at the release site and open voltage-activated $Ca^{2+}$ channels. Once released, enteric neurotransmitters bind to their specific postsynaptic receptors to evoke ionotropic or metabotropic synaptic events. When the receptors are directly coupled to the ionic channel, they are classified as ionotropic. They are metabotropic receptors when their effects to open or close ionic channels are indirectly mediated by guanosine triphosphate-binding proteins and the induction of cytoplasmic second messengers (eg, cAMP).

Synaptic events in the ENS are basically the same as in the brain and spinal cord. Excitatory postsynaptic potentials, inhibitory postsynaptic potentials (IPSPs), and presynaptic inhibition and facilitation are the principal synaptic events in the enteric minibrain. Both slow and fast synaptic mechanisms are operational. Fast synaptic potentials have durations in the millisecond range; slow synaptic potentials last for several seconds or minutes. Fast synaptic potentials are usually EPSPs. The slow synaptic events may be either EPSPs or IPSPs.

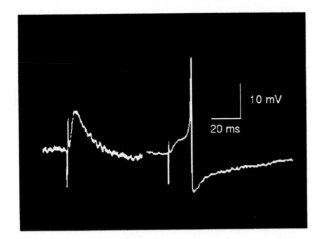

**FIGURE 2.9.** Examples of fast EPSPs. Two fast EPSPs were recorded in a guinea pig myenteric small intestinal neuron with a "sharp" microelectrode in the current clamp mode. The EPSP on the left did not reach threshold for discharge of an action potential; the one on the right did depolarize the membrane potential to spike threshold. The probability for a fast EPSP to trigger action potentials is increased during slow synaptic excitation and presynaptic facilitation and decreased during slow synaptic inhibition and presynaptic inhibition (see Figs. 2.10 and 2.14–2.16).

### Fast Excitatory Postsynaptic Potentials

Fast EPSPs were reported for the earliest intracellular studies of enteric neurons but only in the S type I cells by Hirst and colleagues[3] and Nishi and North.[2] They are membrane depolarizations with durations less than 50 ms (Fig. 2.9). Fast EPSPs were later reported to occur in AH- and S-type neurons in both myenteric and submucous plexuses. They appear to be the sole mechanism of transmission between vagal efferents and enteric neurons. Most of the fast EPSPs are mediated by acetylcholine at nicotinic postsynaptic receptors. The actions of 5-HT at the 5-HT$_3$ receptor subtype and purine nucleotides at P$_{2X}$ purinergic receptors behave much like fast EPSPs, and it is possible that some fast EPSPs are serotonergic or purinergic.[92] Responses mediated by 5-HT$_3$ receptors are found on neurons in both plexuses throughout the gastrointestinal tract, including the gastric corpus.[92] The results of patch clamp recording show that the nicotinic and 5-HT$_3$ receptors are directly coupled to nonspecific cationic channels. The opening of these channels is responsible for the depolarizing event.[93] Rapid desensitization is a characteristic of both the nicotinic and 5-HT$_3$-operated channels, both of which are ionotropic. Purinergic "fast" depolarizing responses are metabotropic and mediated by second-messenger function of phospholipase A and elevation of inositol triphosphate.[92] Amplitudes of nicotinic fast EPSPs in the intestine become progressively smaller when they are evoked repetitively by focal electrical stimulation applied to the surface of the ganglion or interganglionic fiber tract. A decrease in EPSP amplitude occurs at stimulus frequencies as low as 0.1 Hz, and the rate of decline is a direct function of stimulus frequency. A rundown of this nature does not occur at the synapses in the stomach[16,18] or gallbladder.[19] The rundown

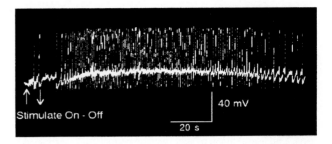

**FIGURE 2.10.** Slow synaptic excitation in an AH-type myenteric neuron in the small intestinal myenteric plexus of the guinea pig in vitro. Electrical stimulation of the synaptic input for 3 s evoked a slowly activating membrane depolarization associated with enhanced excitability that lasted for more than 2 min. Enhanced excitability is reflected by the prolonged train of action potentials that continued for over 2 min after termination of the slow excitatory synaptic input.

phenomenon reflects presynaptic inhibition of acetylcholine release by additional transmitter substances broadly released by the electrical stimulus or by negative feedback involving autoinhibition of acetylcholine release (see section on presynaptic inhibition below). Rundown cannot be attributed to postsynaptic changes because no decrease in the amplitude of the EPSPs occurs during repetitive applications of acetylcholine from microejection pipettes.

Fast EPSPs function in the rapid transfer and transformation of neurally coded information between the elements of the enteric microcircuits. They are the bytes of information in the information-processing operations of the logic circuits. One of the fast EPSPs in Figure 2.9 reached threshold for discharge of an action potential, whereas the other EPSP did not reach threshold. Fast EPSPs do not reach threshold when the neuronal membranes are hyperpolarized during slow IPSPs. They are most likely to reach spike threshold when the membranes are depolarized during slow EPSPs. This fits the definition of neuromodulation, whereby the input-output relations of a neuron to one input are modified by a second synaptic input.

### Slow Synaptic Excitation

Slow EPSPs are evoked experimentally by focal electrical stimulation of interganglionic fiber tracts or the surfaces of ganglia in both myenteric and submucosal neurons and in both AH- and S-type neurons. They are most dramatic in AH neurons, in which conversion from hypo- to hyperexcitability is involved. Neurons with slow EPSPs are found in the small and large intestine and gastric antrum but not the gastric corpus or gallbladder. They seem to be associated with specialized regions where peristaltic motility is a significant function.

Slowly activating membrane depolarization continuing for several seconds to minutes after termination of release of the neurotransmitter from the presynaptic terminal identifies the slow EPSP (Fig. 2.10). Enhanced excitability reflected by a long-lasting train of action potentials, like those seen in extracellular recordings from tonic-type mechanosensitive neurons, is the hallmark of the event. Enhanced excitability is apparent experimentally as repetitive spike discharge during depolarizing current pulses and as anodal break excitation at the offset of hyperpolarizing current pulses. AH neurons, which fire only a single spike at the beginning of a depolarizing current pulse in the inactivated state, will fire repetitively in response to depolarizing pulses when the slow EPSP is in effect. When activated by slow synaptic inputs, the behavior of AH neurons is much like S neurons and may be confused, as such, if they happen to be in an activated state because of ongoing release of the transmitter. Mechanical distortion in the vicinity of AH neurons releases mediators that evoke slow EPSP-like elevation of excitability reminiscent of that in extracellular records from tonic-type neurons.[94]

Postspike hyperpolarization in AH neurons is suppressed during slow EPSPs. Suppression of the after-hyperpolarization is part of the mechanism that permits repetitive spike discharge at increased frequencies during the enhanced state of excitability.

The ionic mechanism for slow EPSPs includes changes in several ionic conductances. The depolarizing phase occurs when $Ca^{2+}$ channels, normally open at rest, are closed.[69,72,95]

This lowers intraneuronal $Ca^{2+}$, which, in turn, leads to closure of $Ca^{2+}$-activated $K^+$ channels. Closure of the $K^+$ channels accounts for the increased input resistance seen in the neuron during the depolarization of the slow EPSP. $Ca^{2+}$ currents during the spike, which in the resting state would lead to a postspike increase in $Ca^{2+}$-activated $K^+$ conductance, are suppressed. This accounts for suppression of the after-hyperpolarization during the EPSP. Enhanced excitability, seen as repetitive spike discharge and anodal break excitation during the EPSP, is probably related to suppression of A-type and delayed rectifier $K^+$ currents.[84]

Slow EPSPs are a mechanism for long-lasting activation or inhibition of gastrointestinal effector systems. The prolonged discharge of spikes during a slow EPSP drives the release of neurotransmitter from the neuron's axon for the duration of the spike discharge. Prolonged inhibition, or excitation at neuronal synapses in the processing circuits and at neuroeffector junctions, is the functional outcome of the slow EPSP. This governs the functional behavior of the effector systems. Compared to twitches of skeletal muscles, contractile responses of the gut musculature are sluggish events that last for several seconds from start to completion. The prolonged train-like discharge of spikes during slow EPSPs is the neural correlate of long-lasting excitatory or inhibitory responses of the muscle groups in the functioning gastrointestinal tract. Prolonged secretory responses in the intestinal crypts are also related to the sustained discharge during slow EPSPs.

Several messenger substances found in neurons and endocrine or immune cells of the brain and gut mimic slow EPSPs when applied experimentally to enteric neurons. Receptors for more than one of the messenger substances may be present on the same neuron. Table 2.1 shows the current list of substances, together with receptor subtypes.

**TABLE 2.1.** Slow EPSP Mimetics

| | |
|---|---|
| Acetylcholine (muscarinic/$M_1$) | Vasoactive intestinal peptide |
| Cholecystokinin (A) | Cerulein |
| Bombesin | Gastrin-releasing peptide |
| Calcitonin gene–related peptide | Tachykinins ($NK_3/NK_1$) |
| Thyrotropin-releasing hormone | Corticotropin-releasing hormone |
| 5-Hydroxytryptamine ($5\text{-}HT_{1P}$) | $\gamma$-Aminobutyric acid |
| Norepinephrine | Motilin |
| Pituitary adenylate cyclase–activating peptide | Glutamate (group 1 metabotropic) |
| Interleukin-1$\beta$ | Interleukin-6 |
| Tumor necrosis factor | Platelet activating factor |
| Adenosine ($A_2$) | Bradykinin ($B_2$) |
| Histamine ($H_2$) | |

Substance P (a tachykinin), 5-HT, and acetylcholine fulfill the criteria for function as a neurotransmitter in the enteric microcircuits. The other substances are implicated mainly by their presence in enteric neurons and/or by mimicry of the slow EPSP when applied experimentally. Receptors for these substances, as well as combinations of receptors for other substances on the list, can be found colocalized on the same enteric neuronal cell body.

Histamine and interleukin-1$\beta$ are examples of signal substances of paracrine origin. Histamine and interleukin-1$\beta$ are released from intestinal mast cells to become a neuromodulatory signal that is decoded by the enteric microcircuits. Mast cells have both detector and signal functions in enteric neuroimmune communication.[90] They use the specificity and memory of the immune system to detect the presence of threatening antigens in the gut and, after doing so, release histamine to signal the ENS to reprogram its output for secretory and motor behavior that effectively eliminates the antigenic threat from the intestinal lumen.[90]

The evidence for 5-HT is as complete as for any known neurotransmitter, including synthesis, storage, and release from enteric neurons. Nevertheless, the strongest evidence is that agents such as N-acetyl-5-hydroxytryptophyl-5-hydroxytryptophan amide, renzapride, and anti-idiotypic antibodies to 5-HT block both the slow EPSP-like actions of 5-HT and the slow EPSP in the same AH neurons.[96] Aside from its role as a putative enteric neurotransmitter, 5-HT also has a paracrine signaling function. A large fraction of the body's 5-HT is stored in enterochromaffin cells in the intestinal mucosa. Mechanical stimulation (shearing forces) of the mucosa releases the 5-HT, which may then reach receptors on AH neuronal projections in the mucosa, other enteric neural elements, and spinal and vagal sensory afferents.[96]

Bornstein and colleagues reviewed five criteria for transmitter function that were fulfilled by substance P: (1) pharmacologic evidence suggests the intramural release of substance P within intestinal segments; (2) the $K^+$ conductance decrease produced by substance P and the slow EPSP is the same; (3) chymotrypsin, which digests substance P, reduces both the response to the peptide and the slow EPSP; (4) the widespread occurrence of slow EPSPs implies that terminals of the responsible axons synapse with most cell bodies in the ganglion, as is the case for the multipolar (AH/Dogiel type II) neurons that contain substance P; and (5) slow EPSPs were evoked in myenteric neurons with ganglia that contained substance P but no immunocytochemically demonstrable 5-HT-containing fibers.[97] Slow EPSPs can be initiated by substance P released from AH/Dogiel type II neurons or from collateral projections of spinal afferents inside the intestinal wall.[98]

An early obstacle in identifying substance P as a neurotransmitter in the enteric microcircuits was the unavailability of suitable antagonists. There are no reports of an effective antagonist for the actions of substance P on the neurons. The putative peptidergic substance P antagonists (D-PRO2, D-PHE7, D-TRP9-substance P; D-PRO2, D-TRP7,9-substance P; and D-ARG1, D-PRO2, D-TRP7,9, LEU11-substance P) did not block the excitatory action of substance P.[99,100] Instead, these putative antagonists behaved like agonists and excited the neurons. The putative nonpeptide antagonist CP-96,345[101] has no specific blocking action on substance P responses in small intestinal myenteric neurons.[102]

Neurokinin-3 receptors appear to be mediators of the action of substance P.[103] The slow EPSP-like action of 5-HT is related to the 5-HP$_{1p}$ receptor, so named by Mawe and his coworkers.[104] This receptor subtype is blocked by the drug renzapride, which is a substituted benzamide compound with promotor effects in the gut.[96] The slow EPSP mimetic action of acetylcholine is mediated by the M$_1$ muscarinic receptor subtype,[105,106] and the action of histamine involves the H$_2$ receptor subtype.[107,108]

Slow EPSP-like actions of acetylcholine result from activation of muscarinic receptors as indicated by blockade of the responses by atropine, hyoscine, pirenzepine, and telenzepine and mimicry by McNeil A343, oxotremorine, and muscarine.[106] The pharmacologic profile of the receptors fits the M$_1$ subtype. Blockade of stimulus-evoked slow EPSPs by muscarinic antagonists has been reported consistent with muscarinic mediation of some of the EPSPs.[106]

Motilin is a slow excitation mimetic of particular interest because it is implicated as a messenger substance in the initiation of the migrating motor complex in the interdigestive period.[109] Additional interest emerges from findings that macrolide antibiotics (eg, erythromycin) act at motilin receptors to facilitate gastric emptying in disorders such as diabetic gastroparesis.[110] Slow EPSP-like actions of motilin are prominent in AH neurons of the gastric antrum.[111]

## Slow EPSP Signal Transduction

Slow activation and the prolonged nature of the responses are characteristics of stimulus-evoked slow EPSPs and the actions of slow EPSP mimetics that offer clues to the mechanism of signal transduction. A 30-ms "puff" of a slow EPSP mimetic or electrical stimulation of synaptic inputs will often evoke changes in excitability that last for several minutes.[4,112] This happens in experiments in which the exposure is virtually lim-

ited to the duration of the puff because of high rates of superfusion in small-volume tissue chambers. Although the mimetics act transiently at discrete sites on the somal membrane, the membrane around the entire cell body is involved in the closure of Ca$^{2+}$-activated K$^+$ channels. This suggests involvement of an intraneuronal second-messenger system in the transduction process that connects localized surface receptors (ie, metabotropic receptors) to the entire cell body. Receptor occupancy by the messenger substance in this case stimulates intraneuronal synthesis or release of a second messenger, which then initiates the neurochemical reactions and molecular conformational changes responsible for transformation of the somal membrane from hypo- to hyperexcitability. Several lines of evidence indicate that receptor-mediated activation of adenylate cyclase and elevation of intraneuronal cAMP are a signal transduction mechanism for the slow EPSP.

Forskolin, a substance that activates adenylate cyclase, is a useful tool for the study of signal transduction in enteric neurons. Application of forskolin elevates cAMP in the ganglia[38] and mimics the slow EPSP in AH- but not in S-type neurons.[113] Likewise, other treatments that elevate cAMP, such as intraneuronal injection of cAMP, application of membrane-permeant analogs of cAMP, and treatment with phosphodiesterase inhibitors all produce slow EPSP-like effects.[87] Treatment of enzymatically dissociated myenteric ganglia with substance P,[114] 5-HT,[115] or histamine[116] stimulates the formation of cAMP. Stimulation of cAMP formation by 5-HT is mediated by 5-HT$_{1p}$ receptors, whereas the histamine action is mediated by the H$_2$ receptor subtype. The combined evidence supports a role for cAMP as an intracellular second messenger in the process of signal transduction in AH neurons. Occupancy of receptors for the slow EPSP activates adenylate cyclase, which, in turn, leads to synthesis of cAMP, phosphorylation of protein kinases, and/or membrane channel proteins and eventually to the dramatic changes in neuronal excitability that occur during slow synaptic excitation. Receptors for several different kinds of mediators are coupled by G proteins to adenylate cyclase to initiate a single post receptor cascade of events that culminates in the slow EPSP.

The experimental use of forskolin has improved insight into the behavior of enteric neurons with low excitability that were described as AH type II and type III in earlier work on neuronal properties determined by intracellular recording.[117] The cell bodies of AH, as well as the type III neurons, are often found in states of inexcitability. In this condition, they have high resting membrane potentials close to the potassium equilibrium potential and low input resistance indicative of high resting potassium conductance. Injection of depolarizing current does not evoke action potentials in this state, whereas synaptic potentials in response to inputs from other neurons in the circuit may be present. The synaptic potentials do not evoke spikes in this state.

Application of forskolin or one of the endogenous slow EPSP mimetics often restores excitability to the AH and type III neurons. When this occurs, the cells may discharge action

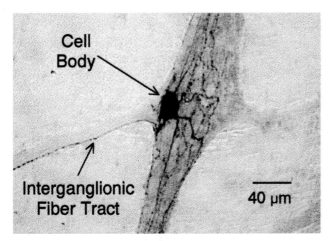

**FIGURE 2.11.** Morphology of an AH/Dogiel type II myenteric neuron revealed by the injection of the intraneuronal marker biocytin from an intracellular "sharp" recording microelectrode in the guinea pig small intestine. The projection of the neuron's processes ramifies extensively within the ganglion and into interganglionic connectives, leading out of the ganglion and into neighboring ganglia, as well as out of the ganglion in the direction of the mucosa (see Fig. 2.13).

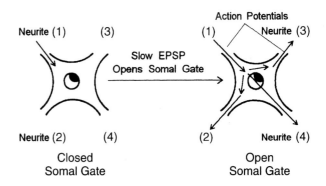

**FIGURE 2.12.** Slow EPSPs in the cell bodies of AH/Dogiel morphologic type II neurons are part of a mechanism for gating the directional spread of excitation (ie, action potential transmission) among neurons in the microcircuits of the enteric plexuses. Slow EPSPs underlie the gating mechanism by which the spread of spike information between neurites, which arise from opposite poles of the cell body, is controlled. When the neuron is in the resting state shown on the left, the excitability of the cell body is low, and the probability that inbound spike information arriving at the soma in neurite 1 will fire the cell body is low. In the event that the somal membrane does fire, the discharge is limited to one or a few spikes by the postspike hyperpolarizing afterpotentials. In this state, the somal gate is totally or partly closed, and no or a restricted amount of information is relayed to the neurites at the opposite poles of the cell body. During a slow EPSP (diagrammed on the right), the probability that the somal membrane will be fired by inbound spikes in neurite 1 and that it will fire repetitively at an increased frequency is greatly increased during a slow EPSP when excitability is enhanced, membrane resistance is increased, and hyperpolarizing after-potentials are suppressed. The slow EPSP opens the somal gate so that inbound activity is transferred to neurites 2, 3, and 4 and relayed on to synapses with neighboring neurons.

potentials with hyperpolarizing after-potentials if the concentration of the agent is low, or they may discharge repetitively like an S-type neuron if exposed to higher concentrations. These neurons are interpreted as interneuronal circuit elements that are not used continuously by the system. When the state of the gut does not require operation of that section of circuitry (eg, reverse peristalsis), the circuit is inactivated by the low excitability state of its component neurons. The circuit is called to activity by chemical modulators that act to boost the excitability of its neurons.

### Significance of Slow EPSPs in the Integrated System

The functional significance of slow synaptic excitation in AH neurons is twofold. The first aspect relates to the significance intuitively attributed to an excitatory synapse. This is an increased probability of spike discharge in the postsynaptic neuron that is then transformed into excitation or inhibition at either the next order neuron or an effector such as the musculature. Intestinal peristalsis, for example, requires sustained discharge by some type of element in the microcircuit to account for the delays of several seconds between stimulus and coordinated responses and for sustained neural drive for several seconds at the circular or longitudinal muscle coat. The behavior of AH neurons during slow EPSPs fits the requirements for a neuronal element, functional significance of which in the circuit would be production of either prolonged excitation or inhibition of the intestinal circular or longitudinal muscle layers. The putative neurotransmitters for the slow EPSP stimulate the release of acetylcholine, tachykinins, vasoactive intestinal peptide, and nitric oxide from myenteric and submucous plexuses.[118–120] This is consistent with the suggestion that AH neurons are the interneuronal source of

coordinated synaptic drive to the excitatory and inhibitory motor innervation of the musculature. The extensive ramifications of the processes of the AH/Dogiel type II neurons to innervate large numbers of neurons in the same and neighboring ganglia (Fig. 2.11) and the localization of substance P in these neurons[121,122] are consistent with this function.

Slow EPSPs also underlie a gating mechanism that controls the spread of action potentials between the neurites arising from opposite poles of the cell body of a multipolar neuron. Figure 2.12 illustrates how slow synaptic gating works in AH/Dogiel type II neurons. Intracellular recording in AH neurons in the low excitability shows that action potentials propagating toward the cell body in one of its processes usually do not fire the membrane of the cell soma. If the invading spike should fire the somal membrane, the action potential of the cell body will be followed by the characteristic afterhyperpolarization, which acts to prevent firing of the cell body by any additional incoming spikes. The probability for the cell body to be fired by inbound spikes is greatly increased during the slow EPSP when excitability is enhanced, membrane resistance is increased, and after-hyperpolarization is suppressed. The membrane of the cell body behaves like a closed gate to the transfer of spike signals between its neurites when it is in

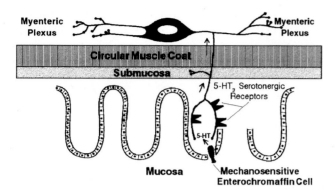

**FIGURE 2.13.** Heuristic model for the functional significance of the properties of AH/Dogiel morphologic type II neurons in the neural networks of the ENS. The projectional geometry of the neurites identifies the significance of the cell body as a gating determinant of neurite-to-neurite communication across the cell soma. Most of the AH neurons project one or more neurites to the mucosa. This expands the functional significance because the projections in the mucosa fire in response to acidic pH and in response to serotonin released by mechanical stimulation of mucosal enterochromaffin cells. As elements in a neural network, AH neurons are stimulated to fire repetitively by slow synaptic inputs. Firing of the neuronal cell body is transformed into slow synaptic output at synapses with neighboring AH neurons in the network. The somal gate is closed in the absence of slow synaptic input. In this state, inbound information from the mucosa is not gated to neurites across the cell body but may become the afferent arm of an axon reflex. In circumstances in which the somal gate is opened by either slow synaptic or paracrine excitatory input (see Fig. 2.12), information from the mucosa is gated in the direction of slow synaptic outputs and the axon reflex path shown on the model.

the low-excitability state. In this state, spike information, such as inbound information from the mucosa (Fig. 2.13), is confined to a single neurite (eg, neurite 1 in Fig. 2.12). The gate is opened, and signals are transferred across the somal membrane to other neurites during the slow EPSP. A closed somal gate isolates the initial segments of each neurite such that spike discharge in one initial segment does not influence another neurite elsewhere around the cell body.

The increase in membrane resistance during the slow EPSP increases the space constant of the somal membrane and facilitates electrotonic spread of the action potential from the neurites into the cell body. This, together with the enhanced excitability, opens the somal gate, resulting in transfer of signals across the cell body to neurites at other poles of the neuron. When this happens, all neurites fire synchronously with the cell body, and the action potentials are conducted away to be distributed in regions of the enteric networks lying further along or around the intestine. Somal gating within a pool of interconnected multipolar neurons is believed to underlie the rapid build-up of action potential discharge in the neuronal pool. This results in simultaneous spike discharge, characteristic of the slow EPSP, in a population of neurons around the circumference and along the length of an intestinal segment. This is a mechanism for synchronizing the behavior of the musculature around the circumference of the bowel within a confined length.[123,124]

The projectional geometry of the neurites identifies the significance of the cell body of AH/Dogiel type II neurons as a gating determinant of neurite-to-neurite communication across the cell soma. Almost all myenteric AH/Dogiel type II neurons project one or more neurites to the mucosa (see Fig. 2.13). This adds to the functional significance because the projections in the mucosa fire in response to acid pH and in response to serotonin released by mechanical stimulation of mucosal enterochromaffin cells.[66,67,125] Figure 2.13 models the functional significance of the properties of AH/Dogiel type II neurons. As coupled elements in muscle control circuits, they are stimulated by slow synaptic inputs to fire prolonged trains of impulses. This kind of activity in the cell body is transformed into slow synaptic output to neighboring AH/Dogiel type II neurons in the circuit. In the absence of slow synaptic input, the somal gate is closed (see Fig. 2.12). In this state, inbound information from the mucosa is not gated to neurites across the cell body but may become the afferent arm of an axon reflex. In circumstances in which the cell body is activated by slow synaptic input, the somal gate is open, and the transformed information from the mucosa is gated in the direction of slow synaptic output and the axon reflex path illustrated in Figure 2.13.

Some authors have applied the term "primary afferent neuron" in reference to AH/Dogiel type II neurons because they respond when mechanical or chemical stimuli are applied to the mucosa.[66,67] This is inappropriate because the complex functions of the AH/Dogiel type II neurons do not fit the classic neurophysiologic descriptions of primary afferent neurons (ie, spinal and vagal afferents); consequently, the term becomes a confusing misnomer for students making an effort to learn enteric neurophysiology. AH/Dogiel type II neurons are unique among the various neuronal types found in the vertebrate nervous system and would best be called simply "AH/Dogiel type II neurons" to retain the original terminology used by those who first described their electrophysiologic behavior[2,3] and to convey their functional significance in the neural networks that control propulsive motility.

## Inhibitory Postsynaptic Potentials

Inhibitory postsynaptic potentials are hyperpolarizing synaptic potentials found in both myenteric and submucous ganglion cells of the small and large intestine and in myenteric neurons of the gastric antrum.[4,18,126–128] They can be evoked by electrical stimulation of either interganglionic fiber tracts or the surface of the ganglion. Stimulus-evoked IPSPs activate relatively slowly and continue for several seconds after termination of the stimulation (Fig. 2.14). The characteristics of slow synaptic inhibition are inverse to those of slow EPSPs in that the hyperpolarization is associated with decreased input resistance and suppression of excitability. Reduction in the membrane resistance and excitability, together with membrane hyperpolarization, decreases the probability of action potential discharge that might occur spontaneously in response to excitatory synaptic inputs or to inbound action potentials in a neurite.

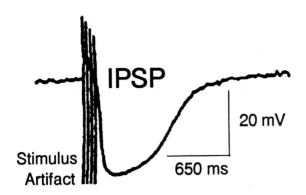

**FIGURE 2.14.** Slow inhibitory postsynaptic potentials (IPSPs) are hyperpolarizing potentials in the ENS that can be recorded with "sharp" microelectrodes in the current clamp mode. Their functional significance is hyperpolarization of the membrane potential away from the action potential threshold and a decrease in the probability of action potential discharge.

**TABLE 2.2.** Slow IPSP Mimetics

| | |
|---|---|
| Acetylcholine | Opioid peptides |
| 5-Hydroxytryptamine 5-HT$_{1A}$ | Norepinephrine ($\alpha_2$) |
| Neurotensin | Cholecystokinin |
| Somatostatin | Adenosine triphosphate |
| Adenosine (A$_1$) | Galanin |
| Nociceptin | |

Inhibitory postsynaptic potentials are more readily demonstrated in the submucous than in the myenteric plexus of in vitro preparations. In earlier studies, slow IPSPs were found in less than 10% of small intestinal myenteric neurons,[4,129] whereas over 80% of submucous neurons show IPSPs in response to electrical stimulation.[127] Interaction of slow excitatory inputs that counteract the inhibitory inputs is a factor accounting for the low incidence of IPSPs in the myenteric plexus studies. Experimental stimulation of interganglionic connectives activates both excitatory and inhibitory inputs, and the excitatory inputs usually predominate to a variable degree. Selective blockade of slow synaptic inputs by adenosine A$_1$ receptor agonists uncovers and enhances stimulus-evoked slow IPSPs in the myenteric plexus.[91]

The decrease in input resistance observed during slow synaptic inhibition reflects increased conductance in potassium channels.[33,36,130,131] Of the variety of potassium channels found in the membranes of enteric neurons, the inwardly rectifying potassium channels appear to be the ones opened by a variety of inhibitory neurotransmitters to account for the increased conductance and hyperpolarization of the membrane potential during the IPSP.[33,130,131] The calcium-activated potassium channels that both contribute to the resting membrane potential and account for postspike hyperpolarization are not involved in the generation of the slow IPSPs.[36,130,132,133] Guanosine triphosphate–binding proteins are suggested to be involved in direct coupling of the receptors to the potassium channels.[130,133]

Several putative neurotransmitters evoke responses similar to slow IPSPs when experimentally applied to enteric neurons. Some of these substances are peptides, others are purine compounds, and another is norepinephrine. The receptors for two or more of these substances may be localized to the cell body of the same neuron. Table 2.2 is a list of the substances that may be found in enteroendocrine cells, as well as enteric neurons. These substances, which are present both in the brain and gastrointestinal tract, sim-

ulate slow synaptic inhibition when applied experimentally to enteric neurons.

Enkephalins, dynorphin, and morphine all mimic the IPSPs in enteric neurons. This is mediated by opiate receptors and limited to subpopulations of neurons. Opiate receptors of the mu subtype predominate on myenteric neurons, whereas the receptors on submucosal neurons are the delta opioid subtype.[134] The effects of opiates and opioid peptides are prevented by naloxone; however, naloxone has not been found to block any of the experimentally evoked IPSPs. Dependence on morphine may be seen in enteric neurons with withdrawal observed as high-frequency spike discharge on the addition of naloxone during chronic exposure of the neurons to morphine.[135,136] Inhibitory postsynaptic potentials–like actions of nociceptin involve an opioid receptor-like receptor that is distinct from typical naloxone-sensitive opioid receptors.[137]

Norepinephrine binds to $\alpha_{2a}$-adrenoceptors to produce IPSPs in enteric neurons. This occurs primarily in neurons of the intestinal submucosal plexus.[127,130] The noradrenergic inputs come from postganglionic fibers of the sympathetic nervous system that are involved with inhibition of secretomotor neurons in the submucosal plexus.

Galanin is a 29 amino acid polypeptide that mimics slow synaptic inhibition in almost all of the neurons of the intestinal myenteric and submucous plexuses.[138] Cholecystokinin does this also, but the effect is seen only in a subpopulation of 10 to 15% of myenteric neurons in the small intestine or gastric antrum.[139–141]

The application of adenosine, ATP, and other purine analogues simulates the slow IPSP in intestinal myenteric neurons.[75] This is seen in nearly all AH neurons and appears to result from the suppression of the enzyme adenylate cyclase and the reduction in intraneuronal levels of cAMP.[142] Both the degradative enzyme adenosine deaminase and a selective adenosine A$_1$ receptor antagonist potentiate slow synaptic excitatory responses.[91] This is thought to reflect the presence and ongoing inhibitory action of endogenous adenosine in in vitro conditions.

Somatostatin is implicated by several kinds of indirect evidence as the endogenous inhibitory transmitter responsible for the intrinsic inhibitory inputs to submucous ganglion cells. Hirst and Silinsky described IPSPs in the submucous plexus that persisted after sympathectomy and could therefore not be attributed to activation of norepinephrine release from sympathetic postganglionic fibers.[143] This IPSP, unlike the noradrenergic IPSPs, usually requires repetitive stimulation and occurs with a more slowly developing time course.[144]

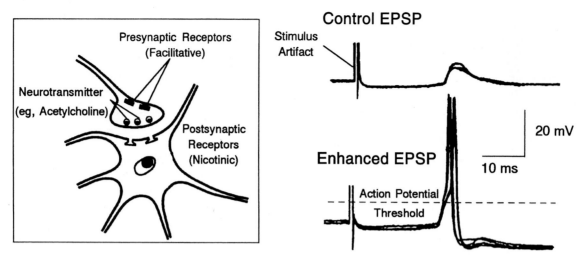

**FIGURE 2.15.** Presynaptic facilitation enhances the release of neurotransmitter and increases the amplitudes of excitatory postsynaptic potentials (EPSPs) in the ENS. The top trace shows a fast nicotinic EPSP recorded with a "sharp" microelectrode. Activation of presynaptic facilitative receptors increased the release of acetylcholine to elevate the amplitude of the EPSP to action potential threshold shown in the bottom trace. Presynaptic facilitative receptors may be activated by neurotransmitters or endocrine and paracrine messenger substances.

Neither naloxone nor adrenergic blocking drugs affect the putative somatostatin-mediated IPSP.[145] Somatostatin-containing nerve terminals and the nonadrenergic slow IPSPs disappear in parallel after destruction of the myenteric plexus and its projections to the submucous plexus.[145]

## Functional Significance of Slow IPSPs

A reduction in the membrane resistance and excitability of the somal membranes, together with membrane hyperpolarization during the slow IPSPs, decrease the probability of action potential discharge. The probability is reduced that the somal membrane will be fired during electrotonic invasion by spikes in the initial axonal segment or during excitatory synaptic input (see Figs. 2.12 and 13). This influence is the inverse of the slow EPSP and acts to close the gate for transfer of spike information across the multipolar soma of AH neurons.

Slow synaptic inhibition probably functions to terminate the excitatory state of slow synaptic excitation and re-establishment of the low excitability state in the ganglion cell soma of AH neurons. This may be a step in the control of sequentially occurring motor events such as the conversion from inhibition to excitation in the circular muscle of an intestinal segment during propagation of propulsive peristalsis. In the intact animal, there may also be inhibitory substances of endocrine or paracrine origin that function in particular situations to lock the somal membranes in a low-excitability state.

## Presynaptic Facilitation

Presynaptic facilitation refers to enhancement of synaptic transmission resulting from actions of chemical mediators at neurotransmitter release sites on enteric axons. This is known to occur at fast excitatory synapses in the myenteric plexus of the small intestine and gastric antrum and at noradrenergic inhibitory synapses in the submucous plexus. It is also seen as an action of cholecystokinin in gallbladder ganglia.[20] Presynaptic facilitation is evident as an increase in amplitude of fast EPSPs at the nicotinic synapses and reflects enhanced release of acetylcholine from axonal release sites (Fig. 2.15). At noradrenergic inhibitory synapses in the submucous plexus, it appears as enhancement of the hyperpolarizing responses to stimulation of sympathetic postganglionic fibers and is associated with elevation of cAMP in the sympathetic nerve terminals.[128]

## Presynaptic Inhibition

Presynaptic inhibition refers to mechanisms that suppress the release of neurotransmitters from axons (Fig. 2.16). It involves binding of chemical messengers to inhibitory receptors at transmitter release sites on the axon. Intracellular electrophysiologic recording with "sharp" microelectrodes in the ENS has established presynaptic inhibition as another significant synaptic event within the enteric microcircuits of the gastric corpus and antrum, as well as the small and large intestine and rectum of the guinea pig.[13,16,18,68,146,147] It is found at fast and slow excitatory synapses, inhibitory synapses, and neuromuscular junctions.

In some cases, presynaptic inhibition involves axo-axonal transmission, whereby release of a neurotransmitter from one axon acts at receptors on another to suppress the release of transmitter from the second axon (see Fig. 2.16). In other cases, it takes the form of autoinhibition and can occur at both neural synapses and neuroeffector junctions. Autoinhibition occurs when the transmitter released from the same enteric neuron accumulates in the vicinity of the release site and activates presynaptic inhibitory receptors to

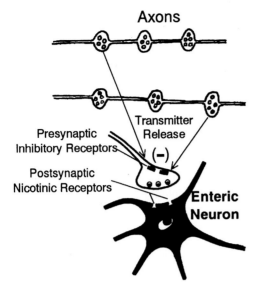

**Axons**

Transmitter
Release

Presynaptic
Inhibitory Receptors

(−)

Postsynaptic
Nicotinic Receptors

**Enteric
Neuron**

**FIGURE 2.16.** Presynaptic inhibition is a form of neurocrine transmission whereby the neurotransmitter released from one axon acts at receptors on a second neuron to suppress the release of neurotransmitter from the second axon. Presynaptic inhibition in the ENS may also involve actions of paracrine or endocrine release of mediators that act at presynaptic inhibitory receptors to suppress synaptic transmission.

suppress further release. It functions in this way as a negative feedback mechanism that automatically regulates the concentration of neurotransmitter within the synaptic or junctional space. Presynaptic inhibition is also mediated by paracrine or endocrine release of substances from non-neuronal cells into the milieu surrounding the synaptic circuits. Mast cells and enteroendocrine cells are sources of non-neuronal messages picked up by presynaptic receptors.

Several messenger substances found in neurons or enteroendocrine or immune cells of the gut produce presynaptic inhibition when applied experimentally to enteric synapses (Table 2.3).

Norepinephrine acts at presynaptic $\alpha_{2a}$-receptors to suppress transmission at both slow and fast excitatory synapses and at excitatory neuroeffector junctions.[130] The presynaptic inhibitory actions of norepinephrine are significant because it is the neurotransmitter released at the synaptic interface between postganglionic sympathetic axons and the

**TABLE 2.3.** Mimetics for Presynaptic Inhibition

1. Norepinephrine ($\alpha_{2a}$)
2. Histamine ($H_3$)
3. Opioid peptides
4. Neuropeptide Y
5. Peptide YY adenosine ($A_1$)
6. Dopamine
7. 5-Hydroxytryptamine ($5\text{-}HT_{4?}$)
8. Acetylcholine (muscarinic)
9. Pancreatic polypeptide
10. Cytokines

ENS.[64] Electrical stimulation of sympathetic postganglionic fibers in the periarterial mesenteric nerves suppresses fast EPSPs in myenteric ganglion cells without altering the responses to exogenously applied acetylcholine.[2,147] Likewise, norepinephrine fulfills the criteria for a presynaptic action by suppressing stimulus-evoked slow EPSPs without affecting the postsynaptic actions of substance P, serotonin, or acetylcholine.[148] As expected for a presynaptic action, norepinephrine does not abort a slow EPSP in progress but blocks the ability to evoke subsequent EPSPs by electrical stimulation of interganglionic connectives.[148]

Norepinephrine reduces the release of 5-HT and substance P from isolated intestinal segments, consistent with presynaptic suppression of slow synaptic excitation.[149,150] Electronmicrographs show axo-axonal synapses with vesicular profiles characteristic of noradrenergic synapses in the guinea pig myenteric plexus.[151] Suppressive effects of norepinephrine on acetylcholine release from intestinal segments in vitro are well documented as supporting evidence for a presynaptic action.[152–154]

Histamine, interleukin-1β, interleukin-6, tumor necrosis factor, and platelet-activating factor receive attention because of their role in neuroimmune communication between mast cells and the enteric program circuits. Histamine, like the other immune/inflammatory messengers on the list, acts at presynaptic receptors on cholinergic axons to suppress fast EPSPs at nicotinic synapses and at sympathetic nerve terminals to suppress the release of norepinephrine in the enteric microcircuits.[89,107,144] This action of histamine is blocked by selective $H_3$ receptor antagonists and mimicked by selective $H_3$ agonists, which is supporting evidence that the presynaptic action of histamine is at the $H_3$ receptor subtype.[144–155] Histamine released during antigenic degranulation of intestinal mast cells acts in a similar manner.[156,157]

Application of 5-HT to enteric synapses reduces the amplitude of the fast EPSPs without effects on nicotinic postsynaptic responses to acetylcholine, thereby fulfilling criteria for presynaptic inhibition.[146] The receptor for the presynaptic inhibitory action is not unequivocally identified but fits the profile of the $5\text{-}HT_1$ receptor in the gastric antrum and small intestine[158–160] or the putative $5\text{-}HT_4$ receptor subtype in the colon.[161]

The presynaptic action of acetylcholine on fast EPSPs occurs at muscarinic receptors in the myenteric and submucous plexuses of the small and large intestine[13,106] and at the synapses in the gastric antrum.[18] Muscarinic receptors are present also on axons of myenteric neurons in culture.[162] The affinity of the presynaptic receptors for selective agonists and antagonists is suggestive of the $M_2$ class of muscarinic receptor.[106]

The presynaptic muscarinic receptors at fast nicotinic synapses are components of autoinhibitory mechanisms that function in negative feedback regulation of the amount of acetylcholine released by the arrival of the action potential at the release site. The inhibition of acetylcholine esterase by drugs such as eserine results in the suppression of stimulus-evoked fast EPSPs, and this effect is reversed by application of atropine. In this situation, the inhibition of acetylcholine esterase permits accumulation of acetylcholine, which feeds back on the presynaptic muscarinic receptors to suppress further release of acetylcholine. Atropine blocks this presynaptic influence of the esterase and restores the EPSP.[13,68] In experiments of this nature, neither the anticholinesterase nor muscarinic antagonist alters the amplitude of postsynaptic depolarizations evoked by microapplication of acetylcholine.

Members of the pancreatic polypeptide family of messenger peptides (eg, NPY, PYY, and PP) act presynaptically to suppress transmission at nicotinic synapses in the microcircuits of the stomach and probably in other regions as well.[163] The presynaptic inhibitory action of NPY is significant because it is colocalized with norepinephrine in sympathetic postganglionic axons, as well as being found in intrinsic neurons. This suggests that both the central nervous system and the local minibrain may use the long-lasting inhibitory action of this mediator to selectively inactivate synapses within the microcircuits. Presynaptic NPY receptors appear to be present on vagal efferent fibers in the gastric corpus and participate in circuit functions by which the microcircuitry of the corpus may elect to turn off its vagal input.[163]

Presynaptic inhibition by adenosine occurs at the $A_1$ type of the $P_1$ purinoreceptor.[91,164,165] This occurs at fast nicotinic synapses, slow excitatory synapses, and noradrenergic inhibitory synapses. The suppression of fast EPSPs occurs in the gastric and intestinal microcircuits, whereas presynaptic inhibition of IPSPs is seen in the intestinal submucous plexus.

## CONCLUSIONS

Many lines of evidence now implicate dysfunction in the ENS as a significant factor underlying symptomatology in patient complaints that fit the criteria for motility disorders. This underscores the need for future attention to the neural factors underlying patient symptoms that fit criteria for functional gastrointestinal motility disorders and also justifies accelerated expansion of research that fits under the umbrella of the subspecialty of neurogastroenterology.

Consideration that the ENS is an independent integrative nervous system with most of the neurophysiologic complexities found in the central nervous system stimulates the premonition that functional motor disorders may reflect neuropathies in the brain-in-the-gut.[166] A lack of understanding of how subtle malfunctions may occur in the synaptic microcircuits of the ENS is undoubtedly the basis of "functional" as the description of some forms of disordered gastrointestinal motility. This is reminiscent of neurologic disorders such as parkinsonian tremors, ballisms, and choreas, which were classified as "functional" prior to an understanding of neurotransmission in microcircuits of somatic motor centers in the brain. Parkinson's disease is a classic example of a functional somatic motor disorder that was ultimately explained as malfunction of dopaminergic neurotransmission

in localized brain centers. Like the status of understanding of somatic motor control centers in the brain a half-century ago, now as we enter the twenty-first century, the ENS remains a virtual "black box" that will need to be opened scientifically to understand gastrointestinal motor disorders. Acquisition of new knowledge of the neurobiology of the enteric minibrain will require application of the methods laid out in this chapter. These are the same methodologies that unified functional concepts for the central nervous system. Electrophysiologic and synaptic behavior of individual enteric neurons, identification of neurotransmitters, identification of how specific neuronal types are wired into synaptic circuits, and the emergent properties of microcircuits in the programming of motor and secretory behavior are areas open to innovative investigation.

### Acknowledgment
The opinions expressed in this review are my own. Nevertheless, they are based on work and interactions in my laboratory with a progression of outstanding students and visiting scientists whose discoveries have helped shape the current concepts of neurogastroenterology. The work on enteric neurophysiology in my laboratory has been supported continuously by the National Institutes of Health's National Institute of Diabetes and Digestive and Kidney Diseases since 1973.

### REFERENCES

1. Wood JD. Electrical activity from single neurons in Auerbach's plexus. Am J Physiol 1970;219:159–69.
2. Nishi S, North RA. Intracellular recording from the myenteric plexus of the guinea-pig ileum. J Physiol (Lond) 1973;231:471–91.
3. Hirst GDS, Holman ME, Spence I. Two types of neurones in the myenteric plexus of duodenum in the guinea-pig. J Physiol (Lond) 1974;236:303–26.
4. Wood JD, Mayer CJ. Intracellular study of electrical activity of Auerbach's plexus in guinea-pig small intestine. Pflugers Arch 1978;374:265–75.
5. Gershon MD. The second brain. New York: HarperCollins Publishers; 1998.
6. Wood JD, Alpers DH, Andrews PLR. Fundamentals of neurogastroenterology. Gut 1999;45:1–44.
7. Wood JD, Alpers DH, Andrews PLR. Fundamentals of neurogastroenterology: basic science. In: Drossman DA, Talley NJ, Thompson WG, et al, editors. The functional gastrointestinal disorders: diagnosis, pathophysiology and treatment: a multinational consensus. McLean (VA): Degnon Associates, 2000. p. 31–90.
8. Grundy D. The changing face of gastrointestinal motility. J Gastrointest Motil 1993;5:231–2.
9. Surprenant A. Slow excitatory synaptic potentials recorded from neurones of guinea-pig submucous plexus. J Physiol (Lond) 1984;351:343–61.
10. Surprenant A. The two types of neurones lacking synaptic input in the submucous plexus of guinea-pig small intestine. J Physiol (Lond) 1984;351:363–78.
11. Wade PR, Wood JD. Electrical behavior of myenteric neurons in guinea-pig distal colon. Am J Physiol 1988;254:G522–30.
12. Messenger JP, Bornstein JC, Furness JB. Electrophysiological and morphological classification of myenteric neurons in the proximal colon of the guinea-pig. Neuroscience 1994;60:227–44.
13. Tamura K, Wood JD. Electrical and synaptic properties of myenteric plexus neurones in the terminal large intestine of the guinea-pig. J Physiol (Lond) 1989;415:275–98.
14. Tamura K. Morphology of electophysiologically identified myenteric

neurons in the guinea-pig rectum. Am J Physiol 1992;262:G545–52.

15. Schemann M, Wood JD. Electrical behavior of myenteric neurones in the gastric corpus of the guinea-pig. J Physiol (Lond) 1989;417:501–18.

16. Schemann M, Wood JD. Synaptic behavior of myenteric neurones in the gastric corpus of the guinea-pig. J Physiol (Lond) 1989;417:519–35.

17. Tack JF, Wood JD. Electrical behaviour of myenteric neurones in the gastric antrum of the guinea-pig. J Physiol (Lond) 1992;447:49–66.

18. Tack JD, Wood JD. Synaptic behavior in the myenteric plexus of the guinea-pig gastric antrum. J Physiol (Lond) 1992;445:389–406.

19. Mawe GM. Intracellular recording from gall-bladder neurones of the guinea-pig gall bladder. J Physiol (Lond) 1990;429:323–38.

20. Mawe GM. The role of cholecystokinin in ganglionic transmission in the guinea-pig gall bladder. J Physiol (Lond) 1991;439:89–102.

21. Bauer AJ, Hanani M, Muir TC, Szurszewski JH. Intracellular recordings from gallbladder ganglia of opossums. Am J Physiol 1991;260:G299–306.

22. Hillsley K, Mawe GM. Correlation of electrophysiology, neurochemistry and axonal projections of guinea-pig sphincter of Oddi neurones. Neurogastroenterol Motil 1998;10:235–44.

23. Liu MT, Kirchgessner AL. Guinea pig pancreatic neurons: morphology, neurochemistry, electrical properties, and response to 5-HT. Am J Physiol 1997;36:G1273–89.

24. Love JA. Electrical properties and synaptic potentials of rabbit pancreatic neurons. Auto Neurosci 2000;84:68–77.

25. Wood JD. Intracellular study of effects of morphine on electrical activity of myenteric neurons in cat small intestine. Gastroenterology 1980;79:1222–30.

26. Furukawa K, Taylor GS, Bywater BAR. An intracellular study of myenteric neurons in the mouse colon. J Neurophysiol 1986;55:1395–406.

27. Cornelissen W, DeLaet A, Kroese ABA, et al. Electrophysiological features of morphological Dogiel type II neurons in the myenteric plexus of pig small intestine. J Neurophysiol 2000;84:102–11.

28. Thomsen L, Pearson GT, Larsen EH, Skadhauge E. Electrophysiological properties of neurones in the internal and external submucous plexuses of newborn pig small intestine. J Physiol (Lond) 1997;498:773–85.

29. Brookes SJH, Ewart WJ, Wingate DL. Intracellular recordings from myenteric neurones in the human colon. J Physiol (Lond) 1987;390:305–18.

30. Sato T, Takayanagi I, Takagi K. Pharmacological properties of electrical activities obtained from neurons in Auerbach's plexus. J Pharmacol (Japan) 1973;23:665–71.

31. Dingledine R, Goldstein A. Effects of narcotic opiates and serotonin on the electrical behavior of neurons in the guinea-pig Auerbach's plexus. Life Sci 1979;14:2299–309.

32. Wood JD. Neuronal interactions within ganglia of Auerbach's plexus of the small intestine. In: Bülbring E, Shuba MF, editors. Physiology of smooth muscle. New York: Raven Press; 1976. p. 321–30.

33. Hirst GDS, Johnson SM, van Helden DF. The calcium current in a myenteric neurone of the guinea pig ileum. J Physiol (Lond) 1985;361:297–314.

34. Mihara S, North RA, Surprenant A. Somatostatin increases an inwardly rectifying potassium conductance in guinea-pig submucous plexus neurones. J Physiol (Lond) 1987;390:335–55.

35. Baidan LV, Zholos AV, Wood JD. Modulation of calcium currents by G-proteins and adenosine receptors in myenteric neurones cultured from guinea-pig small intestine. Br J Pharmacol 1995;116:1882–6.

36. Shen K-Z, North RA, Surprenant A. Potassium channels opened by noradrenaline and other transmitters in excised membrane patches of guinea-pig submucosal neurones. J Physiol (Lond) 1992;445:581–99.

37. Willard AW, Nishi R. Enteric neurons in culture. In: Wood JD, editor. Handbook of physiology: the gastrointestinal system, motility and circulation. Bethesda (MD): American Physiological Society; 1989. p. 331–47

38. Xia Y, Baidan LV, Fertel RH, Wood JD. Determination of levels of

39. cyclic AMP in the myenteric plexus of guinea-pig small intestine. Eur J Pharmacol 1991;206:231–6.

39. Hanani M, Emilov LB, Schmalz PF, et al. The three-dimensional structure of myenteric neurons in the guinea-pig ileum. J Auton Nerv Syst 1998;71:1–9.

40. Obaid AL, Koyano T, Lindstrom J, et al. Spatiotemporal patterns of activity in an intact mammalian network with single-cell resolution: optical studies of nicotinic activity in an enteric plexus. J Neurosci 1999;19:3073–93.

41. Neunlist M, Peters S, Schemann M. Simultaneous multisite optical recording of excitability in the enteric nervous system using voltage sensitive dye. In: Krammer H-J, Singer MV, editors. Neurogastroenterology: from the basics to the clinics. Boston: Kluwer Academic; 2000. p. 163–74.

42. Ohkawa H, Prosser CL. Electrical activity in myenteric and submucous plexuses of the cat small intestine. Am J Physiol 1972;222:1412–9.

43. Wood JD, Mayer CJ. Patterned discharge of six different neurons within a single enteric ganglion. Pflugers Arch 1973;338:247–56.

44. Yokoyama S. Aktionspotentiale des ganglienzelle des Auerbachschen plexus in Kaninchendunndarm. Arch Ges Physiol 1966;288:95–102.

45. Nozdrachev AD, Katchalov UP, Bentov AF. Spontaneous discharge of neurons in myenteric plexus of the intestine of rabbits. Fiziol Zh 1975;61:725–30.

46. Hardy JD, Bard P. Body temperature regulation. In: Mountcastle BV, editor. Medical physiology. St. Louis: CV Mosby; 1974. p. 1305–42.

47. Wood JD. Effects of elevated magnesium on discharge of myenteric neurons of cat small bowel. Am J Physiol 1975;229:657–62.

48. Athey GR, Cooke AR, Wood JD. Synaptic activation of erratic bursttype myenteric neurons in cat small intestine. Am J Physiol 1981;240:G437–41.

49. Erwin DN, Ninchoji T, Wood JD. Effects of morphine on electrical activity of single myenteric neurons in cat small bowel. Eur J Pharmacol 1978;47:401–5.

50. Wood JD. Neurophysiology of ganglia of Auerbach's plexus. Am Zool 1974;14:973–89.

51. Wood JD. Excitation of intestinal muscle by atropine, tetrodotoxin and Xylocaine. Am J Physiol 1972;222:118–25.

52. Edwards AV, Andersson P-O, Jarhult J, Bloom SR. Studies of the importance of the pattern of autonomic stimulation in relation to alimentary effectors. Q J Exp Physiol 1984;69:607–14.

53. St Jarne L. New paradigm: sympathetic neurotransmission by lateral interaction between secretory units. News Physiol Sci 1986;1:103–6.

54. Willard AL, Nishi R. Neuropeptides mark functionally distinguishable cholinergic enteric neurons. Brain Res 1987;422:163–7.

55. Mayer CJ, Wood JD. Properties of mechanosensitive neurons within Auerbach's plexus of the small intestine of the cat. Pflugers Arch 1975;357:35–49.

56. Davison JS. Response of single vagal afferent fibers to mechanical and chemical stimulation of the gastric and duodenal mucosa in cats. J Exp Physiol 1972;57:405–16.

57. Iggo A. Gastrointestinal tension receptors with unmyelinated afferent fibers in the vagus of the cat. Q J Exp Physiol 1957;42:130–43.

58. Ranieri F, Mei N, Groussilat J. Les afferences splanchniques provenant des mechanorecepteurs gastrointestinaux et peritoneaux. Exp Brain Res 1973;16:276–90.

59. Hillsley K, Kirkup AJ, Grundy D. Direct and indirect actions of 5-hydroxytryptamine on the discharge of mesenteric afferent fibres innervating the rat jejunum. J Physiol (Lond) 1998;506:551–61.

60. Berthoud HR, Powley TL. Vagal afferent innervation of the rat fundic stomach-morphological characterization of the gastric tension receptor. J Comp Neurol 1992;319:261–76.

61. Zheng HY, Berthoud HR. Functional vagal input to gastric myenteric plexus as assessed by vagal stimulation-induced Fos expression. Am J Physiol 2000;279:G73–81.

62. Raybould HE. Does your gut taste? Sensory transduction in the gastrointestinal tract. News Physiol Sci 1998;13:275–80.

63. Andrews PLR, Davis CJ, Bingham S, et al.The abdominal visceral innervation and the emetic reflex—pathways, pharmacology, and plasticity. Can J Physiol Pharmacol 1990;68:325–45.

64. Wood JD. Neurotransmission at the interface of sympathetic and enteric divisions of the autonomic nervous system. Chin J Physiol 1999;42:201–10.

65. Iyer V, Bornstein JC, Costa M, et al. Electrophysiology of guinea-pig myenteric neurons correlated with immunoreactivity for calcium binding proteins. J Auton Nerv Sys 1988;22:141–50.

66. Kirchgessner AL, Tamir H, Gershon MD. Identification and stimulation by serotonin of intrinsic sensory neurons of the submucosal plexus of the guinea pig gut—activity-induced expression of Fos immunoreactivity. J Neurosci 1992;12:235–48.

67. Furness JB, Kunze WAA, Bertrand PP, et al. Intrinsic primary afferent neurons of the intestine. Prog Neurobiol 1997;54:1–18.

68. Wood JD. Electrical and synaptic behavior of enteric neurons. In: Wood JD, editor. Handbook of physiology: the gastrointestinal system, motility and circulation. Bethesda (MD): American Physiological Society; 1989. p. 465–517.

69. Grafe P, Mayer CJ, Wood JD. Synaptic modulation of calcium-dependent potassium conductance in myenteric neurons. J Physiol (Lond) 1980;305:235–48.

70. Tatsumi H, Hirai K, Katayama Y. Measurement of the intracellular calcium concentration in guinea-pig myenteric neurons by using fura-2. Brain Res 1988;451:371–5.

71. Akasu T, Tokimasa T. Potassium currents in submucous neurones of guinea-pig caecum and their synaptic modification. J Physiol (Lond) 1989;416:571–88.

72. North RA, Tokimasa T. Persistent calcium-sensitive potassium current and the resting properties of guinea-pig myenteric neurones. J Physiol (Lond) 1987;386:333–53.

73. Morita K, North RA, Tokimasa T. The calcium-activated potassium conductance in guinea-pig myenteric neurones. J Physiol (Lond) 1982;329:341–54.

74. Morita K, North RA. Opiate activation of potassium conductance in myenteric neurons: inhibition by calcium ion. Brain Res 1982;242:145–50.

75. Palmer JM, Wood JD, Zafirov DH. Purinergic inhibition in the small intestinal myenteric plexus of the guinea-pig. J Physiol (Lond) 1987;387:357–69.

76. Johnson SM, Katayama Y, North RA. Multiple actions of 5-hydroxytryptamine on myenteric neurones of the guinea-pig ileum. J Physiol (Lond) 1980;304:459–70.

77. Katayama Y, North RA, Williams JT. The action of substance P on neurons of the myenteric plexus of the guinea-pig small intestine. Proc R Soc Lond B Biol Sci 1979;206:191–208.

78. Starodub AM, Wood JD. Selectivity of omega-Cg-Tx-MCVIIC toxin from *Conus magus* on calcium currents in enteric neurons. Life Sci 1999;64:305–10.

79. Baidan LV, Zholos AV, Shuba MF, Wood JD. Patch clamp recording in myenteric neurons of guinea-pig small intestine. Am J Physiol 1992;262:G1074–8.

80. Morita K, North RA. Clonidine activates membrane potassium conductance in myenteric neurons. Br J Pharmacol 1981;74:419–28.

81. Hirst GDS, Spence I. Calcium action potentials in mammalian peripheral neurones. Nature 1973;243:54–6.

82. North RA. The calcium-dependent slow after-hyperpolarization in myenteric plexus neurons with tetrodotoxin-resistant action potentials. Br J Pharmacol 1973;49:709–11.

83. Zholos AV, Baidan LV, Starodub AM, Wood JD. Potassium channels of myenteric neurons in guinea-pig small intestine. Neuroscience 1999;89:603–18.

84. Starodub AM, Wood JD. A-type potassium current in myenteric neurons of guinea-pig small intestine. Neuroscience 2000;99:389–96.

85. North RA, Tokimasa T. Depression of calcium-dependent potassium conductance of guinea-pig myenteric neurones by muscarinic agonists. J Physiol (Lond) 1983;342:253–66.

86. Hirst GDS, Johnson SM, van Helden DF. The slow calcium-dependent current in a myenteric neurone of the guinea pig ileum. J Physiol (Lond) 1985;361:315–37.

87. Palmer JM, Wood JD, Zafirov DH. Elevation of cyclic adenosine monophosphate mimics slow synaptic excitation in myenteric neurones of the guinea-pig. J Physiol (Lond) 1986;376:451–60.

88. Frieling T, Cooke HJ, Wood JD. Histamine receptors on submucous neurons in the guinea-pig colon. Am J Physiol 1993;264:G74–80.

89. Wood JD. Histamine signals in enteric neuroimmune interactions. Neuroimmunophysiology of gastrointestinal mucosa. Ann N Y Acad Sci 1992;664:275–83.

90. Wood JD. Allergies and the brain-in-the-gut. Clin Perspect Gastroenterol 2000;3:343–8.

91. Christofi FL, Wood JD. Presynaptic inhibition by adenosine A1 receptors on guinea-pig small intestinal myenteric neurons. Gastroenterology 1993;104:1420–9.

92. Galligan JJ, LePard KJ, Schneider DA, Zhou XP. Multiple mechanisms of fast excitatory synaptic transmission in the enteric nervous system. J Auton Nerv Syst 2000;81:97–103.

93. Derkach V, Surprenant A, North RA. 5-HT3 receptors are membrane ion channels. Nature 1989;339:706–9.

94. Kunze WAA, Furness JB, Bertrand PP, Bornstein JC. Intracellular recording from myenteric neurons of the guinea-pig ileum that respond to stretch. J Physiol (Lond) 1998;506:827–42.

95. Morita K, Katayama Y. Substance P inhibits activation of calcium-dependent potassium conductances in guinea-pig myenteric neurones. J Physiol (Lond) 1992;447:293–308.

96. Gershon MD. Roles played by 5-hydroxytryptamine in the physiology of the bowel. Aliment Pharmacol Ther 1998;13:15–30.

97. Bornstein JC, North RA, Costa M, Furness JB. Excitatory synaptic potentials due to activation of neurons with short projections in the myenteric plexus. Neuroscience 1984;11:723–31.

98. Takaki M, Nakayama S. Effects of mesenteric nerve stimulation on the electrical activity of myenteric neurons in the guinea pig ileum. Brain Res 1988;442:351–3.

99. Nemeth PR, Ewart WR, Wood JD. Effects of the putative substance P antagonists (D-pRO2, D-PHE7, D-TRP9 and D-PRO2, D-TRP7,9) on electrical activity of myenteric neurons. J Auton Nerv Syst 1983;8:165–9.

100. Surprenant A, North RA, Katayama Y. Observations on the actions of substance P and (D-Arg1,D-Pro2,D- Trp7,9,Leu11) substance P on single neurons of the guinea pig submucous plexus. Neuroscience 1987;20:189–99.

101. Snider RM, Constantine JW, Lowe JA, et al. A potent nonpeptide antagonist of the substance P (NK1) receptor. Science 1991;251:435–7.

102. Tamura K, Mutabagni K, Wood JD. Analysis of a nonpeptide antagonist for substance P on myenteric neurons of guinea-pig small intestine. Eur J Pharmacol 1993;232:235–9.

103. Schemann M, Kayser H. Effects of tachykinins on myenteric neurones of the guinea-pig gastric corpus: involvement of NK-3 receptors. Pflugers Arch 1991;419:566–71.

104. Mawe GM, Branchek TA, Gershon MD. Peripheral neural serotonin receptors: identification and characterization with specific antagonists and agonists. Proc Natl Acad Sci U S A 1986;83:9799–803.

105. Christofi FL, Palmer JM, Wood JD. Neuropharmacology of the muscarinic antagonist telenzepine in myenteric ganglia of the guinea-pig small intestine. Eur J Pharmacol 1991;195:333–9.

106. North RA, Slack BE, Surprenant A. Muscarinic $M_1$ and $M_2$ receptors mediate depolarization and presynaptic inhibition in guinea-pig enteric nervous system. J Physiol (Lond) 1985;368:435–52.

107. Wood JD. Physiological and pathophysiological paracrine functions of intestinal mast cells in enteric neuro-immune signaling. In: Singer MF, Zigler R, Rohr G, editors. Gastrointestinal tract and endocrine system. London: Kluwer Academic; 1995. p. 254–63.

108. Nemeth PR, Ort CA, Wood JD. Intracellular study of effects of histamine on electrical behavior of myenteric neurons in guinea-pig small intestine. J Physiol (Lond) 1984;355:411–25.

109. Vantrappen G, Peeters TL, Bloom SR, et al. Motilin and the interdigestive migrating motor complex in man. Am J Dig Dis 1979;24:497–500.

110. Tack J, Janssens J, Vantrappen G, et al. Effect of erythromycin on gastric motility in controls and diabetic gastroparesis. Gastroenterology 1992;103:72–9.

111. Wood JD, Tack JF. Motilin excites myenteric neurons in the gastric antrum of the guinea-pig [abstract]. Gastroenterology 1990;99:A1236.

112. Clerc N, Furness JB, Kunze WA, et al. Long-term effects of synaptic activation at low frequency on excitability of myenteric AH neurons. Neuroscience 2000;90:279–89.

113. Nemeth PR, Palmer JM, Wood JD, Zafirov DH. Effects of forskolin on electrical behavior of myenteric neurones in guinea-pig small intestine. J Physiol (Lond) 1986;376:439–50.

114. Baidan LV, Fertel RH, Wood JD. Effects of brain-gut related peptides on cAMP levels in myenteric ganglia of guinea-pig small intestine. Eur J Pharmacol 1992;225:21–7.

115. Xia Y, Fertel RH, Wood JD. Stimulation of formation of cAMP by 5-hydroxytryptamine in myenteric ganglia isolated from guinea pig small intestine. Life Sci 1994;55:685–92.

116. Xia Y, Fertel R, Wood J. Stimulation of formation of adenosine 3′,5′-phosphate by histamine in myenteric ganglia isolated from guinea-pig small intestine. Eur J Pharmacol 1996;316:81–5.

117. Wood JD. Application of classification schemes to the enteric nervous system. J Auton Nerv Syst 1994;48:17–29.

118. Vizi VA, Vizi ES. Direct evidence for acetylcholine releasing effect of serotonin in the Auerbach's plexus. J Neural Transm 1978;42:127–38.

119. Yau WM, Youther ML. Direct evidence for a release of acetylcholine from myenteric plexus of guinea pig small intestine by substance P. Eur J Pharmacol 1982;81:665–8.

120. Javed NH, Cooke HJ. Acetylcholine release from colonic submucous neurons in the guinea pig associated with Cl secretion. Am J Physiol 1992;262:G1331–6.

121. Jenkinson KM, Mann PT, Southwell BR, Furness JB. Independent endocytosis of the NK(1) and NK(3) tachykinin receptors in neurons of rat myenteric plexus. Neuroscience 2000;100:191–9.

122. Jenkinson KM, Morgan JM, Furness JB, Southwell BR. Neurons bearing NK(3) tachykinin receptors in the guinea-pig ileum revealed by specific binding of fluorescently labelled agonists. Histochem Cell Biol 1999;112:233–46.

123. Wood JD. Physiology of the enteric nervous system. In: Johnson LH, Alpers DH, Christensen J, et al, editors. Physiology of the gastrointestinal track. 3rd ed. New York: Raven Press; 1994. p. 423–482.

124. Thomas EA, Bertrand PP, Bornstein JC. Genesis and role of coordinated firing in a feedforward network: a model study of the enteric nervous system. Neuroscience 1999;93:1525–37.

125. Bertrand PP, Kunze WAA, Bornstein JC, et al. Analysis of the responses of myenteric neurons in the small intestine to chemical stimulation of the mucosa. Am J Physiol 1997;36:G422–35.

126. Hirst GDS, McKirdy HC. Synaptic potentials recorded from neurones of the submucous plexus of guinea-pig small intestine. J Physiol (Lond) 1975;249:369–85.

127. North RA, Surprenant A. Inhibitory synaptic potentials resulting from $alpha_2$ adrenoceptor activation in guinea-pig submucous plexus neurones. J Physiol (Lond) 1985;358:17–33.

128. Zafirov DH, Cooke HJ, Wood JD. Elevation of cAMP facilitates noradrenergic transmission in submucous neurons of guinea-pig ileum. Am J Physiol 1993;262:G442–6.

129. Johnson SM, North RA. Slow synaptic potentials in neurones of the myenteric plexus. J Physiol (Lond) 1980;301:505–16.

130. Surprenant A, North RA. Mechanism of synaptic inhibition by noradrenaline acting at alpha 2-adrenoceptors. Proc R Soc Lond B Biol Sci 1988;234:85–114.

131. Mihara S, North RA. Opioids increase potassium conductance in submucous neurones of guinea-pig caecum by activating delta receptors. Br J Pharmacol 1986;88:315–82.

132. Surprenant A, North RA. Inhibitory receptors and signal transduction in submucosal neurones. In: Holle GE, Wood JD, editors. Advances in the innervation of the gastrointestinal tract. Amsterdam: Elsevier Scientific Press; 1992. p. 239–50.

133. Mihara S, Hirai K, Katayama Y, Nishi S. Mechanisms underlying intracellular signal transduction of the slow IPSP in submucous neurones of the guinea-pig caecum. J Physiol (Lond) 1991;436:621–41.

134. North RA, Tonini M. The mechanism of action of narcotic analgesics in the guinea-pig ileum. Br J Pharmacol 1977;61:541–9.

135. North RA, Karras PJ. Opiate tolerance and dependence induced in vitro in single myenteric neurones. Nature 1978;272:73–5.

136. North RA, Sieglgansberger W. Opiate withdrawal signs in single myenteric neurones. Brain Res 1978;144:208–11.

137. Liu S, Hu H-Z, Ren J, et al. Pre- and postsynaptic inhibition by nociceptin in guinea pig myenteric plexus in vitro. Am J Physiol 2001;281:G237–46.

138. Palmer JM, Schemann M, Tamura K, Wood JD. Galanin mimics slow synaptic inhibition in myenteric neurons. Eur J Pharmacol 1986;124:379–80.

139. Nemeth PR, Zafirov DH, Wood JD. Effects of cholecystokinin, caerulein and pentagastrin on electrical behavior of myenteric neurons. Eur J Pharmacol 1985;116:263–9.

140. Schutte IW, Akkermans LM, Kroese AB. CCKA and CCKB receptor subtypes both mediate the effects of CCK-8 on myenteric neurons in the guinea-pig ileum. J Auton Nerv Syst 1997;67:51–9.

141. Schutte IW, Hollestein KB, Akkermans LM, Kroese AB. Evidence for a role of cholecystokinin as neurotransmitter in the guinea-pig enteric nervous system. Neurosci Lett 1997;236:155–8.

142. Xia Y, Fertel RH, Wood JD. Suppression of cAMP formation by adenosine in myenteric ganglia of guinea-pig small intestine. Eur J Pharmacol 1997;32:95–101.

143. Hirst GDS, Silinsky EM. Some effects of 5-hydroxytryptamine, dopamine and noradrenaline on neurones in the submucous plexus of guinea-pig small intestine. J Physiol (Lond) 1975;251:817–32.

144. Liu S, Xia Y, Hu H-Z, et al. Histamine H3 receptor-mediated suppression of inhibitory synaptic transmission in the guinea-pig submucous plexus. Eur J Pharmacol 2000;397:49–54.

145. Surprenant A. Synaptic transmission in neurons of the submucous plexus. In: Singer MV, Goebell H, editors. Nerves and the gastro-intestinal tract. Falk Symposium 50. Boston: MTP Press; 1989. p. 253–63.

146. North RA, Henderson G, Katayama Y, Johnson SM. Electrophysiological evidence for presynaptic inhibition of acetylcholine release by 5-hydroxytryptamine in the enteric nervous system. Neuroscience 1980;5:581–6.

147. Hirst GDS, McKirdy HC. Presynaptic inhibition at a mammalian peripheral synapse. Nature 1974;250:430–1.

148. Wood JD, Mayer CJ. Adrenergic inhibition of serotonin release from neurons in guinea-pig Auerbach's plexus. J Neurophysiol 1979;42:594–603.

149. Bartho L, Holzer P, Lembeck F. Sympathetic control of substance P releasing enteric neurones in the guinea pig ileum. Neurosci Lett 1983;38:291–6.

150. Jonakait GM, Tamir H, Gintzler AR, Gershon MD. Release of [3H] serotonin and its binding protein from enteric neurons. Brain Res 1979;174:55–69.

151. Manber L, Gershon MD. A reciprocal adrenergic-cholinergic axoaxonic synapse in the mammalian gut. Am J Physiol 1979;5:E738–45.

152. Del Tacca M, Soldani G, Selli M, Crema A. Action of catecholamines on release of acetylcholine from human taenia coli. Eur J Pharmacol 1970;9:80–4.

153. Knoll J, Vizi ES. Presynaptic inhibition of acetylcholine release by endogenous and exogenous noradrenaline at high rate of stimulation. Br J Pharmacol 1970;40:400–12.

154. Paton WDM, Vizi ES. The inhibitory action of noradrenaline and adrenaline on acetylcholine output by guinea-pig ileum longitudinal muscle strip. Br J Pharmacol 1969;35:10–28.

155. Tamura K, Palmer JM, Wood JD. Presynaptic inhibition produced by histamine at nicotinic synapses in enteric ganglia. Neuroscience 1987;25:171–9.

156. Frieling T, Cooke HJ, Wood JD. Neuroimmune communication in the submucous plexus of guinea-pig colon after sensitization to milk antigen. Am J Physiol 1994;267:G1087–93.

157. Frieling T, Palmer JM, Cooke HJ, Wood JD. Neuroimmune communication in the submucous plexus of guinea-pig colon after infection with *Trichinella spiralis*. Gastroenterology 1994;107:1602–9.

158. Tack J, Janssens J, Vantrappen G, Wood JD. Actions of 5-hydroxytryptamine on myenteric neurons in the guinea-pig gastric antrum. Am J Physiol 1992;263:G838–46.

159. Surprenant A, Crist J. Electrophysiological characterization of functionally distinct 5-hydroxytryptamine receptors on guinea-pig submucous plexus. Neuroscience 1988;24:283–95.

160. Galligan JJ, Surprenant A, Tonini M, North RA. Differential localization of 5-HT1 receptors on myenteric and submucosal neurons. Am J Physiol 1988;255:G603–11.

161. Frieling T, Cooke HJ, Wood JD. Serotonin receptors on submucous neurons in the guinea-pig colon. Am J Physiol 1991;261:G1017–23.

162. Buckley NJ, Burnstock G. Distribution of muscarinic receptors on cultured myenteric neurons. Brain Res 1984;310:133–7.

163. Schemann M, Tamura K. Presynaptic inhibitory effects of the peptides NPY, PYY, and PP on nicotinic EPSPs in guinea-pig gastric myenteric neurones. J Physiol (Lond) 1992;451:79–89.

164. Christofi FL, Tack J, Wood JD. Suppression of nicotinic synaptic transmission by adenosine in myenteric ganglia of the guinea-pig gastric antrum. Eur J Pharmacol 1992;216:17–22.

165. Barajas-Lopez C, Surprenant A, North RA. Adenosine A1 and A2 receptors mediate presynaptic inhibition and postsynaptic excitation in guinea pig submucosal neurons. J Pharmacol Exp Ther 1991;258:490–5.

166. Wood JD. Neuropathy in the brain-in-the-gut. Eur J Gastroenterol Hepatol 2000;12:597–600.

# CHAPTER 3

# Brain–Gut Interactions in Visceral Sensation and Perception

*Michael D. Crowell and Paul Enck*

Pain referred to the abdomen is the symptom most commonly reported by patients evaluated in gastroenterology clinics. Abdominal pain is often acute and resolves relatively quickly with appropriate intervention. Resolution of acute abdominal pain often occurs in the absence of a clear diagnosis. In a subgroup of patients, however, abdominal pain may become chronic and persists as an episodic or recurrent problem with multiple exacerbations over time or as an intractable, persistent, and debilitating symptom. Extensive diagnostic evaluation often fails to reveal an organic cause for chronic abdominal pain. These patients are often diagnosed with one of the functional gastrointestinal disorders, which include disorders of gastrointestinal afferent processes (eg, hypersensitivity and/or hyperreflexia), characteristic of disorders such as irritable bowel syndrome (IBS). This chapter focuses on the physiology and pathophysiology of afferent sensory processes in brain–gut communications and the relationship to chronic abdominal pain and functional gastrointestinal disorders.

The complex nature of pain originating from the viscera can be understood only by analyzing the various components responsible for the transduction, transmission, and central processing of visceral stimuli. These components include the nervous structures that encode, relay, and modify the stimulus and the central processing that produces the perception and interpretation of the sensations arising from a specific stimulus. The gastrointestinal viscera are relatively insensible to most stimuli compared with other somatic structures. The abdominal organs have been shown to be generally insensitive to light touch, pinching, cutting, and even burning.[1-4] The dissociation between injury and pain in the abdominal viscera led investigators to differentiate noxious stimuli from nociceptive stimuli. Cervero suggested that the term noxious should be applied only to stimuli that signal the "relationship between the stimulus and the integrity of the organism," whereas the term nociceptive should define the "relationship between the stimulus and the nervous system of the subject."[5] From these criteria, it can be inferred that a noxious stimulus would produce actual damage to the organ or tissue and may or may not be associated with the perception of pain, whereas a nociceptive stimulus would produce affective and/or autonomic reflex responses and result in the perception of pain or discomfort. A single stimulus can be simultaneously noxious and nociceptive. For example, overdistention of hollow visceral organs produces both pain and tissue damage (noxious), but at lower levels, the same distention produces autonomic reflexes and the perception of pain (nociceptive) without damage to the organ system. Similarly, irradiation can produce severe damage to the visceral organs and tissue (noxious) without producing an immediate perception of pain (nociception). Therefore, visceral nociceptors can be operationally defined as sensory afferents that encode nociceptive stimuli from the periphery and produce autonomic reflexes or pseudoaffective responses and the perception of pain.

## NEUROANATOMY OF VISCERAL PAIN PATHWAYS

Morphologically, visceral nociceptors consist of afferent fibers that terminate in free nerve endings located between the smooth muscle layers of hollow organs, on their serosal surface, in the mesentery, and within the mucosa of the gastrointestinal tract. Most afferent sensory processes are small, nonmyelinated fibers that belong to the C-polymodal class neurons (C-PMNs). C-PMNs are sensitive to mechanical, chemical, and thermal stimulation. A second major group of receptors is fine myelinated Aδ fibers, also called A-mechanoheat receptors. These receptors respond predominantly to mechanical and thermal stimuli, although certain chemicals such as bradykinin and capsaicin are able to activate them.[6] The primary receptive fields of the Aδ fibers lay within the mucosa. In uninflamed tissue, the receptive field of C-PMNs is located in the muscle layer, serosa, and mesentery; however, the receptive field of C-fibers can be extended into the mucosa following inflammation of the gastrointestinal tract.[7,8]

The enteric nervous system (ENS), although not directly involved in the transmission of the sensation of pain, significantly modulates signal transduction from the viscera. The cell bodies are located in the submucosal and myenteric plexuses and are intricately involved in the control of local reflexes, smooth muscle contractile patterns, absorption, and secretion. The ENS integrates motor activity within the gastrointestinal tract. These neurons do not project directly to the central nervous system (CNS) and therefore do not appear to play a major role in the transmission of sensory information from the viscera or the perception of visceral pain. However, the ENS modulates the local environment and may enhance or inhibit the activation of nociceptors through alteration in smooth muscle tone and contractile activity.

### Classic Afferent Pain Pathways

The neuronal pathways that mediate the sensation of visceral pain arising from the gastrointestinal tract involve three distinct levels of neurons between the abdominal viscera and the cerebral cortex (Fig. 3.1). The first-order neurons arise from the visceral organ stimulated and travel to the spinal cord. Second-order neurons link the spinal cord and the brainstem, whereas third-order neurons travel from the brainstem to higher levels of the cerebral cortex. After leaving the viscus they innervate, the first-order nerves pass through the adjacent autonomic nerve plexus. In general, the plexus appears as a web of nerve tissue associated with the major artery supplying the organ (eg,

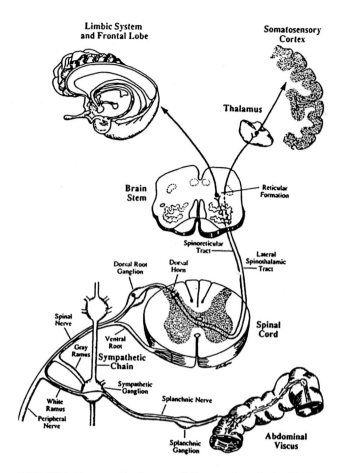

**FIGURE 3.1.**  The neuronal pathways mediating sensations of pain arising from the gastrointestinal tract involve three levels of neurons between the abdominal viscera and the cerebral cortex. First-order neurons arise from the visceral organ stimulated and travel to the spinal cord. Second-order neurons link the spinal cord and the brainstem. Third-order neurons travel from the brainstem to higher levels of the cerebral cortex. After leaving the viscus they innervate, the first-order nerves pass through the adjacent autonomic nerve plexus. Fibers run within the regional splanchnic nerve to the associated sympathetic chain parallel to the spinal cord on either side and then enter the spinal cord and synapse in the dorsal horn. The postsynaptic (ie, second-order) neurons that mediate abdominal visceral sensory processes begin in the superficial laminae of the dorsal horn, cross the midline to the contralateral side, and then travel cephalad within the ventrolateral quadrant of the spinal cord. These neurons run in several ascending pathways (mainly the spinothalamic and spinoreticular tracts) and synapse within several thalamic and reticular formation nuclei of the pons and medulla. Third-order neurons that synapse with spinoreticular tract neurons terminate largely in the limbic system and frontal cortex. Reproduced with permission from Klein KB. Approach to the patient with abdominal pain. In: Yamada T, editor. Textbook of gastroenterology. 2nd ed. Copyright 1995 by Lippincott-Raven Publishers.

celiac, hepatic, superior mesenteric). These plexuses then coalesce to form ganglia, from which the afferent fibers then travel. Fibers run within the regional splanchnic nerve to the associated sympathetic chain parallel to the spinal cord on either side. They then proceed to the spinal nerve via the white ramus communicans, enter the spinal cord, and synapse in the dorsal horn, predominantly in laminae I, II, and V.[9–12] The cell bodies of the first-order neurons lie in the dorsal root ganglia.

Virtually all nerve fibers that carry visceral nociceptive afferent information travel with the sympathetic nervous system (ie, thoracolumbar input).[9,10,13–15] However, many visceral afferents travel via parasympathetic vagal pathways and are thought to primarily serve regulatory autonomic functions, but these pathways may also modulate pain under certain circumstances. These enteroceptors consist of mechanoreceptors that respond to light touch; chemoreceptors that are sensitive to acidity, alkalinity, and nutrients; and osmoreceptors sensitive to changes in the extracellular fluid. Thermoreceptors are also present and under certain conditions may contribute to nociception. Afferent vagal fibers, however, are thought to have little direct effect on pain or pressure perception under normal conditions.[16,17] This observation is based largely on investigations that have demonstrated that stimulation of the splanchnic nerves produced pain, whereas stimulation of the vagus nerve did not.[18] Additionally, inhibition of chronic pain and experimentally induced pain arising from the viscera can be achieved by sectioning the dorsal roots of spinal nerves while the vagus nerve remains intact.[19,20] Recent data, however, have shown that the parasympathetic fibers serve a modulatory role in the transmission of pain from the periphery to the CNS and from the CNS to the periphery, possibly through gating mechanisms. For example, electrical stimulation of the vagus inhibits some and facilitates other spinothalamic tract neurons associated with pain,[21] whereas vagotomy at the cervical level attenuates the antinociceptive effects of analgesics.[22] These observations suggest that spinal visceral afferents interact with vagal afferents at the level of the brainstem and that complex interactions of these two groups of afferents are likely to occur at this level.

The postsynaptic (ie, second-order) neurons that mediate abdominal visceral sensory processes begin in the superficial laminae of the dorsal horn, cross the midline to the contralateral side, and then travel cephalad within the ventrolateral quadrant of the spinal cord. These neurons run in several ascending pathways (mainly the spinothalamic and spinoreticular tracts) and synapse within several thalamic and reticular formation nuclei of the pons and medulla.[9,11] Few data are available regarding the pathways of third-order neurons that transmit visceral pain sensation to higher brain centers, but by analogy to somatic pain pathways, they probably travel widely throughout the brain. By this analogy, pain pathway projections from the spinothalamic tract would travel primarily to the somatosensory cortex, which subserves the sensory-discriminative components of pain perception that are concerned with the quality and localization of the pain. Third-order neurons that synapse with spinoreticular tract neurons terminate largely in the limbic system and frontal cortex and are thought to subserve the motivational-affective aspects of pain perception, known clinically as the aversive or unpleasant features.[23,24]

### Novel Spinal Pathway

The classic models of nociceptive transmission suggest that sensory pathways, either somatic or visceral, are conducted in the anterolateral spinal cord via the spinothalamic and spinomesencephalic tracts. Recently, this view has been seriously challenged with the findings that visceral pain may be relayed in the dorsal spinal column. The dorsal spinal tract has long been held to subserve only the "finer" qualities of sensation, such as joint position sense and two-point discrimination. This postsynaptic dorsal column pathway may be relatively specific to visceral sensation in that it does not appear to play a significant role in cutaneous pain.[25–27] In contrast, both mechanical and chemical irritation of viscera result in stimulation of postsynaptic dorsal column cells and cells of the gracile nucleus.[27] The gracile nucleus, in turn, projects to the contralateral, ventral, posterolateral nucleus in the thalamus. Evidence for the functional importance of this pathway comes from studies in patients with intractable pelvic cancer pain in whom a limited midline myelotomy resulted in complete or near-complete relief of pain.[28–30]

## NEUROPHYSIOLOGY OF VISCERAL AFFERENT PROCESSES

### Encoding of Nociceptive Signals from the Viscera

Numerous hypotheses have evolved regarding the encoding of nociceptive information from the viscera and the processing of this information by the CNS. Three theories of peripheral encoding have emerged at the forefront of debate: the patterning theory, the intensity theory, and the specificity theory. The patterning theory suggests that peripheral afferent neurons fire in highly specific temporospatial patterns that can differentiate between various sensory events.[31] This theory of peripheral encoding has received little electrophysiologic support, however. The intensity theory of pain transmission suggests that both innocuous and noxious stimuli act on the same group of nonspecific afferents and that the different resultant sensations can be distinguished simply by the frequency of neuronal firing.[32,33] Consequently, the intensity of neuronal stimulation would directly correlate with the intensity of neuronal firing, and sophisticated higher CNS processes would act to summate and decode incoming signals. Last, the specificity theory proposes that specific populations of afferent fibers exist that respond only to noxious stimulation and thus represent the recruitment of specific nociceptors.[34] Additional theories involving central and peripheral convergences and peripheral transduction have been proposed to explain the facilitation or inhibition of sensory information from the viscera to the CNS.

After many years of debate, investigators have begun to make significant progress at integrating these theories into a more comprehensive model of peripheral encoding. Recently, three distinct types of afferent mechanoreceptors were identified based on differing discharge frequencies.[17] Functionally, these afferents were described as (a) low-threshold mechanoreceptors that respond to innocuous stimulation, (b) high-threshold mechanoreceptors that respond only to noxious stimulation, and (c) wide-dynamic-range mechanoreceptors that fire to both innocuous and noxious stimuli. All vagal mechanoreceptors were found to be of the low-threshold type, whereas splanchnic afferents were found to be a mixture of the wide-dynamic-range and the high-threshold fibers. Subsequently, these investigators demonstrated that vagal fibers discharged maximally during both peristaltic activity and luminal distention, whereas only a small percentage of splanchnic afferents fired during contractile events. Additionally, splanchnic fibers demonstrated maximal firing rates only during luminal distention. It has been suggested that the wide dynamic range of the splanchnic mechanoreceptors supports the hypothesis of a homogeneous population of visceral afferents responsible for encoding both regulatory information and innocuous and noxious stimuli within the gut.[16] To be effective, this hypothesis requires the progressive recruitment of intensity-encoding afferents and a central mechanism responsible for decoding intensity-summation signals from the periphery.

These electrophysiologic data lend support to the specificity theory by demonstrating the existence of high-threshold populations of afferent fibers that respond only to noxious intensities of stimulation and that involve the recruitment of specific nociceptors. These studies identified a relatively large number of visceral afferent fibers that appear to respond only at levels of abdominal distention associated with pain. These fibers were found to make up approximately 30% of all distention-sensitive fibers.[17,35] Consequently, these observations led proponents of both theories to acknowledge the existence of high-threshold fibers and silent nociceptors, and investigators have now begun attempts to incorporate them into more comprehensive integrative theories of pain transmission.

Cervero and Jaenig have proposed a new model to account for afferent sensory innervation of visceral organs that also rely on three similar types of nociceptive neurons.[36] Under normal circumstances, the low-threshold intensity-coding afferent neurons (LTi) relay information about regulatory function and nonpainful stimulation through specific second-order spinal neurons (Fig. 3.2). These afferents are of the wide-dynamic-range type described by Sengupta and colleagues[17] and respond to stimuli from very low through the high intensities. It has been suggested that these sensory fibers emanating from visceral organs such as the stomach and colon may provide information in a graded manner, such that sensations of mild distention can be distinguished from fullness or intense pain.[37]

If the stimulus intensity in the LTi exceeds a predefined level, these neurons participate in the transmission of nociceptive information to the CNS by activating different second-order neurons in the spinal cord, which results in the perception of pain. At this set point, dedicated nociceptors or high-threshold intensity-coding neurons (HTi) are also activated and transmit nociceptive information to the CNS. A third type of neuron, called silent nociceptors, has recently been identified. These nociceptors are generally quiet and do not participate in the transmission of either vegetative or nociceptive information to the CNS, even during intense stimula-

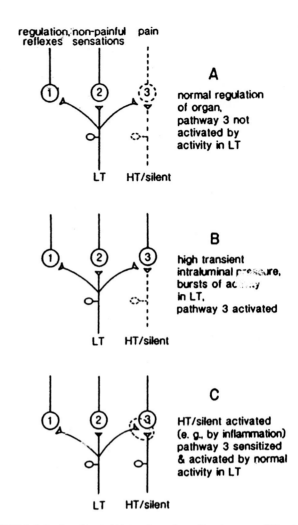

**FIGURE 3.2.** Low-threshold intensity-coding afferent neurons (LTi) relay information about regulatory function and nonpainful stimulation through specific second-order spinal neurons. If the stimulus intensity in the LTi exceeds a predefined setpoint, these neurons then partipate in the transmission of nociceptive information. At higher levels of stimulation, high-threshold intensity-coding neurons dedicated to nociception are activated. Silent nociceptors represent a third type of neuron that is generally quiet but becomes activated through injury, inflammation, and/or central sensitization. Adapted from Jaenig and Häbler.[38]

tion. However, these neurons can become activated through injury, inflammation, and central sensitization. Once sensitized, these fibers transmit pain signals to the CNS during even mild stimulation that occurs with normal regulatory activity in the viscera. These nociceptors may provide the physiologic mechanism for complaints of persistent or chronic abdominal pain in patients without underlying organic pathophysiology.[39–41]

In summary, the data currently available on visceral afferents and the transmission of innocuous and noxious signals to the CNS require a re-evaluation of the functional categories of visceral afferents and nociceptors. The current encoding theories of intensity and specificity need to be integrated into a more realistic model of visceral afferent processing that

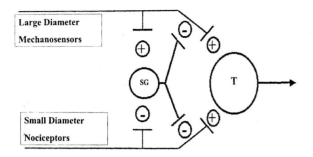

**FIGURE 3.3.** Illustration of the gate control model of pain transmission. Large- and small-diameter sensory afferents from the periphery converge on and activate transmission cell neurons in the dorsal horn opening the gate for the transmission of nociceptive signals from the viscera to the brainstem. Large-diameter mechanosensory afferents from visceral organs deliver excitatory signals to the interneurons and inhibit transmission cell neurons, whereas small-diameter nociceptive sensory afferent fibers deliver inhibitory signals to the interneurons and facilitate the central transmission of nociceptive signals. Finally, interneurons found in the substantia gelatinosa of the dorsal horn can inhibit transmission cell neurons and produce analgesic effects.

accounts for chronic, persistent pain. New models must incorporate recently recognized functional differences in sensory receptors and the coexistence of different neurophysiologic mechanisms in many visceral organs.

## GATING MECHANISMS

The gate control theory of pain transmission proposed by Melzack and Wall[42] states that the perception of pain is dependent on both the interaction of gating mechanisms within the spinal cord (dorsal horn) and in the brainstem. However, the model focuses largely on the interaction of first-order neurons from the viscera with second-order neurons in the dorsal horn of the spinal cord. Figure 3.3 illustrates large- and small-diameter sensory afferents from the periphery that converge on and activate transmission cell neurons in the dorsal horn. This activation opens the gate for the transmission of nociceptive signals from the viscera to the brainstem. Large-diameter mechanosensory afferents from visceral organs deliver excitatory signals to the interneurons and inhibit transmission cell neurons, whereas small-diameter nociceptive sensory afferent fibers deliver inhibitory signals to the interneurons and facilitate the central transmission of nociceptive signals.[43] Finally, interneurons found in the substantia gelatinosa of the dorsal horn can inhibit transmission cell neurons and produce analgesic effects.

The CNS may also directly modulate visceral pain. Descending inhibitory pathways from the medulla and reticular formation converge in the substantia gelatinosa of the dorsal horn, interact with the interneurons, and inhibit transmission cell neurons. This can alter the perception of pain. Specific descending inhibitory inputs have been identified that are associated with abdominal visceral afferents. Additionally, stimulation of the cortex can activate these interneurons, which

may be the neurologic basis for CNS modulation of pain. These observations may also partially explain the mechanisms responsible for the modulation of pain thresholds in patients with anxiety disorders and depression.

Empirical findings suggest that all spinal cord neurons that receive afferents from the viscera also receive afferents from muscle or cutaneous somatic receptors.[44] At the neuronal level, studies have shown that cutaneous stimulation has both facilitator and inhibitory effects on visceral afferents. Simultaneous stimulation of both receptive fields produces a greater response in the spinal neuron, and sequential stimulation produces inhibition in both directions.[45] Clinically, this may be important because pain that occurs simultaneously in both muscle and the colon could produce a lower sensation of pain than would be expected.

The activation of modulatory circuits by somatic stimuli may significantly influence reflex and visceral sensory responses to distention. This hypothesis was recently evaluated in eight healthy human volunteers.[46] Graded isobaric distentions were performed in the stomach and duodenum while transcutaneous electrical stimulation was simultaneously applied to the hand at two different intensities. An intensity-dependent reduction in the perception of gut distention was observed. No significant effect was noted on reflex gastric relaxation to duodenal distention. The authors concluded that somatic stimulation reduces the perception of gut distention without interfering with local reflex responses.

## REFERRED PAIN

Clinical and experimental evidence has clearly shown that visceral pain is poorly localized and temporally dynamic. A stimulus-producing pain, such as noxious balloon distention, within the hollow organs of the gastrointestinal tract may result in widely differing pain reports and referral sites in different patients. Pain may be reported at sites far removed from the organ distended.[47] These observations are collectively defined as referred pain. The mechanisms of referred pain are complex and are thought to involve both peripheral and central processes.

Sensation and perception of pain from the abdominal viscera are largely mediated by sympathetic mechanosensitive afferents. Compared to somatic structures, very few visceral sensory afferents enter the spinal cord at any given level. Additionally, the same splanchnic sensory neuron may originate from multiple visceral organs, and stimulation of a single splanchnic afferent entering the dorsal horn can activate up to 50% of second-order neurons at that level.[44] Consequently, a small number of sensory afferents can activate a significant number of spinothalamic tract neurons and result in poor localization of visceral pain.

As previously discussed, all spinal cord neurons that receive afferents from the viscera also receive afferents from muscle or cutaneous somatic receptors. Afferent fibers from various structures enter the dorsal horn of the spinal cord and then converge with second-order neurons in common spinothalamic projection pathways. Therefore, activation of sensory afferents from different visceral or somatic structures may activate the same second-order spinal neurons. This convergence-projection theory of pain transmission suggests that information from the periphery may be misinterpreted centrally and result in the inability to accurately differentiate the origination of certain nociceptive signals. Therefore, somatic structures, which are more densely innervated and more commonly stimulated than visceral structures, are more likely to be identified as the source of persistent pain. Cutaneous dermatomes offer a clinically useful method of isolating the origin of pain from the abdominal viscera.

Pain originating from the distal esophagus, stomach, proximal duodenum, liver, biliary tree, and pancreas (T5–T6 to T8–T9) is generally referred between the xiphoid process and the umbilicus. The midgut structures (small intestine, appendix, ascending colon, and proximal portions of the transverse colon) are innervated in spinal segments T8–T11 to L1 and have pain referred to the periumbilical region. The distal transverse colon, descending colon, and rectosigmoid colon (T11–L1) are generally referred to dermatomes located between the umbilicus and the pubis and in the perineal regions.[43] Although significant overlap is evident, knowledge of these characteristic landmarks of pain referral may be helpful in clinical practice.

## TRANSMISSION AND CONTROL OF AFFERENT SIGNALS

### Sympathetic and Parasympathetic Contributions to Pain

Although high concentrations of norepinephrine do not directly produce C-fiber activation, there are considerable data to suggest a role of the sympathetic nervous system in peripheral hyperalgesia.[48] Sensitization of nociceptors may occur indirectly via adrenergically mediated release of prostaglandins from nearby cells.[49] However, there are few, if any, studies that have examined the contribution of the sympathetic nervous system to the development of visceral sensitization.

Parasympathetic fibers from the mucosa can also modulate pain transmission but do not appear to mediate pain directly. Of note, electrical stimulation of the abdominal vagus generally induces nausea and vomiting but not pain.[16] It has been shown that electrical stimulation of vagal afferents can activate descending pathways, which inhibit some, and facilitate other, spinothalamic tract neurons in the spinal cord.[22] However, stimulation of vagal afferents more often inhibits, rather than facilitates, pain transmission.[21]

### Smooth Muscle Tone, Motility, and Afferent Transmission

Although correlation between the presence of very-high-amplitude propagated contractions in the colon and reports of abdominal pain have generally been small,[50,51] some episodes of pain may be associated with discrete contractile events.[52] Sensory neurons respond as if in series with smooth muscle fibers.[53] Therefore, many of the neurons in the brainstem that fire to noxious colonic stimuli also fire in response to spontaneous contractions.[54] Atropine reduces smooth muscle tone in the gut and increases the distention volume required to produce pain but does not significantly alter the pressure required to produce pain.[55] Consequently, smooth muscle tone and contractility may influence the threshold for excitation of receptors responsible for pain transmission either directly or indirectly.

Technological advances over the last few years have generated a renewed interest in the clinical evaluation of visceral sensation and perception. These advances have allowed researchers to investigate the influence of more dynamic properties of smooth muscle on visceral perception. Recent evidence has shown that adaptive relaxation of smooth muscle tone occurs in response to rectal balloon distention at a constant pressure.[56] These data suggest that the healthy rectum actively adapts to chronic stretch of the rectal wall, a critical response for the normal, short-term storage function of the rectum. Impaired adaptive relaxation may contribute to symptoms in patient populations with chronic recurrent abdominal pain and urgency. Crowell and Musial compared changes in rectal volume in healthy controls and in patients with irritable bowel syndrome (IBS) during continuous rectal distention at pressures associated with first sensation and a moderate urge to defecate.[57] Therefore, these data suggest that in patients with IBS, symptoms of urgency and lower thresholds for abdominal pain might be caused by impaired adaptive relaxation of the rectum in response to chronic distention, resulting in greater stimulation of visceral mechanoreceptors with luminal distention and increased levels of pain in patients with IBS as compared with normal volunteers.

## CENTRAL PROCESSING OF VISCERAL SENSATION

The complexity of visceral sensory afferent processing and the perception of abdominal pain are only partially revealed in the preceding discussion. Chronic visceral pain is directly influenced by temporal changes in both central and peripheral mechanisms.

Central mechanisms are extremely important in the development of hyperalgesia. Sensitization of tissues adjacent to the area of immediate injury and central hyperexcitability result from secondary hyperalgesia.[58,59] It has been suggested that both primary and secondary hyperalgesia play a role in chronic pain conditions such as the IBS. Considerable clinical evidence exists to support this observation. For example, a significant number of patients with functional gastrointestinal disorders experience pain at distention pressures or volumes that produce, at best, normal internal sensation in healthy volunteers.[39] Furthermore, patients with IBS have significantly lower thresholds for the perception of non-noxious distention

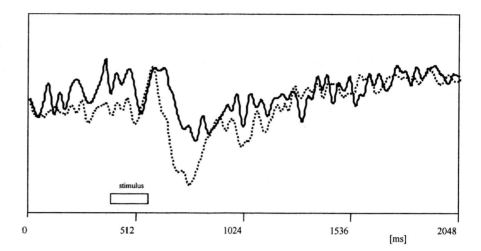

**FIGURE 3.4.** Cortical evoked potentials following mechanochemical (*dashed line*) as compared with only mechanical (*solid line*) stimulation of the esophagus. Note the higher amplitude and shorter latency with chemical stimulation. Reproduced with permission from Roscher S, Renner B, Kuhlbusch R, et al. Cerebral activation after chemical and mechanical stimulation of the esophagus [abstract]. Gastroenterology 1998;114:A168.

of the gut. Mechanisms for both primary (peripheral) and secondary (central) hyperalgesia have been proposed and may be explained through nociceptor sensitization, altered central processing, or central plasticity.[60] Over the past 10 years, significant advances have been made in assessing cortical activation and processing of gastrointestinal stimulation in healthy controls and in patients with functional bowel disorders.

## Cortical Evoked Potentials Following Intestinal Stimulation

Frieling and coworkers used neurophysiologic recordings of evoked potentials (EPs) to directly investigate the gut-brain axis in humans.[61,62] Prior to this work, EPs from visceral organs had been recorded only from the bladder.[63] Numerous studies have since demonstrated the ability of EP recordings to assess the integrity of the gut-to-brain pathways in healthy subjects and in patients with various intestinal and extraintestinal disorders. The specifics of these techniques have been reviewed by Enck and Frieling[64] and others.[65,66] Intestinal EPs have been recorded in response to electrical, mechanical (balloon), and chemical stimulation applied to esophageal mucosa (Fig. 3.4).[67] Stimulation of other intestinal compartments such as the stomach and small intestine has not been successfully completed because of methodologic limitations related to the application of currently available stimuli in a reliable and safe manner. A single study was found that recorded cortical EPs following shock wave treatment of the gallbladder with different lithotripters, but these data remain unclear regarding somatosensory and/or visceral contributions to the EP recorded.[68]

Evoked potentials from the viscera show both similarities and differences compared with those evoked from peripheral somatosensory sites. Evoked potentials from the esophagus and rectum are usually much longer in latency and smaller in amplitude than somatosensory EPs and decrease in size with increased frequency (above 1 Hz) and duration of stimulation. However, similarly to somatosensory EPs, they are positively correlated with the intensity of the stimulus (Fig. 3.5).[69,70] This similarity may help to explain their specific psychophysiologic characteristics. Evoked potentials from the esophagus are

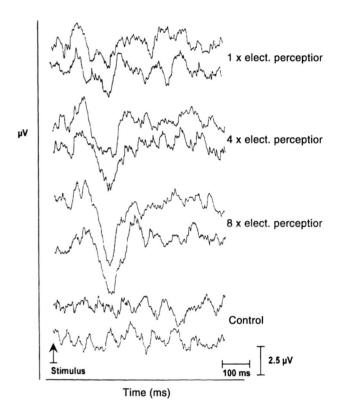

**FIGURE 3.5.** Cortical evoked potentials following esophageal electrical stimulation. Note the increase in evoked potential amplitude with increasing perceived stimulation intensity. Reproduced with permission from Söllenböhmer C, Enck P, Häussinger D, Frieling T. Electrically evoked cerebral potentials during esophageal distension at perception and pain threshold. Am J Gastroenterol 1996;91:970–5.

thought to be transmitted via the vagus nerve since direct vagal stimulation using an electrical pacemaker produces similar responses in the brain as those elicited via esophageal distention.[71] However, the relative contribution of spinal pathways to cortical EP following (painful) stimulation remains unclear since spinal primary and secondary sensitization has been shown to occur following esophageal acid exposure.[72]

One of the primary limitations of EP technology is that it does not provide for precise localization of the cortical regions in which visceral afferent data are processed.[73] A major reason for this limitation is the fact that an electrical field generated by one or more brain dipoles is relatively large, thus limiting the estimate of the dipole numbers and their localization when an electrical field is recorded by multichannel EP. Therefore, the topographic organization of different intestinal compartments (eg, lower and upper esophagus) cannot be reliably determined using EP recordings. However, newer brain mapping techniques are currently being explored that may significantly improve resolution.

To date, evoked potential studies have not been routinely performed in patient populations. The few patient populations that have been studied with EPs include those with autonomic neuropathy caused by diabetes mellitus,[74] chest pain of cardiac and noncardiac origin,[75–78] spinal cord injury,[79] constipation,[80] and dyspepsia.[81] However, the results have generally lacked specificity when compared with EP responses from healthy controls. For example, in patients with diabetic autonomic neuropathy, rather than finding altered EP responses, as would be expected, no EPs could be discerned. In patients with chest pain EPs have been consistently shown to be reduced in amplitude in patients compared to healthy control subjects. These findings were interpreted as indicating changes in central processing of stimuli rather than alterations in the peripheral pathways related to the perception of visceral sensation.

### Brain Mapping of Intestinal Sensory Function

Dynamic brain imaging technologies such as positron emission tomography (PET), functional magnetic resonance imaging (fMRI), magnetoencephalography (MEG), and single-photon emission tomography (SPECT) have recently been applied to the study of the gut-brain axis. Magneto-encephalography provides improved temporal resolution over PET and fMRI but is severely limited by its ability to detect activity only from the superficial cortical surfaces. Activation of brain structures more than 2 cm below the cortical surface requires other approaches, such as PET and fMRI. Most relevant processing of visceral information occurs in deeper brain structures, such as the midbrain and brainstem. Consequently, most recent work has focused on identifying these brain networks activated by visceral sensations using PET and fMRI.

Table 3.1 lists many of the advantages and limitations of different imaging technologies in elucidating central processing of visceral afferent information. The primary limitation of most currently available imaging techniques is their relatively poor temporal resolution. Newer approaches have been developed to improve resolution using event-related processing methodologies but are not in common use.

In spite of the limitations outlined above, a PET study during esophageal stimulation marked the beginning of a series of investigations using imaging techniques in both the upper and lower gastrointestinal tract (Tables 3.2 and 3.3).[82–100] These studies have been recently reviewed by Aziz and Thompson[66] and Aziz and colleagues.[83] For technical details of these methods, the reader is referred to these reviews.

Neuroimaging has also begun to provide evidence of physiologic differences between normal individuals and those suffering from functional gastrointestinal disorders such as IBS in the way visceral stimuli (eg, rectal distention) are processed in the brain. Initial data from PET scans demonstrated increased activation of the anterior cingulate cortex (ACC) among normal individuals compared to patients with IBS. The ACC is a cerebral cortical area that

**TABLE 3.1.** Advantages and Limitations of Different Brain Imaging Techniques

| Technique | Temporal Resolutions | Spacial Resolution | Advantages | Limitations |
| --- | --- | --- | --- | --- |
| EP | High (ms) | Low (cm) | Cheap for multichannel | Cortical surface only |
| MEG | High (ms) | High (mm) | Combination with EP | Cortical surface only |
| PET | Low (min) | High (mm) | Metabolic research | Radiation |
| SPECT | Low (min) | High (mm) | Metabolic research | Radiation |
| fMRI | Low (s) | High (mm) | No radiation | Only functional anatomy |

EP, evoked potential; MEG, magnetoencephalography; PET, positron emission tomography; SPECT, single-photon emission computed tomography; fMRI, functional magnetic resonance imaging.

**TABLE 3.2.** Brain Imaging Studies Following Esophageal Stimulation in Healthy Controls

| Lead Author | Year | Ref. | Technique | Design | Stimulus | Intensity | Position | Controls (n) |
| --- | --- | --- | --- | --- | --- | --- | --- | --- |
| Aziz | 1997 | 82 | PET | Block | Balloon | No pain - pain | Distal | 8 |
| Kern | 1998 | 84 | fMRI | Block | Acid - balloon | Below pain | Distal | 10 |
| Binkofski | 1998 | 85 | fMRI | Block | Balloon | No pain - pain | Distal | 5 |
| Furlong | 1998 | 86 | MEG | ER | Balloon | Below pain | Proximal distal | 34 |
| Schnitzler | 1999 | 87 | MEG | ER | Electrical | Below pain | Distal | 7 |
| Loose | 1999 | 88 | MEG | ER | Balloon | No pain - pain | Proximal distal | 6 |
| Hecht | 1999 | 89 | MEG | ER | Electrical | Below pain | Proximal distal | 9 |
| Aziz | 2000 | 90 | fMRI | Block | Balloon | Below pain | Proximal distal | 6 |

PET, positron emission tomography; fMRI, functional magnetic resonance imaging; MEG, magnetoencephalography; ER, event-related processing.

**TABLE 3.3** Brain Imaging Studies Following Anorectal Stimulation

| Lead Author | Year | Ref. | Technique | Design | Anal | Rectum | Controls (n) | Patients (n) |
|---|---|---|---|---|---|---|---|---|
| Silvermann | 1997 | 91 | PET | Block | No | Balloon | 6 | 6 |
| Baciu | 1999 | 92 | fMRI | Block | No | Balloon | 8 | — |
| Bouras | 1999 | 93 | SPECT | Block | No | Balloon | 10 | — |
| Mertz | 2000 | 94 | fMRI | Block | No | Balloon | 16 | 18 |
| Stottrop | 2000 | 95 | MEG | E-R | Electrical | No | 7 | — |
| Hobday | 2001 | 96 | fMRI | Block | No | Balloon | | — |
| Binkofski | 2001 | 85 | fMRI | Block | Electrical | Electrical | 8 | — |
| Lotze | 2001 | 97 | fMRI | E-R | Balloon | Balloon | 8 | — |
| Kern | 2000 | 84 | fMRI | Block | No | Balloon | 8 | — |
| Nabiloff | 2000 | 98 | PET | Block | No | Balloon | 12 | 12 |
| Ringel | 2000 | 99 | PET | Block | No | Balloon | 6 | 6 |
| Bonaz | 2000 | 99 | fMRI | Block | No | Balloon | — | 8 |

PET, positron emission tomography; fMRI, functional magnetic resonance imaging; SPECT, single-photon emission computed tomography; MEG, magnetoencephalography; ER, event-related processing.

is rich in opiate receptors and is thought to be a major component of cognitive circuits relating to perception and to descending spinal pathways involving pain. More recently, fMRI was used to demonstrate increased activity in the ACC, prefrontal cortex (PFC), and insular cortex (IC) areas and in the thalamus of patients with IBS compared to normal individuals.

Among the first questions to be addressed using advanced imaging techniques was whether intestinal compartments are represented over the primary sensory (S1) cortex—better known as the sensory homunculus—in humans. Because temporal resolution is limited with PET and fMRI, information about the timing of cortical events in S1 could only be addressed using MEG, which has a higher temporal resolution. It was shown that cortical responses from the upper and lower esophagus—in contrast to somatosensory afferents—are directly projected onto the second somatosensory (S2) cortex (Fig. 3.6) but share some of the psychophysiologic characteristics of primary somatosensory (S1) responses (Fig. 3.7).[87,88] A consistent somatotopic pattern of the S2 cortex has not been identified to date. This observation may help

explain the rather diffuse character of visceral, intestinal sensations with respect to localization and referral patterns.

In contrast to the esophagus, stimulation of the anal canal has recently been shown to activate both somatosensory and visceral pathways resulting in activation of both the S1 cortex—halfway between the hand and foot representation—and the S2 cortex (Fig. 3.8).[95] This pattern is unique and has not been reported from any other intestinal segment studied.

The anorectal brain network is summarized in Table 3.4. It includes—besides the S1 and S2 cortices—the IC, anterior cingulate gyrus (ACG), PFC, thalamus (Th), and parieto-orbital cortex (POC). In single studies, activation of the supplementary motor cortex (SMA; for anal stimulation), hippocampus, brainstem (periaqueductal gray and medulla), and cerebellum (for anal but not for rectal stimulation) was observed (Fig. 3.9).

It is obvious from the complex patterns of activation following anorectal stimulation that most of the activated areas in the brain do not serve specific functions but must share responsibility for other afferent processes. It is well known that pain processing, irrespective of its origin, involves dif-

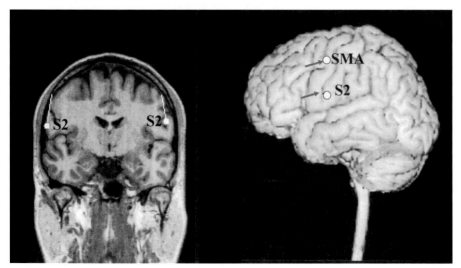

**FIGURE 3.6.** Magnetoencephalographic (MEG) response (MEG dipoles projected onto an individual brain anatomy) after electrical stimulation of the lower esophagus. The early response is located bilaterally in the S2 cortex and the late response in the supplementary motor cortex (SMA). Reproduced with permission from Loose R, Schnitzler A, Sarkar S, et al. Cortical activation during mechanical esophageal stimulation: a neuromagnetic study. Neurogastroenterology 1999;11:163–71.

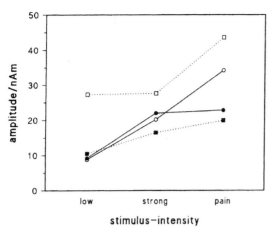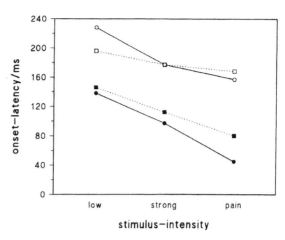

**FIGURE 3.7.** Psychophysiologic characteristics of MEG responses in the S2 cortex following electrical esophageal stimulation with different intensities. Note the decrease in the latency (*right*) and increase in amplitude (*left*) with increasing stimulus intensity. Reproduced with permission from Loose R, Schnitzler A, Sarkar S, et al. Cortical activation during mechanical esophageal stimulation: a neuromagnetic study. Neurogastroenterology 1999;11:163–71.

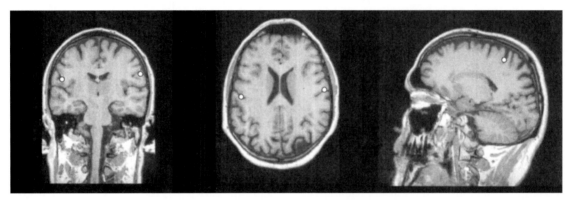

**FIGURE 3.8.** Magnetoelectrical response (MEG dipoles projected onto an individual brain anatomy) after electrical stimulation of the anal canal. Note the unilateral S1 response located halfway between the hand and foot representation area and the bilateral S2 response. Reproduced with permission from Stottrop K, Schnitzler A, Witte OW, Freund HJ, Enck P. Cortical representation of the anal canal. Gastroenterology 1998;114:A167.

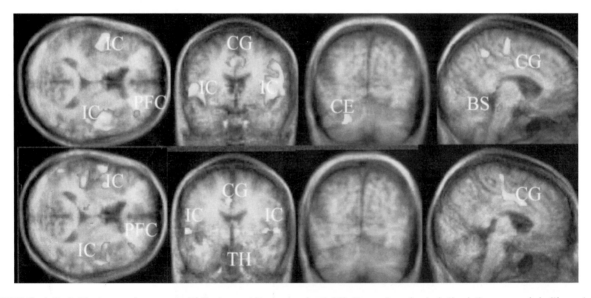

**FIGURE 3.9.** Activated brain areas (group means) following anal (*top row*) and rectal (*bottom row*) mechanical stimulation as recorded with event-related functional magnetic resonance imaging. The sections show the insular cortex (IC), cingulate gyrus (CG), prefrontal cortex (PFC), cerebellum (CE), brainstem (BS), and parieto-orbital cortex (POC). Reproduced with permission from Lotze M, Wietek B, Birbaumer N, et al. Cerebral activation during anal and rectal stimulation. Neuroimage. (In review).

**TABLE 3.4.** Anorectal Brain Network According to Published Studies

| Lead Author | Year | Ref. | S1–S2 | Ins | ACG | CG | PFC | Tha | SMA | CE | POC | BS |
|---|---|---|---|---|---|---|---|---|---|---|---|---|
| Silverman | 1997 | 91 | | | X | (X) | X | | | | (X) | |
| Baciu | 1999 | 92 | | X | X | X | X | | | | X | |
| Bouras | 1999 | 93 | | | X | | X | X | | | | |
| Mertz | 2000 | 94 | | X | X | | X | X | | | | X |
| Stottrop | 2000 | 95 | X | | | | | | | | | |
| Binkofski | 2000 | 85 | X | X | X | X | X | | | X | | X |
| Lotze | 2000 | 97 | X | X | X | X | X | (X) | (X) | (X) | X | (X) |
| Hobday | 2001 | 96 | X | X | X | X | X | | | | | |
| Kern | 2000 | 84 | (X) | | X | | | X | X | | | |
| Nabiloff | 2000 | 98 | | X | X | X | X | X | X | | X | |
| Ringel | 2000 | 99 | | | X | | | | | | | |
| Bonaz | 2000 | 100 | | X | X | | X | | | | X | |

Parentheses indicate nonsignificant activation. S1–S2, somatosensory cortex 1–2; Ins, insular cortex; ACG, anterior cingulate gyrus; CG, cingulate gyrus; PFC, prefrontal cortex; Tha, thalamus; SMA, supplementary motor cortex; CE, cerebellum; POC, parieto-orbital cortex; BS, brainstem.

ferent areas within the CG depending on pain intensity and/or pain quality.[101] Additionally, the PFC is known to be activated by increased vigilance and attention,[102] the POC is activated with interference of body image,[103] and the limbic circuitry (hypothalamus, hippocampus, ACG) plays a central role in the processing of emotions.

Brain imaging of visceral sensory processing has been used extensively for evaluating potential central pathomechanisms in patients with functional bowel disorders. Silverman and colleagues first compared central activation in patients with IBS and healthy controls and demonstrated a poor correlation between ACG activation and perceived stimulus intensity using rectal balloon distention.[91] These investigators further demonstrated increased activation of the PFC in patients with IBS compared to controls. Based on these observations, the authors concluded that alterations in central mechanisms resulted in decreased activation of descending inhibitory pain pathways, thus leading to visceral hyperalgesia in patients with IBS. However, this conclusion may have been premature since other studies[84,94] failed to confirm the proposed alterations in central progressing of visceral pain between IBS patients and controls. A clear quantitative association between brain activation and visceral stimulation remains to be firmly established.

Clearly, our current understanding of brain–gut, gut–brain communications is very limited, and much work remains to be done. The role of brain–gut interactions during voluntary motor functions of the anorectum is at an early stage but may provide extremely useful information for understanding the mechanisms of defecation and continence. Investigations of cortical activation during micturition in health and disease could serve as a recently established example.[104] Cortical representations of efferent motor function during swallowing have been shown to be clinically useful in understanding dysphagia following stroke.[105] Experimental manipulation of cortical processing of visceral afferents by biofeedback and other manipulations of central "states" may also help to further explain abnormalities contributing to functional gastrointesti-

nal disorders.[90,99] Images obtained following stimulation of the stomach[106] should soon allow assessment of cortical activation during the onset and development of nausea[107] and during food ingestion.[108] Finally, PET studies using specific radiolabeled receptor binding agents such as serotonin and histamine in the human brain offer great promise for our future understanding of this exciting area.[85,86,89,92,93,96–98,109,110]

## REFERENCES

1. Hertz AF. The sensibility of the alimentary canal in health and disease. Lancet 1911;1:1051.
2. Ray BS, Neill CL. Abdominal visceral sensation in man. Ann Surg 1947;126:709.
3. Bentley FH. Observations on visceral pain. Ann Surg 1948;128:881.
4. Sherrington CS. Qualitative difference of spinal reflex corresponding with a qualitative difference of cutaneous stimulus. J Physiol (Lond) 1904;30:39.
5. Cervero F. Sensory innervation of the visceral: peripheral basis of visceral pain. Physiol Rev 1994;74:95–138.
6. Rang HP, Bevan S, Dray A. Chemical activation of nociceptive peripheral neurones. Br Med Bull 1991;47:534–48.
7. Ness TJ, Gebhart GF. Visceral pain: a review of experimental studies. Pain 1990;41:167–386.
8. McMahon S, Koltzenburg M. The changing role of primary afferent neurons in pain. Pain 1990;43:269–72.
9. Cervero F. Visceral nociception: peripheral and central aspects of visceral nociceptive systems. Philos Trans R Soc Lond B Biol Sci 1985;308:325–37.
10. Cervero F, Tattersall JEH. Somatic and visceral sensory integration in the thoracic spinal cord. In: Cervero F, Morrison JFB, editors. Visceral sensation. Amsterdam: Elsevier; 1986. p. 189–205.
11. Willis WD Jr. Visceral inputs to sensory pathways in the spinal cord. In: Cervero F, Morrison JFB, editors. Visceral sensation. Amsterdam: Elsevier; 1986. p. 207.
12. Fields HL. Pain from deep tissues and referred pain. In: Fields HL, editor. Pain. New York: McGraw-Hill, 1987. p. 79.
13. Cervero F. Neurophysiology of gastrointestinal pain. Baillieres Clin Gastroenterol 1988;2:183–99.
14. Mayer EA, Raybould HE. Role of visceral afferent mechanisms in functional bowel disorders. Gastroenterology 1990;99:1688–704.
15. White JC, Sweet WH. Pain in abdominal visceral disease. In: White JC, Sweet WH, editors. Pain and the neurosurgeon. Springfield (IL): Charles C Thomas; 1969. p. 560.

16. Grundy D. Mechanoreceptors in the gastrointestinal tract. J Smooth Muscle Res 1993;29:37–46.

17. Sengupta JN, Saha JK, Goyal RK. Stimulus-response function studies of esophageal mechanosensitive nociceptors in sympathetic afferents of opossum. J Neurophysiol 1990;64:796–812.

18. Cannon B. A method of stimulating autonomic nerves in the unanesthetized cat with observations on the motor and sensory effects. Am J Physiol 1933;105:366–72.

19. White JC. Sensory innervation of the viscera. Studies of visceral afferent neurones in man based on neurosurgical procedures for the relief of intractable pain. Res Pub Assoc Res Nerv Mental Dis 1943;23:373–90.

20. Stulrajter V, Pavelasek J, Strauss P, et al. Some neuronal, autonomic, and behavioral correlates of visceral pain elicited by gall-bladder stimulation. Activ Nerv Sup (Praha) 1978;20:203–9.

21. Ren K, Randich A, Gebhart GF. Effect of electrical stimulation of vagal afferents on spinothalamic tract cells in the rat. Pain 1991;44:311–9.

22. Randich A, Thurston CL, Ludwig PS, et al. Antinociception and cardiovascular responses produced by intravenous morphine: the role of vagal afferents. Brain Res 1991;543:256–70.

23. Fields HL. Pain pathways in the central nervous system. In: Fields HL, editor. Pain. New York: McGraw-Hill; 1987. p. 41.

24. Melzack R, Wall PD. Brain mechanisms. In: Melzack R, Wall PD, editors. The challenge of pain. 2nd ed. London: Penguin Books; 1988. p. 122.

25. Giesler GT, Nahin RL, Madsen AM. Postsynaptic dorsal column pathway of the rat. J Neurophysiol 1984;51:260–75.

26. Al-Chaer ED, Lawand NB, Westlund KN, Willis WD. Visceral nociceptive input into the ventral posterolateral nucleus of the thalamus: a new function for the dorsal column pathway. J Neurophysiol 1996;76:2661–74.

27. Al-Chaer ED, Lawand NB, Westlund KN, Willis WD. Pelvic visceral input into the nucleus gracilis is largely mediated by the postsynaptic dorsal column pathway. J Neurophysiol 1996;76:2675–90.

28. Gildenberg PL, Hirshberg RM. Limited myelotomy for the treatment of intractable cancer pain. J Neurol Neurosurg Psychiatry 1984;47:94–6.

29. Hirshberg RM, Al-Chaer ED, Lawand NB, et al. Is there a pathway in the posterior funiculus that signals visceral pain? Pain 1996;67:291–305.

30. Hitchcock ER. Stereotactic cervical myelotomy. J Neurol Neurosurg Psychiatry 1970;33:224–30.

31. Sinclair DC. Cutaneous sensation and the doctrine of specific energy. Brain 1955;78:584.

32. Jaenig W, Koltzenburg M. On the function of spinal primary afferent fibers supplying colon and urinary bladder. J Auton Nerv Syst 1990;30(Suppl):589–96.

33. Ness TJ, Gebhart GF. Characterization of superficial T13–L2 dorsal horn neurons encoding for colorectal distention in the rat: comparison with neurons in deep laminae. Brain Res 1989;8:301–9.

34. Cervero F. Afferent activity evoked by natural stimulation of the biliary system in the ferret. Pain 1982;13:137–51.

35. Cervero F, Sharkey KA. An electrophysiological and anatomical study of intestinal afferent fibers in the rat. J Physiol 1988;401:381–97.

36. Cervero F, Jaenig W. Visceral nociceptors: a new world order? Trends Neurosci 1992;15:374–8.

37. Mayer EM, Gebhart GF. Functional bowel disorders and the visceral hyperalgesia hypothesis. In: Mayer EA, Raybould HE, editors. Basic and clinical aspects of chronic abdominal pain. Pain Research and Clinical Management 1993;9:3.

38. Jaenig W, Habler J-J. Visceral-autonomic integration. In: Gebhart GF, editor. Visceral pain: progress in pain research and management. Vol 5. Seattle: IASP Press; 1995. p.

39. Mayer EA, Gebhart GF. Basic and clinical aspects of visceral hyperalgesia. Gastroenterology 1994;107:271–93.

40. Jaenig W, Koltzenburg M. The neural basis of consciously perceived sensations from the gut. In: Singer MV, Goebell H, editors. Nerves and the gastrointestinal tract. Dordrecht (The Netherlands): Kluwer; 1989. p. 383–98.

41. Jaenig W, Koltzenburg M. Receptive properties of sacral primary afferent neurons supplying the colon. J Neurophysiol 1991;65:1067–77.

42. Melzack R, Wall PD. Gate-control and other mechanisms. In: Melzack R, Wall PD, editors. The challenge of pain. 2nd ed. London: Penguin Books; 1988. p. 165.

43. Klein KB. Approach to the patient with abdominal pain. In: Yamada T, editor. Textbook of gastroenterology. 2nd ed. Philadelphia: JB Lippincott; 1995. p. 750–71.

44. Cervero F, Tattersall JEH. Somatic and visceral sensory integration in the thoracic spinal cord. In: Cervero F, Morrison JFB, editors. Visceral sensation. Amsterdam: Elsevier; 1986. p. 189.

45. Gebhart FR, Randich A. Brainstem modulation of nociception. In: Klemm WR, Vertes RP, editors. Brainstem mechanisms of behavior. New York: Wiley; 1990. p. 315–52.

46. Coffin B, Azpiroz F, Guarner F, Malagelada JR. Selective gastric hypersensitivity and reflex hyporeactivity in functional dyspepsia. Gastroenterology 1994;107:1345–51.

47. Ruch TC. Pathophysiology of pain. In: Ruch TC, Patton JD, Woodbury JW, Lowe AL, editors. Neurophysiology. Philadelphia: WB Saunders; 1961. p. 350.

48. Campbell JN, Mayer RA, Davis KD, Raja SN. Sympathetically maintained pain: a unifying hypothesis. In: Willis WD Jr, editor. Hyperalgesia and allodynia. New York: Raven; 1992. p. 141–50.

49. Taiwo YO, Levine JD. Characterization of the arachidonic acid metabolites mediating bradykinin and noradrenaline hyperalgesia. Brain Res 1988;458:402–6.

50. Crowell MD, Bassotti G, Cheskin LJ, et al. Method for prolonged ambulatory monitoring of high-amplitude propagated contractions from colon. Am J Physiol 1991;26:G263–8.

51. Bassotti G, Crowell MD, Whitehead WE. Contractile activity of the human colon: lessons from 24-hour studies. Gut 1993;34:129–33.

52. Holdstock DJ, Misiewicz JJ, Waller SL. Observations on the mechanism of abdominal pain. Gut 1969;10:19–31.

53. Iggo A. Gastrointestinal tension receptors with unmyelinated afferent fibers in the vagus of the cat. Q J Exp Physiol Cogn Med Sci 1957;42:130–43.

54. Jaenig W. Spinal cord integration of visceral sensory systems and sympathetic nervous system reflexes. In: Cervero F, Morrison JFB, editors. Visceral sensation. Progress in Brain Research. Vol 67. Amsterdam: Elsevier; 1986. p. 255–77.

55. Chapman WP, Jones CM. Variations in cutaneous and visceral pain sensitivity in normal subjects. J Clin Invest 1944;23:81–91.

56. Musial F, Crowell MD, Enck P. Effects of long-term rectal distention on rectal tone. Gastroenterology 1994;106:A546.

57. Crowell MD, Musial F. Rectal adaptation to distention is impaired in the irritable bowel syndrome. Am J Gastroenterol 1994;89:1689.

58. Willis WD. Mechanical allodynia: a role for sensitized nociceptive tract cells with convergent input from mechanoreceptors and nociceptors? Am Pain Soc J 1993;2:23–33.

59. Willis WD Jr. Central sensitization and plasticity following intense noxious stimulation. In: Mayer EA, Raybould HE, editors. Basic and clinical aspects of chronic abdominal pain. Amsterdam: Elsevier; 1993. p. 202–17.

60. Cervero F. Mechanisms of peripheral and central sensitization. Ann Med 1995;27:235–9.

61. Frieling T, Enck P, Wienbeck M. Cerebral responses evoked by electrical stimulation of rectosigmoid in normal subjects. Dig Dis Sci 1989;34:202–5.

62. Frieling T, Enck P, Wienbeck M. Cerebral responses evoked by electrical stimulation of the esophagus in normal subjects. Gastroenterology 1989;97:475–8.

63. Badr G, Carlsson CA, Fall M, et al. Cortical evoked potentials following stimulation of the urinary bladder in man. Electroencephalogr Clin Neurophysiol 1982:54:494–8.

64. Enck P, Frieling T. Human gut-brain interactions. J Gastrointest Motil 1993;5:77–87.

65. Hollerbach S, Tougas G, Frieling T, et al. Cerebral evoked potentials (EP) following electrical and mechanical stimulation of visceral organs in humans. Crit Rev Biomed Eng 1997;25:203–42.

66. Aziz Q, Thompson DG. Brain gut axis in health and disease. Gastroenterology 1998;114:559–78.

67. Roscher S, Renner B, Kuhlbusch R, et al. Cerebral activation after chemical and mechanical stimulation of the esophagus [abstract]. Gastroenterology 1998;114:A168.

68. Schneider TC, Hummel T, Janowitz P, et al. Pain in extracorporeal shock-wave lithotripsy: a comparison of different lithotripsers in volunteers. Gastroenterology 1992;102:640–6.

69. Söllenböhmer C, Enck P, Häussinger D, Frieling T. Electrically evoked cerebral potentials during esophageal distension at perception and pain threshold. Am J Gastroenterol 1996;91:970–5.

70. Hollerbach S, Kamath MV, Chen Y, et al. The magnitude of the central response to esophageal electrical stimulation is intensity dependent. Gastroenterology 1997;112:1137–46.

71. Tougas G, Hudoba P, Fitzpatrick D, et al. Cerebral evoked responses following direct vagal and esophageal electrical stimulation in humans. Am J Physiol 1993;264:G486–91.

72. Sarkar S, Hobson A, Woolf CJ, et al. Oesophageal cortical evoked potentials are potentiated following acid induced hypersensitivity. Gut 1999;44(Suppl 1):A111.

73. Aziz Q, Furlong PL, Barlow J, et al. Topographic mapping of cortical potentials evoked by distension of the human proximal and distal oesophagus. Electroencephalogr Clin Neurophysiol 1995;96:219–28.

74. Rathmann W, Enck P, Frieling T, Gries FA. Visceral afferent neuropathy in diabetic gastroparesis. Diabetes Care 1991;14:1086–9.

75. Smout AJP, DeVore MS, Dalton CB, Castell DO. Cerebral potentials evoked by oesophageal distension in patients with non-cardiac chest pain. Gut 1992;33:298–302.

76. Frobert O, Arendt-Nielsen L, Bak P, et al. Pain perception and brain evoked potentials in patients with angina despite nomal coronary angiograms. Heart 1995;75:436–41.

77. DeVault KR, Castell DO. Esophageal balloon distention and cerebral evoked potential recording in the evaluation of unexplained chest pain. Am J Med 1992;92:20–6.

78. Hollerbach ST, Bulat R, May A, et al. Abnormal cerebral processing of oesophageal stimuli in patients with noncardiac chest pain. Neurogastroenterology 2000;12:555–66.

79. DeVault KR, Beacham S, Castell DO, et al. Esophageal sensation in spinal cord-injured patients: balloon distension and cerebral evoked potential recording. Am J Physiol 1996;271:G937–41.

80. Loening-Baucke V, Yamada T. Is the afferent pathway from the rectum impaired in children with chronic constipation and encopresis? Gastroenterology 1995;109:397–403.

81. Kanazawa M, Nomura T, Fukodo S, Hono M. Abnormal visceral perception in patients with functional dyspepsia: use of cerebral potentials by electrical stimulation of the esophagus. Neurogastroenterology 2000;12:87–94.

82. Aziz Q, Andersson J, Valind S, et al. Identification of the brain loci processing human oesophageal sensation using positron emission tomography. Gastroenterology 1997;113:50–9.

83. Aziz Q, Schnitzler A, Enck P. Functional neuro-imaging of visceral sensation. J Clin Neurophysiol 2000;17:604–12.

84. Kern MK, Arndoerfer RC, Shaker R. Cerebral cortical registration of rectal distension below perception threshold. Gastroenterology 2000;118:A445.

85. Binkofski F, Schnitzler A, Enck P, et al. Somatic and limbic cortex activation in esophageal distention: a functional magnetic resonance imaging study. Ann Neurol 1998;44:811–5.

86. Furlong PL, Aziz Q, Singh KD, et al. Cortical localization of magnetic fields evoked by esophageal distension. Electroencephalogr Clin Neurophysiol 1998;108:234–43.

87. Schnitzler A, Volkmann J, Enck P, et al. Differential cortical organization of visceral and somatic sensation in humans: a neuromagnetic study. Eur J Neurosci 1999;11:305–15.

88. Loose R, Schnitzler A, Sarkar S, et al. Cortical activation during mechanical esophageal stimulation: a neuromagnetic study. Neurogastroenterology 1999;11:163–71.

89. Hecht M, Kober H, Claus D, et al. The electrical and magnetical cerebral responses evoked by electrical stimulation of the esophagus and the location of their cerebral sources. Electroencephalogr Clin Neurophysiol 1999;110:1435–44.

90. Aziz Q, Phillips ML, Gregory LJ, et al. Modulation of the brain processing of human oesophageal sensations by emotions: a functional magnetic resonance imaging study. Gastroenterology 2000;118:A385.

91. Silverman DHS, Munakata JA, Ennes H, et al. Regional cerebral activity in normal and pathological perception of visceral pain. Gastroenterology 1997;112:64–72.

92. Baciu MV, Bonaz BL, Papillon EP, et al. Central processing of rectal pojn: a functional MRI imaging study. AJNR Am J Neuroradiol 1999; 20:1920–24.

93. Bouras EP, O'Brien TJ, Camilleri M, et al. Cerebral topography of rectal stimulation using single photon emission computed tomography. Am J Physiol 1999;277:G687–94.

94. Mertz H, Morgan V, Tanner G, et al. Regional cerebral activation in irritable bowel syndrome and control subjects with painful and nonpainful rectal distention. Gastroenterology 2000;118:842–8.

95. Stottrop K, Schnitzler A, Witte OW, et al. Cortical representation of the anal canal. Gastroenterology 1998;114:A167.

96. Hobday DI, Aziz Q, Thacker N, et al. A study of the cortical processing of ano-rectal sensation using functional MRI. Brain 2001;124: 361–8.

97. Lotze M, Wietek B, Birbaumer N, Cerebral activaton during anal and rectal stimulation. NeuroImage [in Review].

98. Nabiloff BD, Derbyshire SW, Munaka J, et al. Evidence for decreased activation of central fear circuits by expected adversive visceral stimuli in IBS patients. Gastroenterology 2000;118:A137.

99. Ringel Y, Drossman DA, Turkington TG, et al. Anterior cingulate cortex (ACC) dysfunction in subjects with sexual/physical abuse. Gastroenterology 2000;118:A80.

100. Bonaz BL, Papillon E, Baciu M, et al. Central processing of rectal pain in IBS patients: an fMRI study. Gastroenterology 200;118:A615.

101. Tölle TR, Kaufmann T, Siessmeier T, et al. Region-specific encoding of sensory and affective components of pain in the human brain: a positron emission tomography correlation analysis. Ann Neurol 1999;45:40–7.

102. Frith C, Dolan R. The role of the prefrontal cortex in higher cognitive functions. Brain Res Cogn Brain Res 1996;5:175–81.

103. Halsband U, Weyers M, Schmitt J, et al. Recognition and imitation of pantomimed motor acts after unilateral parietal and premotor lesions: a perspective on apraxia. Neuropsychologia 2000;39:200–16.

104. Nour S, Svarer C, Kristensen JKI, et al. Cerebral activation during micturition in normal men. Brain 2000;123:781–9.

105. Hamdy S, Aziz Q, Rothwell JC, et al. Explaining oropharyngeal dysphagia after unilateral hemisperic stroke. Lancet 1997;350:686–91.

106. Ladabaum U, Minoshima S, Hasler WL, et al. Gastric distension correlates with activation of multiple cortical and subcortical regions. Gastroenterology 2001;120:369–76.

107. Faas F, Feinle C, Enck P, et al. Central modulation of gastric motor activity. Am J Physiol 2001;280:G850–7.

108. Liu Y, Gao JH, Liu GL, Fox PT. The temporal response of the brain after eating revealed by functional MRI. Nature 2000;405:1058–62.

109. Fukudo S, Kano M, Hamaguchi T, et al. Role of histaminergic neurons in gut-distension induced brain activation in human. Gastroenterology 2000;118:A630.

110. Diksic M, Nakai A, Kumakura Y, et al. Regional brain serotonin synthesis in male and female irritable bowel syndrome (IBS) patients. Gastroenterology 2000;118:A80.

# PART II

# Motility Tests for the Gastrointestinal Tract

CHAPTER 4

# Pharyngeal Manometry

*William J. Ravich*

## TECHNIQUE OF PHARYNGEAL MANOMETRY

Two major problems confront the pharyngeal manometrist. First, the rapid pressure changes that characterize pharyngeal motor function exceed the capacity of even the best water-perfusion systems to record.[1] Solid-state catheters with miniaturized transducers contained within the catheter itself, although optional for esophageal manometric studies, are mandatory for the accurate measurement of pharyngeal pressure changes. Solid-state catheters, not available in many esophageal function laboratories, are expensive to buy and easily damaged. Second, there are substantial differences in equipment characteristics and procedure protocols used by different groups reporting on pharyngeal manometry. The

catheter diameter and configuration, placement of the transducers along the catheter length, use of unidirectional side-ports versus circumferential transducers, positioning of the pressure recording sensors relative to the pharyngeal structures, patient's body and head position while the studies are performed, and type and volume of swallowed bolus may all affect the pressure recordings.[2] Data therefore must be compared to normative values developed specifically for the catheter type, diameter, and configuration used.

The optimal configuration of recording sites for pharyngeal manometry has not been established. As the pharynx is usually less than 10 cm long, a catheter with recording sites relatively close together (eg, 2–3 cm apart) seems appropriate. Some laboratories have experimented with catheters in which the recording sites are at irregular intervals. Computerized analysis, available with newer manometric systems, adapts easily to catheter modifications and provides detailed data on wave characteristics and the timing of wave progression that in the past using paper tracings could only be obtained with great difficulty, if at all (Fig. 4.1).

Accurate recording of the upper esophageal sphincter (UES) poses a number of difficulties. The asymmetry of resting UES pressure is much greater than that of the lower esophageal sphincter.[3,4] Attempts to deal with this asymmetry have included averaging multiple radially arrayed pressure sensors located at or near the same level of the catheter, ovoid or D-shaped catheters intended to maintain the pressure ports in a relatively fixed and reproducible radial orientation, and water-perfused sleeves or oil-filled cuffs around solid-state transducers designed to integrate the circumferentially applied sphincter pressure into a single value.[5] It is important to recognize that the asymmetry is to some extent a result of compression of the catheter by the surrounding structures. During bolus transit, the pressure within the distended lumen is, and by the laws of physics must be, symmetric (ie, uniform).[6]

Even more challenging is the axial movement of the sphincter segment during deglutition. This has been approach-

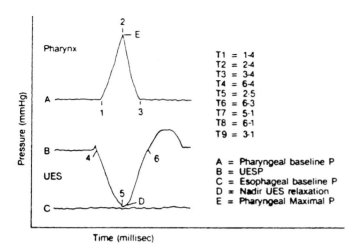

**FIGURE 4.1.** Schema for detailed analysis of pharyngeal manometry. Castell and coworkers have proposed that detailed analysis of pharyngeal and UES function, examining a series of pressure events and intervals, might improve the discriminating capabilities of pharyngeal manometry. As the measurements involved would be too time consuming for manual data analysis, they have developed a computerized system for semiautomatic data analysis. A number of the available computer-based manometric systems are capable of providing this type of information relatively easily. Although the schema uses intraesophageal pressure as a reference for UES relaxation, it may make more sense to use intrapharyngeal atmospheric pressure for this purpose. Reproduced with permission from Castell JA, Dalton DB, Castell DO. Pharyngeal and upper esophageal sphincter manometry in humans. Am J Physiol 1990;258:G173–8.

ed by careful positioning of the sensor at the upper margin of the UES in an attempt to compensate for sphincter movement or by use of specially adapted water-perfused sleeve pressure sensors.[7] The problem of dealing with asymmetry of recorded pressure is not restricted to the sphincter segment. The amplitude and configuration of pharyngeal contractions vary with both radial orientation and longitudinal sensor location,[8] factors that must be controlled for if consistent and meaningful measurements are to be obtained.

Dynamic contrast radiography (ie, barium studies using video-recording systems) remains the first and best means of assessing pharyngeal motor function. Careful simultaneous videoradiographic and manometric studies (also referred to as videofluoromanography) have provided important insights into the interpretation of manometric events. These studies, however, are cumbersome and time consuming to perform, requiring the combined efforts of the radiologist and the manometrist. They are unlikely to become routinely available procedures.

## INDICATIONS FOR PHARYNGEAL MANOMETRY

There are a number of possible indications for pharyngeal manometry (Table 4.1). It is most often used as a research tool to evaluate the physiology of pharyngeal motor function and as a test to confirm the findings of barium studies. The clinical implications of quantifying the strength of pharyngeal contractions remains uncertain, as is the significance of

**TABLE 4.1.** Indications for Pharyngeal Manometry

Assessment of normal pharyngeal physiology
Correlation with results of video barium studies
Quantification of pressures in the pharynx and UES
Confirmation of incomplete or incoordinated UES relaxation
Detection of abnormalities not detected by video barium studies
Assessment of esophageal function as an underlying cause of pharyngeal or UES dysfunction

UES, upper esophageal sphincter.

"abnormalities" of pharyngeal contraction waves and coordination in a patient with normal videoradiographic studies.

Perhaps the best recognized application in clinical practice is the confirmation of UES dysfunction in the presence of radiographic evidence of an incompletely opening or prematurely closing pharyngoesophageal (PE) sphincter. For years, it had been recognized that manometric studies often failed to detect UES dysfunction suggested by barium studies. Although this supported the concept that PE opening was a consequence of factors other than sphincter relaxation alone (eg, distention by the bolus and elevation by the larynx), the infrequency with which manometric evidence of UES dysfunction was found was disturbing. Newer concepts of sensor positioning and of the significance of intrabolus pressure have improved the yield of manometry and now offer the prospect of helping selected patients who might be expected to benefit from cricopharyngeal myotomy (see below).

## NORMAL PHARYNGEAL PERISTALSIS

The medical literature offers confusing data on normal manometric measurements. Studies differ substantially in the instrumentation and protocols used.[2,9–14] Although most followed the lead of Dodds and coworkers' recommendations[9] in using solid-state transducers, there are reports using side-port perfusion systems and sleeve perfusion catheters for the evaluation of UES resting pressure and function. Studies also vary in the diameter of the catheters, placement of the sensors, and type of bolus swallowed. It is difficult to draw firm conclusions about which methods to follow.

Mean pharyngeal pressure using solid-state catheters with outer diameters of 4 to 5.5 mm is about 100 mm Hg, and the mean duration of contractions is about 0.5 seconds. However, the range of pressures seen in normal controls is wide. Dodds and coworkers described a value of 600 mm Hg in the hypopharynx,[9] and the authors have seen hypopharyngeal pressures of over 1,000 mm Hg, possibly representing the combined effect of pharyngeal constrictors and compression by the epiglottis. Dodds and coworkers suggested that pharyngeal

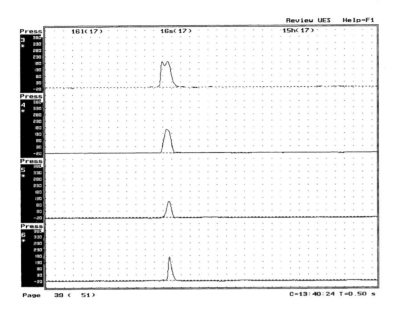

Page  39 ( 51)                    C=13:40:24 T=0.50 s

**FIGURE 4.2.** Normal progressive pharyngeal pressure wave. The normal response of the hypopharynx to swallowing involves a rapid, high-amplitude pressure upstroke ending in a single, sharp peak, followed by a rapid return to baseline. The pressure wave is produced by the contractions of the middle and inferior pharyngeal constrictors. A preliminary step-like pressure increase just preceding the beginning of the high-pressure contraction (barely noticeable in sensors 3 and 5) reflects distention by the bolus entering the pharynx, compressed by the tongue and the advancing peristaltic wave. This pressure increase may be minimal and difficult to appreciate, especially if a liquid bolus is used, but may become pronounced in the presence of increased resistance to flow (see Fig. 4.10).

**TABLE 4.2.** Normal Values for Pharyngeal Manometry: Composite Data

| Measurement | Mean Value | Approximate range for 67% of Controls |
|---|---|---|
| Pharyngeal contraction amplitude (mm Hg) | 71–134 | 45–240 |
| Pharyngeal contraction duration (s) | 0.37–0.63 | 0.3–0.8 |
| UES resting pressure (mm Hg) | 73–114 | 45–130 |
| Nadir of UES relaxation (mm Hg)* | (-)0.8–(+)4 | (-)0.9–(+)2 |

* Upper esophageal sphincter (UES) relaxations based on reports of "dry" swallows. Unlike pharyngeal contractions, "wet" swallows substantially increase the nadir of UES relaxation.

The table provides information representing a composite of data from studies using solid-state catheters with outer diameters of 4.0–5.4 mm.[9–14]

contraction amplitude was higher in the upper and lower pharynx than in the mid-pharynx; however, they did not pay attention to the radial asymmetry of pharyngeal contractions.[9] Sears and colleagues, in a study on the effect of sensor position and orientation on pharyngeal pressure measurements, found that contraction amplitude appeared to be substantially higher in the anterior and posterior orientations than when the sensors were directed laterally.[8] Axial asymmetry may reflect the augmenting effect of tongue thrust and epiglottic tilt in the upper and lower pharynx, respectively. In the previously mentioned study, Dodds and colleagues found that the pharyngeal pressure and duration did not differ between dry and wet swallows; however, the volume of the wet swallows used is not specified in their report.[9]

Pharyngeal function is complex and difficult to interpret. The events are rapid, passing through the length of the pharynx in less than a second (Fig. 4.2). The actual contour of the wave is not as stereotypic as that of the esophageal contraction, varying from swallow to swallow and along the length of the pharynx. A sensor located in the oropharynx often detects a biphasic wave, reflecting a combination of pharyngeal contraction and compression of the base of the tongue against the posterior pharynx (Fig. 4.3). Although the pharyngeal constrictors contract in a progressive manner on videoradiography, the compression of the epiglottis against the posterior wall of the mid-pharynx can create the impression of a focally simultaneous or biphasic contraction without necessarily signifying incoordination (Fig. 4.4). The complex nature of the pharyngeal contraction poses substantial methodologic problems in terms of determining the onset and coordination of the contraction wave.

## NORMAL UPPER ESOPHAGEAL SPHINCTER FUNCTION

As with the pharynx proper, the results of UES pressure differ substantially between studies. A number of studies using catheters with an outer diameter of 4 to 5.5 mm have found that the normal mean UES pressure is about 100 mm Hg (Table 4.2). Upper esophageal sphincter pressure appears to be particularly affected by catheter diameter and sensor characteristics. Smaller-diameter sensors produce lower UES resting pressure values. Like the pharynx, UES resting pressures are quite asymmetric.[4,5] Unidirectional sensors may produce dramatically different values, with higher values in the anterior and posterior orientation and lower values in the right and left lateral projections. This can be controlled for by averaging a number of radially arrayed directional sensors, careful and consistent orientation of the sensor as it is pulled through the sphincter consistently using a single (usually the posterior) orientation to determine UES pressure, or use of a circumferential sensor that provides pressure measurements that integrate the pressures applied to the sensor from all directions.

Traditionally, UES relaxation has been evaluated by positioning the sphincter in the middle high-pressure zone. Placed in this location, relaxation appears prolonged, characterized by

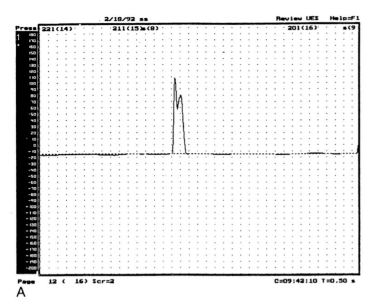

A

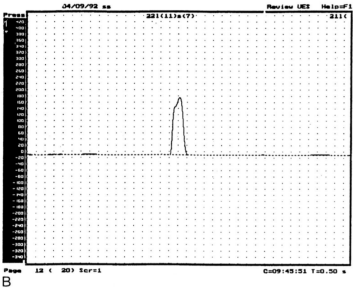

B

**FIGURE 4.3.** Biphasic pressure wave of the upper pharynx. The normal response of the oropharynx to swallowing often involves two distinct components (sensor 2) in which a rapid, high-amplitude pressure increase usually ending in a sharp peak is followed by a secondary high-amplitude increase with a more rounded peak (**A**). The exact contributions to this configuration may best be determined by simultaneous radiographic and manometric studies; however, from the timing of the events, it would seem likely that the first peak is attributable to the pharyngeal constrictor, whereas the second may reflect the effect of the back of the tongue compressing the manometric catheter against the posterior wall of the pharynx. The relative heights of the first and second components of this biphasic wave may vary or the two may meld into a single, somewhat prolonged pressure wave (**B** and **C**), depending on the force and timing of tongue compression and the axial location of the sensor.

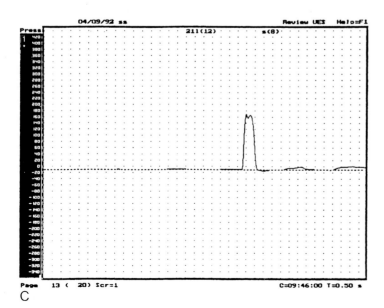

C

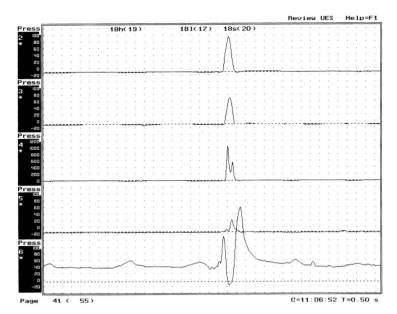

**FIGURE 4.4.** Normal variant contractions in mid-pharynx. Unusually high-pressure amplitude or biphasic contractions are frequently seen in the mid-to-distal pharynx. In the example provided, both features are present (sensor 4) where the contraction amplitude is 1,000 mm Hg. Note that the pressure ranges shown on the scales to the left vary to accommodate the dramatic differences in pressures recorded. Comparison to videoradiographic studies suggests that this pattern and the unusually high pressure may reflect compression by the epiglottis rather than disordered motility. The bottom tracing is obtained with the pressure sensor located within the upper esophageal sphincter (UES). It demonstrates the M-shaped configuration, indicating that it is positioned toward the proximal end of the UES (see Fig. 4.6).

a gradual decrease and return to baseline, and followed by propagation of the pharyngeal contractile wave through the PE segment. Simultaneous videoradiographic and manometric studies have demonstrated that this pattern of "relaxation" actually reflects the UES sensor dropping into the cervical esophagus as the sphincter segment is pulled cephalad by elevation of the larynx during swallowing. Careful analysis has revealed a complicated and dysynchronous movement of the manometry sensor and sphincter segment.[15] An initial elevation of the sensor is followed by a sequence during which the descending sensor passes back into and then through the rising sphincter segment, ending up in the cervical esophagus before returning to its initial resting position (Fig. 4.5).

This information has resulted in a modification of the technique of manometric assessment of UES function. While the resting UES pressure is determined with the sensor in the middle of the high-pressure zone, relaxation is evaluated with the sensor at the upper margin of the UES. Castell and Castell emphasized the importance of looking for an "M-spike" configuration as a marker of proper sensor position.[11] The initial pressure elevation, reflecting the effect of the elevating UES over the sensor, is followed by true UES relaxation and then by a subsequent contractile wave. Upper esophageal sphincter relaxation detected by this technique is of a much shorter duration than that observed with the sensor placed in the middle of the sphincter segment (Fig. 4.6). This adjustment, although logical, may not entirely solve the problems associated with UES and sensor movement as the movement appears to differ substantially between individuals and may be diminished in the neurogenic patient with impaired laryngeal elevation. The extent of movement is volume dependent, increasing as the volume of the swallowed boluses increases.[16,17] Some investigators have used water-perfused, sleeve-catheter devices to avoid the artifacts of UES motion.

Castell and colleagues found that mean residual pressure was –8 mm Hg with dry swallows and was –2 mm Hg with a

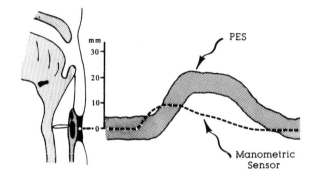

**FIGURE 4.5.** Upper esophageal sphincter and sensor movement during swallowing. The UES is attached to the cricoid cartilage and through that cartilage to other parapharyngeal structures. Movement of the larynx results in movement of the UES segment. Although the catheter placed through either the oral cavity or nasopharynx also moves during swallowing, recording sensor movement is not synchronous with or equivalent to that of the UES. This creates problems for the accurate assessment of UES relaxation. This figure is a schematic representation of movement of the UES and catheter sensor site as measured during simultaneous radiographic and manometric studies. Note that the UES moves a mean of 2.0 cm during swallowing, whereas the sensor moves only a mean of 1.0 cm. Studies suggest that proximal UES movement in normal volunteers may be as great as 2 to 3 cm. As the most prominent segment of the UES (that with >50% of maximum pressure) is < 1.0 cm long, the dissociation of these movements creates technical problems in the assessment of the completeness and timing of UES relaxation. Reproduced with permission from Dodds WJ, Kahrilas PJ. Considerations about pharyngeal manometry. Dysphagia 1987;1:209–14.

5-cc bolus of water.[10] Olsson and colleagues, using a similar but not identical catheter design, found higher mean residual pressure, +4 mm Hg with dry swallows and +7 mm Hg with a wet swallow using a 10-cc bolus of a barium mixture.[13] These differences in residual pressure have important physiologic implications. Cerenko and coworkers postulated that the negative pressure at the nadir of relaxation provides an important suction effect on the swallowed bolus, helping to

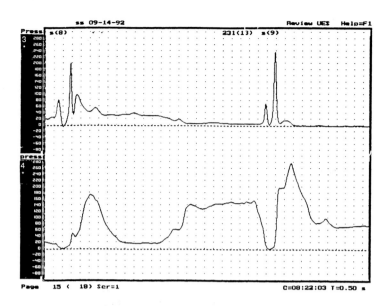

**FIGURE 4.6.** Two views of UES relaxation. In the past, UES relaxation has been evaluated with the sensor position in the middle of the area of high resting pressure. Recent information about the movement of the UES during swallowing suggests that placement at the proximal end of the sphincter segment should be used to compensate for the discrepancy between UES and recording site movement. In the distal tracing (sensor 4), with the sensor in the traditional location in the middle of the high-pressure zone, a slow decrease in pressure begins well before the start of peristalsis. With the sensor at the upper margin of the sphincter (sensor 3), the initial pressure is just barely above intrapharyngeal baseline. After swallowing, there is an initial low-amplitude pressure increase, followed by a rapid drop to baseline, and then by a second, taller peak. This pattern produces the desired M-shaped configuration and a shorter duration of relaxation.

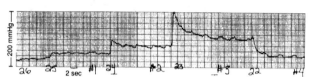

**FIGURE 4.7.** Effect of catheter movement on UES resting pressure. Upper esophageal sphincter pressure is affected by the movement of the manometric catheter. In this tracing, there is a sharp increase in pressure with each movement of the catheter, with a gradual return to a stable resting pressure that takes 15 seconds or longer. Upper esophageal sphincter measurements should therefore be obtained by a slow, stepwise pull-through technique, with at least 20 to 30 seconds between each swallow. Because the segment of UES high-pressure zone is so short, the pull-through should be performed in ½-cm increments. Reproduced with permission from Castell JA, Dalton DB, Castell DO. Pharyngeal and upper esophageal sphincter manometry in humans. Am J Physiol 1990:258:G173–8.

pull the bolus into the esophagus.[18] If a neutral or slightly positive residual pressure is within normal limits, then this suction effect is not essential to bolus transit.

The UES is a highly reactive muscle. Esophageal balloon distention, especially when applied to the upper esophagus, increases UES pressure.[19,20] Elevated UES pressure could result from increased downstream resistance, caused by motor or structural esophageal disorders, through its effect on increasing intraesophageal pressure. Rapid pull-through of the pressure catheter through the PE segment also transiently increases UES pressure (Fig. 4.7), a response that gradually returns to a lower and more stable resting pressure if the catheter is left undisturbed for 20 to 30 seconds.[3] It is therefore important to pull the manometry catheter through the PE segment in stepwise increments, allowing adequate time for the transient pressure increases to return to baseline before obtaining the resting pressure.

Given the discrepancies found in the medical literature, what should an individual manometry laboratory use as its reference values? The best approach is to establish normative values for an individual laboratory by studying a set of normal individuals. If literature controls are used, it will be important to refer to data derived from instrumentation and protocols that closely approximate those used in the individual laboratory.

## THE AGING PHARYNX

A number of investigators have found that UES resting pressure declines with age.[21–23] The onset of UES relaxation is delayed and the intrabolus pressure is increased in the elderly, suggesting an increased resistance to flow through the sphincter segment.[24] Some studies indicate that the hypopharyngeal contraction amplitude may increase with age.[22,25] A study of pharyngeal retention in the elderly reported that retention was associated with weakness of the base of the tongue and of the pharyngeal constrictor muscles but normal UES relaxation.[26]

## PATTERNS OF DYSMOTILITY

In light of our current understanding of equipment requirements for pharyngeal manometry, older studies demonstrating specific pharyngeal manometric abnormalities associated with swallowing disorders must be accepted with caution. Systematic descriptions of characteristic manometric abnormalities using appropriate instrumentation on even a modest sample of patients with specific disorders are virtually nonexistent. However, a few basic patterns of dysfunction can be detected.

## PHARYNGEAL PARESIS

The most common abnormality in the neurologically impaired (neurogenic) pharynx is diffusely decreased pharyngeal contraction amplitude (Fig. 4.8). This is often associated with a

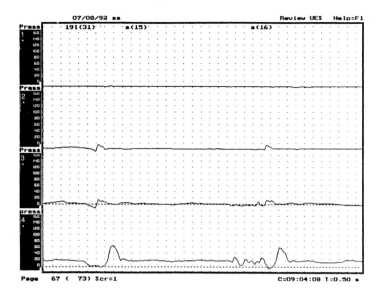

**FIGURE 4.8.** Diffuse pharyngeal paresis. The most common abnormality in the neurologically impaired (neurogenic) pharynx is a generalized decrease in the amplitude of pharyngeal contraction. This is often associated with a loss of progressive peristalsis, the latter resulting when the contraction of the pharyngeal constrictors fails to occlude the pharynx. The figure shows a manometric tracing in a patient with a history of a brainstem stroke. Videoradiography demonstrated diffuse pharyngeal weakness, pharyngeal retention, and aspiration. Although the video study showed a hypopharyngeal bar, the UES resting pressure, detected with a circumferential sensor in the middle of the sphincter segment, demonstrates low UES resting pressure and apparently normal relaxation (see Figs. 4.6 and 4.7 for the probable explanation for this discrepancy).

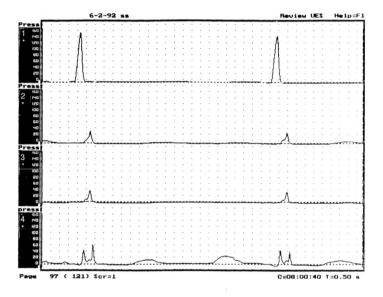

**FIGURE 4.9.** Focal pharyngeal paresis. This study demonstrates good pharyngeal contraction amplitude at the sensor placed in the upper pharynx (sensor 1), with weak contractions in the mid- and lower pharynx (sensors 2 and 3). The patient presented with a chronic swallow-induced cough of many years duration. Videoradiography confirmed that pharyngeal paresis was localized to the mid- to lower pharynx. Although the findings suggest a neurogenic process with focal pharyngeal involvement, neurologic evaluation did not establish a specific diagnosis.

loss of pharyngeal wave progression, the latter resulting when the contraction of the pharyngeal constrictors fails to occlude the pharynx. The finding of diffuse pharyngeal paresis suggests a neurogenic-type process but does not provide information about the specific diagnosis. Neurologic, neuromuscular, or myogenic disorders, including cerebrovascular accidents, amyotrophic lateral sclerosis, myasthenia gravis, polymyositis, and both hypo- and hyperthyroidism, can all produce similar effects. Disorders affecting the pharyngeal soft tissue may cause a similar appearance. On occasion, pharyngeal contraction weakness can appear focal (Fig. 4.9). This pattern suggests a patchy distribution of neurologic injury. Most often, there is preservation of the pressures recorded in the proximal sensor, a finding that may reflect preservation of pressure applied by the tongue thrust against the posterior pharynx. Segmental loss of pharyngeal constrictor function over prominent cervical osteophytes may also cause localized dysfunction.

## UPPER ESOPHAGEAL SPHINCTER DYSFUNCTION

Although hypopharyngeal bars are commonly seen on barium radiography, incomplete UES relaxation often is not confirmed on pharyngeal manometry. This discrepancy suggests either that the opening of the PE segment seen radiographically involves more than UES relaxation alone or that technical limitations prevent the reliable detection of UES dysfunction. With the UES sensor positioned at the upper portion of the UES high-pressure zone to compensate for UES movement during swallowing, manometric studies more often detect incomplete UES relaxation (Fig. 4.10).

The interpretation of the manometric evidence of incomplete relaxation has been called into question. According to Dantas and colleagues, the findings reflect an increase in intrabolus pressure within the sphincter segment rather than

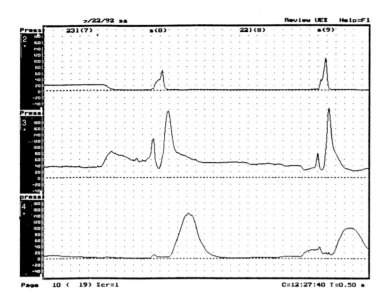

**FIGURE 4.10.** Failure of UES relaxation. The figure shows incomplete UES relaxation, with the nadir of relaxation demonstrating a residual pressure of 29 mm Hg above the intrapharyngeal resting pressure. The patient had a hypopharyngeal bar (ie, incomplete opening of the pharyngeal segment) on videoradiography. The tracing was obtained with the middle sensor placed at the upper end of the UES, where an M-shaped pressure wave is seen. The drop in pressure between the two peaks of the "M-spike" corresponds to the PE segment opening as seen on videoradiography. Note the increased prominence of the early (intrabolus) phase of pharyngeal contraction, a feature interpreted as a manifestation of increased resistance to flow, in this case from failure of UES relaxation.

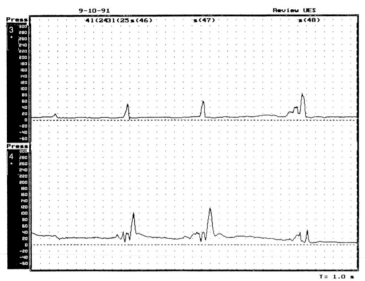

**FIGURE 4.11.** Manometric findings in Zenker's diverticulum. A manometric tracing using a water-perfusion system with the distal sensor (sensor 4) placed at the upper margin of the UES and the proximal sensor (sensor 3) in the mid-pharynx. The onset of pharyngeal contraction should be associated with complete relaxation of the UES sensor. Instead, there is incomplete relaxation. The use of a water-perfusion system in this patient was dictated by the need to use a manometric catheter with a central channel, permitting the catheter to be introduced over an endoscopically placed guidewire.

the direct effect of muscle contraction on the recording transducer.[27] If so, this finding could actually result from a combination of factors, including the size of the swallowed bolus, strength of pharyngeal contractions, and compliance of the sphincter segment. Brasseur and Dodds have suggested the potential value of the evaluation of intrabolus pressure as reflected in a prominent hump during the initial upstroke of the pharyngeal contraction as a reflection of UES dysfunction (see Fig. 4.10).[28] In a study of the biomechanics of the radiologic finding of a cricopharyngeal bar, patients with cricopharyngeal bars had higher intrabolus pressures than normal volunteers.[29] The difference was sustained throughout a range of swallowed bolus volumes and increased as the bolus volume increased. In summary, UES dysfunction might result in incomplete UES relaxation, increased intrabolus pressure, or both. Conceptually, downstream obstruction owing to esophageal pathology also could cause similar manometric findings.

## ZENKER'S DIVERTICULUM

The concept that a Zenker's diverticulum is a consequence of incomplete UES relaxation is the basis of the inclusion of cricopharyngeal myotomy for the surgical treatment for this condition (Fig. 4.11). Manometric studies of patients with Zenker's diverticula, however, have led to conflicting findings, with some studies demonstrating incomplete or uncoordinated UES relaxation,[30,31] whereas others have found no difference between patients with Zenker's diverticula and normal controls.[32] Unfortunately, studies on both sides of the issue suffer from one or more methodologic deficiencies (eg, outdated instrumentation with slow pressure response rates, lack of normal controls, and improper positioning of the UES sensor). A recent study with simultaneous videoradiography and manometry using a water-perfused sleeve catheter suggests that an increased intrabolus pressure is associated with incomplete opening of the PE segment.[33] Catheter placement in patients with Zenker's diverticula is difficult and potentially dangerous. Intubation is best executed using endoscopic or fluoroscopic guidance.

## MANOMETRY IN NEUROGENIC AND MYOGENIC DISORDERS

The diagnosis of neurogenic dysphagia is often made when a videoradiographic study demonstrates abnormal pharyngeal function in the absence of any structural disease. The term is less specific than it may appear. The same findings are often seen in a variety of neurologic, neuromuscular, and myogenic disorders. There are very few reports of the manometric findings in well-defined patient groups with neurogenic dysphagia.

In a study of patients with Parkinson's disease, mid-pharyngeal, but not hypopharyngeal, contraction amplitudes were significantly lower in patients with dysphagia than in age-matched controls.[34] Intrabolus pressure was significantly increased in both dysphagic and nondysphagic patients with Parkinson's disease, a finding that appeared to correlate with a decreased maximal UES diameter found in both groups. Only 21% (4/19 patients) of patients had abnormal UES relaxation; 3 of these 4 patients complained of dysphagia.

In a study of 13 patients with amyotrophic lateral sclerosis, no significant differences were found in pharyngeal and UES pressure manometric measurements when compared to age-matched controls.[35] Those with dysphagia, however, had significantly lowering post–relaxation contraction amplitude through the UES with water swallow. This difference increased with a bread bolus.

A number of studies of patients with oculopharyngeal muscular dystrophy (OPMD) have been reported in the literature. In a study of patients with OPMD dysphagia, the mean pharyngeal pressure amplitude was significantly lower, and the duration of pharyngeal contraction was increased in patients over controls.[36] Resting UES pressure and UES relaxation were not different. In another study of patients with OPMD, again all with at least some degree of dysphagic symptoms, the majority had one or more abnormalities of pharyngeal or UES function, including low LES, prolonged pharyngeal contraction duration, and incoordination of pharynx and UES.[37]

## CONCLUSION

Compared to the esophagus, the application of manometric techniques to the pharynx remains in a primitive state of development. Although a number of studies of pharyngeal motor function have been published since the first edition of this atlas, the gaps in our knowledge remain large. Most studies provide information about normal volunteers. Studies of manometric findings in patients with pharyngeal disorders are few, generally involve a limited number of highly selected patients, and often use outdated methodologies. Perhaps the greatest potential lies in the ability of pharyngeal manometry to assess UES function, particularly in those being considered for cricopharyngeal myotomy. However, the predictive value of this technique for the outcome of myotomy has not been firmly established.

### REFERENCES

1. Orlowski J, Dodds WJ, Linehan JH, et al. Requirements for accurate manometric recording of pharyngeal and esophageal peristaltic pressure waves. Invest Radiol 1982;17:567–72.
2. Wilson JA, Pryde A, MacIntyre CCA, Heading RC. Normal pharyngoesophageal motility: a study of 50 healthy subjects. Dig Dis Sci 1989;34:1590–9.
3. Winans CS. The pharyngoesophageal closure mechanism. A manometric study. Gastroenterology 1972;63:768–77.
4. Welch RW, Luckmann K, Ricks PM, et al. Manometry of the normal upper esophageal sphincter and its alteration in laryngectomy. J Clin Invest 1979;63:1036–41.
5. Salassa JR, DeVault KR, McConnel FMS. Proposed catheter standards for pharyngeal manofluorography (videomanometry). Dysphagia 1998;13:105–10.
6. McConnel FMS, Guffin TN Jr, Cerenko D. The effect of asymmetric pharyngoesophageal pressures on manofluorographic measurements. Laryngoscope 1991;101:510–5.
7. Castell JA, Dalton DB, Castell DO. Pharyngeal and upper esophageal sphincter manometry in humans. Am J Physiol 1990;258:G173–8.
8. Sears VW, Castell JA, Castell DO. Radial and longitudinal asymmetry of human pharyngeal pressures during swallowing. Gastroenterology 1991;101:1559–63.
9. Dodds WJ, Hogan WJ, Lydon SB, et al. Quantitation of pharyngeal motor function in normal human subjects. J Appl Physiol 1975;39:692–6.
10. Castell JA, Dalton CB, Castell DO. Effects of body position and bolus consistency on the manometric parameters and coordination of the upper esophageal sphincter. Dysphagia 1990;5:179–86.
11. Castell JA, Castell DO. Modern solid-state computerized manometry of the pharyngoesophageal segment. Dysphagia 1993;8:270–5.
12. Olsson R, Nilson H, Ekberg O. Simultaneous videoradiography and pharyngeal solid state manometry (videomanometry) in 25 nondysphagic volunteers. Dysphagia 1995;10:36–41.
13. Olsson R, Castell JA, Castell DO, Ekberg O. Solid-state computerized manometry improves diagnostic yield in pharyngeal dysphagia: simultaneous videoradiography and manometry in dysphagia patients with normal barium swallows. Abdom Imaging 1995;20:230–5.
14. DiRe C, Shi G, Manka M, Kahrilas P. Manometric characteristics of the upper esophageal sphincter recorded with a microsleeve. Am J Gastroenterol 1991;1383–9.
15. Dodds WJ, Kahrilas PJ. Considerations about pharyngeal manometry. Dysphagia 1987;1:209–14.
16. Kahrilas PJ, Dodds WJ, Dent J, et al. Upper esophageal sphincter function during deglutition. Gastroenterology 1988;95:52–62.
17. Cook IJ, Dodds WJ, Dantas RO, et al. Opening mechanisms of the human upper esophageal sphincter. Am J Physiol 1989;257:G748–59.
18. Cerenko D, McConnel FMS, Jackson RT. Quantitative assessment of pharyngeal bolus driving forces. Otolaryngol Head Neck Surg 1989;100:57–63.
19. Andreollo NA, Thompson DG, Kendall GPN, Earlam RJ. Functional relationships between cricopharyngeal sphincter and oesophageal body in response to graded intraluminal distension. Gut 1988;29:161–6.
20. Shafik A. Effect of esophageal distension on pressure and electromyographic activity of the pharyngoesophageal sphincter, with identification of the esophagopharyngeal reflex. J Thorac Cardiovasc Surg 1997;114:968–74.

21. Fulp SR, Dalton CB, Castell JA, Castell DO. Aging-related alterations in human upper esophageal sphincter function. Am J Gastroenterol 1990;85:1569–72.

22. Shaker R, Lang IM. Effect of aging on the deglutitive oral, pharyngeal, and esophageal motor function. Dysphagia 1994;9:221–8.

23. McKee GJ, Johnston BT, McBride GB, Primrose WJ. Does age or sex affect pharyngeal swallowing? Clin Otolaryngol 1998;23:100–6.

24. Shaw DW, Cook IJ, Gabb M, et al. Influence of normal aging on oral-pharyngeal and upper esophageal sphincter function during swallowing. Am J Physiol 1995;31:G3889-G396.

25. Wilson JA, Pryde A, MacIntyre CCA, et al. The effects of age, sex, and smoking on normal pharyngoesophageal motility. Am J Gastroenterol 1990;85:686–91.

26. DeJaeger E, Pelemans W, Ponette E, Joosten E. Mechanisms involved in postdeglutition retention in the elderly. Dysphagia 1997;12:63–7.

27. Dantas RO, Kern MK, Massey BT, et al. Effect of swallowed bolus variables on oral and pharyngeal phases of swallowing. Am J Physiol 1990;258:G675–81.

28. Brasseur JG, Dodds WJ. Interpretation of intraluminal manometric measurements in terms of swallowing mechanics. Dysphagia 1991;6:100–19.

29. Dantas RO, Cook IJ, Dodds WJ, et al. Biomechanics of cricopharyngeal bars. Gastroenterology 1990;99:1269–74.

30. Ellis FH Jr, Schleel JF, Lynch VP, Payne WS. Cricopharyngeal myotomy for pharyngo-esophageal diverticulum. Ann Surg 1969;170:340–9.

31. Zaninotto G, Costantini M, Boccu C, et al. Functional and morphological study of the cricopharyngeal muscle in patients with Zecker's diverticulum. Br J Surg 1996;83:1263–7.

32. Knuff TE, Benjamin SB, Castell DO. Pharyngoesophageal (Zecker's) diverticulum: a reappraisal. Gastroenterology 1982;82:734–6.

33. Cook IJ, Gabb M, Panagopoulos V, et al. Pharyngeal (Zecker's) diverticulum is a disorder of upper esophageal sphincter opening. Gastroenterology 1992;103:1229–35.

34. Ali GN, Wallace KL, Schwartz R, et al. Mechanisms of oral-pharyngeal dysphagia in patients with Parkinson's disease. Gastroenterology 1996;110:383–92.

35. MacDougall G, Wilson JA, Pryde A, Grant R. Analysis of the pharyngoesophageal pressure profile in amyotrophic lateral sclerosis. Otolaryngol Head Neck Surg 1995;112:258–61.

36. Fradet G, Pouliot D, Lavoie S, St-Pierre S. Inferior contrictor myotomy in oculopharyngeal muscular dystrophy: a clinical and manometric evaluation. J Otolaryngol 1988;17:68–73.

37. Castell JA, Castell DO, Duranceau A, Topart P. Manometric characteristics of the pharynx, upper esophageal sphincter, esophagus, and lower esophageal sphincter in patients with oculopharyngeal muscular dystrophy. Dysphagia 1995;10:22–6.

CHAPTER 5

# Esophageal Manometry

*June A. Castell, R. Mathew Gideon and Donald O. Castell*

Esophageal manometry has been used as a diagnostic test in esophageal disease for over 20 years. It provides both a qualitative and quantitative assessment of esophageal pressures, coordination, and motility.

## INDICATIONS

Manometric studies are used in the evaluation of patients with symptoms suggestive of esophageal origin such as dysphagia, odynophagia, heartburn, and unexplained chest pain. A manometric study is also indicated in the evaluation of reflux and should always be done prior to antireflux surgery. In addition, it can be useful in determining possible esophageal involvement in systemic disorders such as scleroderma and chronic idiopathic intestinal pseudo-obstruction (Table 5.1).

**TABLE 5.1.** Clinical Indications for Esophageal Manometry

Evaluation of patients with dysphagia
    Primary esophageal motility disorders
    Achalasia
    Spastic disorders
        Diffuse esophageal spasm
        Hypertensive LES
        Nutcracker esophagus
        Nonspecific esophageal motility disorders
    Secondary esophageal motor disorders
    Scleroderma
Evaluation of patients with possible gastroesophageal reflux disease
    Support diagnosis in a complex patient
    Atypical symptoms
    Failed medical therapy
    Evaluate defective peristalsis prior to fundoplication
    Exclude scleroderma
    Assist in placement of pH probe
Evaluation of patients with noncardiac chest pain
    Primary motility disorder
    Pain response to provocative testing (edrophonium chloride, balloon)
Exclude generalized gastrointestinal tract disease
    Scleroderma
    Chronic idiopathic intestinal pseudo-obstruction
Exclude esophageal etiology for suspected anorexia nervosa

LES, lower esophageal sphincter.

**TABLE 5.2.** Normal Values: LES Pressures

| Infused Manometry (Mean of 4 Orifices at 90) | mm Hg; mean ± SD |
|---|---|
| RPT | 29.0 ± 12.1 |
| SPT | |
| End-inspiration | 39.7 ± 13.2 |
| Mid-respiration | 24.2 ± 10.1 |
| End-expiration | 15.2 ± 10.7 |
| Solid-state circumferential ("sphincter") transducer | |
| SPT | 26.0 ± 9.4 |

RPT, rapid pull-through technique; SPT, station pull-through technique.

## TECHNIQUE

Esophageal manometry is most often performed by passing a flexible catheter through the nose into the esophagus. Pressures are sensed either directly, by solid-state transducers in the catheter, or indirectly, by external transducers connected to a water-perfused catheter. These pressures are then transmitted to a recording device for interpretation and storage. Many laboratories are now using a computer to record their esophageal manometry studies, although some laboratories still use a physiograph.

Water-perfusion systems require an external water supply and pump, which makes the equipment bulky and difficult to transport. In addition, since the pressure measurement is relative to the height of a column of water, studies are performed with the patient supine to ensure that the external transducers

**TABLE 5.3.** Normal Values for Esophageal Peristalsis (mm Hg; mean ± SD)

| Recording Site (cm above LES) | Wet Swallows | Dry Swallows | p Value |
|---|---|---|---|
| Amplitude (mm Hg; mean ± SD) | | | |
| 18 | 62 ± 29 | 44 ± 25 | < .001 |
| 13 | 70 ± 32 | 48 ± 27 | < .001 |
| 8 | 90 ± 41 | 63 ± 32 | < .001 |
| 3 | 109 ± 45 | 79 ± 33 | < .001 |
| Mean: 8/3 | 99 ± 40 | 71 ± 28 | < .001 |
| Duration (s; mean ± SD) | | | |
| 18 | 2.8 ± 0.8 | 2.6 ± 0.7 | NS |
| 13 | 3.5 ± 0.7 | 3.4 ± 0.6 | NS |
| 8 | 3.9 ± 0.9 | 3.8 ± 0.8 | NS |
| 3 | 4.0 ± 1.1 | 4.2 ± 0.8 | NS |
| Mean: 8/3 | 3.9 ± 0.9 | 4.1 ± 0.8 | NS |
| Velocity (cm/s; mean ± SD) | | | |
| Proximal | 3.0 ± 0.6 | 4.0 ± 0.4 | < .001 |
| Distal | 3.5 ± 0.9 | 4.0 ± 0.3 | < .001 |

LES, lower esophageal sphincter; NS, not significant.

are at the same level as the esophagus. Solid-state transducers are used for all ambulatory monitoring of esophageal pressures and are now commonly used for stationary manometry studies as well. Circumferential transducers, which measure pressures over 360 degrees, have improved the reliability of pressure measurements in asymmetric structures such as sphincters. Long-term monitoring of sphincter pressures is usually done with a sleeve device. This is a 6-cm segment at

**TABLE 5.4** Manometric Features of Esophageal Motility Disorders

| | LES | Esophageal Body |
|---|---|---|
| *Primary disorders* | | |
| Achalasia | Elevated (> 45 mm Hg) | Baseline elevated |
| | Relaxation incomplete (residual pressure > 8 mm Hg) | Peristalsis absent |
| Incoordinated motility (DES) | May be abnormal | Simultaneous contractions (≥ 20% wet swallows) |
| | | Intermittent peristalsis |
| | | Repetitive contractions (≥ 3 peaks) |
| | | Prolonged duration (> 6 s) |
| | | Retrograde contractions |
| Hypercontracting | | |
| Hypertensive peristalsis ("nutcracker") | May be elevated | Increased distal peristaltic amplitude (>180 mm Hg) |
| | | Increased distal peristaltic duration (> 6 s) |
| Hypertensive LES | Resting LES elevated (> 45 mm Hg) | May be high amplitude |
| | May be incomplete relaxation (> 8 mm Hg) | |
| Hypocontracting (may be secondary to chronic GERD) | | |
| Ineffective motility (IEM) | | ≥ 30% low-amplitude distal contractions (<30 mm Hg) |
| Hypotensive LES | Resting LES pressure < 10 mm Hg | |
| *Secondary Disorders* | | |
| Systemic sclerosis | Hypotensive | Loss of smooth muscle peristalsis |
| | | Normal striated muscle |
| Chagas' disease | Same as achalasia | Same as achalasia |
| Idiopathic intestinal pseudo-obstruction | | Loss of distal motility |
| Chronic GERD | Hypotensive LES | Ineffective motility (IEM) |

LES, lower esophageal sphincter; DES, diffuse esophageal spasm; GERD, gastroesophageal reflux disease; IEM, ineffective esophageal motility.

the distal end of a water-infusion catheter that is covered with a thin, flexible membrane so that the entire length is pressure sensitive. This device is not affected by small displacements of the sensor relative to the high-pressure zone of the resting sphincter. A sleeve device, however, cannot be used to accurately measure sphincter relaxations.

Manometric assessment of the esophagus usually begins with the lower esophageal sphincter (LES). Both the resting pressure of the LES and sphincter relaxation during deglutition are measured. A manometric study of the esophageal body is used to assess the strength and duration of the muscular contraction, evaluate peristaltic activity, and detect any motility abnormality. A complete evaluation should include measurements of both the smooth muscle of the distal esophagus and the striated muscle of the proximal esophagus. Three transducers, spaced at 5-cm intervals, are used. The distal esophagus is evaluated by locating the distal transducers 3 cm above the proximal border of the LES. Ten to 15 5-mL wet swallows are given at 30-second intervals. The proximal esophagus is evaluated in a like manner, with the proximal transducer located 1 cm below the distal border of the upper esophageal sphincter (UES).

Measurements are made of at least the following peristaltic parameters: amplitude, duration, and velocity. Amplitude is a measure of the strength of the contraction and is expressed in millimeters of mercury. Duration of the contraction is expressed in seconds. Velocity is the rate of progression of the contraction down the esophagus and is expressed in centimeters per second.

Normal values for LES parameters as measured by two different techniques are given in Table 5.2. Normal values for esophageal parameters are given in Table 5.3. Table 5.4 lists the common manometric features of esophageal disorders.

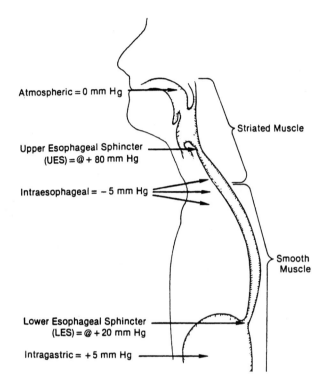

## NORMAL FUNCTION
### Resting Pressure Relationships

**FIGURE 5.1.** Normal pressure relationships. This schematic illustrates the normal pressure relationships of the stomach, LES, esophageal body, UES, and pharynx. Using atmospheric pressure at zero as a reference, the UES maintains a resting pressure of about 80 mm Hg. Intraesophageal pressure is about 5 mm Hg below atmospheric pressure, the LES resting pressure is about 20 mm Hg above atmospheric pressure, and intragastric pressure is about 5 mm Hg above atmospheric pressure. Note that intraesophageal pressure is *lower* than both intragastric and atmospheric pressure, which emphasizes the importance of the sphincters in the prevention of abnormal movement of fluids and air.

### Manometric/Videographic Comparison

**FIGURE 5.2.** Manometric/videographic comparison. This schematic relates manometric pressure measurements to bolus movement as shown videographically. The tracings from the video images on the *right* show the distribution of the barium column at the times indicated above the individual tracings and by *arrows* on the manometric record. In this example, a single peristaltic sequence completely cleared the barium bolus from the esophagus, resulting in 100% volume clearance. Pharyngeal injection of barium into the esophagus occurs at the 1.0-second mark. The entry of barium causes distention and a slightly increased intraluminal pressure, as indicated by the *downward pointing arrow* marked 1.0 s. Shortly thereafter, esophageal peristalsis is initiated. During esophageal peristalsis, luminal closure and hence the tail of the barium bolus passed each recording site concurrent with the onset of the manometric pressure wave. Hence, at 1.5 seconds, the peristaltic contraction had just reached the proximal recording site, and barium had

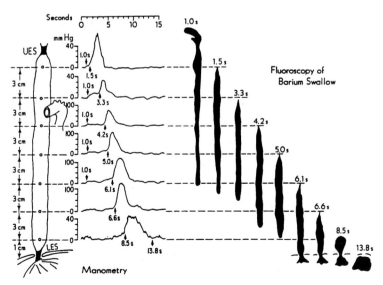

been stripped from the esophagus proximal to that point. Similarly, at 4.2 seconds, the peristaltic contraction was beginning at the third recording site, and, correspondingly, the tail of the barium bolus was located at the third recording site. Finally, after completion of the peristaltic contraction (time 13.8 seconds), all of the barium had been cleared into the stomach. Reproduced with permission from Kahrilas PJ, Dodds WJ, Hogan WJ. Effect of peristaltic dysfunction on esophageal volume clearance. Gastroenterology 1988;94:73–80.

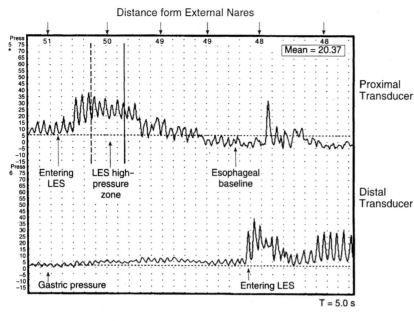

### Lower Esophageal Sphincter

**FIGURE 5.3.** Lower esophageal sphincter: station pull-through. In this example of a station pull-through of a normal LES, both transducers are solid-state circumferential transducers. Any asymmetry in the sphincter pressure will be averaged by the transducer, and it is not necessary to consider orientation. As the catheter is advanced orad, the proximal transducer enters the sphincter, with a resulting rise in pressure. The distal transducer is still recording gastric pressure. This position is marked on the tracing as 51 and represents the distance from the most distal transducer to the tip of the nares in centimeters. At 50 cm, the sphincter pressure rises even higher and reaches its highest pressure. About 20 seconds of resting sphincter pressure are bracketed by the cursors, and the resting LES pressure is calculated as the mean pressure during this time. This mean pressure corresponds to a mid respiratory pressure. As the catheter is advanced even further, the proximal transducer moves from the sphincter into the distal esophagus and measures esophageal pressures that, in normal subjects, are lower than gastric pressure. The distal transducer has begun to enter the LES.

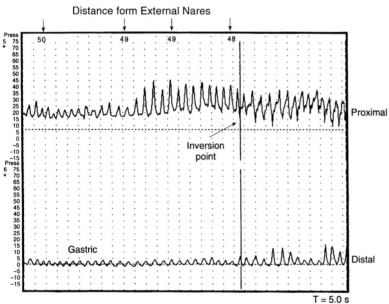

**FIGURE 5.4.** Lower esophageal sphincter pull-through: inversion point. In this example of a station pull-through of a normal LES, the cursor is positioned at the *inversion point* in the proximal channel. It is at this point in the sphincter pull-through that the transducer moves from the abdomen into the chest. Note that to the left of the cursor pressure increases with inspiration, whereas to the right of the cursor pressure decreases with inspiration. The inversion point does not mark the end of the sphincter but rather is a landmark within the sphincter. As shown here, the high-pressure zone of the sphincter is usually found just distal to the inversion point.

**FIGURE 5.5.** Lower esophageal sphincter: rapid pull-through. In this example of a rapid pull-through of a normal LES, the catheter has been rapidly advanced from the stomach through the sphincter into the esophagus in both the proximal and the distal transducers. The sphincter pressure is seen as a single high-pressure peak in each channel. The *dotted horizontal line* is the gastric baseline, and the *solid horizontal line* is at the apex of the LES pressure. Note that esophageal pressure is below gastric baseline. Rapid movement of the catheter through the sphincter may cause the sphincter to contract and create an artifact that results in a higher value for the resting sphincter pressures than those recorded by the station pull-through technique. Table 5.2 includes a comparison of sphincter pressures as measured by the two techniques.

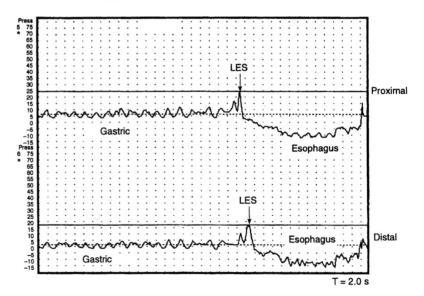

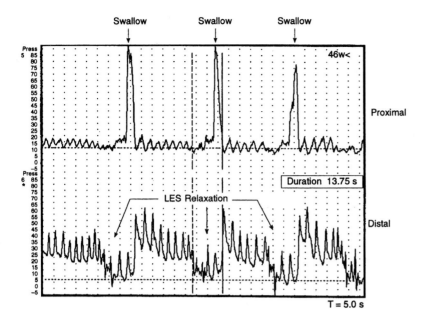

**FIGURE 5.6.** Lower esophageal sphincter relaxation. In this tracing, which shows a normal or complete relaxation of the LES during deglutition, the proximal channel is recording in the esophagus and the distal channel is recording in the high-pressure zone of the sphincter. At the initiation of the swallow, the sphincter relaxes to gastric baseline (zero residual pressure) and remains open until the peristaltic wave clears the esophagus. The cursors have marked the relaxation interval for the second wet swallow and show a duration of 13.75 seconds.

## Esophageal Peristalsis

**FIGURE 5.7.** Normal esophageal peristalsis. In this tracing, three transducers are positioned in the esophagus, with the most distal transducer (channel 6) 3 cm above the proximal boundary of the LES and the next two transducers at 5-cm intervals. At the initiation of a swallow, a peristaltic wave sweeps the length of the esophagus, sealing the lumen behind the bolus. Two such peristaltic waves are shown here. For the first swallow the cursors are marking the beginning and end of each wave as it passes each transducer. The maximum pressures are shown for each wave. A minimum pressure of about 30 mm Hg is required to prevent retrograde bolus escape. Table 5.3 presents normal values for the amplitude and duration of peristaltic contractions in 95 normal volunteers.

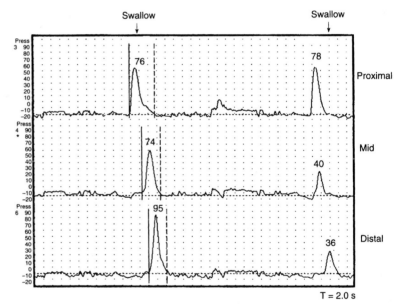

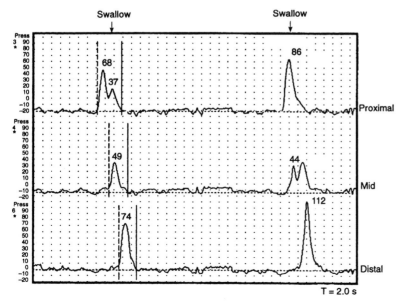

**FIGURE 5.8.** Esophageal peristalsis: normal variant. In this example of normal esophageal peristalsis, each of the two swallows contains one wave that has a double peak (swallow one in channel 3 and swallow two in channel 4). Double-peaked waves are a common finding in manometric tracings of esophageal peristalsis in normal subjects and should not be considered a manometric abnormality.

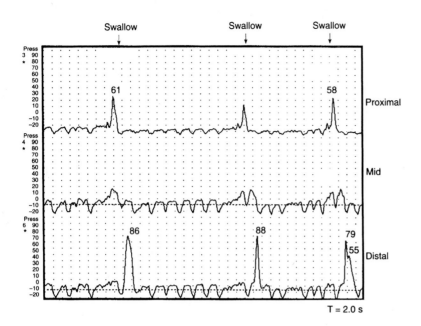

**FIGURE 5.9.** *Proximal esophageal peristalsis. In this example of peristalsis in the proximal esophagus, the proximal transducer is positioned 1 cm below the distal border of the UES with the two distal transducers at 5-cm intervals. Note particularly the absence of peristalsis in the middle channel (channel 4). This transducer is positioned in the transition zone between the striated muscle portion and the smooth muscle portion of the esophagus. A "pressure trough," or area of low pressure, exists in this zone, and this does not represent an abnormal finding.*

## ACHALASIA
### Lower Esophageal Sphincter

**FIGURE 5.10.** Lower esophageal sphincter: achalasia. This tracing shows an example of a station pullthrough of the LES of a patient with achalasia. The LES high-pressure area is identified by the cursors, and the mean resting pressure (46.6 mm Hg) is higher than that normally found (see Table 5.2). Note also that once the catheter is withdrawn out of the sphincter into the esophagus, the esophageal resting pressure is elevated. Normally (see Fig. 5.3), esophageal resting pressure is *lower* than gastric pressure. This elevation of resting esophageal pressure is due to fluid retention in the distal esophagus.

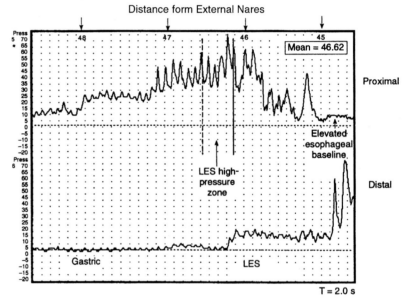

**FIGURE 5.11.** Lower esophageal sphincter relaxation: achalasia. This tracing shows the incomplete relaxation of the LES during deglutition in a patient with achalasia. The proximal transducer is in the esophagus. Note again the elevated esophageal baseline pressure relative to gastric baseline (*dotted line*). The distal transducer is in the high-pressure zone of the LES. Wet (5-mL water) swallows are marked at the top of the tracing. During the five swallows shown on this tracing, the LES never relaxes to gastric baseline (residual pressure 20–30 mm Hg).

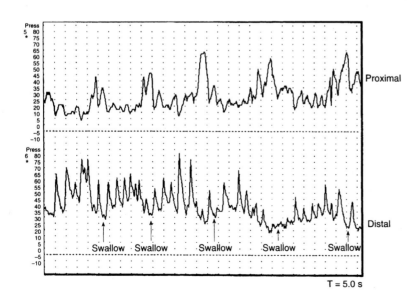

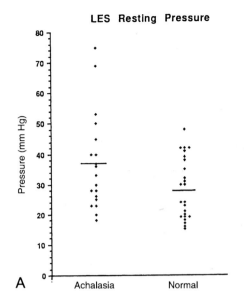

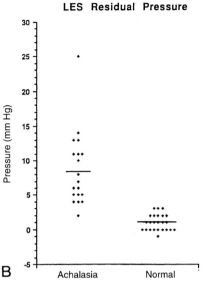

**FIGURE 5.12.** Lower esophageal sphincter: normal versus achalasia. These two graphs compare LES measurements in a group of patients with achalasia to LES measurements in an age-matched group of normal volunteers. **A** compares LES resting pressure and shows that, although patients with achalasia tend to have higher LES resting pressures than do normal subjects, there is considerable overlap. In contrast, **B** shows that patients with achalasia have residual pressures (pressure at the nadir of the LES relaxation) that are much higher than those found in normal subjects.

## Esophageal Body

**FIGURE 5.13.** Distal esophagus: achalasia. This tracing shows a typical manometric study of the distal esophagus of a patient with achalasia. There is no *peristaltic activity*. The initiation of a swallow generates isobaric or "mirror image" wave forms. These wave forms are the result of a common cavity effect. They may be low amplitude, as in this example, or they may be more vigorous, with high amplitudes and multiple peaks, but they are never peristaltic.

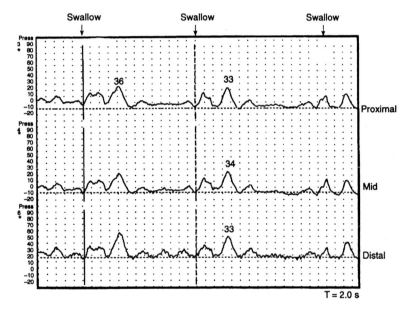

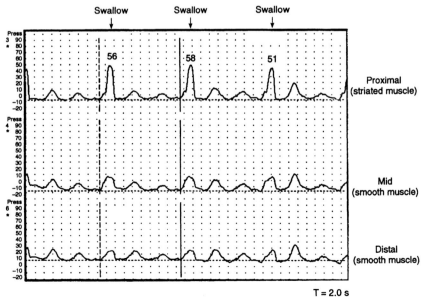

**FIGURE 5.14.** Proximal esophagus: achalasia. The proximal esophagus of the patient with achalasia does not show the typical isobaric waves seen in the distal esophagus. The most proximal transducer in this tracing is located 1 cm below the UES and is recording contractions in the striated muscle portion of the esophagus. Although striated muscle shows contractivity, there is still no peristalsis.

## Upper Esophageal Sphincter

**FIGURE 5.15.** Upper esophageal sphincter: achalasia. This is a tracing of a station pull-through of the UES of a patient with achalasia. The cursors mark the high-pressure zone, with the resting pressure calculated as the mean value between the cursors. A resting UES pressure of 110 mm Hg, although high, is within the normal range.

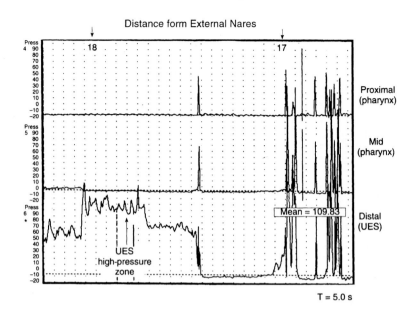

**FIGURE 5.16.** UES relaxation: achalasia. **A** is a tracing of one swallow showing normal UES relaxation. This study was done with a solid-state circumferential transducer so that orientation is not critical. To avoid artifacts due to sphincter elevation during deglutition, the transducer is placed just proximal to the high-pressure zone. When the swallow is initiated, the first pressure rise is caused by the elevation of the still tonic sphincter onto the transducer. As the sphincter relaxes, the pressure drops and then rises again as the sphincter regains tone. Finally, the pressure drops once more as the sphincter returns to its original position distal to the transducer. In the normal subject, residual pressure (pressure at the nadir of the relaxation) is negative. **B** is a tracing of two swallows showing *abnormal* UES relaxation in a patient with achalasia. The residual pressure (pressure at the nadir of the relaxation) is about 10 mm Hg. Normal volunteers have a mean residual pressure of −6 mm Hg with a standard deviation of 7 mm Hg.

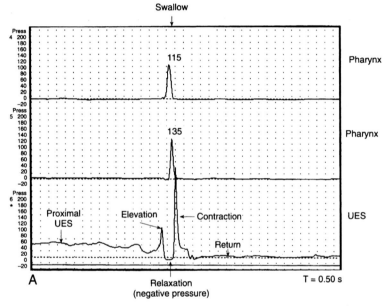

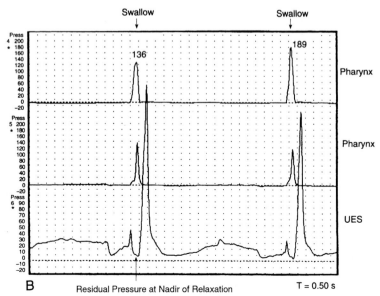

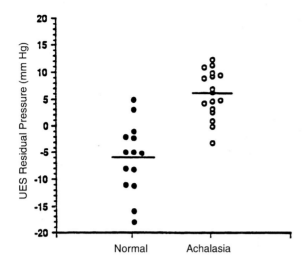

**FIGURE 5.17.** UES residual pressure: normal versus achalasia. This graph compared UES residual pressure for 17 patients with achalasia to that of a group of 14 normal volunteers. Normal mean UES residual pressure is –6 mm Hg, whereas the mean UES residual pressure for achalasia patients is +6 mm Hg. The difference between these values is statistically significant.

## INCOORDINATED MOTILITY
### Diffuse Esophageal Spasm

**FIGURE 5.18.** Diffuse esophageal spasm. This tracing shows an esophageal motility pattern typical of the patient with esophageal spasm. The cursor marks the beginning of the contraction wave initiated by the swallow. This wave is followed by multiple spontaneous, simultaneous contractions. The amplitudes of these contractions, however, are not particularly high. There is also a great deal of contractile activity between swallows.

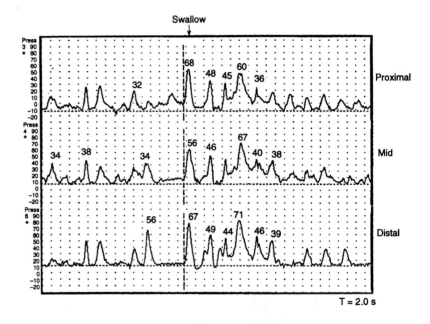

**FIGURE 5.19.** Diffuse esophageal spasm: variant. This tracing shows another pattern common to patients with spasm. Their motility study will show a variety of wave types. Here the *solid cursor* marks a peristaltic wave, whereas the *dotted cursor* marks a simultaneous wave. Note that these simultaneous contractions are quite different in appearance from the isobaric waves typical in achalasia (see Fig. 5.13).

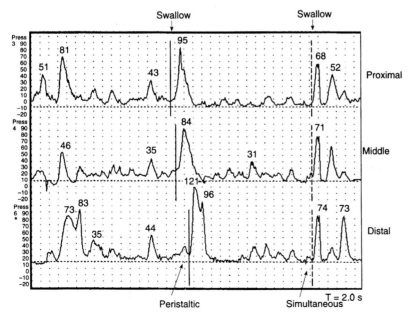

## HYPERCONTRACTING ESOPHAGUS
**Nutcracker Esophagus**

**FIGURE 5.20.** Distal esophagus: nutcracker esophagus. This tracing illustrates the most typical manometric feature, high-amplitude distal peristalsis, of the nutcracker esophagus. The cursors mark the beginning of the wave and show clear peristalsis; however, the amplitudes are well in excess of the normal range as shown in Table 5.3.

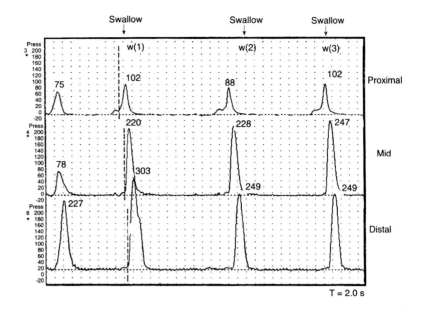

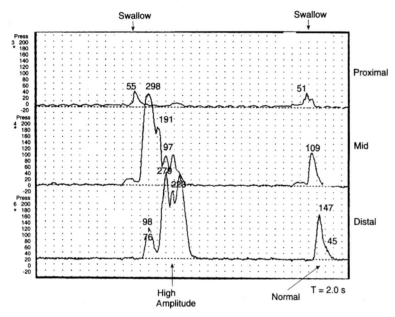

**FIGURE 5.21.** Distal esophagus: nutcracker esophagus variant. This illustration of a nutcracker esophagus shows some of the variability that can be expected in manometric studies of these patients. The wave associated with the first swallow shows the high amplitudes in the distal transducers common in these patients. The wave associated with the second swallow is normal.

**FIGURE 5.22.** Distal esophagus: nutcracker esophagus variant. This tracing further illustrates the variation seen in manometric studies of patients with a nutcracker esophagus. The second of the two swallows on this tracing clearly shows long-duration, multiple peaked waves that are, however, in contrast to similar waves seen with spasm, peristaltic. In addition, there is none of the contractile activity seen between swallows during spasm.

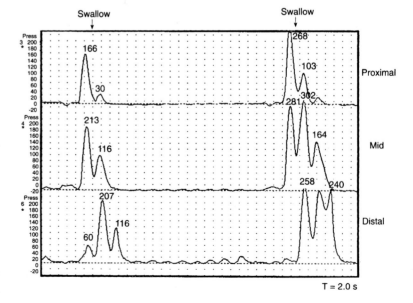

## Hypertensive LES

**FIGURE 5.23.** Hypertensive LES: baseline pressure. This tracing shows a station pull-through of a patient with a hypertensive LES. The resting pressure of the LES, calculated as the mean pressure between the cursors, is 54 mm Hg, which is more than 2 standard deviations above normal (see Table 5.2).

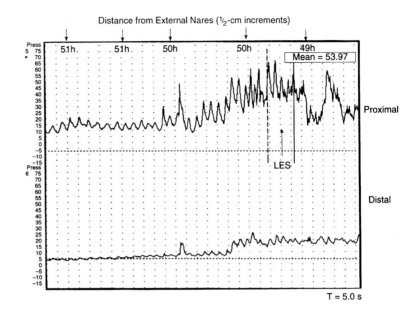

**FIGURE 5.24.** Hypertensive LES: relaxation. The hypertensive LES most commonly does not relax to gastric baseline following a swallow, as shown in this tracing. These four swallows show a residual pressure of about 7 mm Hg. Peristaltic activity above the LES is normal.

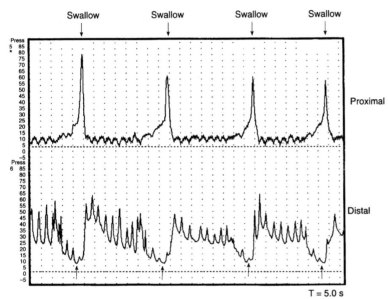

## HYPOCONTRACTING ESOPHAGUS
### Ineffective Esophageal Motility

**FIGURE 5.25.** Distal esophagus: ineffective esophageal motility (IEM). This tracing shows the response of a patient with IEM to three wet swallows. In the first, (w(4)), the peristaltic wave is not transmitted; in the second, the wave is normal; and in the third, the wave drops out in the two distal transducers.

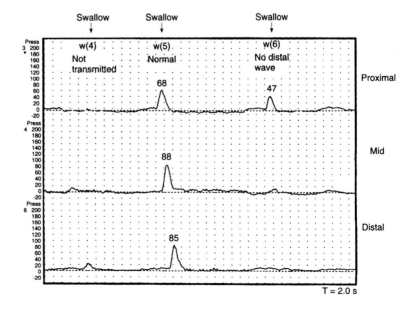

**FIGURE 5.26.** Distal esophagus: IEM. In this tracing there is a dropout of peristalsis in the two proximal transducers with a normal contraction in the distal transducer.

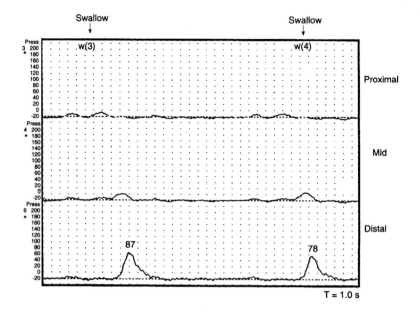

**FIGURE 5.27.** Distal esophagus: IEM. This tracing shows yet another manometric feature of IEM. The response to wet swallows is a low-amplitude peristaltic wave. Radiographic studies have shown that a peristaltic amplitude of greater than 30 mm Hg is necessary to prevent retrograde bolus escape.

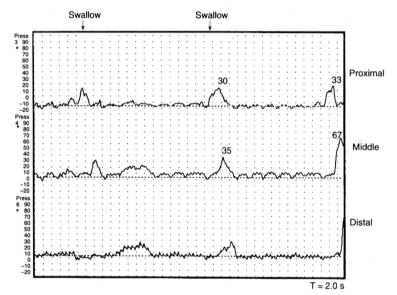

## Manometric Features

**FIGURE 5.28.** Distribution of manometric disorders. This graph details the distribution of various manometric disorders in patients evaluated for noncardiac chest pain and patients evaluated for dysphagia. Of 910 patients evaluated for noncardiac chest pain over a 3-year period, 255 (28%) were found to have some manometric abnormality (*left*). By far the largest single manometric abnormality in this group was the nutcracker esophagus (48%), followed by NEMD (36%). The remaining 16% were divided among diffuse esophageal spasm (DES) (10%), hypertensive LES (4%), and achalasia (2%). Of 251 patients referred for evaluation of dysphagia, 132 (53%) had an esophageal motility disorder. About an even number of patients had either NEMD (39%) or achalasia (36%), with the remaining 25% split among DES (13%), nutcracker (10%), and hypertensive LES (2%). The manometric disorder NEMD would be reclassified as IEM by the criteria we are using today.

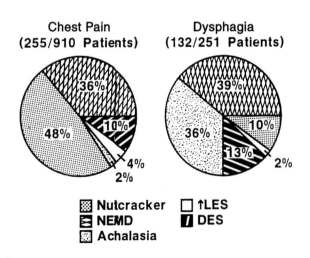

## SCLERODERMA
## LES Pull-through

**FIGURE 5.29.** Lower esophageal sphincter: scleroderma. This tracing shows a typical LES station pull-through for a patient with scleroderma. The LES is quite low, with a mean resting pressure shown here of 9 mm Hg.

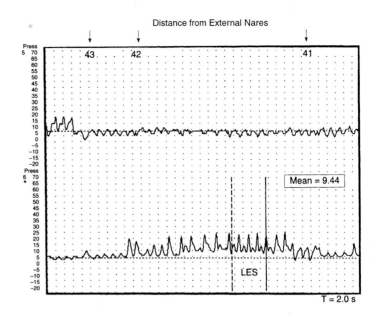

**FIGURE 5.30.** Lower esophageal sphincter relaxation: scleroderma. In this tracing, the distal transducer is located in the high-pressure zone of the LES of a patient with scleroderma. The proximal transducer is 3 cm higher, in the distal esophagus. During the time the tracing was recorded, the patient was given four wet swallows (marked at the top of the tracing). Although the LES shows some relaxation, it does not relax to gastric baseline, and there is no peristalsis in the distal esophagus.

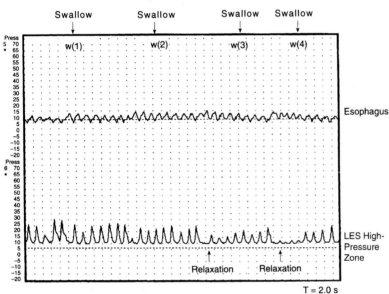

## Absent Distant Peristalsis

**FIGURE 5.31.** Distal esophagus: scleroderma. During the time this tracing was recorded, the patient was given two wet swallows (5 mL of water). There is no peristaltic contraction in the distal esophagus in response to a swallow in the patient with scleroderma.

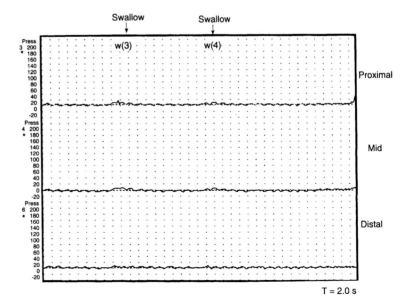

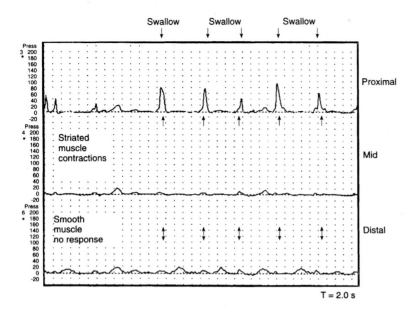

T = 2.0 s

### Normal Proximal Esophagus

**FIGURE 5.32.** Proximal esophagus: scleroderma. In this tracing, the proximal transducer is located 1 cm below the distal border of the UES, in the striated muscle portion of the esophagus. The other two transducers are 5 and 10 cm distal. In response to a wet swallow, the striated muscle contracts, but there is no peristaltic continuation of the contraction through the smooth muscle of the distal esophagus.

## GASTROESOPHAGEAL REFLUX DISEASE
### Relationship of Esophagitis to LES Pressure

**FIGURE 5.33.** Lower esophageal sphincter: relationship to esophagitis. **A** is a station pull-through of the LES of the reflux patient with esophagitis. The cursors are bracketing the high-pressure zone of the LES, and the mean pressure shown is 9 mm Hg. **B** is a graph showing LES pressures in 177 subjects divided into 5 groups. Patients with severe esophagitis had a significantly lower ($p < .01$) mean LES pressure than normal volunteers, although there is a considerable amount of overlap. However, no normal volunteer or patient control (nonreflux patient) had an LES pressure ≤10 mm Hg, whereas 1 patient with noninflammatory gastroesophageal reflux disease (GERD), 4 patients with mild esophagitis, and 8 patients with severe esophagitis fell below this cutoff. **B** Reproduced with permission from Kahrilas PJ, Dodds WJ, Hogan WJ, et al. Esophageal peristaltic dysfunction in peptic esophagitis. Gastroenterology 1986;91:897–904.

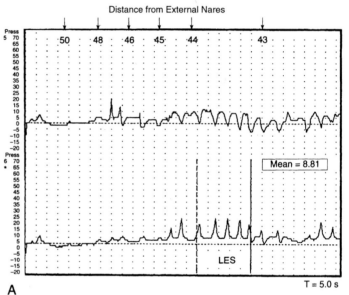

Distance from External Nares

Mean = 8.81

LES

T = 5.0 s

A

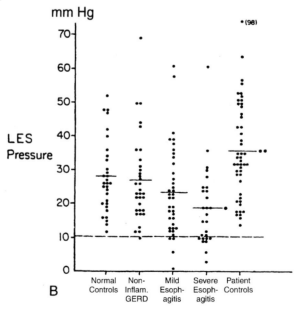

mm Hg

LES Pressure

B

Normal Controls · Non-Inflam. GERD · Mild Esoph-agitis · Severe Esoph-agitis · Patient Controls

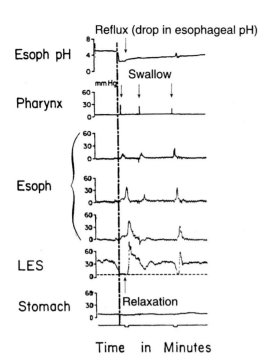

Reflux (drop in esophageal pH)

Esoph pH

Pharynx

Swallow

Esoph

LES

Relaxation

Stomach

Time in Minutes

**FIGURE 5.34.** Lower esophageal sphincter: relationship of transient relaxations to reflux. This figure shows an event of reflux occurring during a transient relaxation of the LES. Before acid reflux, resting LES pressure was stable at about 30 mm Hg above intragastric pressure (*broken line*). Reflux of acid into the esophagus occurred during a relaxation of the LES that was not related to swallowing. The reflux event was followed by three swallow-induced peristaltic clearing waves. In controls, 94% of reflux episodes were related to transient sphincter relaxations. In patients with reflux esophagitis, 65% of reflux episodes accompanied transient sphincter relaxations. Reproduced with permission from Dodds WJ, Dent J, Hogan WJ, et al. Mechanism of gastroesophageal reflux in patients with reflux esophagitis. N Engl J Med 1982;307:1547–52.

## Relationship of Esophagitis to Peristaltic Amplitudes

**FIGURE 5.35.** Distal esophagus: relationship of peristaltic amplitudes to esophagitis. **A** is a tracing showing a low-amplitude peristaltic response of the distal esophagus to three wet swallows of a GERD patient with esophagitis. **B** is a graph comparing peristaltic amplitudes for five groups of subjects: normal volunteers, noninflammatory GERD patients, patients with mild esophagitis, patients with severe esophagitis, and patient controls (non-GERD patients). The mean amplitude was significantly lower in all GERD patient groups than in either control group. The *dashed horizontal line* indicates the 95% cutoff level for control subjects. Ten percent of patients in each of the GERD groups fell below this cutoff. **B** Reproduced with permission from Kahrilas PJ, Dodds WJ, Hogan WJ, et al. Esophageal peristaltic dysfunction in peptic esophagitis. Gastroenterology 1986;91:897–904.

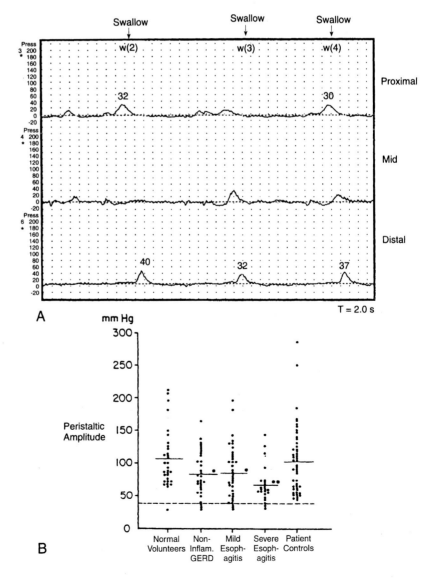

## Relationship of Esophagitis to Failed Peristalsis

**FIGURE 5.36.** Distal esophagus: relationship of failed peristalsis to esophagitis. The tracing in **A** shows failed peristalsis in a GERD patient with esophagitis. **B** is a graph comparing the failure rate of primary peristalsis for water swallows as a function of degree of esophagitis. Compared to the control groups, the mean failure rate of primary peristalsis was significantly greater for the patients with mild and severe esophagitis. The *horizontal dashed line* indicates the 95% confidence interval. Thirteen subjects with non-inflammatory GERD or esophagitis had failed primary peristalsis above this level. **B** Reproduced with permission from Kahrilas PJ, Dodds WJ, Hogan WJ, et al. Esophageal peristaltic dysfunction in peptic esophagitis. Gastroenterology 1986;91:897–904.

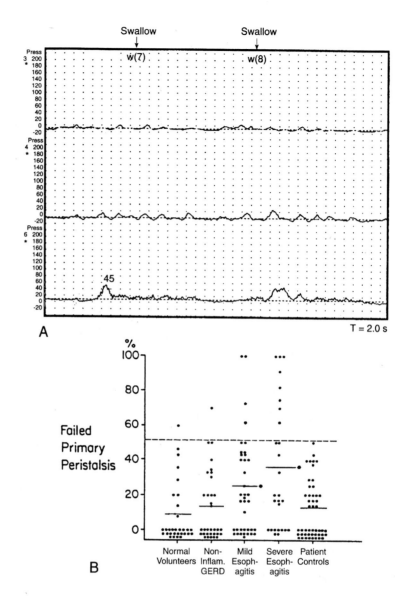

A

B

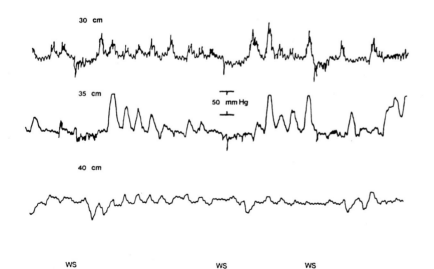

## DIABETES MELLITUS

**FIGURE 5.37.** Distal esophagus: diabetes mellitus. This is an esophageal motility tracing from a patient with diabetes mellitus. The recordings were located at 30, 35, and 40 cm from the nares (top to bottom). Although 50% or more of patients diagnosed with this disease may exhibit DES-like activity (repetitive, simultaneous waves) in response to wet swallows, most do not have esophageal symptoms.

## CONCLUSION

Esophageal manometry presents the clinician and clinical investigator with a powerful tool for quantitating intra-esophageal pressure dynamics. These dynamics provide a useful guide in the diagnosis and evaluation of a variety of disorders that affect the muscles of the esophagus. Current technology is reliable and easy to use. Computer analysis has removed much of the drudgery from reading tracings. Of course, no technology can ever replace careful attention to detail while doing the study and a complete knowledge of the patterns that are associated with a given disorder.

These examples are meant to acquaint the reader with the possibilities inherent in the use of esophageal motility and to show some of the atypical and not so typical wave forms and the disorders with which they are associated. Variations in equipment and technique can produce variations in results, and this should be considered when comparing studies from different laboratories.

### SELECTED READINGS

Allen ML, Orr WC, Mellow MH, Robinson MG. Water swallows versus food ingestion as manometric tests for esophageal dysfunction. Gastroenterology 1988;95:831–3.

Arndorfer RC, Stef JJ, Dodds WJ, et al. Improved infusion system for intraluminal esophageal manometry. Gastroenterology 1977;73:23–7.

Bombeck CT, Vaz O, DeSalvo J, et al. Computerized axial manometry of the esophagus. Ann Surg 1987;206:465–72.

Bonavina L, Evander A, DeMeester TR. Length of the distal esophageal sphincter and competency of the cardia. Am J Surg 1986;151:25–34.

Castell DO. Clinical applications of esophageal manometry. Dig Dis Sci 1982;27:769–71.

Castell DO, Dubois A, Davis CR, et al. Computer-aided analysis of human esophageal peristalsis. Dig Dis Sci 1984;29:65–72.

Castell JA, Castell DO. Computer analysis of human esophageal peristalsis and lower esophageal sphincter pressure II. An interactive system for online data collection and analysis. Dig Dis Sci 1986;31:121–6.

Castell JA, Dalton CB, Castell DO. On-line computer analysis of human lower esophageal sphincter relaxation. Am J Physiol 1988;255:G794–9.

Castell JA, Dalton CB. Esophageal manometry. In: Castell DO, editor. The esophagus. Boston: Little, Brown & Co; 1992. p. 143–60.

Dent J, Chir B. A new technique for continuous sphincter pressure measurement. Gastroenterology 1976;71:263–7.

DeVault K, Castell JA, Castell DO. How many swallows are required to establish reliable esophageal peristaltic parameters in normal subjects? An on-line computer analysis. Am J Gastroenterol 1987;82:754–7.

Dodds WJ, Hogan WJ, Reid DP, et al. A comparison between primary esophageal peristalsis following wet and dry swallows. J Appl Physiol 1973;35:851–7.

Dooley CP, Schlossmacher B, Valenzuela JE. Effects of alterations in bolus viscosity on esophageal peristalsis in humans. Am J Physiol 1988;254:G8–11.

Hogan WJ, Dodds WJ, Stewart ET. Comparison of roentgenology and intraluminal manometry for evaluating oesophageal peristalsis. Rend Gastroenterol 1973;5:28–33.

Hollis JB, Castell DO. Amplitude of esophageal peristalsis as determined by rapid infusion. Gastroenterology 1972;63:417–22.

Hollis JB, Castell DO. Effect of dry swallows and wet swallows of different volumes on esophageal peristalsis. J Appl Physiol 1975;38:1161–4.

Katz PO, Dalton CB, Richter JE, et al. Esophageal testing of patients with non-cardiac chest pain and/or dysphagia. Results of a three year experience with 1161 patients. Ann Intern Med 1987;106:593–7.

Kaye MD, Wexler RM. Alteration of esophageal peristalsis by body position. Dig Dis Sci 1981;26:897–901.

Kraus BB, Wu WC, Castell DO. Comparison of lower esophageal sphincter manometrics and gastroesophageal reflux measured by 24-hour pH recording. Am J Gastroenterol 1990;85:692–6.

Lydon SB, Dodds WJ, Hogan WJ, Arridorfer RC. The effect of manometric assembly diameter on intraluminal esophageal pressure recording. Dig Dis Sci 1975;20:968–70.

Leite LP, Johnston BT, Barrett J, et al. Ineffective esophageal motility (IEM): the primary finding in patients with nonspecific esophageal motility disorder. Dig Dis Sci 1997;42:1859–65.

Mellow MH. Esophageal motility during food ingestion: a physiologic test of esophageal motor function. Gastroenterology 1983;85:570–7.

O'Sullivan GC, DeMeester TR, Joelsson BE. Interaction of lower esophageal sphincter pressure and length of sphincter in the abdomen as determinants of gastroesophageal competence. Am J Surg 1982;143:40–7.

Pope CE. A dynamic test of sphincter strength: its application to the lower esophageal sphincter. Gastroenterology 1967;52:770–86.

Pryde A, Wilson JA, Heading RC. GR800 manometric equipment. Gullet 1991;1:145–7.

Rex DK, Hast JL, Lehman GA, et al. Comparison of radially sensitive and circumferentially sensitive microtransducer esophageal manometry probes in normal subjects. Am J Gastroenterol 1988;83:151–4.

Richter JE, Blackwell JN, Wu WC, et al. Relationship of radionuclide liquid bolus transport and esophageal manometry. J Lab Clin Med 1987;109:217–24.

Richter JE, Wu WC, Johns DN, et al. Esophageal manometry in 95 healthy adult volunteers. Dig Dis Sci 1987;32:583–92.

Sears VW, Castell JA, Castell DO. Comparison of effects of upright versus supine body position and liquid versus solid bolus on esophageal pressures in normal humans. Dig Dis Sci 1990;35:857–64.

Stef JJ, Dodds WJ, Hogan WJ, et al. Intraluminal esophageal manometry: an analysis of variables affecting recording fidelity of peristaltic pressures. Gastroenterology 1974;67:221–30.

Tijskens G, Janssens J, Vantrappen G, DeBondt F. Validation of a fully automated analysis of esophageal body contractility and lower esophageal sphincter function: a study on the effect of the PGE1 analogue Rioprostil on human esophageal motility. J Gastroenterol Motil 1989;1:21–8.

Wilson JA, Pryde A, Macintyre CC, Heading RC. Computerized manometric recording: an evaluation. Gullet 1991;1:87–91.

Winans CS, Harris LD. Quantitation of lower esophageal sphincter competence. Gastroenterology 1966;52:754–60.

# CHAPTER 6

# Sensory Testing

*Kenneth R. DeVault and Sami R. Achem*

Major symptoms felt to arise in the esophagus include heartburn (pyrosis) and chest pain. Although many patients with heartburn can be diagnosed based on conventional testing (endoscopy and ambulatory pH testing) and therapeutic trials, others will be more challenging. Attempts to replicate heartburn (and hence solidify the diagnosis) by the instillation of acid into the esophagus have been used for many years. Esophageal chest pain is more difficult to diagnose. The majority of patients with chest pain will have a normal endoscopy, and over half will have a negative ambulatory pH test. Several methods have been developed to replicate this pain, including intraesophageal balloon distention, acid perfusion, and pharmacologic manipulation of esophageal pressure. Finally, several new techniques have been devised to estimate the tone of the esophageal muscle in vivo, which has been very difficult using standard techniques.

## Esophageal Sensory Physiology

There has been extensive study of the mechanisms that underlie gastrointestinal pain, yet the actual defect that makes one person experience pain whereas another either does not feel anything or interprets a sensation as nonpainful is not known. This holds for both general gastrointestinal pain and for esophageal pain in particular. We know that there are receptors in the esophagus that are sensitive to acid and to pressure. Some of these may be pain specific, whereas others may result in pain when stimulated in a certain way and not result in pain at other times. Once registered in these receptors, pain from the esophagus is carried in the spinal nerves to the spinal cord and then to the brain via the spinothalamic tracts. The understanding that a majority of fibers in the vagus nerve are sensory in nature has challenged this concept, although conventional thought is that these nerves are involved more in visceral reflexes than in pain conveyance.

Pain can be evoked from the gastrointestinal tract using several stimulus modalities. Receptors sensitive to mucosal stimulation have been isolated in the gastrointestinal tract.[1] Theoretically, these receptors underlie the pain produced with esophageal acid both in gastroesophageal reflux and with acid infusion in the Bernstein test. Although these receptors produce a brief burst of impulses with mechanical stimulation of the gastrointestinal tract, another set of receptors responds to mechanical changes in the esophageal wall.[2] These receptors are located in the muscle layers of the viscera and are activated by tension in the wall produced by distention, contraction, or compression of the viscus (Table 6.1).[3,4] Most visceral organs, including the esophagus, are compliant within physiologic pressure ranges, although further increases in distention beyond this physiologic range may result in sharp increases in

**TABLE 6.1.** Mechanisms of Esophageal Pain

| Mechanism | Clinical Example | Method for Testing |
|---|---|---|
| Distention | Pain with swallowing large bolus or cold water | Esophageal balloon distention |
| Spasm | Chest pain with diffuse spasm and nutcracker esophagus | Edrophonium testing |
| Chemical exposure | Chest pain or pyrosis with acid reflux | Acid perfusion testing |

**TABLE 6.2.** Method for Performing the Bernstein Test

1. Perfusion port localized 10–15 cm proximal to lower esophageal sphincter (perfusing through a manometry catheter is okay).
2. 0.1 Normal saline perfused at 6–8 mL/min
3. If patient experiences pain with saline, test is concluded (*diagnosis: nonspecific hyperalgesia*).
4. After 30 minutes, saline is stopped.
5. 0.1 Normal HCl perfused at 6–8 mL/min
6. If patient experiences pain with acid, test is concluded (*diagnosis: acid-induced symptom*).
7. If no symptoms by 30 minutes, perfusion is stopped (*diagnosis: normal study*).

**TABLE 6.3.** Summary of Published Studies Indicating Reproduction of Chest Pain Following Acid Infusion

| Year | Lead Author/ Reference | Patients Positive (n) | Positive Test (%) |
|------|------------------------|----------------------|-------------------|
| 1987 | Vantrappen[13] | 11/33 | 33 |
| 1988 | De Caestecker[7] | 21/60 | 35 |
| 1988 | Peters[11] | 7/20 | 35 |
| 1989 | Koch[17] (patients with mitral valve prolapse and chest pain) | 5/19 | 26 |
| 1989 | Soffer[12] | 2/20 | 10 |
| 1989 | Hewson[18] | 35/71 | 49 |
| 1989 | Berezin[19] (study done in children with atypical chest pain) | 45/60 | 75 |
| 1990 | Hewson[9] | 15/45 | 33 |
| 1990 | Hewson[20] | 8/159 | 5 |
| 1990 | Ghillebert[8] | 18/50 | 36 |
| 1990 | Humeau[21] | 4/40 | 10 |
| 1991 | Nevens[10] | 14/37 | 37 |
| 1991 | Hewson[22] | 18/95 | 18 |
| 1991 | Richter[23] | 15/75 | 20 |
| 1992 | Rokkas[24] | 29/110 | 26 |
| 1994 | Rose[25] | 11/55 | 20 |
| 1995 | Mehta[26] | 3/25 | 12 |
| 1995 | Ghillebert[27] | 106/270 | 39 |
| 1996 | Frobert[28] | 10/63 | 15 |
|  | Total | 381/1307 | 29 |

pressure and mechanoreceptor discharge.[2] Intraganglionic laminar nerve endings found in the myenteric plexus may function as the receptor organ for this type of sensation. To stimulate these receptors, pharmacologic agents have been administered to patients (ergonovine, edrophonium, bethanechol) to increase the amplitude and duration of esophageal contractions in the hope of evoking a pain response. Direct mechanical stimulation of the specific organ may also provide a physiologic and specific form of afferent sensory stimulation. This is particularly effective since distention affects the circular muscle and, perhaps more importantly, stretches the longitudinal muscle.

## Acid Perfusion Testing (Bernstein Test)

The acid perfusion test was introduced by Bernstein and Baker over 40 years ago.[5] This test was not originally intended to diagnose heartburn but was an attempt to find an objective method to reproduce esophageal pain and to differentiate it from cardiac angina. We attempt to replicate the original test as closely as possible by applying a 15- to 30-minute control period of intraesophageal saline infusion at a rate of 6 to 8 ml/min followed by an infusion of 0.1-N hydrochloric acid (HCl) administered at the same rate for a period of 30 minutes or until symptoms occur (Table 6.2). If the acid perfusion provokes the familiar angina-like chest pain and saline solution does not induce the pain, the test suggests an esophageal origin of the pain. Patients who get pain with the saline are difficult to interpret but probably have a form of visceral hyperalgesia that is not acid related.

Although the test appears to be highly specific,[6] its sensitivity is relatively low, with figures ranging from 5 to 75%.[7–13] A negative test result has little clinical value and does not exclude an esophageal origin of the chest pain. Patients with Barrett's esophagus have been noted to have a decrease in their sensitivity to acid, resulting in even more false negatives.[14] Interestingly, a recent study found that the acid sensitivity in patients with Barrett's esophagus returned after their squamous epithelium was re-established using ablative and acid-suppressant therapy.[15] It is important to closely follow a protocol when doing this study since many factors can influence the results. For example, a prior acid

infusion decreases the amount of acid required to produce symptoms in normal controls.[16] Table 6.3 presents the results of the majority of studies published to date.[7–13,17–28]

Because of low sensitivity compared to 24-hour pH monitoring with symptom assessment, some authors have considered the acid perfusion test to be obsolete.[18,23] The test is easy to perform and has almost no side effects; therefore, it is reasonable to include it in the diagnostic evaluation of patients with noncardiac chest pain. The test has little to offer in the patient with typical reflux symptoms, which are highly specific for reflux,[29] or in the patient with esophagitis, for whom endoscopy is a much more reliable way to make the diagnosis.

## Edrophonium Test

Higher than normal peristaltic pressures have been suggested to cause esophageal pain in nutcracker esophagus. This suggestion led to the development of provocation tests designed to produce pain by inducing increases in esophageal pressures and esophageal motility disorders. The parasympathomimetic agents bethanechol and edrophonium, the sympathomimetic agent ergonovine, and pentagastrin have all been used. Edrophonium hydrochloride is a rapid-acting cholinesterase inhibitor used in the evaluation of myasthenia gravis that seems to offer the best results in esophageal provocation with the lowest level of side effects.

The standard edrophonium (Tensilon) test involves the intravenous injection of 80 µg/kg of edrophonium, which reproduces

**TABLE 6.4.**  Studies Evaluating Edrophonium in Chest Pain

| Year | Lead Author/Reference | Positive Tests | % |
|------|----------------------|----------------|---|
| 1981 | London[36] | 10/10 | 100 |
| 1985 | Richter[31] | 15/50 | 30 |
| 1987 | Katz[37] | 210/910 | 23 |
| 1987 | VanTrappen[13] | 6/12 | 50 |
| 1987 | Nasrallah[38] | 19/51 | 39 |
| 1987 | Lee[33] | 48/120 | 40 |
| 1988 | De Caestecker[7] | 12/60 | 20 |
| 1989 | Koch[17] | 3/17 | 18 |
| 1989 | Soffer[12] | 0/20 | 0 |
| 1989 | Hewson[18] | 15/78 | 19 |
| 1990 | Hewson[9] | 26/159 | 16 |
| 1990 | Hewson[20] | 24/44 | 55 |
| 1990 | Ghillebert[8] | 16/50 | 32 |
| 1990 | Humeau[21] | 6/40 | 15 |
| 1990 | Breumelhof[39] | 2/44 | 5 |
| 1990 | Dalton[30] | 25/75 | 33 |
| 1991 | Nevens[10] | 7/87 | 19 |
| 1991 | Goudot-Pernot[40] | 19/78 | 24 |
| 1992 | Rokkas[24] | 26/110 | 24 |
| 1994 | Rose[25] | 8/55 | 15 |
| 1995 | Mehta[26] | 10/25 | 40 |
| 1995 | Ghillebert[27] | 58/220 | 26 |
| 1996 | Frobert[28] | 9/63 | 14 |
|  | Total | 574/2378 | 24 |

*10-mg dose.

**TABLE 6.5.**  Advantages and Disadvantages of Edrophonium (Tensilon) Testing

Advantages

A positive test suggests (but not proves) that the esophagus is the source of pain

Pain does not occur in healthy controls or irritable bowel syndrome

Can be used as office infusion test since manomety monitoring is not indispensable

Safe: no evidence of coronary artery flow restriction

Widely available

Inexpensive ($1.52/dose in our laboratory)

Antidote: atropine widely available (rarely needed)

Rapid onset of action and relatively short half-life (approx. 2 h)

Disadvantages

Variable sensitivity and uncertain specificity (no available gold standard)

Positive test may not help in therapeutic selection (acid suppression, muscle relaxant, or other)

Positive test may not predict clinical outcome or therapeutic response

Subject to variability in reporting: relies on patient's "replication" of chest pain

Occasional side effects (light-headedness, nausea, cramps)

Manometric changes do not help discriminate between patients and controls

Must include a placebo control infusion

esophageal manometric changes and chest pain in 20 to 30% of patients with noncardiac chest pain.[30,31] This medication has a very rapid onset of action and a relatively brief half-life of 1.8 ± 0.6 hours.[32] We currently use a 10-mg dose in all patients to simplify our protocol. This slightly higher dose is easier to use but has not demonstrated a significant improvement in sensitivity.[33] The pain occurs on swallowing, within 5 minutes after the administration of the drug, and disappears quickly as the drug is rapidly metabolized. Edrophonium has shown no effect on coronary artery diameter and actually decreases cardiac workload.[31] Edrophonium is known to increase esophageal contraction amplitude and duration as well as the number of repetitive contractions after swallowing in both patients and normal control subjects (Fig. 6.1). This increase is not greater in patients with chest pain with a positive (pain) response as compared with patients in whom the test did not induce pain. The changes in contractions observed in patients with chest pain are similar to those in healthy control subjects who never experience pain during the test.[30] This indicates that we do not clearly understand the mechanism by which edrophonium induces pain in the positive-response patients. Some investigators have argued that the high-amplitude esophageal contractions generated by edrophonium may result in decreased blood flow to the esophagus, which induces chest pain. Recent evidence does not support that theory and suggests that spasm owing to vigorous esophageal contractions is a more likely explanation for chest pain.[34] Studies by de Caestecker and colleagues suggested that the pain receptors involved in edrophonium-induced noxious stimuli reside in mechanoreceptors located in the esophageal longitudinal muscle.[35] This also suggests that when a subjective parameter such as pain is the end point for a positive test result, a placebo control is necessary to interpret the test correctly. We give a saline placebo followed by the active drug and base the interpretation of the test on the patient's symptoms only. Seeing an increase in pressure and bizarre waveforms in a patient without pain suggests that the pain is not related to problems with pain from intermittent high pressure or dysmotility.

The results of the published studies are outlined in Table 6.4.[7,10,12,13,17,18,20,21,24,28,31,33,36–40] It is clear that there is a wide range of positive response. Certainly, there are great differences in patient selection and considerable potential for referral bias in these studies. Investigators have attempted to correlate the results of a positive edrophonium test in predicting acid- and motility-induced pain without success.[27] Thus, a positive edrophonium test suggests the presence of esophageal origin of the chest pain but does not identify the specific physiologic mechanism involved during spontaneous pain episodes. The advantages and disadvantages of this test are presented in Table 6.5.

## INTRAESOPHAGEAL BALLOON DISTENTION

Intraesophageal balloon distention (IEBD) has been used in health and disease states to stimulate mechanoreceptors in the esophagus. This technique has been validated in animal models in which IEBD has been shown to activate tension-

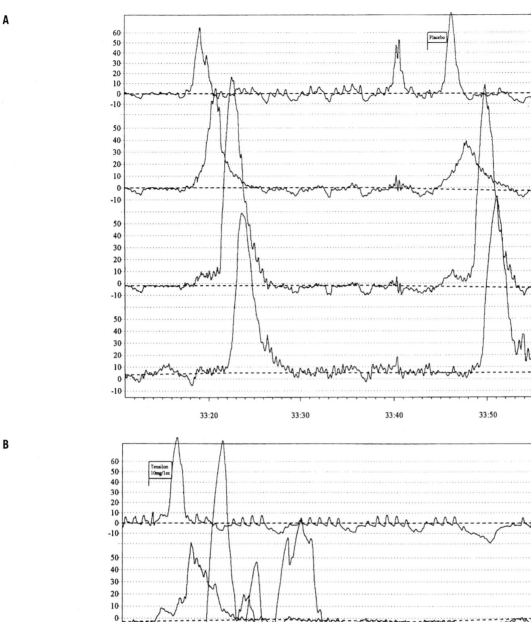

**FIGURE 6.1.** Esophageal manometry tracing showing pressures before (**A**) and after (**B**) edrophonium 10 mg intravenously. This patient experienced pain with the increased pressure (positive test), but the actual manometric tracing does not predict symptoms.

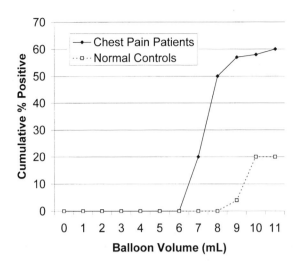

**FIGURE 6.2.** Graphic representation of data from Richter et al.[43] Patients with chest pain were both more likely to experience pain and to experience it at a lower distention volume. Sixty percent of patients with chest pain experience pain with balloon volumes less than 10 cc, whereas this was rare in control subjects.

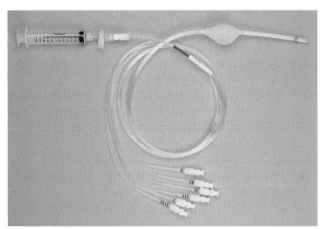

**FIGURE 6.3.** Combined balloon provocation/manometry catheter (Wilson-Cook, Winston-Salem, NC).

sensitive mechanoreceptors associated with vagal afferents that are located in the longitudinal and circular muscle layers.[41] Although this technique has been used since 1955 to distinguish esophageal from cardiac pain,[42] it was not until 1986 that the test acquired wide popularity in the evaluation of patients with chest pain. In a seminal study, Richter and colleagues reported that balloon distention reproduced chest pain in 28 (56%) of 50 patients with noncardiac chest pain and 6 (20%) of 30 healthy controls ($p < .005$).[43] Twenty-four of 28 patients experienced chest pain at $\leq 8$ mL, whereas all of the volunteers experienced chest pain at volumes $\geq 9$ mL (Fig. 6.2).[43] Intraesophageal balloon distention has been demonstrated to be reproducible in both normal controls and patients.[44,45] The finding that there is a lowered threshold to distention in the colon in patients with irritable bowel syndrome and in the stomach in patients with

nonulcer dyspepsia suggests that there may be some common disruption in visceral sensation in these three so-called functional disorders.[46,47]

There is no one technique for performing these studies that has been studied well enough and validated to be declared superior. Early studies used handmade balloons fashioned from rubber condoms, finger cots, and even surgical gloves. Recently, a commercially available balloon catheter has been developed (Wilson-Cook, Winston-Salem, North Carolina (Fig. 6.3). Comparative studies of both latex and silicone have shown that the latex balloon offers the better diameter volume and pressure volume characteristics at the low volumes often required to induce pain. Placement of the balloon should take into consideration the variable differences in regional sensory perception through the esophagus.[3] Most of the available publications shown in Table 6.6 have chosen to locate the balloon 10 cm above the lower esophageal sphincter.[8,10,21,27,35,40,43,48–51] A number of other variables in methodology should also be considered when performing IEBD. For instance, rapid balloon inflation may result in sensation being perceived at lower volumes. Since it is difficult to produce consistent inflation rates manually, some investigators have used an automated mechanical pump to inflate the balloon. Some investigators have used a stepwise increase in volume, whereas other authors have deflated the balloon between each increase in volume. Randomization of the inflation is important to avoid an anticipatory response. Sham inflations should be included as part of the protocol as a means to control for objective reporting. The dwell time (time balloon remains inflated) can affect the results of the test since prolonged inflation increases sensation intensity. When designing a protocol, there are several factors to be considered. This is a test of visceral sensitivity only, and motility disorders or changes produced by the balloon inflation do not seem to have a role in distinguishing pathology. Measuring intraballoon pressures also does not seem to distinguish between control subjects and patients, although more sophisticated techniques, which will be discussed below, may reveal something about the pathology of these disorders. Some patients with irritable bowel syndrome and with fibromyalgia have a lower pain threshold to esophageal distention, suggesting a common alteration in visceral receptor sensitivity or modulation but also the possibility of false-positive tests in patients with multiple complaints.[52,53] Females have a lower esophageal pain threshold than do males, independent of body size, but the difference is small enough to not be clinically significant.[54] Caution must be used in interpretation of balloon distention testing in older patients since both visceral sensation from the esophagus and the ability of an inflated balloon to induce secondary peristalsis seem to diminish with aging in normal subjects.[55,56] Taller individuals have a blunted pain response when compared with those of shorter stature. The advantages and disadvantages of this technique are presented in Table 6.7.

The response to balloon distention in individual patients can be modulated with pharmacologic interventions. Imipramine has been demonstrated to improve symptoms in

**TABLE 6.6** Outcome of Studies Evaluating Balloon Distention in Noncardiac Chest Pain

| Year | Lead Author/ Reference | Type Balloon | Inflation Method | Positive Response Definition | Positive Response | % |
|------|------------------------|--------------|------------------|-----------------------------|-------------------|---|
| 1986 | Richter[43] | Polyvinyl | Syringe | Pain at 8 mL | 18/30 | 60 |
| 1986 | Barish[48] | Polyvinyl | Syringe | Pain at 8 mL | 28/50 | 56 |
| 1990 | Deschner[49] | Latex | Syringe | Pain and spasm | 38/62 | 61 |
| 1990 | Ghillebert[8] | Polyvinyl | Syringe | Pain at 8 mL | 1/20 | 5 |
| 1990 | Humeau[21] | Polyvinyl | Syringe | Pain at 8 mL | 13/45 | 35 |
| 1991 | Nevens[10] | Not described | Syringe | Pain at 8 mL | 3/12 | 29 |
| 1991 | Goudot-Pernot[40] | Polyvinyl | Syringe | Pain at 9 mL | 33/78 | 42 |
| 1991 | Clouse[50] | Polyvinyl | Syringe | Pain at 8 mL | 29/65 | 45 |
| 1992 | De Caestecker[35] | Latex | Syringe | Pain at any volume | 8/13 | 61 |
| 1993 | Gignoux[51] | Not described | Syringe | Pain at 7 mL | 13/54 | 24 |
| 1995 | Ghillebert[27] | Not described | Not described | Not described | 26/220 | 14 |
| | | | | Total | 210/649 | 32 |

**TABLE 6.7.** Advantages and Disadvantages of Balloon Provocation Testing

Advantages

    A positive test suggests (but not proves) that the esophagus is the source of pain

    Pain does occur at high volumes in healthy controls

    Can be used as office test since manomety monitoring is not indispensable

    Safe: no documented perforation

    Widely available

    Highest yield of all provocative tests

Disadvantages

    Variable sensitivity and uncertain specificity (no available gold standard)

    Positive test does not always help in therapeutic selection

    Positive test does not predict clinical outcome or therapeutic response

    Subject to variability in reporting: relies on patient's "replication" of chest pain

    More difficult intubation owing to size of balloon

    Must include a placebo inflation

    Requires a second intubation if the laboratory uses solid-state equipment

patients with noncardiac chest pain[57] and also has been suggested to increase both pain and sensation thresholds to balloon distention in a group of normal controls.[58] A preliminary report found octreotide to improve both sensory and pain thresholds in a group of patients with chest pain.[59] Nifedipine has been studied using both standard balloon distention and barostat testing and has not been found to reliably improve this response.[60,61]

## COMBINED STIMULTION

Several studies have used multiple stimuli in an attempt to increase the diagnostic yield in the evaluation of patients with noncardiac chest pain. Barish and colleagues found that

esophageal balloon distention was superior to the combination of acid perfusion and edrophonium tests in replicating chest pain.[48] Whereas the combined use of acid and edrophonium induced chest pain in 8 of 50 patients, esophageal balloon distention replicated chest pain in 24 of 50 patients. Other investigators have found discrepant results. Ghillebert and colleagues noted that the combined use of acid and edrophonium stimulation resulted in 49% of their patients replicating their chest pain, whereas balloon distention alone had a 14% yield.[27] The reasons for these differences are not entirely certain. Care must be exercised when performing multiple provocation studies during the same session. Recent information suggests that perfusion of acid prior to balloon distention in patients with normal esophageal tests lowers their threshold for esophageal balloon distention.

### New Techniques

*Barostat*

Barostat testing is another form of balloon distention that has been used to measure wall tone in several visceral organs. In these studies, the volume of intraballoon air is varied to maintain a set pressure. The balloon or bag attached to the barostat is large enough to essentially allow infinite distensibility at the volume required to fill the given viscera. This results in a change in volume needed to maintain the set pressure even with quite small changes in wall tone. The use of this technology is well described in both the stomach and colon but has only recently been applied to the esophagus.[62] Esophageal barostat experiments were able to measure a difference in tone between the smooth and striated esophagus and record changes in tone after application of the smooth muscle relaxant amyl nitrite. A recent study used a barostat device to find a reduction but not a loss of esophageal wall tone in patients with achalasia.[63] A similar technique has been used to both measure esophageal tone and document a fall in esophageal tone, which commenced with deglutition and persisted until passage of the peristaltic wave.[64]

**TABLE 6.8.** Motility and Balloon Provocation May Guide Therapy

| Motility Finding | Balloon Provocation | Initial Treatment Trial |
| --- | --- | --- |
| Normal | Abnormal | Agents that lower visceral sensation |
| Normal | Normal | Consider psychology referral for behavior treatment |
| Hypertensive peristalsis (nutcracker) | Abnormal | Combination of agent that lowers visceral sensation and agent that lowers peristaltic pressures |
| Hypertensive peristalsis (nutcracker) | Normal | Agent that lowers peristaltic pressures |
| Hypotensive peristalsis (IEM) | Abnormal | Reconsider reflux along with agent that lowers visceral sensation |
| Hypotensive peristalsis (IEM) | Normal | Reconsider reflux |

IEM, ineffective esophageal motility.

### Impedance Testing

A recent study has suggested previously unreported abnormalities in esophageal compliance in a group of patients with chest pain.[65] Impedance planimetry measures a cross-sectional area of the esophagus from which wall tension can be indirectly calculated. The researchers were able to determine the esophagus to be less distensible and stiffer in patients with chest pain compared to normal controls. It is unclear if studies of this type will become more than an interesting research tool.

## Clinical Applications of Sensory Testing

### Gastroesophageal Reflux Disease

Most of the current clinical approaches to the diagnosis of gastroesophageal reflux disease (GERD) do not include provocative testing. Perhaps we have discarded a useful test prematurely. Endoscopy and ambulatory pH testing have become the de facto gold standard for the diagnosis of GERD. Although the finding of esophagitis on endoscopy is very specific for GERD, the lack of esophagitis is not sensitive in excluding GERD.[66] Ambulatory pH testing is also not a perfect standard. Normal acid exposure was reported in up to 29% of patients with documented esophagitis, and differences were found in the simultaneous acid exposure recorded by two attached probes.[67,68] Patients with symptomatic but not excessive gastroesophageal reflux have persistence of symptoms and requirements for therapy similar to patients with excessive reflux but are less likely to have endoscopic findings.[69,70] This "endoscopic negative" form of GERD produces symptoms and illness behavior identical to that of GERD with endoscopic findings.[71] Many authors are also advocating a high-dose trial of proton pump inhibitor as a "test" for GERD.[72]

A Bernstein test may help in the diagnosis of reflux in patients with unclear symptoms and testing. For example, if a patient who has had a fundoplication but continues to complain of reflux symptoms despite a lack of response to therapy and a pH testing showing physiologic amounts of esophageal acid exposure is demonstrated to have a heightened sensitivity to acid, a drug that lowers sensitivity (trazodone perhaps) may be added to his/her acid suppression. We are currently studying whether a lowered sensitivity to acid perfusion or balloon distention in patients referred for antireflux surgery might predict a poor outcome owing to increased esophageal sensitivity to all forms of stimulation.

### Noncardiac Chest Pain

Most studies with balloon distention and other forms of sensory provocation of the esophagus have been directed at noncardiac or unexplained chest pain. Many patients with chest pain may have normal coronary arteries and no evidence of a cardiac or pulmonary cause for their pain. In some centers, this may represent more than half of all patients evaluated for chest pain.[73] The esophagus has been extensively examined as a potential point of origin for that pain. One of the major challenges in the evaluation of patients with noncardiac chest pain is the lack of a biologic marker or a gold standard that can be confidently used to identify the esophagus as a source of the patient's chest pain. Gastroesophageal reflux has been suggested as the most common, treatable cause of noncardiac chest pain. We agree that an empiric course of reflux therapy is a reasonable first step after cardiac, major life-threatening, and musculoskeletal causes of pain have been excluded.

Since antireflux medications are very effective, easy to prescribe, and widely available, the majority of patients referred to a gastroenterologist for chest pain may have already had at least some trial of therapy. If this has been insufficient, it can be increased or extended, but many patients will still have chest pain after an appropriate trial. Esophageal spasm and other forms of dysmotility were once thought to be important in the genesis of these symptoms. Modern studies have shown that the majority of patients with chest pain have normal motility and that the more common disorders (nutcracker esophagus and nonspecific disorders) found are very nonspecific.[37] It seems likely that many patients with these symptoms have a degree of enhanced visceral pain perception from the esophagus, heart, or both.[74] Esophageal provocative testing has evolved as a method to reproduce esophageal pain in a similar analogy as chest pain may be induced when performing a stress test for the heart. We feel that the knowledge of the patient's esophageal manometry along with the demonstration of altered visceral sensibility allows us to tailor the therapy of the patient (Table 6.8). Others favor sequential trials of combinations of medicine, which is a reasonable approach but often leaves the patient with a great deal of confusion about the diagnosis. It has been suggested and we have also observed that patients (and their health care providers) are more satisfied with a more definitive diagnosis that can occasionally be suggested by the results of these tests.

## REFERENCES

1. Mayer EA, Raybould HE. Role of visceral afferent mechanisms in functional bowel disorders. Gastroenterology 1990;99:1688–704.

2. Iaenig W, Morrison JFB. Functional properties of spinal visceral afferents supplying abdominal and pelvic organs, with special emphasis on visceral nociception. In: Cervero F, Morrison JFB, editors. Progress in brain research. Vol 67. New York: Elsevier; 1986. p. 189–205.

3. Grundy D, Scratcher T. Sensory afferents from the gastrointestinal tract. In: Schultz SG, Wood JD, Rauner BB, editors. Handbook of physiology. Vol 1. New York: Oxford University Press; 1989. p. 593–620.

4. Leek BF. Abdominal and pelvic visceral receptors. Br Med Bull 1977;33:163–8.

5. Bernstein LM, Baker LA. A clinical test for esophagitis. Gastroenterology 1958;34:760–81.

6. Richter JE. Provocative tests in esophageal diseases. In: Scarpignato C, Galmiche JP, editors. Functional evaluation in esophageal disease. Frontiers of gastrointestinal research. Vol 22. Basel: Karger; 1994. p. 188.

7. De Caestecker JS, Pryde A, Heading RC. Comparison of intravenous edrophonium and esophageal acid perfusion during esophageal manometry in patients with non-cardiac chest pain. Gut 1988;29:1029–34.

8. Ghillebert G, Janssens J, Vantrappen G, et al. Ambulatory 24-hour intraesophageal pH and pressure recordings v. provocation tests in the diagnosis of chest pain of esophageal origin. Gut 1990;31:738–44.

9. Hewson EG, Dalton CB, Richter JE. Comparison of esophageal manometry, provocative testing, and ambulatory monitoring in patients with unexplained chest pain. Dig Dis Sci 1990;35:302–9.

10. Nevens F, Janssens J, Piessens J, et al. Prospective study on prevalence of esophageal chest pain in patients referred on an elective basis to a cardiac unit for suspected myocardial ischemia. Dig Dis Sci 1991;36:229–35.

11. Peters L, Maas L, Petty D, et al. Spontaneous noncardiac chest pain: evaluation by 24-hour ambulatory esophageal motility and pH monitoring. Gastroenterology 1988;94:878–86.

12. Soffer EE, Scalabrini P, Wingate DL. Spontaneous noncardiac chest pain: value of ambulatory esophageal pH and motility monitoring. Dig Dis Sci 1989;34:1651–5.

13. Vantrappen G, Janssens J, Ghillebert G. The irritable esophagus: a frequent cause of angina-like chest pain. Lancet 1987;1:1232–4.

14. Johnson DA, Winters C, Spurling TJ, et al. Esophageal acid sensitivity in Barrett's esophagus. J Clin Gastroenterol 1987;9:23–7.

15. Fass R, Yalam JM, Camargo L, et al. Increased esophageal chemoreceptor sensitivity to acid in patients after successful reversal of Barrett's esophagus. Dig Dis Sci 1997;42:1853–8.

16. Siddiqui MA, Johnston BT, Leite LP, et al. Sensitization of esophageal mucosa by prior acid infusion: effect of decreasing intervals between infusions. Am J Gastroenterol 1996;91:1745–8.

17. Koch KL, Davidson WR Jr, Day FP, et al. Esophageal dysfunction and chest pain in patients with mitral valve prolapse: a prospective study utilizing provocative testing during esophageal manometry. Am J Med 1989;86:32–8.

18. Hewson EG, Sinclair JW, Dalton CB, et al. Acid perfusion test: does it have a role in the assessment of non cardiac chest pain. Gut 1989;30:305–10.

19. Berezin S, Medow MS, Glassman M, Newman LJ. Use of the intraesophageal acid perfusion test in provoking nonspecific chest pain in children. J Pediatr 1989;115:709–12.

20. Hewson EG, Dalton CB, Hackshaw BT, et al. The prevalence of abnormal esophageal test results in patients with cardiovascular disease and unexplained chest pain. Arch Intern Med 1990;150:965–9.

21. Humeau B, Cloarec D, Simon J, et al. Pseudo-angina pain of esophageal origin. Results of functional study and value of the balloon distention test. Gastroenterol Clin Biol 1990;14:334–41.

22. Hewson EG, Sinclair JW, Dalton CB, Richter JE. Twenty-four-hour esophageal pH monitoring: the most useful test for evaluating noncardiac chest pain. Am J Med 1991;90:576–83.

23. Richter JE, Hewson EG, Sinclair JW, Dalton CB. Acid perfusion test and 24-hour esophageal pH monitoring with symptom index: comparison of tests for esophageal acid sensitivity. Dig Dis Sci 1991;36:565–71.

24. Rokkas T, Anggiansah A, McCullagh M, Owen WJ. Acid perfusion and edrophonium provocation tests in patients with chest pain of undetermined etiology. Dig Dis Sci 1992;37:1212–6.

25. Rose S, Achkar E, Easley KA. Follow-up of patients with noncardiac chest pain. Value of esophageal testing. Dig Dis Sci 1994;39:2063–8.

26. Mehta AJ, De Caestecker JS, Camm AJ, Northfield TC. Sensitization to painful distention and abnormal sensory perception in the esophagus. Gastroenterology 1995;108:311–9.

27. Ghillebert G, Janssens J, Vantrappen G. Esophageal testing in 287 patients with noncardiac chest pain: the Leuven experience [abstract]. Gastroenterology 1995;108:A605.

28. Frobert O, Funch-Jensen P, Bagger JP. Diagnostic value of esophageal studies in patients with angina-like chest pain and normal cornonary angiograms. Ann Intern Med 1996;124:959–69.

29. Klauser AG, Schindbeck NE, Muller-Lissner SA. Symptoms in gastroesophageal reflux disease. Lancet 1990;335:205–8.

30. Dalton CB, Hewson EG, Castell DO, Richter JE. Edrophonium provocation test in noncardiac chest pain. Dig Dis Sci 1990;35:1445–51.

31. Richter JE, Hackshaw BT, Wu WC, Castell DO. Edrophonium: a useful provocative test for esophageal chest pain. Ann Intern Med 1985;103:14–21.

32. Hollis JB, Castell DO. Effects of cholinergic stimulation on human esophageal peristalsis. J Appl Physiol 1976;40:40–3.

33. Lee CA, Reynolds JC, Ouyang A, et al. Esophageal chest pain: value of high dose provocative testing with edrophonium chloride in patients with normal manometrics. Dig Dis Sci 1987;32:682–8.

34. Gustafsson U, Tibling L. The effect of edrophonium chloride-induced chest pain on esophageal flow and motility. Scand J Gastroenterol 1997;32:104–7.

35. De Caestecker JS, Pryde A, Heading RC. Site and mechanism of pain perception with esophageal balloon distension and intravenous edrophonium in patients with esophageal chest pain. Gut 1992;33:580–6.

36. London RL, Ouyang A, Snape WJ Jr, et al. Provocation of esophageal pain by ergonovine or edrophonium. Gastroenterology 1981;81:10–4.

37. Katz PO, Dalton CB, Richter JE, et al. Esophageal resting of patients with noncardiac chest pain or dysphagia: results of three years' experience with 1161 patients. Ann Intern Med 1987;106:593–7.

38. Nasrallah SM, Hendrix EA. Comparison of hypertonic glucose to other provocative tests in patients with noncardiac chest pain. Am J Gastroenterol 1987;82:406–9.

39. Breumelhof R, Nadorp JH, Akkermans LM, Smout AJ. Analysis of 24-hour esophageal pressure and pH data in unselected patients with noncardiac chest pain. Gastroenterology 1990;99:1257–64.

40. Goudot-Pernot C, Champigneulle B, Bigard MA, et al. [A comparative prospective study of an edrophonium test and an esophageal balloon distension test in 78 patients with non-coronary angina and 12 healthy controls.] Ann Gastroenterol Hepatol (Paris) 1991;27:41–8.

41. Sengupta JN, Kauvar D, Goyal RK. Characteristics of vagal esophageal tension-sensitive afferent fibers in the opposum. J Neurophysiol 1989;61:1001–10.

42. Bayliss JH, Komitz R, Trounce JR. Observation on distension of the lower end of the esophagus. QJM 1955;94:143.

43. Richter JE, Barish CF, Castell DO. Abnormal sensory perception in patients with esophageal pain. Gastroenterology 1986;81:845.

44. Hazan S, Steinberg A, Morris N, et al. Long-term reproducibility of intraesophageal balloon distention studies in patients with unexplained chest pain [abstract]. Gastroenterology 1997;112:A145.

45. Lasch H, Devault KR, Castell DO. Intraesophageal balloon distention in the evaluation of sensory thresholds: studies on reproducibility and comparison of balloon composition. Am J Gastroenterol 1994;89:1185–90.

46. Lemann M, Dederding JP, Flourie B, et al. Abnormal perception of visceral pain in response to gastric distention in chronic idiopathic dyspepsia. The irritable stomach syndrome. Dig Dis Sci 1991;36:1249–54.

47. Ritchie J. Pain from distention of the pelvic colon by inflating a balloon in the irritable colon syndrome. Gut 1973;14:125–32.

48. Barish CF, Castell DO, Richter JE. Graded esophageal balloon distention. A new provocative test for noncardiac chest pain. Dig Dis Sci 1986;31:1292–8.

49. Deschner WK, Maher KA, Cattau EL Jr, Benjamin SB. Intraesophageal balloon distention versus drug provocation in the evaluation of noncardiac chest pain. Am J Gastroenterol 1990;85:938–43.

50. Clouse RE, McCord GS, Lustman PJ, Edmundowicz SA. Clinical correlates of abnormal sensitivity to intraesophageal balloon distension. Dig Dis Sci 1991;36:1040–5.

51. Gignoux C, Bost R, Hostein J, et al. Role of upper esophageal reflex and belch reflex dysfunctions in noncardiac chest pain. Dig Dis Sci 1993;38:1909–14.

52. Costantini M, Sturniolo GC, Zaninotto G, et al. Altered esophageal pain threshold in irritable bowel syndrome. Dig Dis Sci 1993;38: 206–12.

53. Gupta PK, Clauw DJ, Maher KA, et al. Patients with fibromyalgia have lowered thresholds of visceral nociception [abstract]. Am J Gastroenterol 1993;88:1488.

54. Nguyen P, Castell D. Evidence of gender differences in esophageal pain threshold. Am J Gastroenterol 1995;90:901–5.

55. Lasch H, Castell DO, Castell JA. Evidence for diminished visceral pain with aging: studies using graded intraesophageal balloon distention. Am J Physiol 1997;272:G1–3.

56. Ren J, Shaker R, Kusano M, et al. Effect of aging on the secondary esophageal peristalsis: presbyesophagus revisited. Am J Physiol 1995;268:G772–9.

57. Cannon RO, Quyyumi AA, Mincemoyer R, et al. Imipramine in patients with chest pain despite normal coronary angiograms. N Engl J Med 1994;330:1411–7.

58. Peghini P, Katz P, Castell D. Imipramine increases pain and sensation thresholds to esophageal balloon distension in humans [abstract]. Gastroenterology 1997;112:A255.

59. Hazan S, Buckley E, Castell DO, Achem SR. Octreotide improves sensory and pain thresholds in patients with noncardiac chest pain [abstract]. Gastroenterology 1996;110:A132.

60. Smout AJ, Devore MS, Dalton CB, Castell DO. Effects of nifedipine on esophageal tone and perception of esophageal distension. Dig Dis Sci 1992;37:598–602.

61. DeVault KR. Nifedipine does not alter barostat determined esophageal smooth muscle tone [abstract]. Gastroenterology 1995;108:A591.

62. Mayrand S, Diamant NE. Measurement of human esophageal tone in vivo. Gastroenterology 1993;105:1411–20.

63. Gonzalez M, Mearin F, Vasconez C, et al. Oesophageal tone in patients with achalasia. Gut 1997;41:291–6.

64. DeVault KR. Receptive relaxation of the human esophagus demonstrated with in vivo barostat testing [abstract]. Gastroenterology 1995;108:A591.

65. Rao SS, Gregerson H, Hayek B, et al. Unexplained chest pain: the hypersensitive, hyperreactive and poorly compliant esopahgus. Ann Intern Med 1996;124:950–8.

66. Pace F, Santalucia F, Bianchi PG. Natural history of gastroesophageal reflux disease without esophagitis. Gut 1991;32:845–8.

67. Schlesinger PK, Donahue PE, Schmidt B, Layden TJ. Limitations of 24 hour intraesophageal pH monitoring in the hospital setting. Gastroenterology 1985;89:797–804.

68. Murphy DW, Yuan Y, Castell DO. Does the intraesophageal pH probe accurately detect acid reflux? Simultaneous recording with two pH probes in humans. Dig Dis Sci 1989;34:649–56.

69. Trimble KC, Douglas S, Pryde A, Heading RC. Clinical characteristics and natural history of symptomatic but not excessive gastroesophageal reflux. Dig Dis Sci 1995;40:1098–104.

70. Watson RG, Tham TC, Johnston BT, McDougall NI. Double blind cross-over placebo controlled study of omeprazole in the treatment of patients with reflux symptoms and physiological levels of acid reflux—the sensitive esophagus. Gut 1997;40:587–90.

71. Tew S, Jamieson GG, Pilowski I, Myers J. The illness behavior of patients with gastroesophageal reflux disease with and without endoscopic esophagitis. Dis Esophagus 1997;10:9–15.

72. Johnsson F, Weywadt L, Sonhaug JN, et al. One-week omeprazole treatment in the diagnosis of gastro-oesopahgeal reflux disease. Scand J Gastroenterol 1998;33:15–20.

73. Katz PO, Codario R, Castell DO. Approach to the patient with unexplained chest pain. Compr Ther 1997;23:249–53.

74. Achem SR, DeVault KR. Recent developments in chest pain of undetermined origin. Curr Gastroenterol Rep 2000;2:201–9.

# CHAPTER 7

# Scintigraphy

*Alan H. Maurer, Henry P. Parkman and Robert S. Fisher*

## INDICATIONS

Esophageal motility disorders are most often diagnosed based on esophageal manometry, which measures contraction amplitude, peristalsis, and the pressures of the esophageal sphincters. Manometric recording requires tube placement and reflects pressure changes, not the bulk transit of solids or liquids in the esophagus. As manometry is invasive, it is inconvenient, particularly when repeat studies are desired to assess the response to a therapeutic intervention. An alternative technique for evaluating esophageal motility is videoesophagography. Both anatomic and functional information can be obtained from barium videoesophagography, but quantifying the volume of retained solids or liquids in the esophagus is difficult.

Given the limitations of both manometry and videoesophagography, other methods to assess esophageal motility have been sought. Esophageal transit scintigraphy (ETS) is an alternative, noninvasive test for assessing esophageal motor function that addresses some of the problems associated with manometry and barium studies. As many as 50% of patients with dysphagia and normal manometric and barium studies have been reported to demonstrate evidence of esophageal dysmotility with a radiolabeled solid bolus.[1]

Although ETS has been in use for over 25 years, indications for its use are still poorly defined. Early studies demonstrated a high sensitivity for detecting motility disorders,[2] but later studies reported low sensitivity, especially for disorders characterized by high-amplitude contractions or elevated lower esophageal sphincter (LES) pressures.[3,4] Using the methods described in this chapter, we have shown ETS to have similar sensitivity to videoesophagography for detecting achalasia, scleroderma, and nonspecific motor disorders but less sensitivity for detecting diffuse esophageal spasm (DES) and isolated LES dysfunction (Table 7.1).[5]

Esophageal transit scintigraphy is best used when serial, quantitative studies are required to assess response to a therapeutic intervention, manometric and barium studies are nondiagnostic, the expertise or facilities for manometry or videoesophagography are not available, or conflicting results are obtained with other tests.

**TABLE 7.1.** Sensitivity and Specificity of Esophageal Transit Scintigraphy and Videoesophagography Based on Manometric Diagnoses[*]

| | Sensitivity (%) | Specificity (%) | Positive Predictive Value (%) |
|---|---|---|---|
| **Esophageal transit scintigraphy** | | | |
| Achalasia | 91 | 98 | 95 |
| DES | 33 | 99 | 67 |
| Scleroderma | 75 | 99 | 75 |
| LES dysfunction | 25 | 99 | 67 |
| NSEMD | 71 | 76 | 48 |
| **Videoesophagography** | | | |
| Achalasia | 100 | 98 | 96 |
| DES | 67 | 100 | 100 |
| Scleroderma | 75 | 100 | 100 |
| LES dysfunction | 25 | 98 | 50 |
| NSEMD | 62 | 85 | 57 |

[*]Adapted from Parkman et al.[5]

DES, diffuse esophageal spasm; LES, lower esophageal sphincter; NSEMD, nonspecific esophageal motility disorder.

## TECHNIQUE

The patient is fasted, preferably overnight, or for at least 3 hours before beginning the study. Esophageal transit scintigraphy is recorded using a large field of view nuclear medicine camera that encompasses the distance from the oropharynx to the stomach within its field of view. A standard low-energy, all-purpose collimator is most commonly used to record the images. Since obtaining high counts for quantitation is more important than spatial resolution, a high-sensitivity, low-energy collimator, if available, is useful.

The nuclear medicine camera must be interfaced to a computer capable of dynamic (cine) image acquisition, generation of time-activity curves, and quantitative region-of-interest analysis. The computer must also be capable of playback of the cine images for physician review and interpretation. Today, such equipment is readily available in most nuclear medicine laboratories.

Because of its favorable energy (140 keV) and short half-life (6 hours), technetium 99m ($^{99m}$Tc)–labeled radiopharmaceuticals are used to perform ETS. These radiopharmaceuticals limit radiation exposures to values well below those received for similar fluoroscopic radiographic examinations (Table 7.2). Any radiopharmaceutical that is nonabsorbable within the gastrointestinal tract, such as $^{99m}$Tc-sulfur colloid (SC) or $^{99m}$Tc-diethylenetriamine pentaacetic acid (DTPA), can be used.

Numerous methods for performing and analyzing ETS have been proposed using solid, semisolid, and liquid boluses. For liquid boluses, the radiopharmaceutical is simply mixed with water. Ham and colleagues found transit to be faster for 10-mL boluses than for 20-mL boluses in the upright but not the supine position.[6] Tatsch and colleagues reported increased sensitivity for diagnosing a motility disorder when using a viscous medium of baby paste when compared to a liquid only.[7] For a more solid bolus, the radiopharmaceutical can easily be prepared in gelatin cubes.[8] We routinely use 200- to 300-µCi $^{99m}$Tc-SC in 15 mL of water per swallow. We acquire our images with the camera set on the 140-keV photopeak of $^{99m}$Tc with a 20% window.

The simplest measure of esophageal motility is the esophageal transit time (ETT) for a liquid or solid bolus to traverse the entire esophagus. The images are recorded using a 64 × 64 byte mode matrix. For most clinical studies, we prepare two swallows of 15 mL of water. There is considerable variability from swallow to swallow in both normal subjects and symptomatic patients. Barium studies have shown that up to five swallows are needed to maximize the sensitivity for detecting an abnormal swallow.[10] The desirability of using multiple swallows has similarly been confirmed for ETS.[7]

The camera may be positioned either anteriorly or posteriorly over the chest with the oropharynx at the upper edge of the field of view and the stomach at the lower edge. Posterior imaging is preferred to minimize attenuation effects from the heart as the bolus transits the distal esophagus.[11]

Before beginning the study, it is helpful to use a radioactive point source to confirm proper positioning. A mark is first placed at the mouth at the upper edge of the field of view and then at the stomach at the lower edge of the field of view to ensure that the entire esophagus is within the field of view of the camera. The patient's head is placed in either a left or right lateral position to minimize the camera-to-subject distance.

The patient should first perform a single practice swallow with unlabeled water. The patient is instructed to take up all of the liquid with a straw, hold it in the mouth, and then swallow on command.

Esophageal transit scintigraphy is then performed in two phases. Following a practice swallow, 15 mL of water mixed with $^{99m}$Tc-SC is taken again through a straw and held in the mouth. Immediately prior to giving the command to swallow, the computer-camera acquisition is started. The patient is then directed to perform a single swallow and then relax for 30 seconds, breathing through the mouth to avoid another swallow.

The computer is set to record the transit of the first single swallow using rapid imaging at 0.25 seconds per image for a total of 30 seconds. From these images, Russell and associates demonstrated that regional esophageal transit curves can be generated that appear similar to manometric tracings by dividing the esophagus into upper, middle, and lower thirds (Fig. 7.1A).[3] The time-activity curves do not represent pressure changes but rather the radioactive counts from the esophagus as the volume of the liquid traverses each region. The ETT is calculated from a single supine swallow (see Fig. 7.1A).

Thirty seconds after the initial swallow, the patient is then asked to perform serial dry swallows at 15- to 30-second intervals. Tolin and colleagues proposed analyzing the

**TABLE 7.2** Radiation Exposures*

| | Organ Dose (mrad) | | | | | | |
| Study | Stomach | Small Intestine | Upper Large Intestine | Lower Large Intestine | Ovaries | Testes | Whole Body |
|---|---|---|---|---|---|---|---|
| Esophageal transit | | | | | | | |
| 300-µCi $^{99m}$Tc-sulfur colloid | 28 | 83 | 160 | 97 | 29 | 2 | 5 |
| Gastric emptying | | | | | | | |
| 250-µCi $^{111}$In-DTPA | 110 | 490 | 1,100 | 2,000 | 420 | 27 | 60 |
| 500-µCi $^{99m}$Tc-sulfur colloid | 120 | 120 | 230 | 230 | 42 | 2 | 9 |

*Adapted from Siegel et al.[9]
Tc, technetium; In, indium; DTPA, diethylenetriamine pentaacetic acid.

counts remaining in the esophagus at the end of 10 minutes of repeated swallows.[12] To analyze this second phase of the study, an esophageal region of interest comprising the entire esophagus is defined for computer analysis (Fig. 7.1B). The total number of counts within the esophagus ($E_t$), is plotted as a percentage of the maximal number of counts ($E_{max}$) obtained during the initial swallow (see Fig. 7.1B). The per-

centage of esophageal retention at time (t) is given by the equation:

$$\% \text{ esophageal retention (t)} = E_t/E_{max} \times 100\%$$

The percentage of activity retained at the end of the 10 minutes (E10) can be used as an index of esophageal clear-

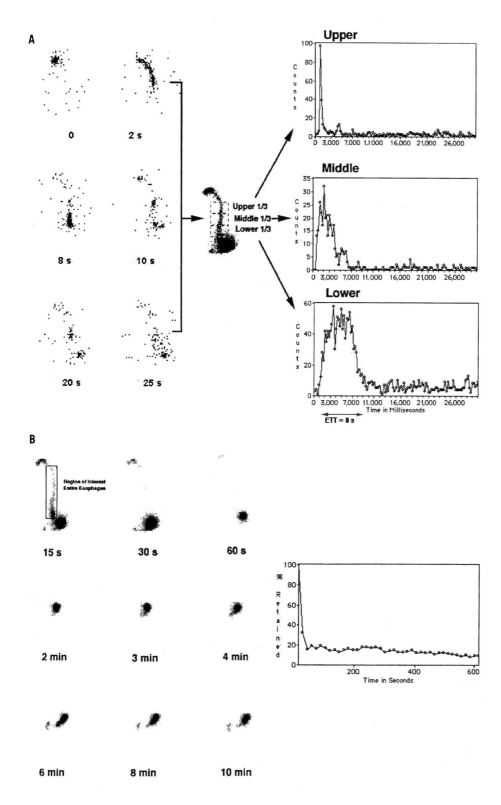

FIGURE 7.1. **A**, Normal esophageal transit scintigraphy: images and analysis. Normal regional esophageal transit (single swallow). Sample dynamic images (*left panel*) demonstrate normal, aboral progression of the bolus through the esophagus. A mild delay in the mid-esophagus at the level of the aortic arch (2-second image) that then clears rapidly may normally be seen. A composite image is produced by summing all of the images from the initial 30 seconds (*center panel*). The regions of interest (*dotted lines*) that define the upper, middle, and lower thirds of the esophagus are shown on a summed composite image. Time-activity curves (*right panel*) generated from these images show the counts recorded in each region as the bolus progresses down the esophagus. The width of the bolus curve increases in the distal third of the esophagus owing to the time required for relaxation of the LES. The esophageal transit time (ETT) (8 seconds) is measured using the leading edge (10% of peak in the upper) and the trailing edge (10% peak in the distal third) of the esophagus. **B**, Normal global esophageal clearance (multiple swallows). The images are reformatted in the computer as 15 seconds per image. Representative images are shown (*left panel*). In the initial 15-second summed image, a region of interest (rectangular box) is drawn to encompass the entire esophagus. From this region, a time-activity curve (*right panel*) is generated showing the percentage of activity retained in the esophagus for each time. The amount of activity retained at 10 minutes (E10) after multiple swallows can be used to characterize primary esophageal motor disorders (Fig. 7.2) or follow therapeutic intervention (Fig. 7.10).

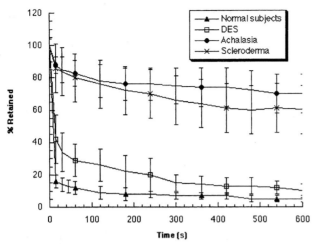

**FIGURE 7.2.** Esophageal clearance for the primary esophageal motility disorders. The mean data for normal subjects are shown compared with data for diffuse esophageal spasm (DES), achalasia, and scleroderma. Normal individuals show very rapid clearance with greater than 80% of the administered activity clearing the esophagus after the first swallow. Achalasia and scleroderma are indistinguishable using only a global clearance curve. They both show, in most cases, greater than 50% retention by the end of 10 minutes. Diffuse esophageal spasm shows mild retention up to 3 to 4 minutes, which then clears with continued swallows. Not shown are summary data on patients with gastroesophageal reflux. In general, the pattern of retention is similar to that of diffuse esophageal spasm. Quantitation of scintigraphic esophageal clearance should always be considered together with the results of a visual review of the dynamic images before coming to any conclusion on a final diagnosis (Table 7.3). Adapted from Tolin et al.[12]

ance. The primary esophageal motor disorders show either moderate to severe retention at 10 minutes (achalasia or scleroderma) or only mild retention (diffuse esophageal spasm) (Fig. 7.2). Patients with reflux esophagitis usually demonstrate either mild retention similar to DES or values intermediate with DES and achalasia or scleroderma (Fig. 7.3).

As gastroesophageal reflux (GER) is common and often associated with esophageal dysmotility, we routinely perform GER scintigraphy in all patients referred for ETS who are suspected of having GER. Following the ETS study, the patient drinks 300 μCi of $^{99m}$Tc-SC suspended in an additional 150 mL of orange juice that has been mixed with an equal volume of 0.1-N HCl.[13] The weak acidification decreases the LES pressure and delays gastric emptying, which increases the likelihood of detecting reflux. The patient is imaged in a supine position under a gamma camera, and an abdominal binder is used to increase abdominal pressures in 20-mm increments (0–100 mm Hg). At each level of binder pressure, computer images are recorded for 30 seconds. In normal individuals, no reflux of gastric contents is seen. In patients with GER, reflux can be seen (see Fig. 7.3C).

Some investigators favor summing the serial dynamic images from ETS into a single condensed image. For interested readers, an excellent review on this method has been published by Klein.[14] This method has the advantage of summarizing the study in a single image. However, proponents of the composite image acknowledge the importance of always reviewing the cine images as a movie on the computer screen.

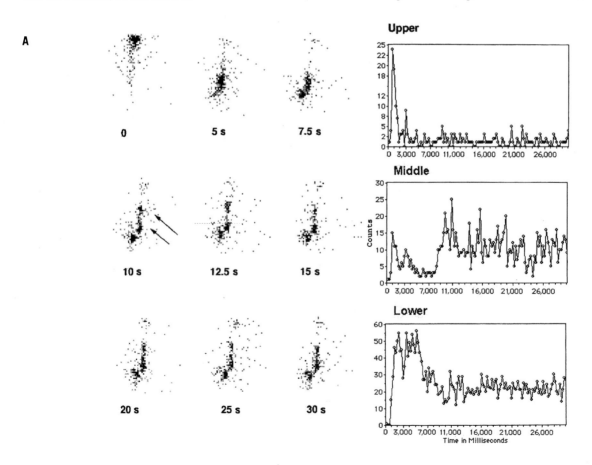

**B**

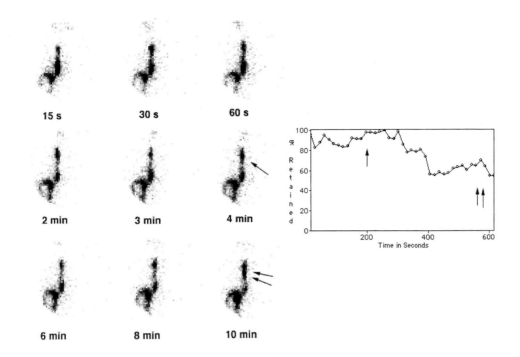

**C**

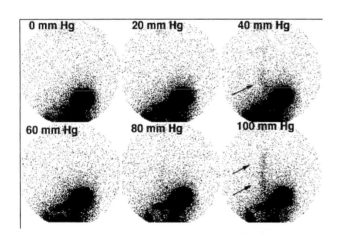

**FIGURE 7.3.** Reflux esophagitis. **A,** Dynamic single swallow—supine. The left panel images are selected frames from the initial single swallow. These images demonstrate retrograde movement of the bolus from the distal esophagus back up into the middle esophagus (*arrows*). In patients with nonspecific esophageal motility disorders, such retrograde contractions clear rapidly, but in patients with reflux esophagitis, there may be delayed clearance from the esophagus. The retrograde bolus movements can also be seen in the time-activity curve for the middle esophagus (*arrows*). **B,** Global clearance (multiple swallows)—supine. The images show retention in the middle and distal esophagus. Review of the multiple swallows in cine mode clearly identified several episodes of gastroesophageal reflux (*arrows*). The global clearance curve shows retention (E10 = 55%), which is at the high range of that typically seen with reflux esophagitis. **C,** Gastroesophageal reflux scintigraphy study. The initial image prior to inflation of the abdominal binder (0 mm Hg) shows no activity in the esophagus. With increasing abdominal binder pressure, mild reflux is seen at 40 mm Hg (*single arrow*). The activity clears, and a second, large reflux episode is seen at 100 mm Hg pressure (*double arrows*).

## RESULTS AND INTERPRETATION

Our approach to interpreting ETS includes reviewing all components of the study, including (1) visual, cinematic review of the bolus transit from the initial supine and erect swallows; (2) visual, cinematic review of the clearance of esophageal activity during the subsequent 10 minutes of swallowing, noting any episodes of GER (see Fig. 7.3B); (3) review of the time-activity curves generated from the upper, middle, and lower thirds of the esophagus and calculation of the ETT; and (4) calculation of the esophageal retention at 10 minutes (E10). Our diagnostic criteria for the major esophageal motor disorders based on this analysis are summarized in Table 7.3. With this approach, we have found good correlation with manometry (see Table 7.1). Using a similar approach, Blackwell and colleagues also demonstrated agreement between scintigraphy and manometry in 84% of patients.[15]

It is particularly important to review the cine images to appreciate normal variants. Some otherwise normal patients may show a prolonged ETT. This is most commonly caused by transient hang-up of the bolus from an enlarged left atrium or left ventricle compressing the esophagus. In these cases, the ETT may be prolonged, but there is an otherwise normal, smooth aboral progression of the bolus through the esophagus. Other patients may show transient antegrade and retrograde bolus movements in the mid- to distal esophagus followed by rapid clearance. These antegrade-retrograde bolus movements should be considered normal variants when the ETT and E10 values are also normal. When associated with an increase in the E10 or evidence of reflux, these may be attributable to localize reflux esophagitis or (in the absence of any reflux) a nonspecific motility disorder.

**TABLE 7.3.** Diagnostic Criteria for Interpreting Esophageal Transit Scintigraphy

| | Single Swallow ETT (s) | Esophageal Retention at 10 Min (%) | Visual Review | |
|---|---|---|---|---|
| | | | Single-Swallow Images and Curves | Multiple Swallows Over 10 Min |
| Normal | ≤ 14 | ≤ 18 | Normal aboral progression of bolus in upper, middle, and lower thirds of esophagus; may see 1–2 mild retrograde/antegrade bolus movements that clear quickly; smooth transition across LES | Rapid progressive clearance of activity from esophagus; may see mild focal retention at mid-esophagus (level of aortic arch); no visualization of GER during successive swallows |
| Achalasia | > 30 | > 50 | Aperastaltic esophagus; may see normal bolus movement in upper third of esophagus from oropharyngeal push, severe delay in transit mild and distal thirds; no improvement in upright position | Severe retention in mid- to distal third of esophagus; may have typical bird's peak appearance, no GER episodes |
| Scleroderma | > 30 | 18 ≥ E10 ≤ 30 | Normal bolus movement in upper third of esophagus; delay in transit in mid and distal thirds in supine position that significantly improves with upright swallow | Moderate to severe retention in mid- and distal thirds of esophagus in supine position that clears significantly with upright swallow; GER episodes variably seen |
| Diffuse esophageal spasm | > 14 | 18 ≥ E10 ≤ 30 | Repetitive retrograde/antegrade transit throughout entire esophagus; because of intermittent nature may need to perform > 2 swallows to detect or use a semisolid bolus | Usually normal; may see mild retention |
| Lower esophageal sphincter dysfunction | 14 | ≤ 30 | Normal transit in upper and mid-esophagus with localized delay in transit across LES; difficult to differentiate from normal when only mild elevation in ETT (15–16 s) | Usually normal; may see mild retention; no GER episodes |
| NSEMD | > 14 | ≤ 30 | Localized episodes of abnormal retrograde/ antegrade transit in ≥ 2 swallows; difficult to differentiate from normals; use of semisolid/solid bolus may be helpful[17] | May see mild retention |
| Reflux/ esophagitis | > 20 | ≤ 30 | Normal transit in upper and mid-esophagus with mild delay in distal third of esophagus | Mild retention in distal esophagus; may see 1 or more spontaneous reflux episodes |

ETT, esophageal transit time; GER, gastroesophageal reflux; LES, lower esophageal sphincter; NSEMD, nonspecific esophageal motility disorder.

We routinely analyze a minimum of two swallows: the first is upright and the second is supine. Quantification is performed only on the supine swallow to avoid the effect of gravity. If there is significant retention in the first upright swallow, the patient can be given multiple sips of unlabeled water to clear residual activity before proceeding to the supine swallow. An improvement in regional transit and global retention in the erect position compared to the supine is most helpful to differentiate achalasia (no significant change with position) (Fig. 7.4) from scleroderma, which improves when the patient is upright (Fig. 7.5).

Normal values for ETT have been determined by several investigators and appear to be reproducible. Kazem reported a normal ETT of a single swallow of 10 to 20 mL of water as up to 8 seconds, with an observed delay in the distal esophagus of up to 5 seconds for relaxation of the LES.[2] Russell and associates[3] and Blackwell and associates[15] reported similar values of 7.2 ± 1.7 and 7.3 ± 2.3 (mean ± SD) seconds, respectively. Holloway and coworkers reported a slightly longer normal ETT of 9.6 seconds (with a range of 6–15 seconds).[4] Our normal ETT for a supine swallow is 9.3 ± 2.1 seconds (upper limit of normal = 13.5 seconds, mean + 2 SD).[5]

Russell and colleagues found prolonged radionuclide ETT in 100% of patients with dysphagia and abnormal manometric findings. Of greater interest was the fact that 9 (64%) of 14 patients with dysphagia and normal manometric findings had abnormal esophageal transit detected with ETS.[3] Our results in diagnosing the major esophageal motility disorders based simply on measurement of ETT alone are summarized in Figure 7.6.

By analyzing the global retention at 10 minutes after multiple swallows (E10), Tolin and colleagues reported 100% sensitivity for detecting primary motor disorders and good separation of the primary motor disorders based on the severity of impaired clearance (see Fig. 7.2).[12] Our normal value for E10 is 11.3 ± 3.5% (upper limit of normal = 18.3%, mean + 2 SD). Using a similar analysis, Klein has reported an upper limit of normal of 19.8%.[14] Our results for diagnosing the major esophageal motility disorders based only on measurement of E10 are shown in Figure 7.7.

Esophageal transit scintigraphy is less sensitive than manometry for disorders characterized by high-amplitude progressive contractions. Styles and coworkers reported a

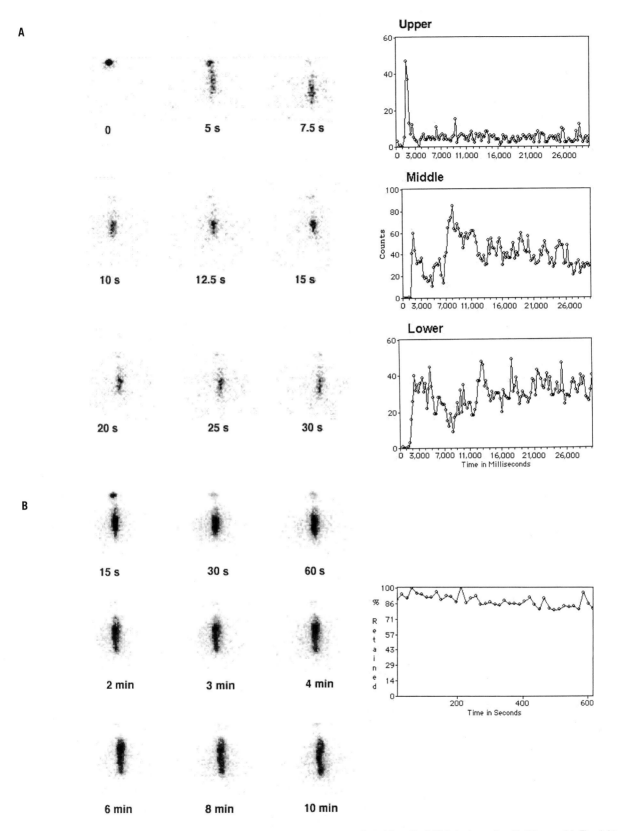

**FIGURE 7.4. A**, Achalasia. Dynamic single swallow. The *left panel* images are selected from the initial single swallow (0–30 seconds). The right side curves show the resulting time-activity curves for regions of interest placed over the upper, middle, and lower thirds of the esophagus. In achalasia, the oropharynx propels the bolus through the upper third, and transit may appear normal. The curves then demonstrate poor bolus transit owing to aperistalsis in the middle and distal thirds. **B**, Achalasia–global clearance (multiple swallows). The *left panel* images show marked retention in the middle to distal esophagus (1–10 minutes) with no passage of activity through the LES. The clearance curve shows marked retention with 85% of administered activity in the esophagus at 10 minutes. There was no improvement in esophageal emptying when the patient was imaged upright.

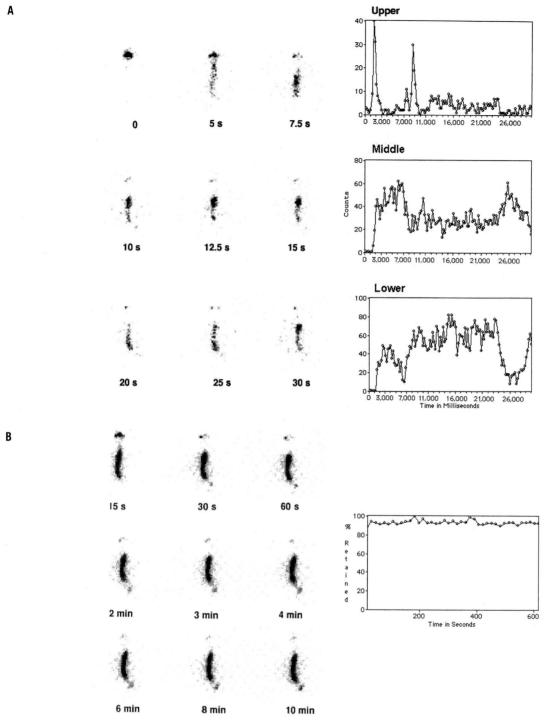

**FIGURE 7.5.** Scleroderma. Dynamic single swallow—supine. The *left panel* images are selected from the initial single swallow (0–30 seconds). The curve on the right shows the resulting time-activity curves for regions of interest placed over the upper, middle, and lower thirds of the esophagus. There is normal initial bolus transit through the upper third of the esophagus. An incidental retrograde contraction from the middle esophagus back into the upper third occurs at 8 seconds. The curves then demonstrate delayed bolus transit owing to decreased peristalsis in the middle and distal thirds of the esophagus. This pattern, supine, is similar to that seen with achalasia (see Fig. 7.4A). **B**, Global clearance (multiple swallows)—supine. The *left panel* images show marked retention in the middle to distal esophagus (1–10 minutes) with no passage of activity through the LES into the stomach. The global clearance curve shows marked retention with 95% of administered activity in the esophagus at 10 minutes. This pattern is indistinguishable from achalasia in the supine position. **C**, Dynamic single swallow—upright. The *left panel* images are selected from a single swallow (0–30 seconds) from the same patient in **A** repeated upright. The curves on the right show marked improvement in the upper, middle, and lower thirds of the esophagus. This change to more normal transit upright is typical of that seen in scleroderma. As the disease progresses, there may be residual delay in transit upright, but, in general, transit significantly improves when compared with the supine swallow. **D**, Global clearance from multiple swallows—supine. The *left panel* images, repeated in this same patient, show marked improvement (E10 = 95%) when the patient is supine, which improves (E10 = 20%) in the upright position. This improvement in the upright position is characteristic of scleroderma.

C

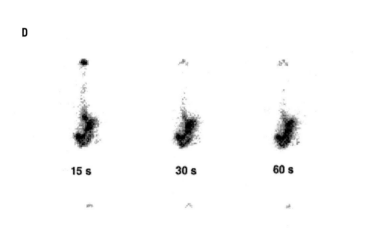

Upper

Middle

Lower

Time in Milliseconds

D

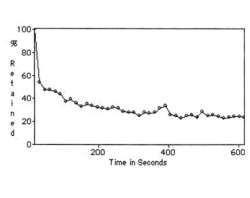

Time in Seconds

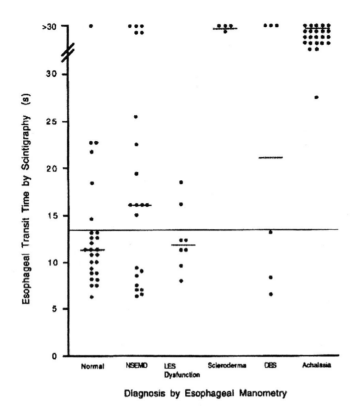

**FIGURE 7.6.** Esophageal transit time (ETT) versus manometric diagnoses. Normal and individual patient values of ETT are plotted grouped according to the patients' final manometric diagnoses. Reproduced with permission from Parkman HP, Maurer AH, Caroline DF, et al. Optimal evaluation of patients with nonobstructive esophageal dysphagia: manometry, scintigraphy, or video-esophagography. Dig Dis Sci 1996;41:1355–68. These data show that a single measurement of ETT is not helpful for making the diagnosis of a specific esophageal motor disorder. Similar to the measurement of global clearance (Fig. 7.2), achalasia and scleroderma tend to show the largest delay in transit with most patients having an ETT of greater than 30 seconds. The results for diffuse esophageal spasm (DES), lower esophageal sphincter (LES) dysfunction, and nonspecific esophageal motility disorders (NSEMD) are more variable. Just as with scintigraphic measurement of esophageal clearance, quantitation of ETT must be considered together with the results of a visual review of dynamic images before making any conclusion on a final diagnosis (Table 7.3).

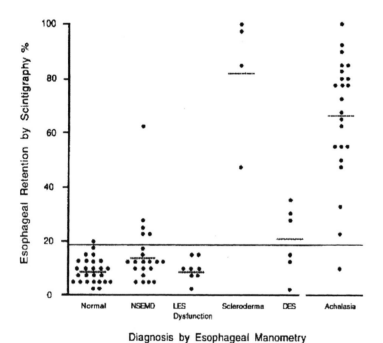

**FIGURE 7.7.** Esophageal retained activity at 10 minutes (E10) versus manometric diagnoses. The individual patient values for E10 are plotted grouped according to the patients' final manometric diagnoses. Reproduced with permission from Parkman HP, Maurer AH, Caroline DF, et al. Optimal evaluation of patients with nonobstructive esophageal dysphagia: manometry, scintigraphy, or videoesophagography. Dig Dis Sci 1996;41:1355–68. These more recent data show results similar to that in Fig. 7.2 and include the findings of patients with nonspecific esophageal motility disorders (NSEMD) and lower esophageal dysfunction (LES). Achalasia and scleroderma again show the greatest amount of retention. There is no significant retention in LES and considerable overlap with normals in NSEMD and DES.

---

**FIGURE 7.8.** Diffuse esophageal spasm (DES). **A**, Dynamic single swallow—supine. The representative cine images shown do not demonstrate as dramatically the multiple antegrade and retrograde contractions that occur in DES, which are better appreciated in viewing the images as a movie on the computer screen. The regional transit curves also help to demonstrate the to and fro movements of the bolus (seen as multiple peaks) as the bolus moves antegrade and retrograde within the esophagus. **B**, Global clearance (multiple swallows)—supine. Despite the marked antegrade and retrograde movement of the bolus within the esophagus, the clearance (E10 = 3%) is normal.

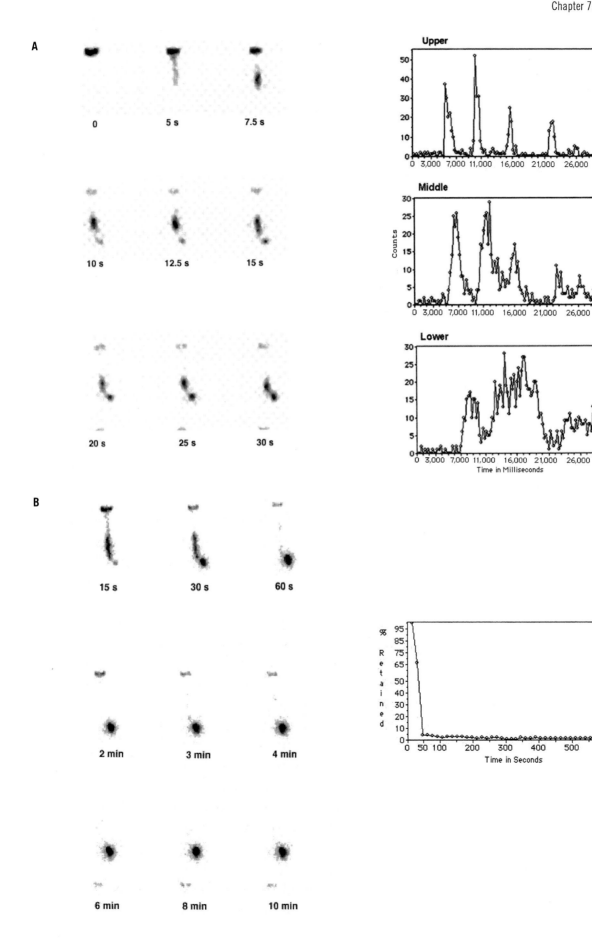

**A**

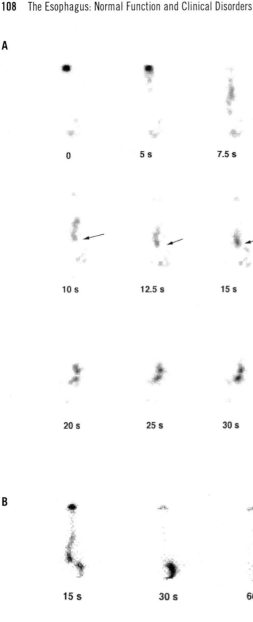

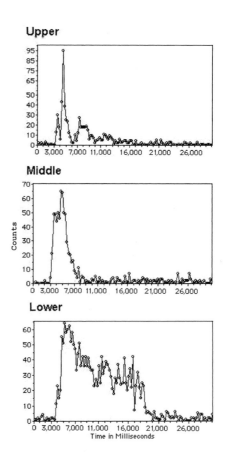

**Upper**

**Middle**

Counts

**Lower**

Time in Milliseconds

**B**

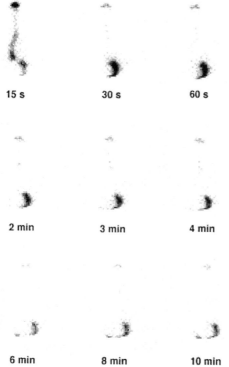

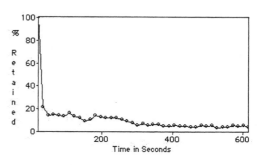

% Retained

Time in Seconds

**FIGURE 7.9.** Hypertensive LES. **A**, Dynamic single swallow—supine. The *left panel* images are selected images from the initial single swallow. The curves on the right show normal initial bolus transit through the upper and middle thirds of the esophagus. There is slowing of transit across the lower esophageal sphincter (*arrow*), resulting in prolongation of the ETT (16 seconds). **B**, Global clearance (multiple swallows)—supine. The *left panel* images show early retention within the esophagus, which clears within 3 to 4 minutes. The clearance curve confirms only mild retention at 3 to 4 minutes and a normal E10 of 4% at 10 minutes.

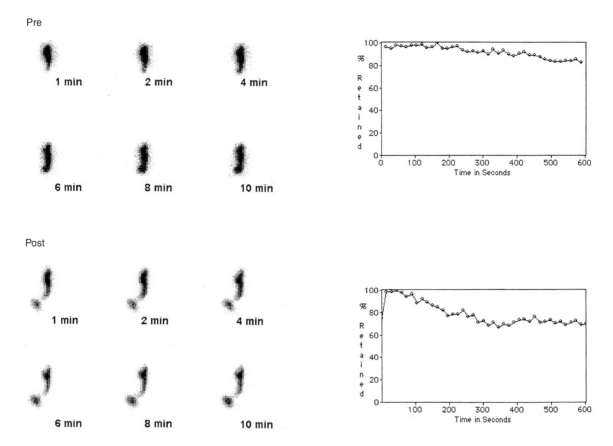

**FIGURE 7.10.** Achalasia pre and post therapy. Pretherapy summed, multiple swallow images (1–10 min) are shown (*top*) as well as the corresponding esophageal clearance curve for a 52-year-old male with achalasia. Prior to dilatation there was 84% retained at 10 minutes. The patient underwent treatment with pneumatic balloon dilation of the LES. Post dilatation his symptoms were difficult to evaluate, so repeat ETS was performed (*bottom*). The images and curves confirmed incomplete dilatation with 72% retention at 10 minutes. Based on the results of quantitative ETS, the patient underwent repeat dilation with subsequent improvement in symptoms.

correlation between ETS and manometry in only 22 (52%) of 42 patients with dysphagia and high-amplitude contractions. There was disagreement in 6 (14%) patients and equivocal studies in 14 (33%) patients.[16] Only a measure of ETT was used in that study. Drane and colleagues evaluated ETT and the percentage of retained esophageal activity. They found that the results of scintigraphy agreed with manometry in 13 (81%) of 16 patients with high distal esophageal pressure greater than 120 mm Hg but in only 3 (20%) of 15 patients with pressures less than 120 mm Hg.[17]

Similar to the above, we found the lowest sensitivities for ETS in detecting diffuse esophageal spasm and isolated LES dysfunction (see Table 7.1). When present, the diffuse nature of the abnormalities seen in DES during the cine imaging of the single swallow is similar to that of manometry (Fig. 7.8A). There is usually no significant retention seen in the global clearance (Fig. 7.8B) (See also Figs. 7.2 and 7.7). As DES may occur intermittently, it is helpful to use more than two swallows or to use a semisolid (gelatin) when performing ETS, especially when there is a clinical suspicion of DES.[17] In isolated LES dysfunction, there may be only a mild increase in ETT. Visually, this is characterized by slowing of the bolus

when passing through the LES (Fig. 7.9A). The global clearance curve will usually show some mild retention early but no significant retention by 10 minutes (Fig. 7.9B). As with DES, it may be helpful to use more that two swallows or to use additional swallows with a sold or semisolid to detect this.

Nonspecific esophageal motility disorders are characterized by one or more minor manometric abnormalities. Mughal and coworkers concluded that ETS is not useful as a screening test for esophageal dysmotility because of the high prevalence of nonspecific esophageal motility disorders and low sensitivity for detecting this disorder.[19]

The ease with which ETS can be used to quantitate esophageal emptying makes it an important tool for assessing the response to therapeutic interventions, particularly in achalasia (Fig. 7.10). Treatment of achalasia is usually directed at lowering pressures of the LES by mechanical dilation or surgery. It has been shown that measurement of LES pressures is not sufficient to determine the response to treatment because patients may report subjective improvement while emptying abnormalities persist.[20,21] The effect of drugs such as nifedipine and isosorbide dinitrate has also been studied with ETS in achalasia and DES.[22,23]

## CONCLUSIONS

Sensitivity for detecting abnormal esophageal motility with ETS can be maximized if multiple criteria are used for interpretation including visual analysis of the bolus transit and quantification of ETT and esophageal retention (E10). It is important to play back and visually review in a cine loop a dynamic display of the swallows. Although most studies have relied on analysis of a single swallow, up to five swallows may be needed to achieve good correlation with the results of manometry. Use of both liquid and solid or semisolid boluses can be helpful. Use of ETS will vary depending on local experience and expertise, but its ability to quantitatively assess the response to therapy remains one of its most useful applications.

### REFERENCES

1. Kjellen G, Svedberg JB, Tibbling L. Solid bolus transit by esophageal scintigraphy in patients with dysphagia and normal manometry and radiography. Dig Dis Sci 1984;29:1–5.
2. Kazem I. A new scintigraphic technique for the study of the esophagus. AJR Am J Roentgenol 1972;115:681–8.
3. Russell COH, Hill LD, Holmes ER, et al. Radionuclide transit: a sensitive screening test for esophageal dysfunction. Gastroenterology 1981;80:887–92.
4. Holloway RH, Lange RC, Plankey MW, McCallum RW. Detection of esophageal motor disorders by radionuclide transit studies, a reappraisal. Dig Dis Sci 1989;34:905–12.
5. Parkman HP, Maurer AH, Caroline DF, et al. Optimal evaluation of patients with nonobstructive esophageal dysphagia: manometry, scintigraphy, or videoesophagography? Dig Dis Sci 1996;41:1355–68.
6. Ham HR, Piepsz A, Georges B, et al. Quantitation of esophageal transit by means of 81m Kr. Eur J Nucl Med 1984;9:362–5.
7. Tatsch K, Schroettle W, Kirsch C. A multiple swallow test for the quantitative and qualitative evaluation of esophageal motility disorders. J Nucl Med 1991;32:1365–70.
8. Kjellen G, Svedberg JS. Oesophageal transit of a radionuclide solid bolus in normals. Clin Physiol 1983;3:69–74.
9. Siegel J, Wu RK, Knight L, et al. Radiation dose estimates for oral agents used in upper gastrointestinal disease. J Nucl Med 1983;24:835–7.
10. Ott DJ, Chen YM, Hewson EG, et al. Esophageal motility: assessment with synchronous video tape fluoroscopy and manometry. Radiology 1989;173:419–22.
11. Klein HA. The effect of projection in esophageal transit scintigraphy. Clin Nucl Med 1990;15:157–62.
12. Tolin RD, Malmud LS, Reillely J, Fisher RS. Esophageal scintigraphy to quantitate esophageal transit (quantitation of esophageal transit). Gastroenterology 1979;76:1402–8.
13. Fisher RS, Malmud LS, Roberts GS, Lobis IF. Gastroesophageal (GE) scintiscanning to detect and quantitate GE reflux. Gastroenterology 1976;70:301–8.
14. Klein HA. Esophageal transit scintigraphy. Semin Nucl Med 1995;25:306–17.
15. Blackwell JN, Hannan WJ, Adam RD, Heading RC. Radionuclide transit studies in the detection of esophageal dysmotility. Gut 1983;24:421–6.
16. Styles CB, Holt S, Bowes KL, Hooper R. Esophageal transit scintigraphy—a cautionary note. J Can Assoc Radiol 1984;35:31–3.
17. Drane WE, Johnson DA, Hagan DP, Cattau EL. "Nutcracker" esophagus: diagnosis with radionuclide esophageal scintigraphy versus manometry. Radiology 1987;163:33–7.
18. Jadali F, Charkes N, Parkman H, et al. Is a semi-solid swallow a better test of esophageal transit than multiple liquid swallows [abstract]? J Nucl Med 1993;34:169P.
19. Mughal MM, Marples M, Bancewicz J. Scintigraphic assessment of oesophageal motility: what does it show and how reliable is it? Gut 1986;27:946–53.
20. VanTrappen G, Helleman J. Treatment of achalasia and related motor disorders. Gastroenterology 1980;79:144–54.
21. Pope CE. Is LES enough? Gastroenterology 1976;71:328–9.
22. Rozen P, Gelfond M, Zaltzman S, et al. Dynamic, diagnostic, and pharmacological radionuclide studies of the esophagus in achalasia. Radiology 1982;144:587–90.
23. McCallum RW. Radionuclide scanning in esophageal disease. J Clin Gastroenterol 1982;4:67–70.

# CHAPTER 8

# Ultrasonography

*Ravinder K. Mittal and Jianmin Liu*

A number of techniques are currently available to assess the anatomic structure and physiologic functions of the esophagus. These techniques provide information on different aspects of esophageal function. Each of these techniques has strengths and limitations. A barium swallow study of the esophagus, for example, is an important test to determine the gross intraluminal anatomy and motor function of the esophagus. It is a reasonable test to grossly determine the mucosal defect, intraluminal patency, distensibility of the esophagus, esophageal peristalsis, impaired relaxation of the lower esophageal sphincter (LES), transit of a liquid, semiliquid, and solid bolus. Its weakness, however, is that it does not provide information on the fine details of the mucosal abnormalities and does not quantitate the esophageal motor function. The latter is best assessed by esophageal manometry or a pressure recording technique. Manometry, on the other hand, does not provide any information on the anatomy of the esophagus. Radionuclide scintigraphy is probably the best test for quantitation of the transit of liquid bolus. In recent years, a number of other tests have also been used to assess other physiologic functions of the esophagus; for example, the esophageal mucosal potential difference is a test of the integrity of the esophageal mucosa. Impedance planimetry and esophageal barostat can quantitate the compliance and distensibility of the esophagus.

This chapter summarizes the novel and available information on the role of ultrasonography, the newest test available in the assessment of esophageal anatomy, physiology, and pathophysiology. Ultrasonography of the esophagus yields unique information on the muscular anatomy and motor function of the esophagus. Ultrasonographic methods in the assessment of esophageal function have been used since the late 1980s. Two ultrasonographic techniques are currently in use: endoscopic ultrasonography and probe ultrasonography.

In the endoscopic ultrasonography technique, the ultrasound transducer is mounted on the end of an endoscope, and this transducer provides either linear or circumferential cross-sectional images depending on the rotation of the transducer. Earlier studies using this technique focused on the muscle thickness in patients with achalasia of the esophagus compared to normal subjects. Since the endoscope is relatively large in diameter, it cannot be placed into the esophagus for extended periods of time. The probe ultrasonography technique uses a small transducer, which is mounted on a small-diameter catheter, ranging from 1 to 3 mm in size (Fig. 8.1). These catheters are fairly long and thus can be placed transnasally into the esophagus for extended periods of time. We have successfully performed up to 24 hours of continuous recordings of the esophagus and stomach using the probe ultrasonography technique. Since the catheters are relatively small, the technique can be combined with manometry and pH measurements and has the potential to provide important physiologic and pathophysiologic information on the function of the esophagus. Furthermore, the information gained by ultrasonography can be compared with concurrently recorded information from the manometry and pH recordings.

The technique of miniature ultrasonography in the assessment of esophageal motility was first introduced by Tanaguchi and his colleagues at the University of Washington, Seattle. They used M mode ultrasonography and a miniature ultra-

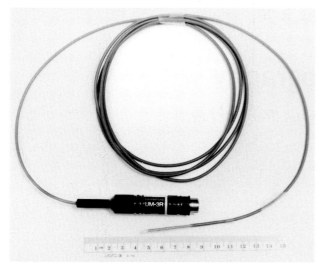

**FIGURE 8.1.** A 20-MHz probe ultrasound catheter (Olympus).

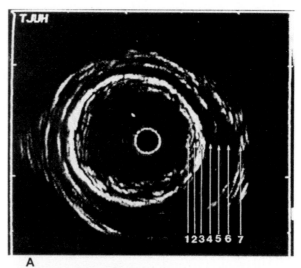

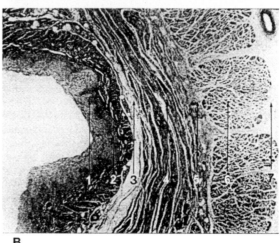

**FIGURE 8.2.** **A**, A cross-sectional sonogram was taken from the distal fluid-filled esophagus of an autopsy specimen in a patient who died of nongastrointestinal-related disease. The first hypoechoic layer represents the mucosa, including the squamous epithelium and lamina propria. The second thin hyperechoic layer represents the muscularis mucosa. The third very bright hyperechoic layer represents the submucosa. The fourth hypoechoic layer represents the circular smooth muscle. The fifth thin hyperechoic layer represents the intermuscular connective tissue. The sixth hypoechoic layer represents the longitudinal smooth muscle. The seventh hyperechoic layer represents the adventitia. **B**, Esophageal histologic section taken at the same level as the image in **A**. All histologic layers correspond with the sonographic layers: 1, mucosa; 2, muscularis mucosae; 3, submucosa; 4, circular smooth muscle; 5, intermuscular connective tissue; 6, longitudinal smooth muscle; 7, adventitia.

sound transducer mounted on a suction catheter to record simultaneous pressure and sonograms. Later, Miller and his colleagues provided a significant amount of information on the baseline anatomy of the esophagus, first in normal subjects and then in patients with achalasia and scleroderma of the esophagus, using probes that rotated 360 degrees and provided cross-sectional images of the esophagus. They also reported the use of simultaneous intraluminal manometry and ultrasonography to determine the temporal relationship between esophageal pressure and changes in muscle thickness. They discovered that changes in the muscle thickness during esophageal contraction correlated in a close temporal relationship with the changes in intraluminal pressure. The increase in muscle thickness of the longitudinal and circular muscles of the esophagus paralleled the increase in pressure and peak thickness correlated with the peak pressure. Since 1994, our group has used this technique in a creative fashion to provide unique information related to the esophageal motor function in health and disease.

This chapter summarizes our ultrasonographic data as well as data from the laboratories of other investigators. We summarize the use of this technique in the study of the physiology of the esophagus and the pathophysiology of various primary esophageal motility disorders. Our observations suggest that this technique is able to identify motor events that may be the cause of esophageal chest pain and heartburn sensation. We speculate that in this millennium, probe ultrasonography will become a powerful tool in the hands of both research and clinical esophagologists to study unique aspects of the esophageal anatomy, physiology, and pathophysiology.

## TECHNIQUE

Probe sonograms were initially developed to study the intravascular anatomy of the coronary blood vessels, specifically the anatomy of the atheromatous plaques. Their use in the gastrointestinal tract was first directed toward its use through the biopsy channel of an endoscope. Miller and col-

leagues were the first to advocate its use as a transnasal ultrasonographic technique. These ultrasound probe catheters are available in different diameters (1–3 mm) and various lengths (95–200 cm) (see Fig. 8.1). The ultrasound frequency of the transducers currently available ranges from 7.5 to 30 MHz. A higher-frequency transducer has a lesser depth of penetration but the ability to provide details of the structures in the field of view. The depth of penetration of 20 MHz is approximately 2 cm, somewhat less with 30 MHz and greater with 7.5, 12, and 15 MHz.

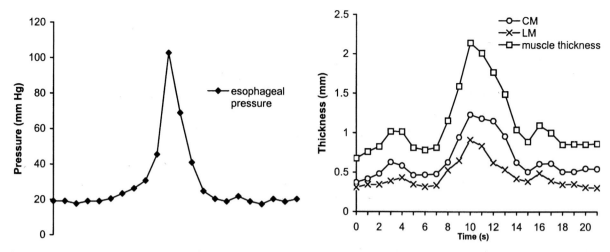

**FIGURE 8.3.** Temporal correlation between intraluminal pressure change and ultrasonographic muscle thickness during a swallow-induced contraction. Sonograms, esophageal pressure, and muscle thickness during a 5-mL water swallow are shown. Before the swallow, the esophageal muscle is thin and the cross-sectional configuration is oblong. During contraction , there is thickening of the muscular wall. The increase in intraluminal pressure is associated with an increase in thickness of both the circular and longitudinal muscles. LM, longitudinal muscle; S, intermuscular septum; CM, circular muscle; US, ultrasound probe; M, mucosa.

These high-frequency probes can provide either linear or cross-sectional images. To obtain the cross-sectional images, the transducer rotates 360 degrees at a speed of 12 to 20 rotations per second. Different layers of the esophagus can be seen on these images; for example, using a 12- or 20-MHz transducer, seven different layers of the esophagus are seen. From the luminal to the serosal surface, these layers are mucosa, submucosa, muscularis mucosa, circular muscle layer, intermuscular septum, longitudinal muscle layer, and adventitia of the esophagus (Fig. 8.2). The anatomy of these layers, especially the two layers of the muscularis propria, changes in a dynamic fashion with muscle contraction. Since images can be recorded in real time at a speed of 12 to 20 frames/second, the ultrasound technique provides a unique way to study the anatomy and physiology of the esophagus. The principle that allows study of the muscle function of the esophagus using this technique is that there is an increase in the thickness of both circular and longitudinal muscle layers during contraction and peristalsis. Detailed analysis of the images along with concurrent pressure recordings reveals that there is a close temporal correlation between the changes in circular and longitudinal muscle thickness and the increase in intraluminal pressure (Fig. 8.3). In fact, it appears that the muscle thickening starts approximately 200 milliseconds earlier than the increase in intraluminal esophageal pressure. Does the increase in thickness of the circular muscle represent contraction of the circular muscle layer, or is it the result of an active contraction of the longitudinal muscle layer? Although we still do not know for sure, the law of mass conservation may suggest that the increase in circular muscle thickness can occur as a result of the contraction of the longitudinal muscle layer. The latter may explain why, in some situations (eg, during a sustained esophageal contraction associated with chest pain and heartburn), the increase in the thickness of circular and longitudinal muscle layers can be seen without any increase in the intraluminal pressure. A

sustained esophageal contraction (SEC) may thus represent a contraction of the longitudinal muscle.

## LOWER ESOPHAGEAL SPHINCTER

The geometric shape, muscle thickness, and opening of the LES during relaxation can be assessed from sonograms and reveal important physiologic information about its function. Studies related to the opening of the LES are in progress; therefore, these data are not presented in this chapter. Data are available on the thickness of the muscle and the geometric shape of the LES. Several studies show that both circular and longitudinal muscles of the LES are much thicker than the respective muscle layers of the esophagus (Fig. 8.4, Table 8.1). This is expected since the LES muscle maintains a higher basal or continuous tone compared with the esophageal muscle. The muscle thickness of the two layers of the muscularis propria in normal subjects and patients with achalasia of the esophagus is shown in Table 8.2. The LES muscle thickness is not fixed in a given subject; it increases and decreases in parallel with the increase and decrease in the LES pressure (Fig. 8.5). Atropine, for instance, decreases LES pressure and muscle thickness (Fig. 8.6). During a swallow-induced LES relaxation, the thickness of both circular and longitudinal muscles first decreases and then increases as the LES pressure decreases and increases, respectively. Following relaxation, a

**TABLE 8.1.** Esophageal Muscle Thickness in Normal Subjects (N = 11)

|  | Circular Muscle (mm) | Longitudinal Muscle (mm) | Total Thickness (mm) | p Value |
|---|---|---|---|---|
| LES | 1.09 ± 0.06 | 0.60 ± 0.03 | 1.69 ± 0.09 | .0001 |
| Esophagus | 0.76 ± 0.05 | 0.49 ± 0.03 | 1.25 ± 0.08 | .001 |

LES, lower esophageal sphincter.

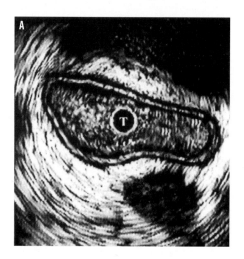
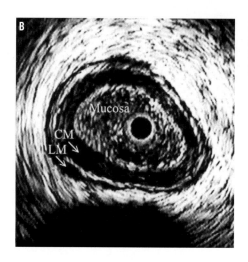

**FIGURE 8.4.** Sonograms of the body of the esophagus (**A**) and the LES (**B**). T, transducer; CM, circular muscle; LM, longitudinal muscle.

normal LES shows a powerful contraction, which is referred to as a post-relaxation hypercontraction. During this contraction, the LES muscle is markedly thicker, and the LES is geometrically circular in shape. The geometric shape of the LES changes in a dynamic fashion along with the changes in pressure. In the resting or baseline state, the LES is not circular; its shape varies markedly, from oval to eclipse, from one indi-

vidual to the other (Fig. 8.7). In a given individual, the asymmetry in shape also changes along with the changes in pressure. The asymmetry in the shape of the LES is the reason for the circumferential asymmetry of the LES pressure. The asymmetry of the pressure decreases markedly during periods of post-relaxation hypercontraction when its shape is also relatively geometrically symmetric and circular (Fig. 8.8). The LES muscle thickness is markedly thicker in achalasia of the esophagus (Fig. 8.9) and in some patients with diffuse esophageal spasm and nutcracker esophagus. Whether this increase in thickness represents an increase in muscle tone or hypertrophy of the LES musculature is not yet clear.

**TABLE 8.2.** Comparison of Mean Esophageal Muscle Width: Achalasia versus Control Subjects

|  | CSM | LSM | TM |
|---|---|---|---|
| Normal controls, cm (mean ± SEM) | 0.124 ± 0.038 | 0.088 ± 0.028 | 0.224 ± 0.049 |
| Achalasia patients, cm (mean ± SEM) | 0.206 ± 0.137 | 0.128 ± 0.077 | 0.317 ± 0.180 |
| Percent difference | 166 | 160 | 142 |
| $p$ value | < .017 | < .041 | < .033 |

CSM, circular smooth muscle thickness; LSM, longitudinal smooth muscle; TM, total muscle thickness.

Adapted from Miller LS et al. Gastrointest Endosc 1995;42:545–9.

## BODY OF THE ESOPHAGUS

The cross-sectional shape of the esophagus, muscle thickness in the resting state, and changes in muscle thickness during contraction provides important physiologic information related to the function of the esophagus. The esophagus is somewhat like a slit in shape in the resting state (Fig. 8.10). The muscle is somewhat thicker in the distal esophagus compared with the proximal esophagus. During contraction, the esophagus assumes an almost geometrically circular shape,

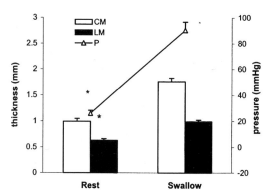

**FIGURE 8.5.** Changes in LES pressure (P) and muscle thickness during swallow-induced contraction. Swallowing causes LES relaxation followed by contraction. Basal LES pressure and muscle thickness were compared with pressure and muscle thickness during contraction. Note the marked increase in LES pressure and thickness of circular and longitudinal muscles during swallow-induced contraction versus during baseline state. *$p$ < .001 (n = 20 in 4 subjects).

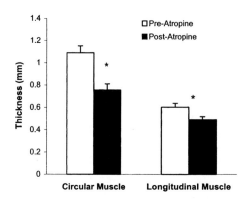

**FIGURE 8.6.** Effect of atropine on the thickness of circular and longitudinal muscles in LES. Atropine resulted in a decrease in the thickness of circular and longitudinal muscles. *$p$ < .01 (n = 6).

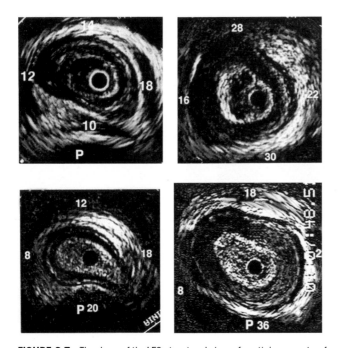

**FIGURE 8.7.** The shape of the LES at rest and circumferential asymmetry of pressure. Images were obtained from four subjects. A cross-section of the LES at the axial site of peak LES pressures is shown, as is LES pressure in each quadrant. Note that the shape of the LES is not circular in any subject. The shape of the mucosal plug is identical to that of the LES. Highest pressures were recorded in the leftward direction. The radius of the LES, as measured from the center of the transducer, was less toward the left side versus the right side. Reproduced with permission from Liu et al. Am J Physiol 1997;272:G1509–17

which is most likely the reason for circumferential symmetry of the esophageal pressures. There is a marked increase in the thickness of both circular and longitudinal muscle layers during esophageal contraction. The detailed analysis of the sonograms and concurrent pressure recordings reveal a close temporal correlation between changes in pressure and muscle thickness during contraction (see Fig. 8.3). This increase in muscle thickness is observed in both the circular and longitudinal muscle layers of the esophagus. Studies of the peristaltic reflex show that distention of the esophagus with a balloon results in an increase in the thickness of both circular and longitudinal muscle layers of the esophagus along with an increase in the pressure proximal to the site of distention (Fig. 8.11). Distal to distention, there is an inhibition of any ongoing motor activity or a reduction in the tone of the esophagus. Sonograms show a decrease in the muscle thickness of both circular and longitudinal muscle layers distal to the site of distention, which is equivalent to inhibition or relaxation (Fig. 8.12). Therefore, an increase in muscle thickness on sonograms represents a muscle contraction or muscle excitation, and a decrease in the muscle thickness is a marker of muscle relaxation or inhibition. Thus, ultrasonography can adequately record contraction and relaxation of the esophageal muscles—the two most important components of a peristaltic reflex. According to Laplace's law, the pressure inside a circular tube and muscle thickness are directly related to the wall thickness. In accordance with this law, in a given subject, there is a direct correlation between the increases in muscle thickness and the

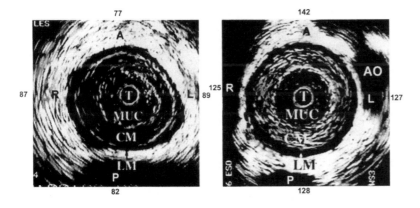

**FIGURE 8.8.** Images of the LES (*left*) and esophagus (*right*) during swallow-induced contraction. Compared with the shape in the basal state (see Fig. 8.4), note that the LES and esophagus are relatively more symmetric during swallow-induced contraction. Also note that LES and esophageal pressures are relatively more symmetric during swallow-induced contraction. Numbers represent pressure in mm Hg. T, transducer; MUC, micro; cm, circular muscle; LM, longitudinal muscle; A, anterior; P, posterior; R, right; L, left.

**FIGURE 8.9.** Images of the LES (*left image*) and the body of the esophagus (*right image*) in achalasia. Both circular and longitudinal muscle layers are thicker in the LES and in the body of the esophagus. The shape of the LES is also more rounded. The lumen of the esophagus is dilated and filled with fluid and air bubbles.

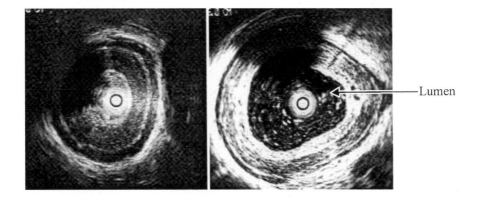

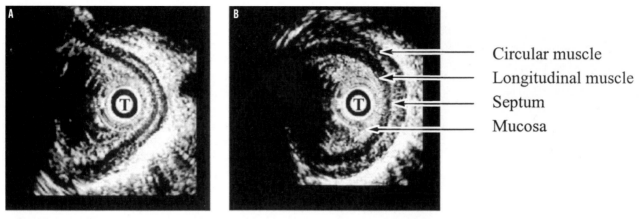

**FIGURE 8.10.** Cross-sectional images of the esophagus: **A**, at resting stage; **B**, at contracting stage. Note the marked increase in thickness of the circular and longitudinal muscle layers during contraction. T, ultrasound transducer.

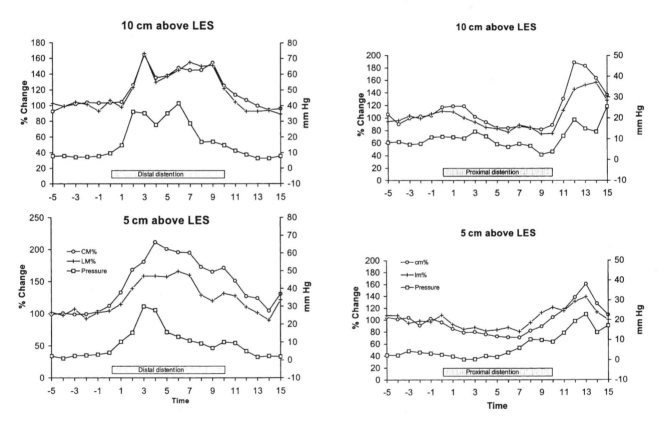

**FIGURE 8.11.** The temporal correlation between changes in esophageal pressure and muscle thickness proximal to distention. The pressure and muscle thickness were recorded at 5 (distal) and 10 cm (proximal) above the LES. Each graph represents mean data from five observations made in five subjects. Note a close temporal correlation between the pressure and muscle wall thickness at proximal and distal esophageal sites. Time scale is in seconds. The onset of muscle thickness started about 0.5 to 1 second before the pressure increase and lasted 2 to 3 seconds after the pressure drop. The changes in circular and longitudinal muscles started at the same time, and during relaxation, the decrease in muscle thickness occurred at the same time as well. Reproduced with permission from Yamamoto et al. Am J Physiol 1998;38:G806–11.

**FIGURE 8.12.** Temporal correlation between pressure and muscle thickness distal to the distention. The balloon inflated with 8-cc air. The pressure and muscle thickness were recorded at 5 (distal) and 10 cm (proximal) above the LES. Each graph represents mean data from five observations made in five subjects. Note that there was either a small (proximal esophagus) or no change in pressure distal to the distention, but the longitudinal and circular muscle thickness was significantly decreased. The decrease in distal muscle thickness in response to esophageal distention represents descending inhibition in the longitudinal and circular muscle layers. The time scale is in seconds. Reproduced with permission from Yamamoto et al. Am J Physiol 1998;38:G806–11.

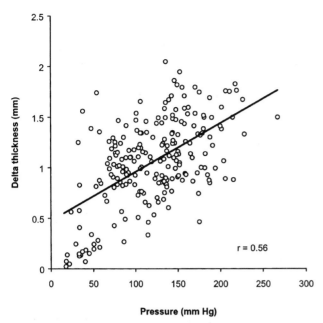

**FIGURE 8.13.** Correlation between the peak contraction pressure and delta esophageal wall muscle thickness. Delta muscle thickness represents the difference between peak and baseline muscle thickness during each swallow-induced contraction. Similar to the relationship of peak pressure and peak muscle thickness, there was also a moderate correlation between the delta muscle thickness and the esophageal contraction amplitude.

amplitude of esophageal contraction (Figs. 8.13 and 8.14). In the same individual, a higher-amplitude esophageal contraction results in a higher muscle thickness as compared with a lower-amplitude esophageal contraction.

## ESOPHAGEAL MUSCLE HYPERTROPHY IN PRIMARY MOTOR DISORDERS OF THE ESOPHAGUS

Autopsy studies show that patients with diffuse esophageal spasm (DES) show hypertrophy of the esophageal musculature. Probe ultrasonography studies reveal an increase in the muscle thickness of both circular and longitudinal muscle layers in patients with DES (Fig. 8.15). However, it is not clear whether this increase in the thickness is the result of hypertrophy or the increase in muscle tone. In patients with DES, the

muscular thickening is greatest in the most distal esophagus, and there is gradual thinning of the muscle toward the proximal esophagus. Interestingly, patients with nutcracker esophagus, similar to DES, also show a thickening of the esophageal musculature in the distal esophagus (Fig. 8.16). Furthermore, a gradient in the muscle thickness from a proximal to the distal direction can also be seen in patients with nutcracker esophagus. However, on average, the muscle appears to be thinner in the nutcracker esophagus compared to patients with DES. What is the significance of this increase in muscle thickness? From a physiologic point of view and in accordance with Laplace's law, the increase in muscle thickness is likely to result in higher-amplitude contraction seen in DES and nutcracker esophagus compared to normal subjects. Interestingly, a similar increase in muscle thickness is also seen in patients with achalasia of the esophagus. In fact, the muscle is thickest in achalasia of the esophagus. However, as a result of esophageal stasis and food retention, the muscle thins as the esophagus becomes distended and the muscle is stretched. Hence, it appears that the thickness of the muscularis propria is a hallmark of primary motility disorders of the esophagus. Patients with scleroderma of the esophagus, on the other hand, have a thinner esophageal musculature compared to normal subjects. Furthermore, the echo pattern of the muscle layers appears to be different in scleroderma of the esophagus, which is suggestive of the fibrosis in the muscle layer.

## IDENTIFICATION OF SUSTAINED ESOPHAGEAL CONTRACTION AS A MARKER OF CHEST PAIN AND HEARTBURN BY ULTRASONOGRAPHY

Perhaps the most important observation made by prolonged ultrasonography is what we have called a SEC, a motor event never described before. Prolonged, simultaneous pressure and sonogram recordings reveal that within a 2-minute period prior to the occurrence of esophageal chest pain, there is a frequent (two-thirds of the time) occurrence of a sustained increase in esophageal muscle thickness (Figs. 8.17 and 8.18). The SEC is defined as an increase in the muscle thickness of greater than the mean + 2 SD above the baseline thickness lasting longer than 18 seconds. The 18-second duration represents the mean + 3 SD of a normal swallow-associated contraction. The unique aspect of this increase in muscle

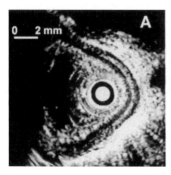
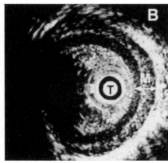
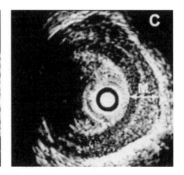

**FIGURE 8.14.** Sonograms of the esophagus: **A**, resting state and during two swallow-induced contractions; **B** and **C**, with corresponding pressures of 132 mm Hg and 226 mm Hg, respectively. Note that the muscle thickness was greater in **C** as compared with **B**. T, ultrasound transducer; M, muscle layer.

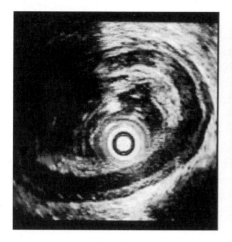
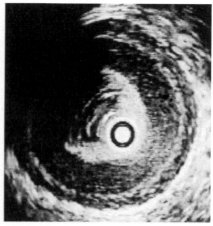

**FIGURE 8.15.** Sonograms from a patient with diffuse esophageal spasm. The esophageal wall is markedly thicker compared to normal subjects both in the LES (*left image*) and the body of the esophagus (*right image*).

**FIGURE 8.16.** Sonograms from a patient with nutcracker esophagus. The esophageal wall is markedly thicker compared to normal subjects both in the LES (*left image*) and the body of the esophagus (*right image*).

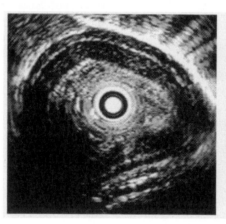
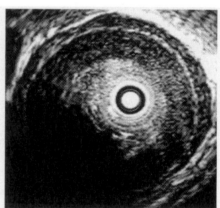

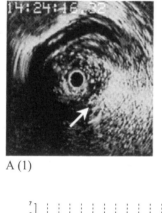
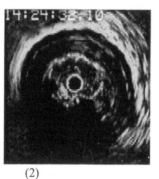
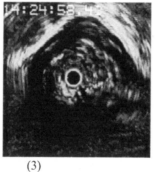
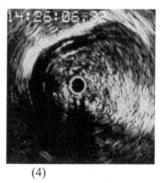

A (1)                    (2)                    (3)                    (4)

B         (1)        (2)        (3)                    (4)

**FIGURE 8.17. A**, A sustained esophageal contraction (SEC) during an acid reflux (+) chest pain event (CP). Note that there was a refluxate (*arrow*) into the esophagus (1) followed by a contraction of the esophagus (2), which lasted for 60 seconds (3) before returning to the baseline thickness (4). **B**, The corresponding esophageal pressure (E2 in mm Hg), pH, and muscle wall thickness (Wall). Note the sustained increase of esophageal wall thickness from 14:24:26 to 14:25:30. Chest pain occurred during SEC. Reproduced with permission from Miller LS, Klenn B et al. Intraluminal ultrasonography of the distal esophagus in systemic sclerosis.

**FIGURE 8.18.** Physiologic record of a sustained esophageal contraction associated with chest pain. Esophageal pH, distal esophageal pressure, and esophageal smooth muscle thickness (wall thickness) are shown during a 2.5-minute recording interval. The *vertical line* shows the onset of chest pain (time = 5.0 s). The onset of SEC occurs approximately 120 seconds before the onset of pain. The esophageal pressure recording shows two nonsustained increases in esophageal pressure accompanied by brief increases in esophageal muscle thickness during the SEC. There is no reflux during the event (pH > 4.0). Reproduced with permission from Balaban et al. Gastroenterology 1999; 116:29–37.

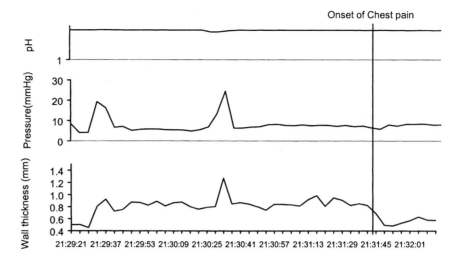

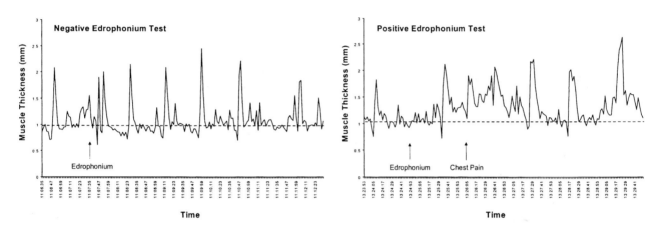

**FIGURE 8.19.** Ultrasound analysis of esophageal muscle thickness during negative and positive edrophonium (Tensilon) tests. The baseline muscle thickness is represented by the *horizontal dashed line*. Peaks in muscle thickness are voluntary 5-mL water swallows performed every 60 seconds. There is no sustained increase in esophageal muscle thickness in a subject who had no chest pain after edrophonium injection (*upper panel*). In contrast, the ultrasonographic record of a subject whose chest pain was reproduced 72 seconds after injection of edrophonium demonstrates a sustained increase in esophageal muscle thickness preceding the onset of pain (*lower panel*). Reproduced with permission from Balaban et al. Gastroenterology 1999;116:29–37.

thickness is that it is not associated with an increase in intra-esophageal pressure. Thus, the traditional pressure recording technique cannot identify this contraction. We speculate that SEC represents contraction of the longitudinal muscle layer. The mean duration of SEC, associated with esophageal chest pain, is approximately 70 seconds. Interestingly, pharmacologically induced chest pain (with edrophonium chloride [Tensilon]) is also associated with a similar contraction (Fig. 8.19). Patients who do not respond to edrophonium chloride with chest pain do not show SEC.

Even more interesting information is the identification of SEC, albeit of lesser duration with heartburn sensation (Fig. 8.20). A number of investigators in the 1960s felt that heartburn sensation was related to a motor event in the esophagus. However, the problem was that, using manometric techniques, they could not reliably identify a motor event in association with heartburn sensation. Similar to esophageal

chest pain, prolonged monitoring of the esophagus with probe ultrasonography and manometry reveals a SEC occurring prior to the onset of heartburn. This contraction is not associated with an increase in intraesophageal pressure and therefore most likely represents a contraction of the longitudinal muscle of the esophagus. The mean duration of this contraction is much smaller than that associated with chest pain, 32 versus 71 seconds. Heartburn induced by acid infusion of the esophagus (Bernstein test) is also associated with a similar contraction, that is SEC (Fig. 8.21). Subjects who do not experience heartburn with acid infusion into the esophagus do not show SEC.

It is clear that probe ultrasonography has yielded unique, novel, and important information related to the physiology and the pathophysiology of the esophagus. We are fairly certain that more information on the esophageal function using this ultrasound technique will most likely emerge in the

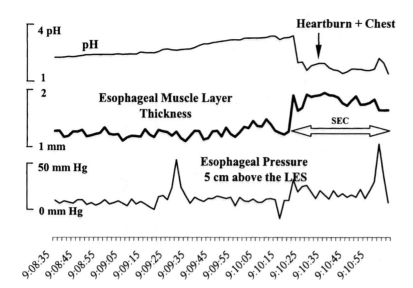

**FIGURE 8.20.** A symptomatic episode (combination of heartburn and chest pain) with acid reflux associated with a sustained esophageal contraction (SEC). The onset of SEC occurred approximately 20 seconds before the onset of heartburn. LES, lower esophageal sphincter. Reproduced with permission from Pehlivanov et al. Am J Physiol 2001; 28:G743–7.

**FIGURE 8.21.** An example of a heartburn episode associated with sustained esophageal contraction (SEC) during the acid perfusion test (Bernstein test). Heartburn occurred 3 minutes after the onset of acid perfusion and 20 seconds after the onset of SEC. Reproduced with permission from Pehlivanov et al. Am J Physiol 2001;28:G743–7.

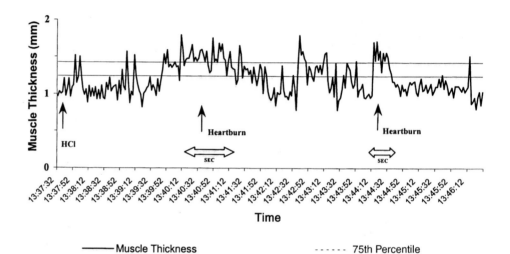

coming years. We strongly believe that the principles of ultrasonography used to study esophageal physiology and pathophysiology can also be applied to study other parts of the gastrointestinal tract.

### Acknowledgment

This work was supported by National Institutes of Health grant R01 DK51604-04A1.

### SELECTED READINGS

Balaban D, Yamamoto Y, Liu J, et al. Sustained esophageal contraction: a marker of esophageal chest pain identified by intraluminal ultrasonography. Gastroenterology 1999;116:29–37.

Barthet M, Mambrini P, Audibert P, et al. Relationships between endosonographic appearance and clinical or manometric features in-patients with achalasia. Eur J Gastroenterol Hepatol 1998;10:559–64.

Bergami GL, Fruhwirth R, Di Mario M, Fasanelli S. Contribution of ultrasonography in the diagnosis of achalasia. J Pediatr Gastroenterol Nutr 1992;14:92–6.

Biancani P, Zabinski MP, Behar J. Pressure, tension, and force of closure of the human lower esophageal sphincter and esophagus. J Clin Invest 1975;56:476–83.

Deviere J. Primary achalasia: analysis of endoscopic ultrasonography features with different instruments. Gastrointest Endosc Clin North Am 1995;5:631–4.

Ferguson TB, Woodbury JD, Roper CL, Burford TH. Giant muscular hypertrophy of the esophagus. Ann Thorac Surg 1969;8:209.

Hatlebakk JG, Odegaard S. Endoscopic ultrasound: a new look at achalasia? Eur J Gastroenterol Hepatol 1998;10:543–5.

Kojima Y, Ikeda M, Nakamura T, Fujino MA. Nonspecific esophageal motor disorder associated with thickened muscularis propria of the esophagus. Gastroenterology 1992;103:333–5.

Liu JB, Miller LS, Goldberg BB, et al. Transnasal US of the esophagus: preliminary morphologic and function studies. Radiology 1992;184:721–7.

Liu J, Miller L, Goldberg BB. Endoluminal ultrasound in gastroenterology: application of new technology. Clin Diagn Ultrasound 1994;29:185–215.

Liu J, Pehlivanov N, Mittal RK. Correlation between esophageal muscle thickness and intraluminal pressures in DES: an ultrasonographic study. Gastroenterology 2000;118:1431.

Liu J, Parashar VK, Mittal RK. Asymmetry of the lower esophageal sphincter pressure: is it related to the shape or the thickness of the muscle? Am J Physiol 1997;272:G1509–17.

Melzer E, Ron Y, Tiomni E, et al. Assessment of the esophageal wall by endoscopic ultrasonography in patients with nutcracker esophagus. Gastrointest Endosc 1997;46:223–5.

Melzer E, Tiomny A, Coret A, Bar-Meir S. Nutcracker esophagus: severe muscular hypertrophy on endosonography. Gastrointest Endosc 1995;42:366–7.

Miller LS, Liu JB, Barbarevech CA, et al. High-resolution endoluminal sonography in achalasia. Gastrointest Endosc 1995;42:545–9.

Miller LS, Liu J, Klenn BC, et al. Intraluminal ultrasonography of the distal esophagus in systemic sclerosis.

Miller LS, Liu JB, Colizzo FP, et al. Correlation of high frequency esophageal ultrasonography and manometry in the study of esophageal motility. Gastroenterology 1995;105:832–7.

Miller LS, Schiano TD. The use of high frequency endoscopic ultrasonography probes in the evaluation of achalasia. Gastrointest Endosc Clin North Am 1995;5:635–47.

Mittal RK, Pehlivanov N, Liu J. The esophageal muscle thickness in patients with hypertensive esophageal peristalsis. Gastroenterology 2000;118:1430.

Nicosia M, Brasseur J, Ji-Bin L, Miller L. Longitudinal shortening in the esophagus [abstract]. Gastroenterology 2000;118(1 Suppl 2):A133.

Pehlivanov N, Liu J, Kassab G, et al. Relationship between esophageal muscle thickness and intraluminal pressure: an ultrasonographic study. Am J Physiol 2001;28:G743–7.

Schiano TD, Fisher RS, Parkman HP, et al. Use of high-resolution endoscopic ultrasonography to assess esophageal wall damage after pneumatic dilation and botulinum toxin injection to treat achalasia. Gastrointest Endosc 1996;44:151–7.

Taniguchi DK, Martin RW, Trowers EA, et al. Change in esophageal wall layer during motility: measurement with a new miniature ultrasound device. Gastrointest Endosc 1993;39:146–52.

Van Dam J. Endoscopic ultrasonography in achalasia. Endoscopy 1994;26:792–3.

Van Dam J, Falk GW, Sivak MV Jr, et al. Endosonographic evaluation of the patient with achalasia: appearance of the esophagus using the echoendoscope. Endoscopy 1995;27:185–90.

Winsinewski R, Yamamoto Y, Liu J, Mittal RK. Characterization of gastric antral contractility using high-frequency intraluminal ultrasonography in normal subjects. Gastroenterology 1997;112:A852.

Yamamoto Y, Liu J, Smith TK, Mittal RK. Distension related responses in the circular and longitudinal muscles of the esophagus: an ultrasonographic study. Am J Physiol 1998;38:G806–11.

Ziegler K, Zimmer T. The role of endoscopic ultrasonography in esophageal motility disorders. Endoscopy 1992;24 Suppl 1:338–41.

CHAPTER 9

# pH Testing

*Mohan Charan, R. Matthew Gideon and Philip O. Katz*

Allison introduced the term "reflux esophagitis" in 1946, acknowledging that irritant gastric juices were refluxed from the stomach to the esophagus.[1] As clinicians became more familiar with the spectrum of gastroesophageal reflux disease (GERD), it became clear that many patients with reflux symptoms did not have pathologic or endoscopic evidence of esophagitis, and another diagnostic approach was needed. A greater understanding of reflux disease came with the development of continuous pH monitoring, which also offered a new method for diagnosis of GERD. Spencer first described the technique of continuous monitoring of intraesophageal pH using a glass electrode.[2] Johnson and DeMeester were the first to study normal volunteers and symptomatic patients and to analyze esophageal acid exposure data quantitatively.[3] Over time, esophageal pH monitoring has evolved into a patient- and physician-friendly technology with multiple applications in the evaluation and management of patients with GERD. This chapter reviews the present uses of ambulatory pH monitoring in GERD and presents examples of some applications of single- and dual-channel pH monitoring.

## INSTRUMENTATION AND METHODOLOGY

Today, pH monitoring is performed in the office of a gastroenterologist or surgeon and in specialized esophageal laboratories at many hospitals. Performance of the study requires a pH catheter containing one or more electrodes, a data logger (recorder), a personal computer, and program software. Several types of pH catheters are available. The catheters measure approximately 2 to 4 mm in diameter and contain either antimony or glass electrodes. Catheters containing antimony electrodes may have one or more pH electrodes; however, catheters with a glass electrode are single channel. Catheters can contain electrodes that are either monopolar, requiring an external reference electrode, or combination electrodes with a built-in (internal) reference. The catheters containing an external reference electrode can produce portions of the tracing that are unreadable (artifact) owing to loose contact with the skin, and perspiration-induced ionic changes in composition with electrode solution can be a source of inaccurate readings.[4–6]

Most pH catheters containing internal reference electrodes are of larger diameter than monopolar catheters to accommodate additional wiring (up to 4.5 mm). Glass electrodes have a long operational life (40 to 50 studies with optimal care) and a more rapid and linear response, with the least recording drift. They are expensive (>$500) and are generally mounted on stiff bulky catheters. The antimony monocrystalline catheters are available with single- and multichannel electrodes, making them more versatile. They are generally smaller, more flexible, and less expensive ($50 to 100) but have an operational life of <10 studies, respond more slowly to sudden pH changes, have greater electrode drift, and have far less linear response than glass electrodes.[5–7] In clinical studies, both types of electrodes appear to provide similar results.[8] Today, antimony pH probes, with their increased versatility, are widely accepted and have become the industry standard for use in clinical practice.

## SET-UP AND CALIBRATION

The pH study actually starts with a two-point calibration of the electrode, which must be performed using an acidic and a neutral buffer (usually pH 1 and pH 7 or pH 4 and pH 7). Antimony electrodes should use buffer solutions provided by the manufacturer, whereas glass electrodes may use any commercially available pH buffer.[6] A poststudy calibration can be repeated to either confirm or deny slow pH drift and to rule out pH electrode failure.

Modern data loggers are battery-powered and lightweight and can be worn on waist belts or shoulder straps. The cost of data loggers ranges from $6,500 to $10,000. The data logger samples esophageal pH every 4 to 5 seconds. Most data loggers are equipped with event markers that can be activated by the patient for the purpose of recording meals and snacks, symptoms, and recumbent periods. The patient also records these events on a diary using a 24-hour clock on the data recorder so that specific symptoms and events can be correlated with the pH tracing and the events marked by the patient. An important reminder to those performing the study is that patients frequently fail to push the event marker sufficiently hard enough to register on the recorder and often neglect to record event times on the diary in conjunction with their activation of event markers. This can result in poor data quality, so careful instructions to the patient are needed.

## ELECTRODE PLACEMENT

The pH catheter is calibrated and connected to the data logger. The catheter is then passed through a nostril and positioned with one electrode 5 cm above the superior margin of the lower esophageal sphincter (LES). This position is selected to avoid possible electrode displacement in the stomach, especially during shortening of the esophagus induced by swallowing. If the electrode is placed too high above the LES, the sensitivity of the test may be compromised. The LES is localized before a pH study by esophageal manometry, which is considered a reference standard. Although this adds time and some expense to study performance and

slightly increases patient discomfort, it continues to be the most accurate measure for proper probe placement. To avoid this, other methods of LES localization have been employed, although their accuracy has been questioned. They include endoscopy, fluoroscopy, and pH step-up using a catheter pull-through across the LES, and LES locator devices, which use a water perfusion port within the pH catheter.[9] We always use manometry as our method of placement and do not recommend any of these other methods other than consideration of an LES locator as endoscopic, fluoroscopic, and step-up techniques are too inaccurate. A few studies have shown that electrodes can be placed accurately using the pull-through technique, whereas others find it prone to error, especially in the presence of a hiatal hernia or free reflux. Lower esophageal reflux locators are more accurate than pull-through techniques but also can result in incorrect placement because of hiatal hernias. Once the LES is located with manometry, the pH electrode is first passed into the stomach to document an acid pH (pH < 4). The pH probe is then pulled back to the desired location placing one electrode 5 cm above the proximal border of the LES. Additional electrodes may be placed above or below the reference electrode depending on the information desired (see below). Following proper placement, the data logger is started and the study begun.

## INDICATIONS

Prolonged ambulatory pH monitoring should be considered to aid in the evaluation of patients as outlined below:

1. Typical symptoms of GERD (heartburn, regurgitation) with normal endoscopy who have not responded to antisecretory therapy
2. Atypical symptoms of GERD (for initial diagnosis or after a trial of therapy):
   • Unexplained chest pain of noncardiac etiology
   • Pulmonary symptoms—cough, asthma, recurrent aspiration pneumonia
   • Otolaryngologic symptoms—hoarseness, laryngitis
   • Other atypical symptoms in which GERD is considered such as nonulcer dyspepsia, belching, hiccups, epigastric pain
3. Failure to respond to medical therapy
4. Preoperative evaluation to confirm GERD
5. Follow-up:
   • Medical therapy—to assess the efficacy of the medical regimen, particularly in Barrett's esophagus
   • Surgical therapy—pre- and postoperative assessment

## DIET AND ACTIVITIES DURING STUDY

The pH of various foods and beverages consumed during a study period is variable. Therefore, in earlier studies, standardization of food intake was recommended. Acidic foods such as pickles, citrus fruit, and tomato-based products, as well as carbonated beverages (particularly colas), were prohibited. It should be noted that the effect of these products on esophageal pH is short lived and can probably be disregarded in most patients.[10] In fact, exclusion of the actual eating period from the overall analysis eliminates the artifact introduced by meals with pH <4 and improves the separation of normal from abnormal.[11] Our current practice is not to restrict patients during the study. Patients are encouraged to maintain their usual diet routine and activity level through the course of the study and to try to bring on their symptoms. Many patients have eliminated certain foods or activities because these tend to give them symptoms. The opportunity to monitor the patient while eating or drinking these symptom-producing foods can be extremely helpful in evaluation.

## DRUGS DURING STUDY

Studies monitoring pH studies are performed to answer two basic questions: (1) Is esophageal acid reflux the cause of the patient's symptoms? and (2) In the patient who remains symptomatic despite medical therapy, has the reflux been controlled, and, if it has not, are the remaining symptoms due to esophageal acid? Therefore, the clinician has the option of performing the pH study with the patient off or on medical therapy. In studies performed off medical therapy, patients should be asked to stop acid-neutralizing drugs (antacids, histamine$_2$ blockers, proton pump inhibitors) and promotility agents. Proton pump inhibitors should be stopped for a minimum of 5 days before a study and promotility agents and histamine$_2$ blockers stopped 48 hours prior. The effect of sucralfate is unknown, so it is our preference to discontinue it for 48 hours prior to study. When pH studies are to be performed on medical therapy, patients should be instructed to take their medication as prescribed. Drugs that decrease LES pressure, such as calcium channel blockers, nitrates, theophylline, or sedatives, should also be discontinued if prescribed on an as-needed basis. Patients who take these types of drugs for a chronic medical condition (calcium blockers for heart disease) should continue their therapy while being studied unless there is concern that these drugs are responsible for the reflux.

## LENGTH OF STUDY

Most clinicians agree that the 24-hour study is the method of choice, but a 16-hour study from 4 pm to 8 am can provide accurate information and improve patient tolerance.[12] Although some investigators have made a case for short-term postprandial recordings rather than a 24-hour study,[13] we have found that shorter studies preclude adequate symptom assessment and do not allow nighttime study, so we strongly prefer a study that includes the sleeping period.[14] Overall patient tolerance has been excellent, with between 90 and

**TABLE 9.1.** Normal Values for pH Monitoring

| Variable | Normal |
| --- | --- |
| Time pH < 4 (%) | |
|    Total period | < 4.2 |
|    Supine period | < 1.2 |
|    Upright period | < 6.3 |
| Duration of longest episode (min) | < 9.2 |
| Number of episodes | |
|    Total | < 50.0 |
|    Longer than 5 min | < 3.0 |

96% of patients completing the study.[8] Our personal experience is at the upper limit of this range. Technical problems such as electrode drift are responsible for a small number of unsuccessful studies, with the remainder attributable to the inability of patients to tolerate the catheter. At the completion of the study, the catheter is removed and recalibrated and the data logger is uploaded to the computer for analysis.

## DEFINING NORMAL

Gastroesophageal reflux is a physiologic phenomenon that occurs in normal individuals, especially in the postprandial period and upright position. Although reflux frequency in controls is not normally distributed, if nonparametric analysis of normal data using the 95th percentile is used, normal values are remarkably similar for controls in different geographic areas. Johnson and DeMeester proposed a scoring system,[15] which is used most commonly and incorporates six variables as outlined in Table 9.1.

pH monitoring carries a sensitivity and specificity of 90%. The cutoff limit of pH 4 has been chosen for the following rationale: the proteolytic enzyme pepsin is inactive above pH 4, and symptomatic patients with reflux only report heartburn when the intraesophageal pH drops below 4.[16] The proportion of time that pH is below 4, called reflux time or acid exposure time, is the variable most widely used. The number of reflux episodes shows a much poorer correlation with the grade of esophagitis than does acid exposure time. In our laboratory, we report the Johnson and DeMeester score but rely on time pH < 4 as the defining variable to determine normalcy, seldom including any other variable other than the symptom correlation (see below). Some define a reflux episode as a rapid fall in pH of more than 1 pH unit, even though the threshold of pH < 4 may not be reached. We do not consider this unless extremely high symptom correlation occurs with these events.

## REPRODUCIBILITY

Studies on reproducibility have demonstrated a wide variability in total reflux time and the number of episodes of reflux on separate days. Studies comparing the esophageal acid exposure time of normal individuals with patients with endoscopically proven esophagitis have 77 to 100% sensitivity and 85 to 100% specificity of esophageal acid exposure values in segregating these populations.[17,18] This observation is of limited clinical value as endoscopic demonstration of esophagitis will establish the diagnosis of GERD, obviating the need for a 24-hour pH study. A slightly lower reproducibility has been noted for patients with pulmonary symptoms or noncardiac chest pain.[19] The clinical value of a normal study, well performed, is quite high; in our experience, patients with normal pH studies seldom respond to antisecretory therapy or surgery.

An attempt to augment the interpretation of the study incorporates the so-called Symptom Index (SI) proposed by Weiner and colleagues to express the relationship between symptoms and reflux episodes.[20] It is defined as the percentage of symptom episodes that are related to reflux:

$$SI = \frac{\text{Number of symptoms with pH} < 4}{\text{Total number of symptoms}} \times 100$$

A value of >50% is considered a usual threshold for considering a high SI as these patients are more likely to respond to therapy. The disadvantage of the SI is that it does not take into account the number of reflux episodes. For this reason, another parameter, the Symptom Sensitivity Index, was proposed by Breumelhof and colleagues[21] and defined as:

$$SSI = \frac{\text{Number of reflux-related symptoms episodes}}{\text{Total number of reflux episodes}} \times 100$$

A value of 10% or greater is considered to be positive. This is a cumbersome calculation that has limited clinical usefulness and is not used in many laboratories. Careful use of the SI adds to the interpretation of the study and should be used routinely, particularly in refractory patients.

### Multichannel Monitoring

Current technology allows both single- and multichannel monitoring using a single catheter. Examples are shown of distal and proximal upright reflux, normal distal and proximal reflux, and recumbent reflux (Figs. 9.1 to 9.3). Probes can be customized as to length, but, currently, the standard is channels 10, 15, and 20 cm apart. This allows monitoring at two simultaneous levels in the esophagus or simultaneous intragastric and intraesophageal monitoring. Dual intraesophageal monitoring is particularly useful in patients with otolaryngologic and pulmonary symptoms and patients in whom proximal esophageal or hypopharyngeal monitoring is desirable to assess the propensity of the patient to aspirate (see Clinical Examples). In addition, abnormal proximal reflux may be the only finding to suggest that otolaryngo-

logic or pulmonary symptoms are attributable to GERD. Further, abnormal proximal reflux time is a valuable prognostic indicator of response of pulmonary symptoms to proton pump inhibitors or surgery. Simultaneous intragastric and intraesophageal monitoring is extremely useful in assessing the response to medical therapy and in evaluation of symptoms appearing to be refractory to proton pump inhibitors. Assessment of intragastric pH control, particularly at night, and the presence of continued esophageal reflux in the setting of a high-dose proton pump inhibitor can be ascertained. Probes are similar in design to single channel, being similar in diameter and offering similar comfort levels and patient tolerance. Studies are successfully completed in 90%, as is the case with single-channel monitoring.

We have recently begun evaluating a three-channel probe, which will allow simultaneous monitoring of distal, proximal esophagus, and hypopharynx using a single catheter and data logger. Initial studies suggest that this is well tolerated and technically satisfactory. Further studies are in progress, but this technical advance will be useful in evaluation of patients with extraesophageal symptoms.

## CLINICAL EXAMPLES

### Unexplained Chest Pain

Noncardiac chest pain is a troublesome symptom for patients and clinicians and one in which pH monitoring is extremely valuable. Traditional diagnostic studies for GERD (barium swallow and endoscopy) are normal in a high percentage of this patient population. The Bernstein test, a useful screening test for acid sensitivity, has good specificity (approximately 85%), but a low sensitivity (30 to 50%) for the diagnosis of acid-associated chest pain is rarely used in clinical practice today.[21,22] Ambulatory pH monitoring can be used in several ways to aid in the diagnosis of reflux in this patient population:

1. Total reflux time can be assessed. Approximately 50% of patients with noncardiac chest pain will have abnormal esophageal acid exposure time on a 24-hour study.
2. Symptoms can be correlated with esophageal reflux (Fig. 9.4). If the symptom index is high (>50%), the likelihood of a response to antisecretory therapy is quite good 50%).
3. Exercise can produce reflux in normal subjects and/or exacerbate reflux in patients with chest pain. In fact, exercise may be the only provoker of a reflux event. Patients with exercise-induced pain and normal coronary arteries can be tested on a treadmill or while performing the specific exercise that triggers the pain. If pain can be correlated with a reflux event during exercise, the diagnosis of GERD can be confirmed.[23] We occasionally will perform combined ambulatory monitoring of esophageal pH and Holter monitoring to assess the contribution of GERD to chest pain in patients with known coronary artery disease.[23]

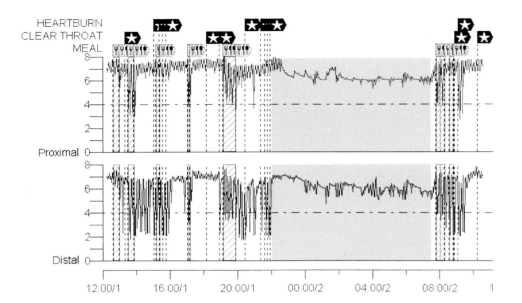

**FIGURE 9.1.** Upright gastro-esophageal reflux before therapy.

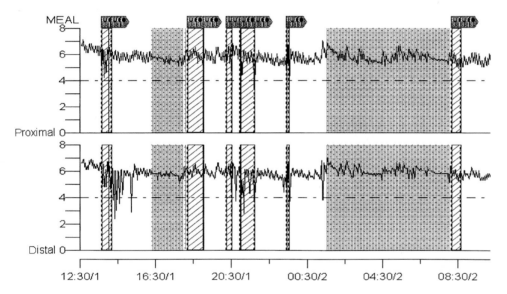

**FIGURE 9.2.** Proximal and distal normal esophageal acid exposure.

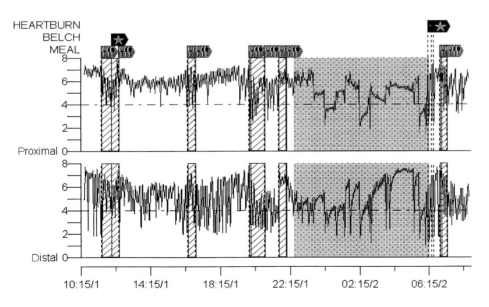

**FIGURE 9.3.** Proximal and distal upright and recumbent gastro-esophageal reflux.

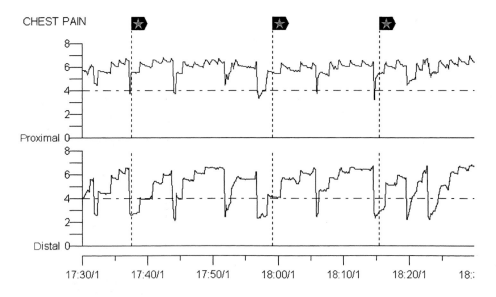

**FIGURE 9.4.** Chest pain proximal and distal (–) cardiac W/U pH probe (+). Chest pain associated with reflux (the association).

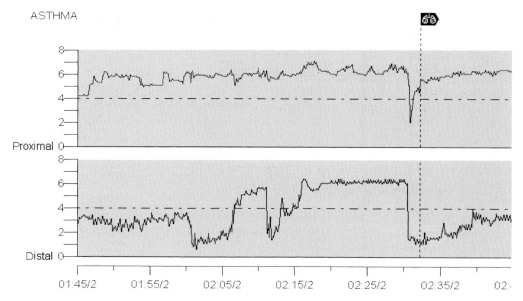

**FIGURE 9.5.** Proximal and distal overnight asthma attack/gastroesophageal reflux.

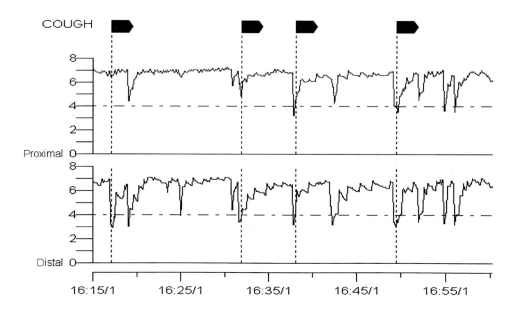

**FIGURE 9.6.** Cough (+) symptoms association. Ambulatory pH monitoring shows reflux episodes preceding cough.

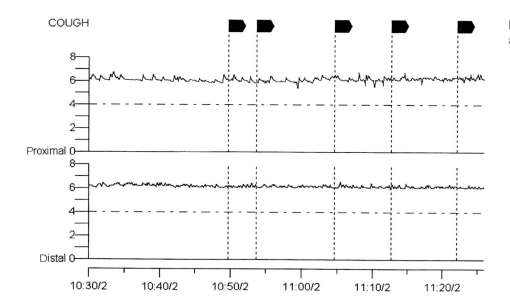

**FIGURE 9.7.** Negative symptom association cough, no reflux.

## PULMONARY DISEASE

The association of reflux and pulmonary disease has long been recognized. Up to 80% of asthmatics will have abnormal acid reflux parameters in both the upright and supine position,[24] and up to 20% of patients with chronic cough will have abnormal pH studies, suggesting that these diseases are, at least in part, GERD related. The judicious use of dual- or three-channel pH monitoring makes it possible to document the presence or absence of reflux as a contributing factor in asthma (Fig. 9.5), chronic cough (Figs. 9.6 and 9.7), chronic bronchitis, idiopathic pulmonary fibrosis, and, rarely, recurrent pneumonia, if there is proximal reflux or acid refluxes above the upper esophageal sphincter, documenting the potential for microaspiration. This is another group of patients with a low prevalence of endoscopic esophagitis yet a high frequency of reflux by 24-hour pH monitor. In general, we use dual monitoring in patients with pulmonary symptoms. If the triple probe proves to be technically easy to perform and interpret, this will become the diagnostic choice as a probe can be placed 2 cm above the upper esophageal sphincter. Modern dual-channel monitoring with the proximal esophageal probe 20 cm above the LES will allow the clinician to assess the potential for aspiration based on the frequency of proximal (high) reflux—a rare occurrence in normal subjects.

## OTOLARYNGOLOGIC SYMPTOMS

Chronic hoarseness, cervical dysphagia, globus, posterior pharyngitis, and laryngitis have all been associated with GERD (Figs. 9.8 and 9.9). This is a group of patients in whom typical esophageal symptoms such as heartburn may not be seen and endoscopic esophagitis is uncommon, making the diagnosis difficult. This is consistent with the finding that patients with ear, nose, and throat disorders appear to be predominantly upright refluxers.[25] When reflux episodes occur in the upright position, they are usually of short duration and do not cause significant esophagitis. The use of multichannel probes, allowing simultaneous distal and proximal esophageal and/or pharyngeal monitoring, allows confirmation that acid refluxes above the upper esophageal sphincter and provides greater certainty of the relationship between an otolaryngologic symptom and reflux. Patients with hoarseness have a high degree of daily variability in reflux frequency, with normal studies seen in as many as 15% if only a distal esophageal probe is used. Several patients with hoarseness have been reported in whom distal esophageal acid exposure time is normal, yet pharyngeal reflux is demonstrated, reinforcing the importance of multichannel monitoring in this patient population.[25]

## SYMPTOMATIC PATIENTS WITH NEGATIVE WORK-UP

Monitoring of pH is particularly useful in patients who have symptoms suggestive of GERD but a negative endoscopy and barium swallow (Fig. 9.10). The diagnostic approach to these patients has been to use a therapeutic trial of high-dose antisecretory therapy. If this fails and the patient has a normal study when monitored off therapy, an alternative diagnosis should be entertained, whereas an abnormal study suggests a need for more intensive medical treatment. There is a subgroup of patients with normal esophageal acid exposure but a very high symptom correlation—the so-called sensitive esophagus, which is only diagnosed by prolonged pH monitoring with calculation of the symptom index. These are very difficult patients to treat and often do not respond to even high doses of proton pump inhibitors; therefore, correlation of esophageal reflux episodes and symptoms is crucial in sorting out the symptoms in these patients.

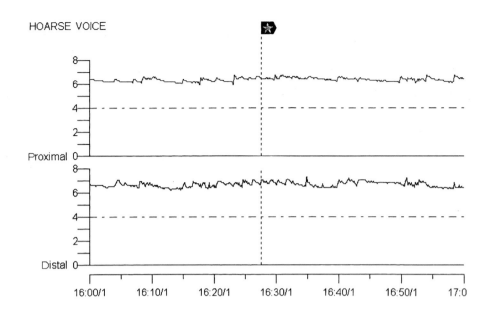

**FIGURE 9.8.** Hoarseness (–) symptom association. No reflux seen prior to symptom.

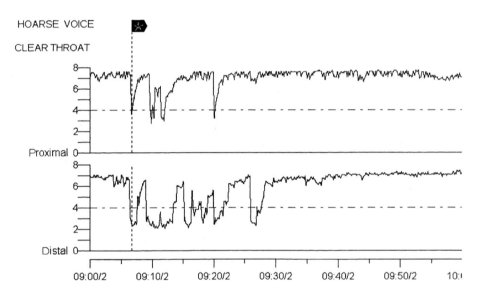

**FIGURE 9.9.** Hoarseness occurs immediately after reflux episode, which is positive (+) symptom association.

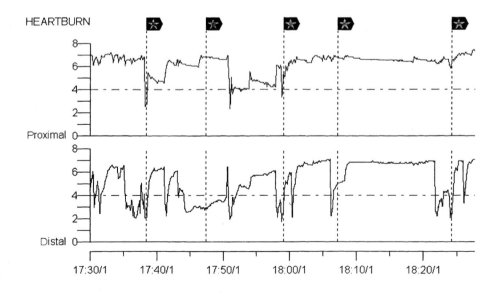

**FIGURE 9.10.** (–) EGD (+) pH probe heartburn. The endoscopy is normal, but the pH study demonstrates frequent reflux with strong symptom correlation.

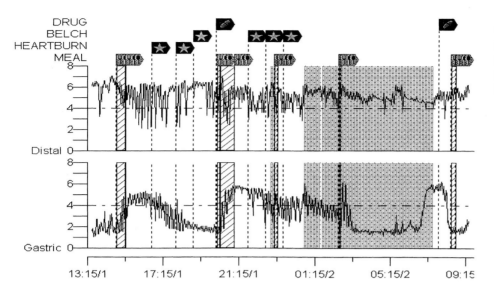

**FIGURE 9.11.** Dual-channel gastric and esophageal pH monitoring shows continued overnight acid reflux on twice-daily proton pump inhibitor before meals.

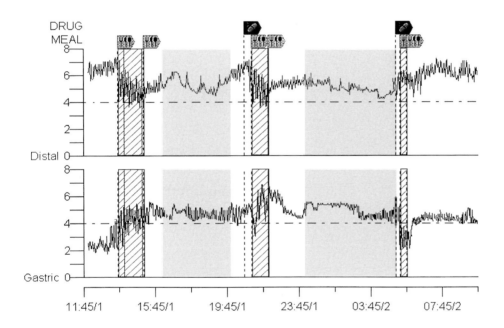

**FIGURE 9.12.** Dual-channel gastric and esophageal pH monitoring shows good gastric acid control on twice-daily proton pump inhibitor therapy before meals.

## ASSESSMENT OF RESPONSE TO THERAPY

Evaluation of patients' response to antisecretory therapy with proton pump inhibitors is rapidly becoming the most common reason for performance of prolonged pH monitoring in our laboratory and of primary importance in the evaluation of the difficult patient with GERD (Figs. 9.11 to 9.15). The most common clinical scenario is the patient with suspected GERD who has failed to have adequate symptom relief with antisecretory therapy, with proton pump inhibitor doses of twice daily or higher. It is not clear whether these patients have been inadequately treated, are taking the proton pump inhibitor incorrectly, or perhaps are resistant, or whether the empiric diagnosis was even correct. We often study these patients while they continue to take their proton pump inhibitor, performing combined intragastric and esophageal monitoring.[17] If reflux continues and symptoms correlate, more therapy is

needed (see Fig. 9.11). If gastric pH is controlled and no reflux occurs, yet the patients still have symptoms, acid reflux is unlikely to be responsible for the symptoms. Some patients with known reflux disease will fail to respond to medical therapy, despite seemingly adequate medication dosage. This may be because the patient continues to produce acid during the sleeping period, even despite receiving a twice-daily proton pump inhibitor. This pharmacologic phenomenon, which we have termed nocturnal gastric acid breakthrough, is seen in 70 to 80% of patients on proton pump inhibitors (see Fig. 9.11).[18] Nocturnal acid breakthrough is defined as a drop in gastric pH <4 for greater than 1 continuous hour overnight and may be associated with esophageal reflux, particularly in patients with Barrett's esophagus.[19] We routinely study these patients with combined gastric and esophageal monitoring while continuing medications and looking for nocturnal breakthrough, continued nocturnal reflux, and symptom correlation

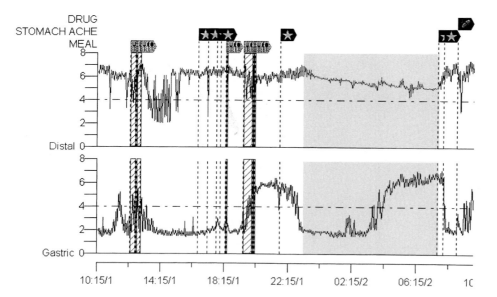

**FIGURE 9.13.** Patient on once-daily proton pump inhibitor therapy before meals in morning shows poor gastric acid control.

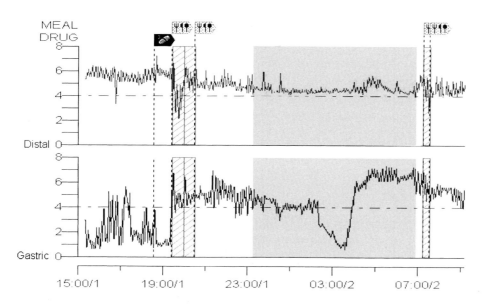

**FIGURE 9.14.** Ambulatory pH monitoring for patient on once-daily proton pump inhibitor therapy before meals in evening shows good gastric acid control and no reflux.

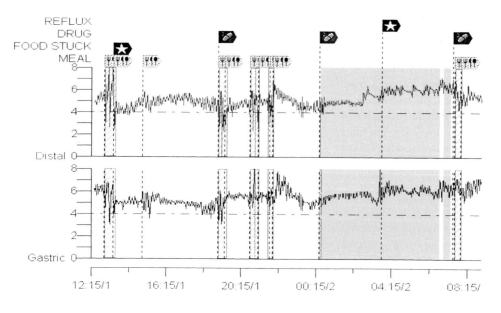

**FIGURE 9.15.** Patient on twice-daily proton pump inhibitor before meals and H$_2$ receptor antagonist at nighttime. Dual-channel pH monitoring shows gastric acid control and no reflux.

to ascertain whether more medication is needed. If nocturnal breakthrough is documented and the patient continues to reflux, an increase in therapy is needed (see Fig. 9.6), and surgery needs consideration.

## ANTIREFLUX SURGERY

Ambulatory pH monitoring should be done in almost all patients in whom antireflux surgery is planned. The diagnosis of abnormal esophageal acid exposure can be confirmed, and the rare patient with an alternative diagnosis such as pill-induced esophagitis or achalasia can be excluded. An abnormal pH study, particularly in the patient with extraesophageal symptoms, is helpful in predicting a successful surgical outcome. Postoperative prolonged esophageal monitoring can be used if needed if the patient has a return of symptoms after surgery.

## CONCLUSION

Esophageal pH monitoring has evolved from a cumbersome, uncomfortable inpatient procedure to a patient- and physician-friendly ambulatory procedure that is invaluable in selected patients with GERD. In particular, we have gained insight into the patterns of reflux—upright, supine, and exercise induced—and the importance of symptom correlation with reflux events and of so-called extraesophageal presentations of the disease, such as chest pain, hoarseness, asthma, and other head and neck symptoms. The patient who appears to have failed medical therapy can now be evaluated effectively and optimally managed. Preoperative evaluation for antireflux surgery confirms that the operation is being performed only in patients with proven GERD. Multichannel pH monitoring is now commonplace, and intragastric pH monitoring can be used to assess proton pump inhibitor therapy.

All of this can be done in the patient's own environment, on an unrestricted diet, and with a minimum of discomfort. Newer techniques are sure to evolve, making this technology even more patient and physician friendly, giving us new insights into the pathogenesis of reflux disease, particularly extraesophageal presentations, allowing us to evaluate the new therapies that are rapidly being developed to treat this very common disease.

### REFERENCES

1. Allison PR. Peptic ulcer of the esophagus. J Thorac Cardiovasc Surg 1946;15:308–17.
2. Spencer J. Prolonged pH recording in the study of gastroesophageal reflux. Br J Surg 1969;56:9–12.
3. Johnson LF, DeMeester TF. Twenty-four hour pH monitoring of the distal esophagus. A quantitative measure of gastroesophageal reflux. Am J Gastroenterol 1974;62:325–32.
4. Emde C, Garner A, Blum A. Technical aspects of intraluminal pH metry in man: current status and recommendations. Gut 1987;28:1177–88.
5. McLauchlan G, Rawlings JM, Lucas ML, et al. Electrodes for 24 hour pH monitoring: a comparative study. Gut 1987;28:935–9.
6. Smout AJPM. Ambulatory monitoring of esophageal pH and pressure. In: Castell DO, Richter JE, editors. The esophagus. 3rd ed. Lippincott Williams & Wilkins; 1999. p. 119–33.
7. Kahrilas PJ, Quigley EMM. Clinical esophageal pH recording: a technical review for practice guideline development. Gastroenterology 1996;110:1982–96.
8. Mattox HE, Richter JE. Prolonged ambulatory esophageal pH monitoring in the evaluation of gastroesophageal reflux disease. Am J Med 1990;89:345–56.
9. Wilder-Smith CH, Gennoni MA, Triller J, et al. Is a fluoroscopic verification of the electrode position necessary in ambulatory intragastric pH monitoring? Digestion 1992;52:1–5.
10. Shoenut JP, Duerksen D, Yaffe CS. Impact of ingested liquids on 24-hour ambulatory pH tests. Dig Dis Sci 1998;43:834–9.
11. Wo JM, Castell DO. Exclusion of meal periods from ambulatory 24-hour pH monitoring may improve diagnosis of esophageal acid reflux. Dig Dis Sci 1994;39:1601–7.
12. Dobhan R, Castell DO. Prolonged intraesophageal pH monitoring with 16-hour overnight recording. Dig Dis Sci 1992;37:857–64.
13. Jorgenson F, Elsborg L, Hesse B. The diagnostic value of computerized short term esophageal monitoring in suspected gastroesophageal reflux. Scand J Gastroenterol 1988;23:363–7.
14. Bianchi Porro G, Pace F. Comparison of three methods of intraesophageal pH recording in the diagnosis of gastroesophageal reflux. Scand J Gastroenterol 1988;23:743–50.
15. Johnson LF, DeMeester TR. Twenty four hour pH monitoring of distal esophagus. Am J Gastroenterol 1974;62:323–32.
16. Tuttle SG, Rufin F, Bettarello A. The physiology of heartburn. Ann Intern Med 1961;55:292–300.
17. Masclee AAM, De Best ACAM, De Graaf R, et al. Ambulatory 24-hour pH-metry in the diagnosis of gastroesophageal reflux disease. Scand J Gastroenterol 1990;25:225–30.
18. Kasapidis P, Xynos E, Mantides A, et al. Differences in manometry and 24-hour pH-metry between patients with and without endoscopic or histologic esophagitis in gastroesophageal reflux disease. Am J Gastroenterol 1993;88:1893–9.
19. Weiner GJ, Morgan TM, Cooper JB, et al. Ambulatory 24-hour esophageal pH monitoring, reproducibility and variability of pH parameters. Dig Dis Sci 1988;33:1127–33.
20. Weiner GJ, Richter JE, Cooper JB, et al. The Symptom Index: a clinically important parameter of ambulatory 24-hour esophageal pH monitoring. Am J Gastroenterol 1988;83:358–61.
21. Breumelhof R, Smout AJPM. The Symptom Sensitivity Index: a valuable additional parameter in 24-hour esophageal pH recording. Am J Gastroenterol 1991;86:160–4.
22. Richter JE, Hewson EG, Sinclair JW, et al. Acid perfusion test and 24 hour pH monitoring with symptom index. Comparison of tests for esophageal acid sensitivity. Dig Dis Sci 1991;36:565–71.
23. Schofield PM, Bennett DH, Whorwell PJ, et al. Exertional gastroesophageal reflux: a mechanism for symptoms in patients with angina pectoris and normal coronary angiograms. BMJ 1987;294:1459–61.
24. Hewson EG, Sinclaire JW, Hackshaw BT, et al. The role of ambulatory Holter/pH monitoring in coronary artery disease patients with refractory chest pain [abstract]. Gastroenterology 1989;96:208.
25. Sontag SJ, O'Connell S, Khandelwal S. Most asthmatics have gastroesophageal reflux with or without bronchodilator therapy. Gastroenterology 1990;99:613–20.

CHAPTER 10

# Manometry

*Brian E. Lacy, Kenneth L. Koch and Michael D. Crowell*

The stomach is a remarkable mixing chamber. From sips of water to large milk shakes, from a dieter's rice cake to a full-course Thanksgiving turkey dinner, the stomach must accommodate ingested foods and then properly mix and empty nutrient suspensions into the duodenum. In addition to these physiologic mixing/emptying activities, the stomach contributes to many pleasurable sensations related to the satisfying epigastric fullness that accompanies the ingestion of a meal. On the other hand, when the neuromuscular apparatus of this sophisticated mixing chamber is dysfunctional, a variety of unpleasant and vague symptoms, ranging from epigastric distress to nausea and vomiting, are experienced.

In this chapter, the normal gastric anatomy and electromechanical activities that produce normal stomach motility are reviewed. Similar to cardiac physiology, the stomach should be viewed as a sophisticated "electromechanical" organ rather than an apparatus that simply contracts. Thus, abnormalities in gastric motility may be understood in terms of myoelectrical dysfunction and contraction/relaxation disorders. Disorders of contractile activity are illustrated and discussed in this chapter.

## NORMAL GASTRIC MOTILITY: ELECTROMECHANICAL ACTIVITY

### Gastric Muscular and Electrical Regions

#### Anatomy

The anatomic and pacemaker regions of the stomach are described in Figure 10.1. The fundic area is considered the proximal stomach, the area that relaxes to accommodate ingested food. The body (corpus) and antrum are considered the distal stomach, where solid foods are mixed and gently broken down by recurrent peristaltic waves.[1] When food particles are < 1 mm in diameter, these nutrient suspensions are emptied into the duodenum by gastric peristaltic contractions.[1]

#### Pacemaker Region/Activity

From an anatomic viewpoint, the pacemaker region is an ill-defined area, as shown in Figure 10.1. The pacesetter potentials are thought to arise from the interstitial cells of Cajal located near the circular muscle layer.[2] (Note that the fundic muscle does not have a 3 cycle per minute (cpm) rhythm but rather is electrically "silent.") The frequency of the pacesetter potential is modulated by ongoing changes in vagal, splanchnic, and hormonal activity. Pacesetter potentials migrate distally from the corpus toward the pylorus at a rate of 3 cpm, with increasing velocity in the antrum.[3] The antrum is the site of most tachygastrias and tachyarrhythmias (abnormal 4–9 cpm electrical waves).[4]

### Methods of Recording Stomach Motility

#### Intraluminal Pressure

Gastric motility may be measured by a number of different methods, as shown in Figure 10.2. Intraluminal pressure recording devices have been the most popular means to quantitate gastric contractions (Fig. 10.3). Barium studies were used previously; however, although radiographic methods demon-

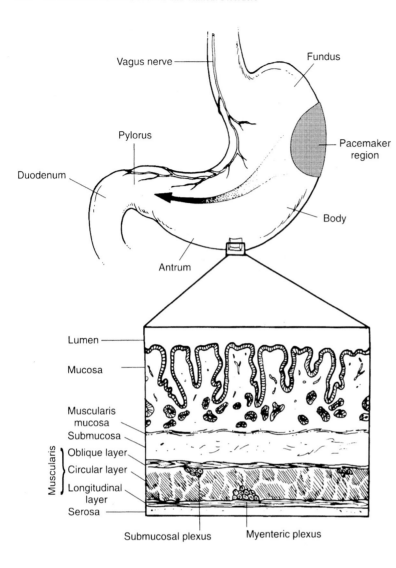

**FIGURE 10.1.** Anatomic regions of the stomach. The major regions of the stomach are the fundus, body, and antrum. The inset shows the layers of the stomach that comprise the inner mucosal layer and the outer muscularis tunica. The majority of the muscularis consists of a circular muscle layer, which is thickest in the area of the antrum, and an outer longitudinal muscle layer. An inner oblique muscle layer is also present in the region of the gastric body-antrum. The major enteric plexi in the stomach are the submucosal (Meissner's plexus) and myenteric (Auerbach's plexus) plexi. Extrinsic innervation to the stomach is derived from the vagus nerve and the splanchnic nerves.

Electrical pacesetter potentials, which coordinate contractions of the gastric smooth muscle, originate in an ill-defined pacemaker region located on the greater curvature near the junction of the fundus and proximal gastric body. As shown by the *arrow*, the pacesetter potentials migrate distally toward the pylorus. Pacesetter potentials occur at 3 cpm (cycles per minute) in humans. The pylorus is a sphincter that separates the stomach from the duodenum.

**FIGURE 10.2** Methods of recording gastric motility. Gastric motility is the result of a series of precisely coordinated muscular contractions and relaxations. These mechanical events are mediated by changes in membrane electrical events, that is, action or spike potentials linked to pacesetter potentials.

Intraluminal pressures may be recorded with water-perfused or solid-state pressure transducers mounted on a variety of catheters. These instruments require lumen-obliterating contractions to activate the pressure transducers. Intragastric balloons attached to catheters or tubes may be used to record pressure or tone. The position of the catheters should be verified by fluoroscopy. In animal experiments, strain gauges are sewn to the serosa of the stomach to record circular or longitudinal muscle contractions.

Gastric myoelectric activity may be measured with Ag-AgCl electrodes positioned on the skin as shown in the figure. Bipolar electrodes may be sewn to the serosa in animal studies; cardiac pacing wires may be used for this purpose in humans. Slow waves and action potentials may be recorded with either serosal or mucosal electrodes; action potentials cannot be recorded directly with cutaneous electrodes. Mucosal electrodes mounted within a catheter may be held against the mucosa with suction or special magnets.

The result of postprandial gastric electrical and mechanical activity is the grinding, mixing, and emptying of gastric contents into the duodenum. The latter can be assessed by scintigraphic methods (see Chapter 7), ultrasonography, or magnetic resonance imaging.

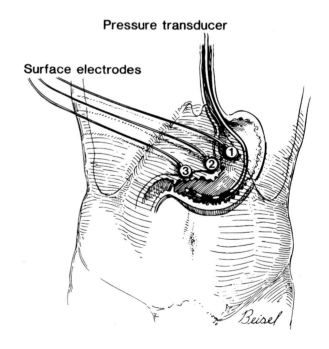

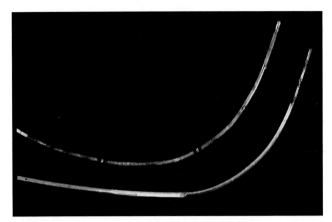

**FIGURE 10.3.** Antroduodenal motility catheters. This figure shows two different types of motility catheters used to record intraluminal pressures. Top Catheter is a solid-state catheter, whereas bottom catheter is a water-perfused catheter.

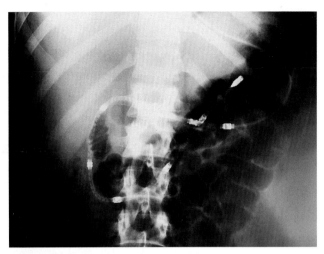

**FIGURE 10.4.** Abdominal flat plate radiograph of antroduodenal catheter in place.

The stomach is a remarkable mixing chamber. From sips of water to large milk shakes, from a dieter's rice cake to a full-course Thanksgiving turkey dinner, the stomach must accommodate ingested foods and then properly mix and empty nutrient suspensions into the duodenum. In addition to these physiologic mixing/emptying activities, the stomach contributes to many pleasurable sensations related to the satisfying epigastric fullness that accompanies the ingestion of a meal. On the other hand, when the neuromuscular apparatus of this sophisticated mixing chamber is dysfunctional, a variety of unpleasant and vague symptoms, ranging from epigastric distress to nausea and vomiting, are experienced.

In this chapter, the normal gastric anatomy and electromechanical activities that produce normal stomach motility are reviewed. Similar to cardiac physiology, the stomach should be viewed as a sophisticated "electromechanical" organ rather than an apparatus that simply contracts. Thus, abnormalities in gastric motility may be understood in terms of myoelectrical dysfunction and contraction/relaxation disorders. Disorders of contractile activity are illustrated and discussed in this chapter.

## NORMAL GASTRIC MOTILITY: ELECTROMECHANICAL ACTIVITY

### Gastric Muscular and Electrical Regions

*Anatomy*
The anatomic and pacemaker regions of the stomach are described in Figure 10.1. The fundic area is considered the proximal stomach, the area that relaxes to accommodate ingested food. The body (corpus) and antrum are considered the distal stomach, where solid foods are mixed and gently broken down by recurrent peristaltic waves.[1] When food particles are < 1 mm in diameter, these nutrient suspensions are emptied into the duodenum by gastric

peristaltic contractions.[1]

*Pacemaker Region/Activity*
From an anatomic viewpoint, the pacemaker region is an ill-defined area, as shown in Figure 10.1. The pacesetter potentials are thought to arise from the interstitial cells of Cajal located near the circular muscle layer.[2] (Note that the fundic muscle does not have a 3 cycle per minute (cpm) rhythm but rather is electrically "silent.") The frequency of the pacesetter potential is modulated by ongoing changes in vagal, splanchnic, and hormonal activity. Pacesetter potentials migrate distally from the corpus toward the pylorus at a rate of 3 cpm, with increasing velocity in the antrum.[3] The antrum is the site of most tachygastrias and tachyarrhythmias (abnormal 4–9 cpm electrical waves).[4]

### Methods of Recording Stomach Motility

*Intraluminal Pressure*
Gastric motility may be measured by a number of different methods, as shown in Figure 10.2. Intraluminal pressure recording devices have been the most popular means to quantitate gastric contractions (Fig. 10.3). Barium studies were used previously; however, although radiographic methods demonstrated a wide variety of lumen- and nonlumen-obliterating contractions, radiographic findings were not easily quantifiable. It is appreciated that a major deficiency in intraluminal pressure recording methods is that nonlumen-obliterating contractions are not detected. Sphincters, either esophageal or pyloric, may be reliably measured with Dent sleeve devices.

Intraluminal pressure recordings require solid-state or perfused catheters, intubation of the stomach, and placement of the catheters in the appropriate regions. Catheters can be placed during upper endoscopy or during fluoroscopy. Proper placement is usually verified with an abdominal radiograph (Fig. 10.4). Catheters are connected to a variety of commercially available recorders through pressure transducers and couplers.

**A**

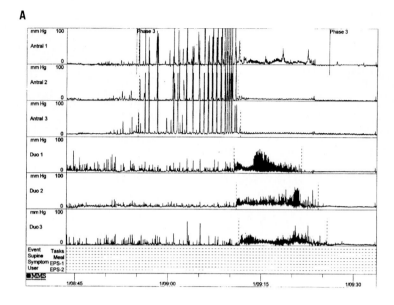

**B**

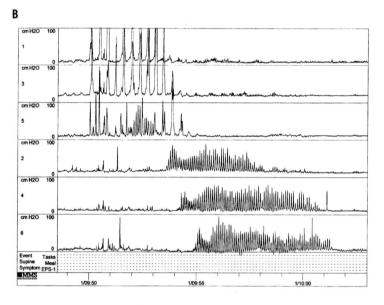

**C**

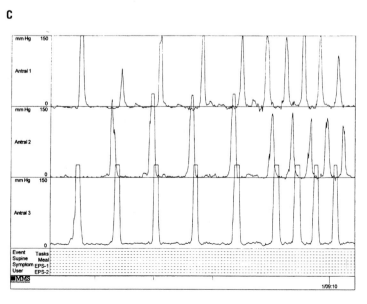

**FIGURE 10.5.** Gastric motility during fasting (the interdigestive state). **A**, Normal antroduodenal manometry—fasting state. Antral activity is recorded in the *top three panels*, whereas duodenal activity is recorded in the *lower three panels*. Time is recorded on the x axis, whereas amplitude of contractions, measured in mm Hg, is measured on the y axis. Gastric motility that occurs during fasting, recorded with intraluminal catheters, is characteristically divided into three distinct phases, as shown in **A**. Phase 1 of the migrating motor complex (MMC) is noted in the antrum in the first part of the tracing. The antrum is quiescent during phase 1 of the MMC (*far left-hand side of the panel*). Phase 1 always follows phase 3 of the MMC and typically lasts 40 to 50 minutes. Irregular, single contractions typify phase 2 of the MMC (see *mark*). This period typically lasts 40 to 50 minutes and culminates in the regular phase 3 contractions of the MMC, which last 3 to 5 minutes. Normal antral activity usually occurs at a frequency of 3 cpm. Phase 3 contractions originate in the antrum approximately 70% of the time and migrate through the duodenum and small intestine. Approximately 30% of the time, phase 3 contractions originate in the duodenum and migrate distally to the ileum. In **A**, the phase 3 front arises in the antrum and propagates normally into the small intestine. The phase 3 activity front in the antrum is then followed by the period of quiescence, phase 1. **B**, Normal antroduodenal manometry—fasting state. High-amplitude phasic antral contractions during phase 3 of the MMC are demonstrated in the *upper two panels*. This activity front propagates distally into the small intestine and initiates a normal-appearing phase 3 activity front in the small intestine at 11 to 12 cpm (*lower three panels*). The tracings in panel 3 were taken as the motility catheter migrated in and out of the pylorus. Visually, these tracings appear to be a composite of antral and duodenal activity. The amplitude of contractions is between that normally seen in the antrum (100 mm Hg) and the duodenum (50 mm Hg), whereas the frequency of contractions is also between that of the antrum (3 cpm) and the duodenum (11–12 cpm). **C**, Normal antral manometry—fasting state. Enlarged view of **B**. Phase 2 contractions are high amplitude, and the frequency is irregular (*left-hand side and middle portion of the panel*). On the *far right side* of the tracings, the contractions become more regular and rhythmic and average 3 cpm. Normal propagation of the wave front from proximal antrum (*top panel*) to lower antrum (*middle panel*) to the prepyloric region (*lower panel*) is demonstrated here. This process of disordered phase 2 contractions developing into more ordered, rhythmic contractions seen in phase 3 of the MMC is often referred to as antral build-up.

Using cutaneous electrodes, gastric myoelectrical activity (EGG) during the interdigestive patterns was studied in humans.[14] The normal 3-cpm myoelectrical rhythm was most stable during phase 1, or motor quiescence. A decrease in gastric frequency occurs during the transition from phase 1 to 2, and the frequency was very unstable during phase 3. Only 44% of phase 3 contractile complexes were reflected in the EGG signal as an increase in power at 3 cpm (see Chapter 13 for details).[14]

## Postprandial Mechanical and Electrical Activity of the Stomach

### Postprandial Mechanical Activities of the Stomach after Solid Meals

A series of gastric motility responses involving relaxation and contraction occurs after the ingestion of solid food.[15] Details of these gastric mechanical responses to solid food are presented in the legend of Figure 10.6.

An example of fundic relaxation in response to a swallow during a meal is shown in Figure 10.7. The rhythmic contractions of the antrum are also shown.[16] The contraction frequency is normally five peristaltic waves per minute in the dog, whereas in humans, three gastric peristaltic contractions per minute are elicited after meals.[17]

Figure 10.8 shows the relationship between intraluminal contractions in the distal antrum, pyloric pressures, and the flow of gastric chyme into the duodenum.[18] Each antral contraction empties 2 to 3 mL of nutrient suspension into the duodenum. When antral contractility is absent, pyloric pressure increases, thereby preventing retrograde flow from the duodenum back into the stomach. As the pressure increases in the antrum with the next peristaltic wave, the flow begins again across the pylorus and into the duodenum. It is in this fashion that solid and liquid meals are emptied over the hours after ingestion. A normal fed response to a meal is seen in Figure 10.9. Figure 10.10 demonstrates an apparently normal fed response and highlights some of the difficulties in interpreting antroduodenal motility studies.

### Postprandial Mechanical Activities of the Stomach after Liquid Meals

The gastric motility response to liquids begins with the rapid movement of liquids from the fundus to the antrum, filling of the gastric antrum, and onset of recurrent gastric peristalses, which empties liquids into the duodenum. The fundus slowly contracts, which creates an additional pressure gradient between the stomach and the duodenum, thereby forcing more liquid into the small bowel. Liquids of increasing caloric density or viscosity are emptied more slowly than non-nutrient liquids.[15] These inhibitory effects on gastric emptying are mediated by the release of hormones such as cholecystokinin in response to fatty liquids or to stimulation of osmoreceptors in the duodenum in response to hyperosmolar liquids. Physiologic delays in gastric emptying can be accomplished by increasing fundic relaxation, decreasing antral contractions, or increasing pyloroduodenal resistance.

### Postprandial Myoelectrical Activities

The key to normal peristaltic coupling is the proper aboral migration of the gastric pacesetter potential or gastric slow wave from the pacemaker region to the distal antrum. The gastric slow wave itself produces only a very tiny contraction in the circular muscle. Contractions of the circular muscle are needed for the work of gastric mixing/emptying and require plateau and action potentials that exceed the threshold for contraction of circular smooth muscle.[1,2] As measured by extracellular electrodes, a series of action potentials linked to the slow waves occurs during depolarization of the circular muscle.[2] Gastric myoelectrical activities are fully described in Chapter 13.

### Postprandial Pyloric Activity

As shown in Figures 10.6 (III) and 10.8, the pylorus is relaxed and open as the antral peristaltic waves empty aliquots of nutrient suspensions into the duodenum. Closure of the pylorus or increasing resistance to antral flow delays gastric emptying. Closure of the pylorus in response to fat in the duodenum may also delay the emptying of nutrients from the stomach.[19]

### Postprandial Antroduodenal Coordination

The duodenal bulb and postbulbar region of the duodenum are crucial mixing chambers in which the nutrient suspension is exposed to a variety of receptors located on the duodenal mucosa. Efficient gastric emptying and subsequent absorption of nutrients require neuromuscular coordination between the stomach and the small intestine, with a normal slow-wave frequency in the small intestine of approximately 12 cpm. Thus, an antral peristaltic wave normally empties a nutrient load into a relaxed bulb. The duodenal bulb then contracts to empty its contents into the more distal duodenum. Muscular resistances in the duodenum may serve as yet another "brake" to modulate the rate of gastric emptying.

The final result of normal gastric myelectrical activity, contractile activity, normal pyloric function, and antroduodenal coordination is the proper emptying of nutrients from the stomach into the duodenum. Thus, the lag phase and the linear phase of gastric emptying, as measured by scintigraphy, are mediated by specific electromechanical events of the stomach.

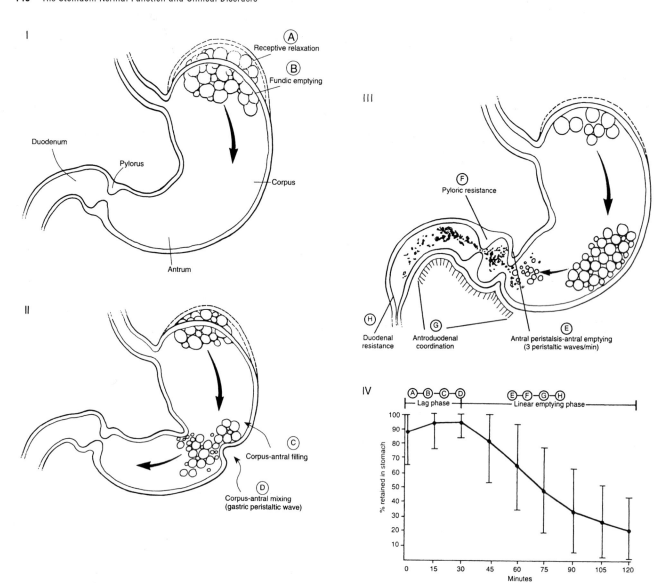

**FIGURE 10.6.** Gastric motility responses to solid food. **I**, Ingested food is received in the gastric fundus, which relaxes as the food bolus enters the proximal stomach (ie, receptive relaxation [**A**]). Receptive relaxation is a property of the proximal stomach—the fundus and proximal gastric body (corpus). Relaxation of the fundus allows for the accommodation of large volumes of food without a concomitant increase in pressure within the stomach. The ingested food is subsequently emptied from the fundus (**B**) into the corpus and antrum. Slow (0.3–1/min) contractions force the ingested food into the more distal stomach, where mixing begins. **II**, The corpus and the antrum fill (**C**) as the food is received from the fundus. Recurrent and gentle peristaltic waves mix the food with secreted acid and pepsin and move the food toward the pylorus (**D**). The peristaltic waves break the food into tiny pieces (1 mm) and mix them into a suspension suitable for emptying. Antral peristalses normally occur at 3 cpm, the rate of the pacesetter potentials. **III**, when the food particles in suspension are less than 1 mm and caloric content and viscosity are appropriate, then antral peristaltic contractions (**E**) occurring at three peristalses per minute sweep aliquots of the nutrient suspension through the pylorus. The pyloric sphincter may offer variable resistance or may close (**F**) during the antral peristaltic wave. Pyloric closure results in retropulsion of larger food particles back into the stomach for further mixing. Normal antro-duodenal coordination (**G**) ensures that antral peristalsis is coordinated with decreased duodenal pressure and resistance (**H**) to ensure efficient emptying with each antral peristalsis.

Abnormalities in any of these postprandial phases of gastropyloroduodenal muscular relaxations or contractions may lead to symptoms (epigastric fullness, epigastric pain, nausea) or altered gastric emptying of the solid foods. **IV**, When gastric motility is normal (as outlined in **A** though **H**), ingested meals are emptied in a normal fashion. This figure shows the gastric emptying rate for two technetium-labeled scrambled eggs as recorded by scintigraphy. The lag phase represents the time of redistribution of food from fundus to antrum and mixing of the contents (**A** to **D**) before the linear phase of emptying of gastric contents into the duodenum takes place (**E**, **F**, and **G**). During the linear emptying period, recurrent gastric peristaltic contractions empty small aliquots, or gushes, of the suspended nutrients into the duodenum. Extragastric factors such as duodenal resistance (**H**) also affect the rate of gastric emptying.

Thus, gastric emptying rates are produced by complex myoelectrical and mechanical (contractile) events coordinated by extrinsic and intrinsic neural activity of the stomach in concert with hormonal, duodenal, and small bowel influences on the rate of gastric emptying.

**FIGURE 10.7.** Fundic relaxation after deglutition and postprandial contraction pattern in the antrum. In response to the ingestion of food, intraluminal pressure recordings show different motor activities in the fundus compared with the antrum or distal stomach. The fundus relaxes in response to the swallowing of food, while the antrum exhibits cyclical contractions in the postprandial period. Antral contractions occur at 5 to 6 cpm, the normal slow-wave frequency in the dog. Reproduced with permission from Lind JF, Duthie HL, Schlegel JF, Code CF. Motility of the gastric fundus. Am J Physiol 1961;201:197–202.

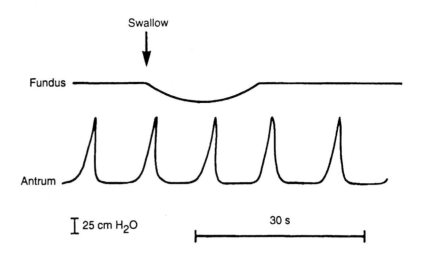

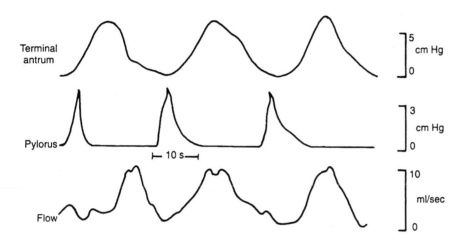

**FIGURE 10.8.** Antral contractions precede the flow of gastric contents into the duodenum. This figure shows terminal antral contractions that occur when the pyloric pressure is zero. During the antral contractions, gastric content is propelled into the duodenum, as recorded by the flow rates. The flow of luminal content into the canine duodenum takes place as 2- to 3-mL gushes. The peak rate of flow is approximately 10 mL/sec. The volume of the gush is determined by the duration of the flow. Reproduced with permission from Malbert CH, Ruckebusch Y. Relationships between pressure and flow across the gastroduodenal junction in dogs. Am J Physiol 1991;260:G653–7.

**FIGURE 10.9.** Normal antroduodenal manometry—fed response. Sporadic irregular contractions are seen in the stomach prior to eating a meal (*far left-hand side of top three panels*). The patient is then given a standard liquid meal, which is ingested over 5 to 10 minutes (see *mark*). After ingestion of a meal, high-amplitude but irregular contractions are seen in the antrum (*top three panels*), and irregular but lower-amplitude contractions are seen in the small intestine (*bottom two panels*).

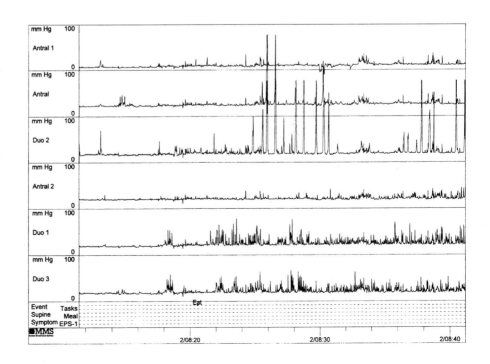

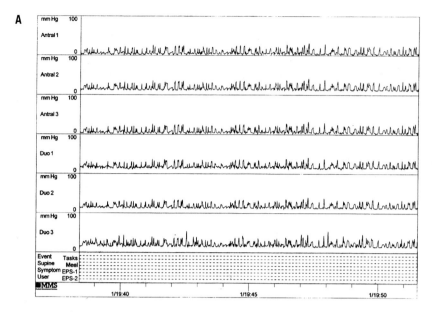

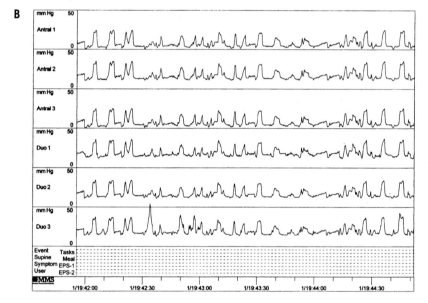

**FIGURE 10.10. A**, Antroduodenal manometry—apparently normal fed response. These tracings are from a woman with complaints of chronic nausea and early satiety. These tracings demonstrate an apparently normal fed response in the stomach and duodenum shortly after a standard liquid meal was ingested. Initial review demonstrates what appears to be a fed response in both the antrum (*top three panels*) and in the duodenum (*bottom three panels*). **B**, Antroduodenal manometry. This is the same tracing as in **A**; however, the scale is changed so that the time (x axis) is slowed down. When this is done, it is easy to see that the "contractions" in all six leads are mirror images of one another. This tracing was captured during an episode of retching and vomiting, and these antral "contractions" and small bowel "contractions" actually represent abdominal wall contractions. Note that these contractions are different from the characteristic retrograde contractions seen during vomiting.

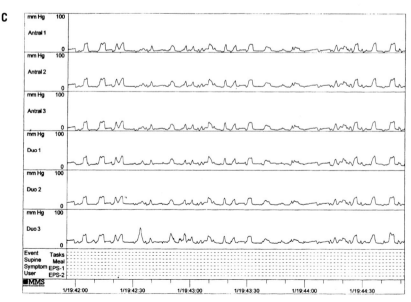

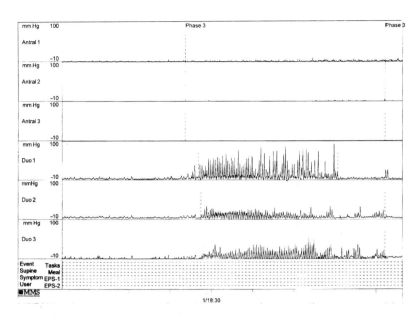

**FIGURE 10.11.** Antroduodenal manometry—fasting state. Severe antral hypomotility. Recordings from this young woman with idiopathic gastroparesis during the fasting part of the study reveal essentially no antral motility (*top three panels*). Placement of the solid-state catheter was confirmed both endoscopically and radiographically. Octreotide injection (50 μg SQ) stimulated a normal phase 3 activity front in the small intestine (*lower three panels*), which indicates that a myopathic process is not present in the small intestine and is unlikely to be present in the stomach, even with such severe antral hypomotility.

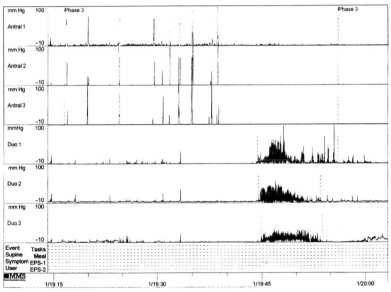

**FIGURE 10.12.** Antroduodenal manometry—fasting state. Severe antral hypomotility (< 1 cpm). Scattered, high-amplitude antral contractions are seen during phase 2 of the MMC (*top three panels*) in these tracings from a woman with idiopathic gastroparesis. However, regular 3-cpm contractions and generation of a normal phase 3 activity front in the antrum do not occur. A spontaneous phase 3 front is initiated in the small bowel and is propagated normally (*bottom three panels*) in an aboral direction (starts at 19:45).

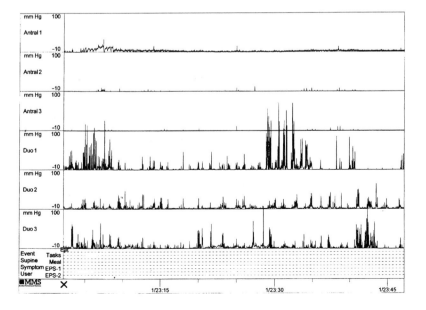

**FIGURE 10.13.** Antroduodenal manometry—absence of fed response. Severe antral hypomotility with absent fed response in the stomach. Essentially no contractile activity is noted in the antrum (*top three panels*). A standard meal was provided at approximately 22:55 (see *mark*). A fed conversion is noted in the small bowel (*lower three panels*); however, it is abnormal, given the presence of repetitive discrete clustered contractions (see Chapter 15 for discussion of small bowel motility). This patient had complaints of early satiety and postprandial nausea.

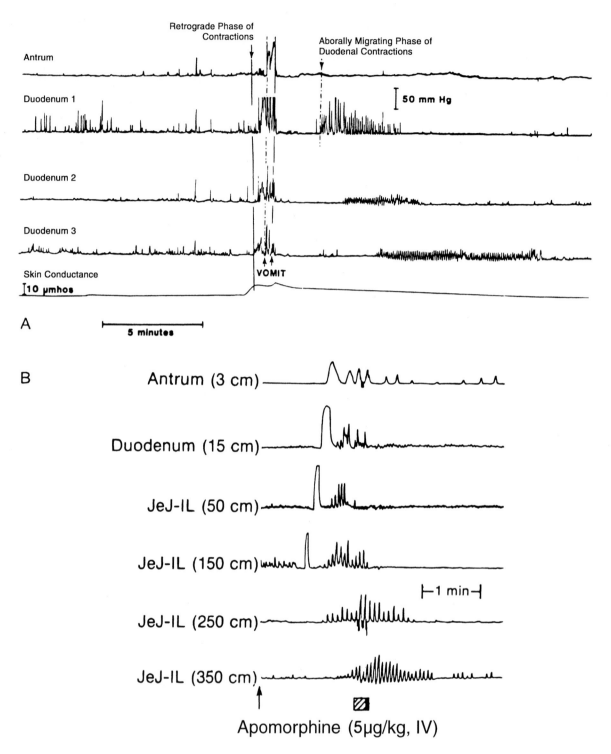

**FIGURE 10.14. A,** Retrograde peristaltic contractions recorded from the duodenum and antrum during vomiting. The retrograde contractions during vomiting were measured with intraluminal catheters. The retrograde contractions began in the duodenum (3) and migrated rapidly in the orad direction into the antrum. These events occurred spontaneously in a fed subject and preceded an episode of vomiting. Within 3 minutes of these events, a phase 3-like contraction complex commenced in the duodenum and migrated aborally from duodenum 1 to duodenum 3 ports. (Reprinted with permission from Thompson DG, Malagedla J-R. Vomiting and the small intestine. Dig Dis Sci 1982;27:1121–5). **B,** Retrograde peristaltic contractions induced by apomorphine in dog. These retrograde contractions begin in the jejunum-ileum (Jej-II [150 cm]), 150 cm from the pylorus, and propagate orally to the antrum (antrum [3 cm]) as recorded with strain gauges sewn to the serosa. Almost simultaneously, a phase 3-like contraction complex begins at JeJ-IL (250 cm) and migrates distally through the area of the strain gauge at JeJ-IL (350 cm). These motor events were associated with retching and illness behavior. The apomorphine-induced retrograde contractions were prevented by vagotomy, which indicates parasympathetic control of the motor events. Reproduced with permission from Lang IM, Sarna SK, Condon RE. Gastrointestinal motor correlates of vomiting in the dog: quantification and characterization as an independent phenomenon. Gastroenterology 1986;90:40–7.

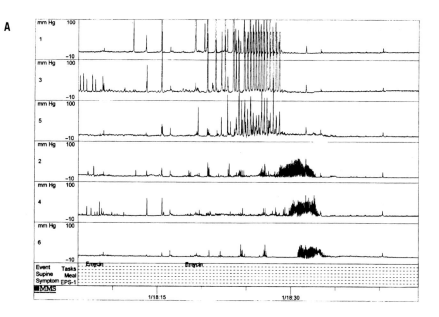

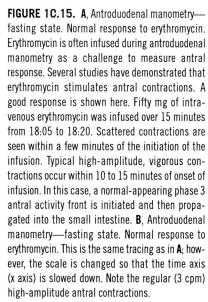

**FIGURE 10.15. A,** Antroduodenal manometry—fasting state. Normal response to erythromycin. Erythromycin is often infused during antroduodenal manometry as a challenge to measure antral response. Several studies have demonstrated that erythromycin stimulates antral contractions. A good response is shown here. Fifty mg of intravenous erythromycin was infused over 15 minutes from 18:05 to 18:20. Scattered contractions are seen within a few minutes of the initiation of the infusion. Typical high-amplitude, vigorous contractions occur within 10 to 15 minutes of onset of infusion. In this case, a normal-appearing phase 3 antral activity front is initiated and then propagated into the small intestine. **B,** Antroduodenal manometry—fasting state. Normal response to erythromycin. This is the same tracing as in **A;** however, the scale is changed so that the time axis (x axis) is slowed down. Note the regular (3 cpm) high-amplitude antral contractions.

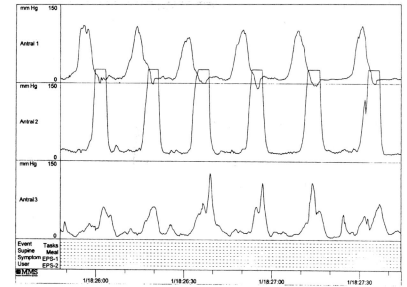

**FIGURE 10.16.** Antroduodenal manometry—fasting state. Normal antral response to intravenous erythromycin without propagation into the small intestine. High-amplitude phasic contractions are seen in the antrum (*top three panels*) approximately 10 minutes after initiation of intravenous erythromycin infusion (50 mg IV). Propagation of a phase 3 front into the small intestine does not occur in this case (*lower three panels*)

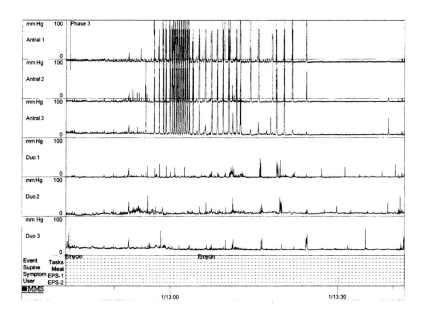

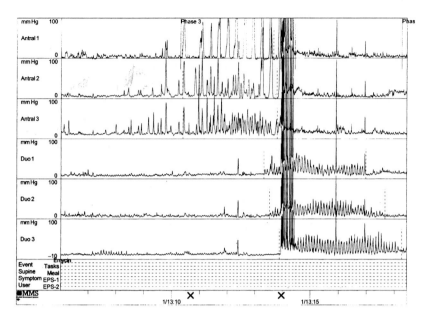

**FIGURE 10.17.** Antroduodenal manometry—fasting state. Exuberant antral response to erythromycin. These tracings are from a woman who was referred for complaints of early satiety. Five minutes after erythromycin infusion (50 mg IV), irregular contractions are noted in the antrum (*top three panels*). These develop into more regular high-amplitude contractions (*mark 1*), which then lead to vomiting (*mark 2*). Vomiting is demonstrated in all six panels as very high-amplitude, closely spaced mirror-image contractions. Despite vomiting, a phase 3 activity front is propagated into the small intestine (tracings 4–6).

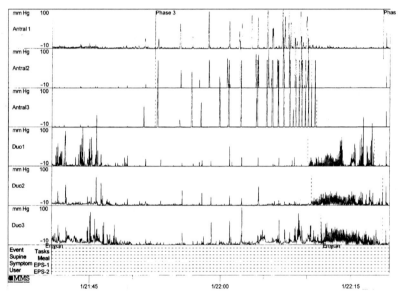

**FIGURE 10.18.** Antroduodenal manometry—fasting state. Abnormal response to erythromycin. These tracings are from a young woman with idiopathic gastroparesis and documented severe antral hypomotility on antroduodenal manometry (see Fig. 10.18 for comparison). Intravenous erythromycin (50 mg) produced some high-amplitude contractions (*top three panels*); however, they were decreased in frequency (< 2 cpm). Interestingly, this antral build-up, although abnormal, was enough to stimulate a normal propagated wave front into the small intestine (*lower three panels*).

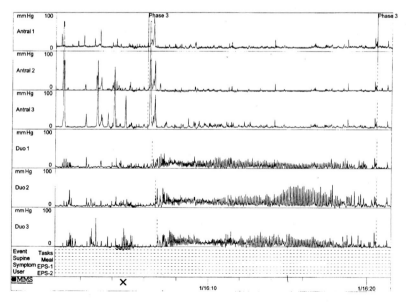

**FIGURE 10.19** Antroduodenal manometry—fasting state. Normal response to octreotide injection. Octreotide is often given during testing to determine the responsiveness of the small intestine. This information can be clinically useful as octreotide is one of only a few agents that reliably stimulate small bowel motility. Octreotide (50 µg sc) was given at approximately 16:05 (see *mark*) and induced a prolonged phase 3 activity front in the small intestine (*lower three panels*). Octreotide normally inhibits antral activity, which is demonstrated here (*upper three panels*).

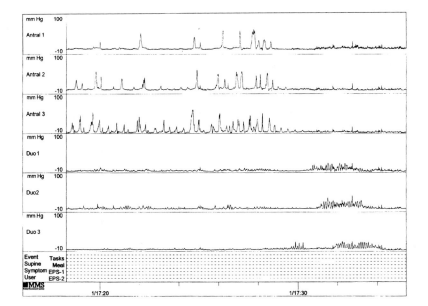

**FIGURE 10.20.** Antroduodenal manometry—fasting state. Scleroderma. Evidence of a myopathic process affecting the small intestine is demonstrated by the very low-amplitude contractions seen in the *bottom three tracings.* Octreotide injection (50 μg SQ) at 17:30 induces a low-amplitude phase 3 activity front that propagates normally in an aboral direction, although the duration is abbreviated. There is no evidence of a severe myopathic process in the stomach, given the normal amplitude of contractions during phase 2 (*top three tracings*). This patient had progressive weight loss with severe abdominal distention and bloating and recurrent episodes of nausea and vomiting.

## GASTRIC MOTILITY DISORDERS: MECHANICAL AND ELECTRICAL DYSFUNCTION

### Gastric Mechanical Dysfunction

#### *Fundus*

In response to the ingestion of liquids and solids, the gastric fundus relaxes to accommodate the volume received. After vagotomy, the fundus does not accommodate or relax normally in response to ingestion of foods.[20] Generally, there is incomplete relaxation or a diminished ability to accommodate ingested foods in the postvagotomy situation.[21] Dysfunction of the fundus has recently been assessed with gastric barostat methods. In patients with dyspepsia, the compliance of the gastric fundus is normal when compared with healthy volunteers.[22] These findings raise the hypothesis that dyspeptic patients have abnormal perceptions of gastric fundic motility. Inadequate fundic relaxation and excessive fundic relaxation are potential disorders that have not been reported in other patient groups.

#### *Body-Antrum*

ANTRAL HYPOMOTILITY: Antral hypomotility is illustrated in Figures 10.18 to 10.20.[23] In contrast to the normal subject with regular, rhythmic, postprandial antral contractions (see Fig. 10.5), the patients shown in Figures 10.11 to 10.13 have marked antral hypomotility, as shown by very low-amplitude and, quite commonly, nearly absent antral contractions. Antral hypomotility is associated with postsurgical gastroparesis, diabetic gastroparesis, and idiopathic gastroparesis. A recent study found antral hypomotility in patients with functional dyspepsia.[24]

ANTRAL TONE: Abnormalities in antral tone are also possible mechanisms of motor dysfunction of the distal stomach. Preliminary studies have shown that balloon distention of the body-antrum precipitates increased symptoms in dyspeptic patients compared with healthy volunteers,[25] but the changes in gastric tone are similar in the patients and controls.

Therefore, it is possible that symptoms of dyspepsia are attributable to altered perception of normal tone or abnormal sensory input from the stomach (ie, electrical abnormalities) rather than abnormalities in contractile function or tone.

#### *Pylorus*

Dysfunction of the pylorus ranges from pylorospasm, an entity that is infrequently diagnosed (but has been associated with diabetic gastroparesis), to pyloric incompetence, which may predispose to bile reflux gastritis. Pyloric stenosis, secondary to fibrous inflammatory changes or tumors, may result in gastric outlet obstruction and symptoms of delayed gastric emptying.

### Nausea and Vomiting

In addition to early satiety, epigastric discomfort, abdominal distention, nausea, and vomiting are common symptoms associated with gastric motility disorders.

#### *Gastric Mechanical Activity during Nausea and Vomiting*

As shown in Figure 10.14, spontaneous vomiting in a healthy subject was associated with a retrograde peristaltic contraction, which began in the duodenum and was followed by phase 3-like contractions in the duodenum.[26] During nausea, antral contractions are not present, but duodenal contractions may occur (personal observations). In response to apomorphine-induced nausea and vomiting, the canine gastrointestinal tract responds with stereotypical contractile activity.[27] As shown in Figure 10.14B, a burst of contractions occurs at approximately 150 cm into the jejunum and migrates in a retrograde manner through the duodenum and into the antrum, while at the strain gauge located at 250 cm, a contraction wave moves distally. These contractile sequences were associated with retching and illness in the dog.

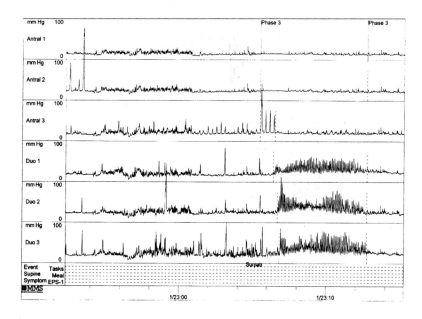

**FIGURE 10.21.** Antroduodenal manometry—fasting state. Normal response to sumatriptan. Approximately 5 minutes after subcutaneous injection of sumatriptan (6 mg), a phase 3 activity front is induced in the small intestine (*lower three panels*). Scattered antral contractions are seen prior to sumatriptan injection (*top three panels*); however, these stop after the injection. Sumatriptan is a 5-hydroxytryptamine agonist that has been shown to stimulate small bowel motility in both normal volunteers (Tack J, Coulie B, Wilmer A, Peeters T, Janssens J. Actions of the 5-hydroxytryptamine-1-receptor agonist sumatriptan on interdigestive gastrointestinal motility in man. Gut 1998; 42:36–41) and in patients with neuropathic disorders of the small intestine (Mathis C, Schettler-Duncan VA, Crowell MD, Lacy BE. The effects of sumatriptan on antroduodenal manometry in patients with gastrointestinal dysmotility. Gastroenterology 2001;120: A1257).

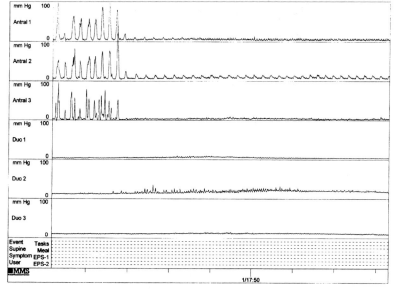

**FIGURE 10.22.** Antroduodenal manometry—fasting period. Polymyositis. This patient has severe polymyositis with recurrent bouts of pseudo-obstruction. A myopathic process is noted in the small intestine, evidenced by nearly flat tracings (*lower three panels*). Correct positioning of the motility catheter was verified during endoscopy and afterward by an abdominal radiography. A spontaneous phase 3 activity front is seen in the stomach (*top three panels*). This appears to propagate into the small intestine, although the amplitude of contractions is severely diminished (*bottom three panels*). In connective tissue disorders, the myopathic process often does not affect the stomach until much later in the course of the disease, and the effects on the stomach are often greatly overshadowed by small intestine symptoms. Note that there is a persistent artifact in the *second panel from the top*.

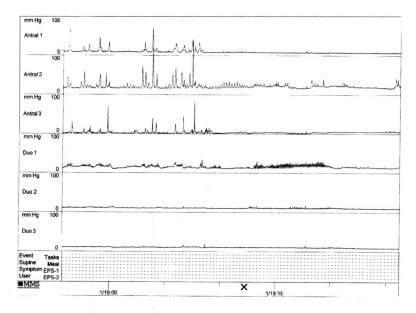

**FIGURE 10.23.** Antroduodenal manometry—fasting state. Systemic lupus erythematosis. These tracings are from a woman with complaints of nausea, vomiting, weight loss, and abdominal bloating and distention. Scattered antral contractions (phase 2) can be seen in the *first half of the top three panels*. Octreotide injection (50 µg SQ) is then given (*see mark*). Antral activity is inhibited; however, essentially no contractile activity is seen in the *lower two panels*, consistent with a myopathic process of the small intestine. Very low-amplitude contractions are seen in the most proximal duodenal port (*third panel from the bottom*).

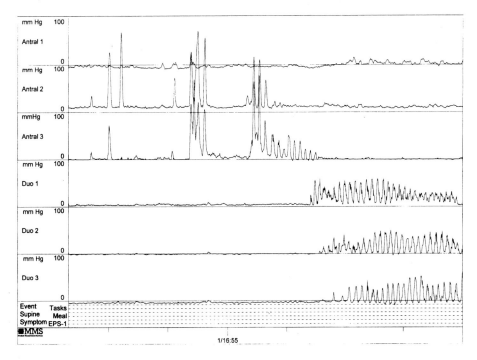

**FIGURE 10.24.** Antroduodenal manometry—fasting period. This patient previously underwent vagotomy and pyloroplasty for recurrent ulcer disease. Irregular disordered contractions are noted in the antrum (*top three panels*). A spontaneous phase 3 activity front is seen in the small intestine, which propagates normally (*bottom three panels*). A phase 3 activity front in the antrum, which usually precedes small bowel phase 3 wave fronts, did not occur in this patients.

### Miscellaneous Stomach Patterns

#### *Gastric Responses to Sham Feeding*

In response to cephalic vagal stimulation of sham feeding, antral contractions increase[30] and EGG waves increase in amplitude at the 3-cpm frequency.[31] Furthermore, atropine blocks sham feeding–induced antral contractions, and patients with previous vagotomies failed to show an increase in 3-cpm electrical activity during sham feeding. These data indicate that cephalic vagal reflexes increase gastric contractile and electrical activity.

#### *Gastric Responses to Cold Pressor Tests*

In response to plunging the hand into 4°C water, gastric emptying is delayed, and antral hypomotility occurs.[32] The amplitude of normal 3-cpm EGG activity decreases in response to the cold pressor test.[33] These data indicate that an increase in sympathetic nervous system activity induced by the cold pressor test decreases gastric contractile and electrical activity.

#### *Gastric Responses to Drug Challenges*

Erythromycin is often used to treat patients with gastroparesis because of its ability to stimulate antral contractions. The effects of erythromycin are demonstrated in normal patients in Figures 10.15, 10.16, and 10.17 and in a patient with idiopathic gastroparesis in Figure 10.18.

Octreotide is known to stimulate small bowel motility. A subcutaneous injection of 50 μg of octreotide usually indicates a phase 3 activity within minutes in normal volunteers (Fig. 10.19). An abbreviated response is seen in a patient with scleroderma. (Fig. 10.20). Sumatriptan has recently been shown to also stimulate small bowel motility;[29] its effects are shown in Figure 10.21.

A number of different disease states often produce characteristic patterns that can be identified during antroduodenal manometry. Patients with scleroderma usually have preserved antral motility even if the small bowel is significantly affected (see Fig. 10.20). Polymyositis also affects the small bowel first, leaving the stomach relatively unaffected (Fig. 10.22). Similar effects may be seen in patients with systemic lupus erythematosis (Fig. 10.23). Patients who have had prior vagotomy and pyloroplasty may demonstrate a number of different motility patterns, depending on the extent of prior surgery. Disordered contractions in the antrum are frequently seen (Fig. 10.24).

### SUMMARY

The study of gastric motility using manometry is the study of stomach movements. Stomach movements involve muscular contractions and relaxations that occur during fasting or postprandial conditions and during a host of environmental and personal stressors. The muscular or mechanical activities of the stomach are modulated and mediated by electrical events. The study of the manometric events of the normal stomach will help us to better understand and treat mechanical dysfunctions in our patients.

## REFERENCES

1. Meyer JE. Motility of the stomach and gastroduodenal junction. In: Johnson LR, ed. Physiology of the gastrointestinal tract. New York: Raven Press, 1987:393–410.

2. Sarna S. *In vivo* myoelectrical activity: methods, analysis, and interpretation. In: Schultz S, Wood JD, eds. Handbook of physiology, the gastrointestinal system. Baltimore: Williams & Wilkins, 1989: 817–863.

3. Hinder RA, Kelly KA. Human gastric pacesetter potential: site of origin, spread and response to gastric transection and proximal gastric vagotomy. Am J Surg 1977;133:29–33.

4. Bortolotti M, Sarti P, Barbara L, Brunelli F. Gastric myoelectrical activity in patients with chronic idiopathic gastroparesis. J Gastrointest Motil 1990;2:104–108.

5. Abell TL, Malagelada J-R. Glucagon-evoked gastric dysrhythmias in humans shown by an improved electrogastrographic technique. Gastroenterology 1985;88:1932–1940.

6. Familoni BO, Bowes KL, Kingma YJ, Cote KR. Can transcutaneous recordings detect gastric electrical abnormalities. Gut 1991;32:141–146.

7. Koch KL, Stewart WR, Stern RM. Effect of barium meals on gastric electromechanical activity in man. A fluoroscopic-electrogastrographic study. Dig Dis Sci 1987;32:1217–1222.

8. Hamilton JW, Bellahsene BE, Reicherlderfer M, et al. Human electrogastrograms. Comparison of surface and mucosal recordings. Dig Dis Sci 1986;31:33–39.

9. Stern RM, Koch KL. Electrogastrography: methodology, validation and applications. New York: Praeger, 1985.

10. Labo G, Bortolotti M, Vezzadini P, et al. Interdigestive gastroduodenal motility and serum motilin levels in patients with idiopathic delay in gastric emptying. Gastroenterology 1986;90:20–26.

11. Vantrappen G, Janssens J, Hellemans J, Ghroos Y. The interdigestive motor complex of normal subjects and patients with bacterial overgrowth of the small intestine. J Clin Invest 1977;59:1158–1166.

12. Cohen S, Snape WJ. Movement of the small intestine and large intestine. In: Sleisenger MH, Fordtran JS, eds. Gastrointestinal disease: pathophysiology, diagnosis, treatment. Philadelphia: WB Saunders, 1989:1088–1105.

13. van der Schee EJ, Grashuis JL. Contraction-related, low-frequency components in canine electrogastrographic signals. Am J Physiol 1983; 245:G470–475.

14. Geldof H, van der Schee EJ, Grashuis JL. Electrogastrographic characteristics of the interdigestive migrating complex in humans. Am J Physiol 1986; 250:G165–171.

15. McCallum RW. Motor function of the stomach in health and disease. In: Sleisenger M, Fordtran J, eds. Gastrointestinal disease: pathophysiology, diagnosis, treatment. Philadelphia: WB Saunders, 1989: 675–713.

16. Lind JF, Duthie HL, Schlegel JF, Code CF. Motility of the gastric fundus. Am J Physiol 1961;201:197–202.

17. Rees WDW, Miller LJ, Malagelada J-R. Dyspepsia, antral motor dysfunction, and gastric stasis of solids. Gastroenterology 1980;78: 360–365.

18. Malbert CH, Ruckebusch Y. Relationships between pressure and flow across the gastroduodenal junction in dogs. Am J Physiol 1991;260: G653–657.

19. Heddle R, Dent J, Read NW, et al. Antropyloroduodenal motor responses to intraduodenal lipid infusion in healthy volunteers. Am J Physiol 1988;254:G671–679.

20. Aune S. Intragastric pressure after vagotomy in man. Scand J Gastroenterol 1969;4:447–454.

21. Azpiroz F, Malagelada J-R. Gastric tone measured by an electronic barostat in health and postsurgical gastroparesis. Gastroenterology 1987;92:934–943.

22. Mearin FO, Cucala M, Azpiroz F, et al. Origin of gastric symptoms in functional dyspepsia. Gastroenterology 1989;96: A337.

23. Malagelada J-R, Stanghellini V. Manometric evaluation of functional upper gut symptoms. Gastroenterology 1985;88:1223–1231.

24. Stanghellini V, Ghidini C, Maccarini MR, et al. Fasting and postprandial gastrointestinal motility in ulcer and nonulcer dyspepsia. Gut 1992;33:184–190.

25. Lemann M, Dederding JR, Jian R, et al. Abnormal sensory perception to gastric distention in patients with chronic idiopathic dyspepsia—the irritable stomach. Gastroenterology 1989;96:A29.

26. Thompson DG, Malagelada J-R. Vomiting and the small intestine. Dig Dis Sci 1982;27:1121–1125.

27. Lang IM, Sarna SK, Condon RE. Gastrointestinal motor correlates of vomiting in the dog: quantification and characterization as an independent phenomenon. Gastroenterology 1986;90:40–47.

28. Tack J, Coulie B, Wilmer A, Peeters T, Janssens J. Actions of the 5-hydroxytryptamine-1-receptor agonist sumatriptan on interdigestive gastrointestinal motility in man. Gut 1998;42:36–41.

29. Mathis C, Schettler-Duncan VA, Crowell MD, Lacy BE. The effects of sumatriptan on antroduodenal manometry in patients with gastrointestinal dysmotility. Gastroenterology 2001;120: A1257.

30. Katschinski M, Dahmen G, Reinshagen M, et al. Cephalic stimulation of gastrointestinal secretory and motor responses in humans. Gastroenterology 1992;103:383–391.

31. Stern RM, Crawford HE, Stewart WR, et al. Sham feeding. Cephalic-vagal influences on gastric myoelectrical activity. Dig Dis Sci 1989; 34:521–527.

32. Thompson DG, Richelson E, Malagelada J-R. Perturbation of upper gastrointestinal function in cold stress. Gut 1983;24:277–283.

33. Stern RM, Hu S, and Koch KL. Effects of cold stress on gastric myoelectrical activity. J Gastrointest Motil 1991;3:225–228.

# CHAPTER 11

# Barostat Measurements

*Fernando Azpiroz and Beatrice Salvioli*

Some parts of the gastrointestinal tract, such as the proximal stomach, have the capability of exerting a tonic, that is, sustained, contraction. This type of contraction has been described on the basis of radiologic studies since the beginning of the century.[1] Toward the end of the 1970s, electrophysiologic studies in smooth muscle strips in vitro demonstrated that both the proximal stomach and the small intestine have a basal tone (Fig. 11.1).[2]

However, gut tonic activity is difficult to detect under physiologic conditions in vivo. For instance, measuring intraluminal pressures in the proximal stomach, either directly or by means of intraluminal bags at different volumes, does not detect tonic changes, probably because pressure changes produced by tonic activity are eclipsed by background noise caused by respiratory artifacts and other movements.[3]

In general, muscular activity in vitro can be measured either by using an isometric system, which maintains a constant length and measures changes in tension, or by means of an isotonic system, which maintains a constant muscle tension and measures changes in length (Fig. 11.2). Given that the isometric approach in the stomach (ie, fixed intraluminal volumes) was ineffective, an isotonic approach was applied, maintaining a constant intraluminal pressure and measuring changes in muscular length, that is, in intraluminal volume. For this purpose, an electronic barostat was developed (Fig. 11.3).

The barostat maintains a constant pressure within an intraluminal bag by injecting or withdrawing air.[4,5] When the pressure falls below the selected level, the system injects air, and when the pressure increases, the system aspirates air (Fig. 11.4). Thus, the volume of air within the intraluminal bag reflects the tonic contraction: a volume reduction reflects a contraction, and a volume expansion reflects a relaxation. Barostats with different types of air pumps have been manufactured (Fig. 11.5).

## THE BAG OF THE BAROSTAT

The function of the intraluminal bag is to isolate a segment of the gut without interfering with its function. The bag has to be oversized and flaccid, without offering resistance to inflation or deflation (Fig. 11.6). Ultrathin polyethylene (sandwich bags) is suitable for that purpose. By using a bag sealer, any shape can be tailored (Fig. 11.7).

The intraluminal bag is connected to the pressure transducer and the air pump of the barostat by a double-lumen catheter. The pressure should be monitored directly within the bag by a separate lumen. To maintain a constant pressure level in the bag, the air pump of the barostat presses and suctions air into and from the bag. Hence, the pressures in the pump and along the inflation line may differ considerably from the pressure level in the bag. If the pressure is not monitored directly within the bag, the system will be dampened,

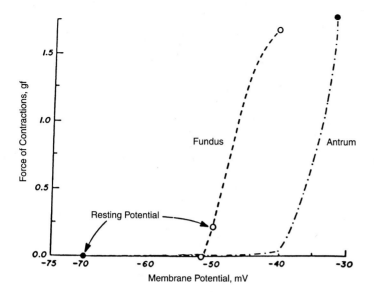

**FIGURE 11.1.** Functional division of the stomach. Comparisons of voltage-tension curves of the fundus and antrum of circular muscle of canine stomach. Inflexion point at approximately −50 mV for the fundus and −40 mV for the antrum represents the threshold for contraction. The resting membrane potential of smooth muscle cells of the proximal stomach is above the threshold for contraction, that is, the muscle maintains a basal tonic contraction. Changes in membrane potential modulate this tonic activity, a hyperpolarization relaxes the muscle, and a partial depolarization increases the tonic contraction. By contrast, in antral smooth muscle cells, the resting membrane potential is below the threshold for contraction, and partial depolarization triggers action potentials with concomitant phasic contractions. Adapted from Szurszewski JH.[2]

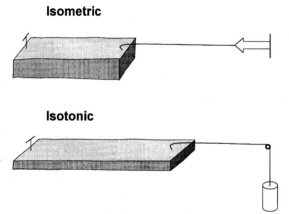

**FIGURE 11.2.** In vitro measurement of muscle activity. The isometric system measures changes in tension at fixed length, and the isotonic system changes in length at constant tension.

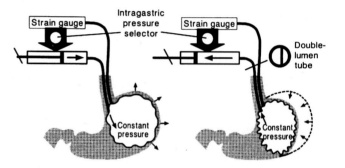

**FIGURE 11.3.** The barostat consists of a pressure transducer connected by an electronic relay to an air pump. A pressure selector allows the desired pressure level to be set. When the stomach relaxes, the system injects air (*left*), and when the stomach contracts, air is aspirated (*right*). Reproduced with permission from Azpiroz F, Malagelada J-R. Gastric tone measured by an electronic barostat in heath and postsurgical gastroparesis. Gastroenterology 1987;92:934–43.

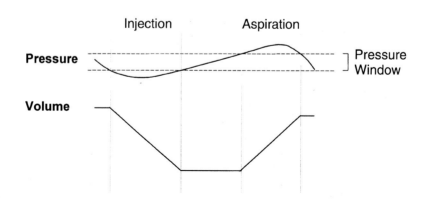

**FIGURE 11.4.** Operation of the barostat. When the pressure falls below the selected level, the system injects air, and when the pressure increases, the system aspirates air. For most purposes, the barostat operates best at a pump speed of 40 mL/s and a pressure window (from injection to aspiration) of 0.3 mm Hg. In some systems, these parameters can be programmed; other systems may require a simple internal adjustment.

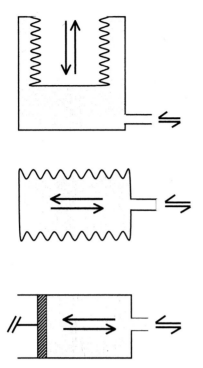

**FIGURE 11.5.** Models of a barostat pump. The pump of the barostat may be either deformable (bellows type) or rigid (piston type), and this is important because it determines the compression factor, that is, the volume change caused by the deformation of the pump and the compression of air produced by a pressure increment. For most bellows-type barostats, the compression factor is approximately 5 to 7 mL/mm Hg, but each barostat should be tested. Other systems are considerably less deformable, but still the compression factor (if only because of the compressibility of air) may be important when intrabag volumes are small, as in the small intestine. The compression factor is calculated by connecting the pressure line to the inflation line in a closed system. With this set-up, volume change produced by an increment in the operating pressure is measured. The volume change should then be divided by the pressure increment to express the compression factor in mL/mm Hg.

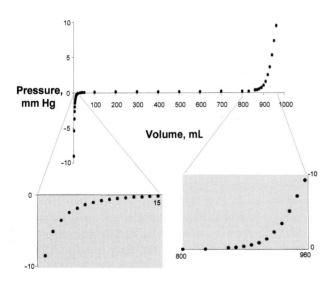

**FIGURE 11.6.** Compliance of the bag. Intrabag pressure measured at different inflation volumes. Data are means of triplicate tests.

**A**

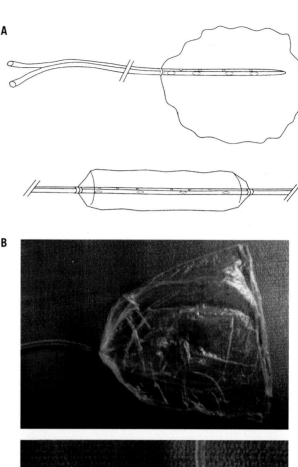

**B**

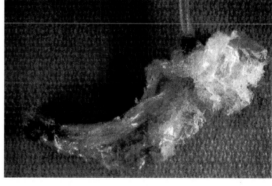

**FIGURE 11.7.** Intraluminal bags. **A**, For reservoir organs like the stomach, the spherical type of bags is appropiate. For tubular regions, such as the small intestine, cylindrical bags can be used with a fixed length and radially oversized. Gastric tone can be recorded with a 700-mL bag, but distention may require a 1,100-mL capacity. Small bowel motor activity can be monitored with 10-cm-long bags; a perimeter of 18 cm will suffice both for recording intestinal tone and to produce distention. The connecting tube can be made of polyvinyl with internal diameters of 0.8 mm for the pressure line and 2 mm for the inflation line. However, the diameter of the inflation line depends on the organ and the type of study. Specifically, the diameter of the tube will be inversely related to the length of the tube and the airflow required (ie, magnitude and velocity of volume changes in the organ studied). For most purposes, the type of double-lumen tubes used for gastric suction, specifically 12 French size, is appropriate. The tube has to be protected, either externally or both lumen internally, so that the bag can be tightly tied without collapsing the tube. Before each study, the probe (bag and connecting catheter) should be tested, under water, for leaks. **B**, Bag before and after recording gastric tone in a dog. The flaccid bag adapts to the gastric wall, and after extubation, it maintains the intragastric shape.

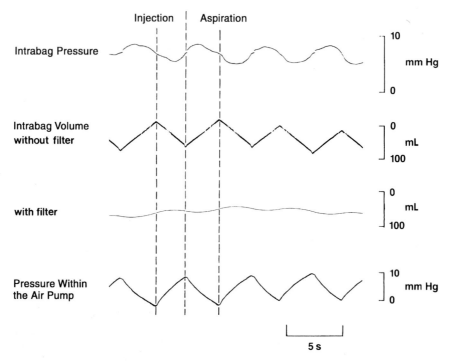

**FIGURE 11.8.** Variations produced by respiratory motion. The bag within the abdominal cavity is subjected to small pressure changes caused by respiratory motion that elicit a rapid and continuous to-and-fro response in the barostat. To press and suction air rapidly through the inflation line, the pressure in the pump increases and decreases considerably. These pressure changes in the pump produce a compression and decompression of the air volume and a deformation of the pump that artificially magnify the respiratory volume variations. The magnitude of the error can be calculated by measuring the pressure within the pump, but, for practical purposes, it is not necessary. The magnitude of the error is fairly constant because it is related to the resistance to airflow through the inflation line and not to the volume of air within the bag. Therefore, when intrabag volumes are large, as in the stomach, the respiratory artifacts do not interfere with the measurements. However, with small volumes, as in the small intestine, the respiratory artifacts may obscure the volume recordings. In this case, the simplest approach is to use an on-line filter that smooths the respiratory oscillations (a 0.5-Hz filter usually clears up the tracing). Reproduced with permission from Rouillon J-M, Azpiroz F, Malagelada J-R. Reflex changes in intestinal tone: relationship to perception. Am J Physiol 1991;261:6280–6.

and the pressure in the bag may not be maintained constant.

Normally, the movements of the gut are fairly slow, and intrabag pressure is maintained constant by the barostat with a relatively slow airflow through the inflation channel. However, respiration induces a motion artifact (Fig. 11.8).[6]

## INTUBATION TECHNIQUE

The bag of the barostat should be finely folded before intubation. Oral intubation is preferred because nasal extubation may be very uncomfortable, particularly using large bags. A wire introduced into the inflation line stiffens the tube and facilitates pharyngeal passage of the bag.[7] Pyloric passage for intestinal studies can be achieved with a weighted tip. Intestinal progression of the tube to the desired location may be speeded using an inflatable tip balloon or alternatively inflating the bag of the barostat once into the intestine. After intubation, the bag has to be unfolded by inflation of air under controlled pressure. A volume of 300 mL may be required for intragastric bags; in the intestine, the volume depends on the length of the bag. Extubation should be performed with the connecting tube open because if a com-

plete suction is performed, the bag becomes rigid, and extubation may be traumatic.

## SELECTION OF THE OPERATING PRESSURE

The abdominal cavity behaves as a water-filled container, and the hydrostatic pressure at each site depends on body position. The operating pressure in the barostat is adjusted in each study at a level 1 to 2 mm Hg above intra-abdominal pressure (Fig. 11.9). It is advisable to position the subjects so that the bag is located in the upper part of the abdominal cavity. Otherwise, the intra-abdominal pressure will be higher, and viscera lying on top of the bag will artificially dampen the responses. Intragastric pressure may vary from 1 to 2 mm Hg upright to 4 to 5 mm Hg in the recumbent position. Furthermore, since air floats within the abdominal cavity, air in the intragastric bag will occupy different areas, depending on the body position. Upright, air will be located in the upper part of the stomach, but in the supine position, air will tend to displace into the antrum, which is located close to the anterior abdominal wall. To record gastric tone, that is, the tonic contraction of the

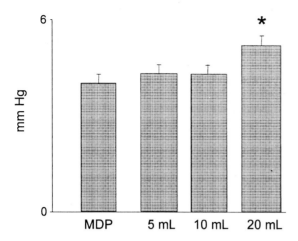

**FIGURE 11.9.** Determination of intra-abdominal pressure. Intra-abdominal pressure can be determined as the minimal distending pressure (MDP) by increasing intrabag pressure in 1-mm Hg steps every minute until the bag starts to inflate and the barostat records changes induced by respiratory motion. Alternatively, small amounts of air can be introduced into the bag while measuring intrabag pressure. With small volumes, such as 5 mL and 10 mL in the stomach, intrabag pressure reflects the intra-abdominal pressure and indeed is similar to the MDP. However, with larger volumes, such as 20 mL in the stomach, intrabag pressure is significantly higher. * $p < .05$ vs MDP. (Data from Distrutti et al.[24])

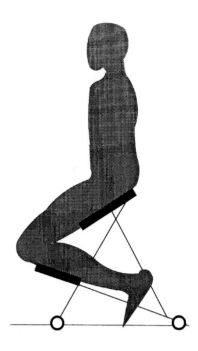

**FIGURE 11.10.** Body position for gastric studies. Ergonomic chairs allow the trunk to remain erect while the person sits comfortably and are useful for prolonged studies recording tone of the proximal stomach.

proximal stomach, the upright position is advised.[7,8] Ergonomic chairs are very useful for this purpose (Fig. 11.10). Small intestinal activity can be adequately recorded in the recumbent position.

## DESCRIPTIVE STUDIES

Using the barostat at a constant, physiologic pressure level (1 to 2 mm Hg above intra-abdominal pressure), changes in intrabag volume reflect variations in gut tone. Furthermore, using this pressure level, the barostat does not disturb the normal physiologic activity of the upper gut.[4] The barostat in the proximal stomach detects variations of baseline volume during the interdigestive motor cycle (Fig. 11.11). Baseline volume is large during motor quiescence (phase 1) and decreases during periods of motor activity (phases 2 and 3). These baseline variations reflect changes in gastric tone. However, superimposed on these baseline changes, the barostat also detects volume waves at a rhythm of about one per minute.[5] In humans, manometry fails to detect any kind of activity in the proximal stomach, but in dogs, the one-per-minute contractions of the proximal stomach are much more vigorous and can be detected by manometry (Fig. 11.12).[3,4] The barostat also detects changes in intestinal tone during the interdigestive motor cycle (Fig. 11.13).[6]

During swallowing, the barostat detects the receptive relaxation of the stomach, which is analogous to the relaxation of the lower esophageal sphincter associated with swallowing (Fig. 11.14).[4,8–10] After meal ingestion, the barostat detects the accommodative relaxation and, subsequently, a progressive contraction that conceivably produces gastric emptying (Fig. 11.15).[9] Hence, the stomach operates as a reservoir of variable capacity (Fig. 11.16).

These descriptive experiments are very illustrative but have limited value, particularly during the postprandial period. Indeed, tone measurements by means of the barostat require that the volume measured within the bag corresponds to the total intragastric volume, which is not true after a meal.

## MEASUREMENT OF REFLEX RESPONSES

The barostat can be used for mechanistic studies in the gut. In these experiments, the gut lumen can be kept empty so that the barostat measures the total intraluminal volume. The barostat can be applied to measure physiologic reflexes, such as the gastric relaxation induced by intestinal nutrients (Fig. 11.17).[11] In a dog model with isolated loops of intestine (Fig. 11.18), it has been shown that this reflex relaxation depends both on the type of nutrients and the area of the gut exposed (Fig. 11.19).[12] However, in humans, the evaluation of nutrient-induced reflexes is limited by the fact that once the nutrients have been infused into the intestine, their fate is uncontrolled in that they may spread and stimulate different areas of the gut.

Other types of better controlled stimuli, such as distention, can also be applied to elicit reflexes. Distention can be produced by means of an inflatable balloon and allows

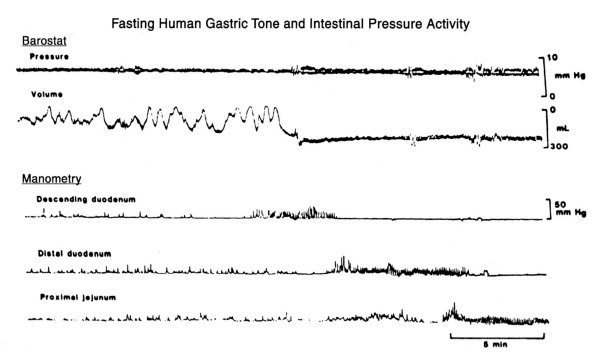

**FIGURE 11.11.** Interdigestive activity of the proximal stomach. During intestinal phases 2 and 3 recorded by manometry, the barostat records a high gastric tone and phasic volume waves. During duodenal phase 1, gastric tone is low without volume waves. Reproduced with permission from Azpiroz F, Malagelada J-R. Gastric tone measured by an electronic barostat in health and postsurgical gastroparesis. Gastroenterology 1987;92:934–43.

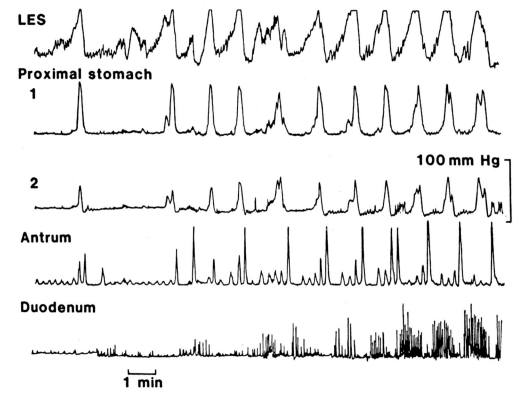

**FIGURE 11.12.** Canine gut pressure activity during fasting recorded by manometry. Note the relationship of funding waves with an increase in lower esophageal sphincter (LES) pressure and antral activity and with a decrease in duodenal phase 3 activity. Reproduced with permission from Azpiroz F, Malagelada J-R. Pressure activity patterns in the canine proximal stomach: response to distension. Am J Physiol 1984;247:265–72.

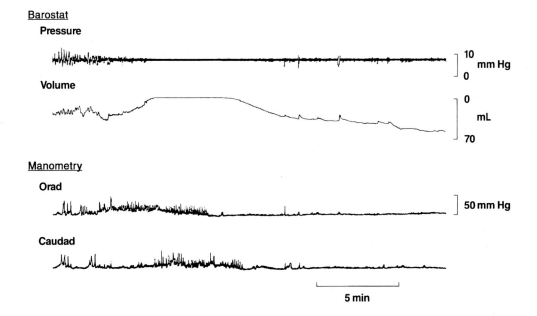

Barostat
**Pressure**

] 10
mm Hg
] 0

**Volume**

] 0
mL
] 70

Manometry

**Orad**

] 50 mm Hg

**Caudad**

5 min

**A**

The Receptive Relaxation of the Stomach

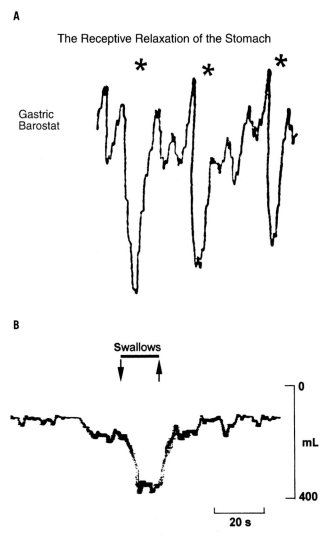

Gastric
Barostat

**B**

Swallows

0

mL

400

20 s

**FIGURE 11.14.** Gastric receptive relaxation. **A**, Example of gastric relaxation in response to swallowing. **B**, This phenomenon (see asterisks) was initially described by Cannon using a hydrostatic barostat. Adapted from Cannon and Lieb.[10]

**FIGURE 11.13.** Interdigestive variations in intestinal tone. Intestinal tone monitored with a 10-cm intraluminal bag and pressure activity recorded 5 cm orad and 5 cm caudad to the bag by manometry. Note barostat volume collapse during phase 3 progression and subsequent relaxation. During phase 1, the intestine progressively relaxed (gradual volume increase undetected by manometry). Reproduced with permission from Rouillon J-M, Azpiroz F, Malagelada J-R. Reflex changes in intestinal tone: relationship to perception. Am J Physiol 1991;261:G280–6.

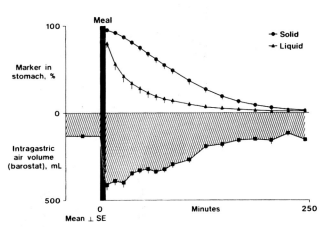

**FIGURE 11.15.** Gastric accommodation. Gastric tone, measured by the barostat, during gastric emptying of a radiolabeled meal, measured by scintigraphy. Before meal ingestion, intragastric volume was small, reflecting the high basal gastric tone. Meal ingestion was associated with a marked volume increase, reflecting a gastric accommodation. Ingestion of the 300-mL meal not only did not collapse the intragastric bag but also caused a marked expansion up to a total volume (air plus meal) close to 700 mL. Subsequently, gastric tone recovered, paralleling gastric emptying. Reproduced with permission from Moragas G, Azpiroz F, Pavía J, Malagelada J-R. Relations among intragastric pressure, postcibal perception and gastric emptying. Am J Physiol 1993;264:G1112–7.

**A**

Gastric Accommodation          Gastric Emptying

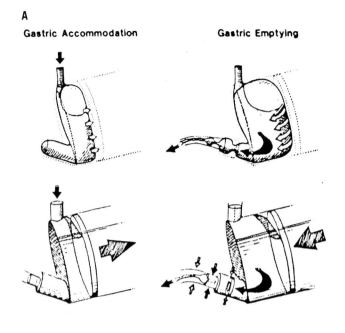

**B**

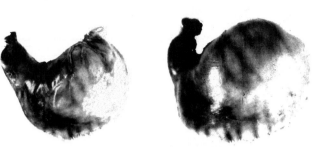

**FIGURE 11.16.** Gastric reservoir function. **A,** The proximal stomach relaxes to accommodate the meal and subsequently contracts to produce gastric emptying. Final gastric outflow is regulated by the resistance of the antroduodenal path. Reproduced with permission from Malagelada J-R, Azpiroz F. Determinants of gastric emptying and transit in the small intestine. In: Schult SG, Wood JD, Rauner BB, editors. Handbook of physiology. Section 6: the gastrointestinal system. Vol 1: motility and circulation. 2nd ed. Bethesda (MD): American Physiology Society; 1989. p. 909–37. **B,** Canine stomach before and during inflation. Note the greater distensibility and storage function of the proximal stomach.

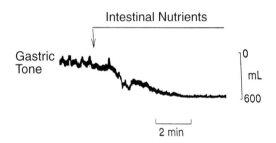

**FIGURE 11.17.** Enterogastric reflex induced by nutrients. Basal gastric tone was high (small volume); a continuous infusion of nutrients into the duodenum, mimicking the postprandial intestinal load, produced a marked gastric relaxation (volume increment).

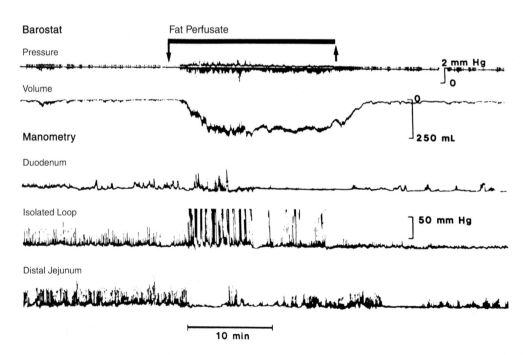

**FIGURE 11.18.** Gastric tone in a canine model with an isolated loop of proximal intestine. Phasic pressure activity was recorded proximal to the loop, within the loop and distal to it, by manometry. Fat infusion into the loop produced a gastric relaxation and stimulated phasic activity in the loop. After washing out the loop with saline, gastric tone recovered. Reproduced with permission from Azpiroz F, Malagelada J-R. Regulation of gastric tone by the proximal and distal small bowel in the dog [abstract]. Surg Forum 1984;35:185.

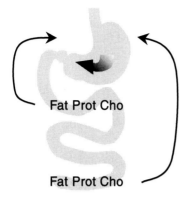

**FIGURE 11.19.** Intestinal control of gastric tone. Gastric tone is regulated depending on the nutrient composition of chyme along the small intestine. In dogs, fat induces a marked gastric relaxation in the proximal intestine, protein (prot) has a weak effect, and carbohydrate (cho) has no effect. By contrast, in the distal intestine, carbohydrate and protein induce a marked gastric relaxation, whereas fat has no effect.

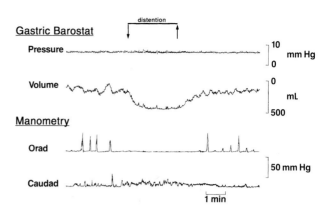

**FIGURE 11.20.** Enterogastric reflex induced by distention. Distention of a duodenal balloon produced a marked gastric relaxation, which reverted after cessation of the stimulus. Phasic pressure activity recorded in the antrum orad to the distending balloon was also inhibited during the distention. Reproduced with permission from Azpiroz F, Malagelada J-R. Perception and reflex relaxation of the stomach in response to gut distention. Gastroenterology 1990;98:1193–8.

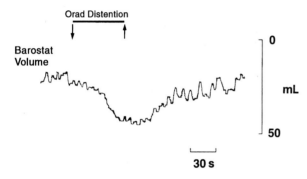

**FIGURE 11.21.** Antegrade intestino-intestinal reflex. Intestinal tone recorded by a 10-cm-long bag. Distention of an 8-cm orad balloon induced an intestinal relaxation that reverted after deflation of the balloon. Reproduced with permission from Rouillon J-M, Azpiroz F, Malagelada J-R. Reflex changes in intestinal tone: relationship to perception. Am J Physiol 1991;261:6280–6.

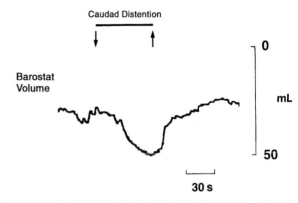

**FIGURE 11.22.** Retrograde intestino-intestinal reflex. Distention of a 20-cm caudad balloon induced an intestinal relaxation. Reproduced with permission from Rouillon J-M, Azpiroz F, Malagelada J-R. Reflex changes in intestinal tone: relationship to perception. Am J Physiol 1991;261:6280–6.

application of brief stimuli (Fig. 11.20).[13] The barostat has proven particularly useful to measure reflex responses, as compared with other methods that measure phasic activity, such as manometry or electromyography. Since phasic activity is intermittent, an inhibitory reflex may be undetected, particularly using brief stimuli. Intestinal distention also elicits intestino-intestinal relaxatory reflexes,[6,14] both antegrade (Fig. 11.21) and retrograde (Fig. 11.22). Using two barostats, enterogastric and intestino-intestinal reflexes can be simultaneously recorded.[15]

Thermal stimuli can also be applied in the gut.[11,16] Warm stimulation either of the stomach or the duodenum elicits a reflex gastric relaxation (Fig. 11.23). By contrast, cold stimulation of the stomach produces a gastric contraction (Fig. 11.24).

The barostat can also record somatovisceral reflexes,[17] such as the gastric reflex relaxation induced by the cold pressure test, that is, hand immersion into iced water (Fig. 11.25).

## PHARMACOLOGIC STUDIES

The barostat is well suited to measure the effect of drugs on gut tone. For instance, glucagon, a drug well known to inhibit gut muscular activity, induces a short lag time and marked relaxation both of the stomach and the small intestine (Fig. 11.26).[6,18,19]

Pharmacologic studies in dogs have demonstrated that the high level of gastric tone during fasting is maintained by a basal cholinergic input that can be suppressed by atropine and that is difficult to further increase by pharmacologic doses of bethanecol (Fig. 11.27).[20] During fasting, adrenergic blockers do not modify gastric tone, suggesting the lack of basal adrenergic input. However, adrenergic stimulation by epinephrine produces a gastric relaxation. Enterogastric relaxatory reflexes, induced either by intestinal nutrients or distention, produce a gastric relaxation via a nonadrenergic, noncholinergic mechanism.[21,22] By combining pharmaco-

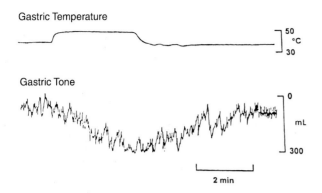

**FIGURE 11.23.** Gastrogastric reflex induced by warm stimulation. Intragastric temperature was maintained by a thermostat that recirculates water at fixed temperatures through an intragastric bag. Gastric warming of the distal stomach produced a relaxation of the proximal stomach measured by the barostat. Reproduced with permission from Villanova N, Azpiroz F, Malagelada J-R. Perception and gut reflexes induced by stimulation of gastrointestinal thermoreceptors in humans. J Physiol [Lond] 1997;502.1:215–22.

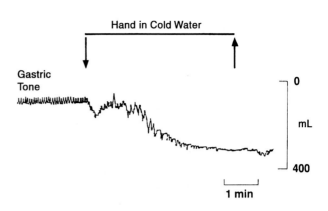

**FIGURE 11.25.** Somatovisceral reflex. After a few minutes, hand immersion into cold water induced a gastric relaxation.

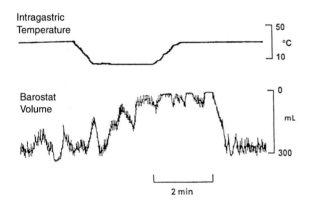

**FIGURE 11.24.** Gastrogastric reflex induced by cooling. Cooling of the distal stomach by means of a thermostat produced a marked contraction of the proximal stomach measured by the barostat. Gastric tone returned to baseline after rewarming of the stomach. Reproduced with permission from Villanova N, Azpiroz F, Malagelada J-R. Gastrogastric reflexes regulating gastric tone and their relationship to perception. Am J Physiol 1997;273:G464–9.

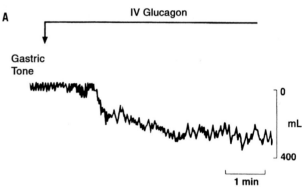

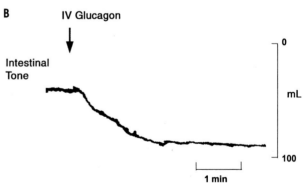

**FIGURE 11.26.** Relaxatory effect of glucagon. Shortly after intravenous administration, glucagon inhibited the tonic contraction of the stomach (**A**) and small intestine (**B**). Reproduced with permission from Notivol R, Coffin B, Azpiroz F, et al. Gastric tone determines the sensitivity of the stomach to distension. Gastroenterology 1995;108:330–6.

**FIGURE 11.27.** Combined pharmacologic and vagal cooling experiments in dogs. During fasting (intravenous saline), gastric tone is high and vagal cooling produces a gastric relaxation, suggesting that fasting tone is maintained by a vagal input. An adrenergic agonist produces a gastric relaxation, which is still further increased by vagal cooling. Adrenergic blockers have no effect on basal gastric tone or tone during cooling. A cholinergic agonist produces an increase in basal gastric tone and abolishes the effect of cooling. Cholinergic blockade produces a gastric relaxation that is not further increased by vagal cooling. Adapted from Azpiroz F, Malagelada J-R. Importance of vagal input in maintaining gastric tone in the dog. J Physiol [Lond] 1987;384:511–24.

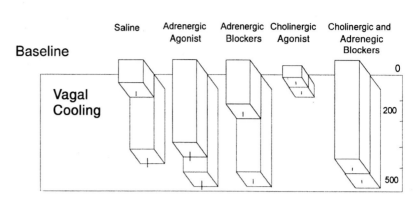

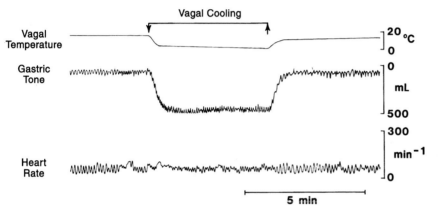

**FIGURE 11.28.** Effect of vagal cooling on canine gastric tone. Experiments were performed in a chronic canine model with an implanted cooling jacket around the supradiaphragmatic vagal nerves. In the fasting conscious and resting animal, vagal cooling produced a complete gastric relaxation without changes in heart rate. After vagal rewarming, gastric tone recovered. Reproduced with permission from Azpiroz F, Malagelada J-R. Importance of vagal input in maintaining gastric tone in the dog. J Physiol [Lond] 1987;384:511–24.

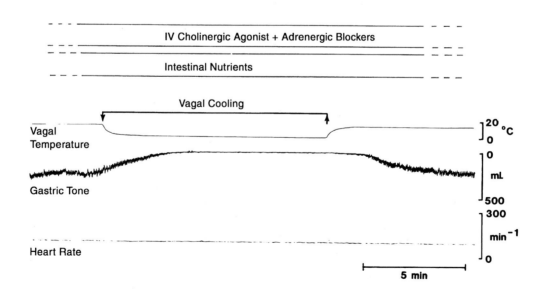

**FIGURE 11.29.** Mechanism of enterogastric reflex induced by nutrients. During intestinal infusion of nutrients and simultaneous intravenous administration of a cholinergic agonist plus adrenergic blockers, gastric tone is low, suggesting that intestinal nutrients relax the stomach by a nonadrenergic, noncholinergic mechanism. During vagal cooling, gastric tone increases, driven by the cholinergic pharmacologic background, and after vagal rewarming, the stomach relaxes again, suggesting that the relaxatory input is driven by the vagus. Reproduced with permission from Azpiroz F, Malagelada J-R. Vagally mediated gastric relaxation induced by intestinal nutrients in the dog. Am J Physiol 1986;251:G727–35.

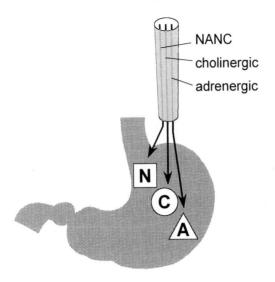

**FIGURE 11.30.** Vagal innervation of the proximal stomach. During fasting, the stomach is maintained by vagal cholinergic input. Nutrients induce gastric relaxation by a vagal nonadrenergic, noncholinergic (NANC) mechanism. During fasting, there is no basal adrenergic input on the proximal stomach, but adrenergic stimulation induces a gastric relaxation.

logic studies with a technique of reversible vagal blockade by cooling, it was further shown that both basal cholinergic input and nonadrenergic, noncholinergic relaxatory reflexes are mediated by the vagus (Figs. 11.28 to 11.30).[20–22]

## MEASUREMENT OF COMPLIANCE

The applications of the barostat so far described are all performed using constant intraluminal pressure and measuring variations in intraluminal volume. However, the barostat can also be used to manipulate intraluminal pressure while measuring the volume response.[5,17,18,23,24]

The barostat at a constant pressure level measures variations in tone but not the absolute tone level. Indeed, comparisons of tone based on absolute volume levels are not reliable because the basal volume depends on the pressure set by the barostat, which is selected based on the determination of the intra-abdominal pressure level. Small errors in the determination of the intra-abdominal pressure or changes attributable to body position may have a major impact on the basal volume recorded by the barostat. Determination of the basal level of tone in different subjects may be achieved by glucagon administration to abolish muscular contraction.

Another alternative to compare tone in different subjects is to measure compliance.[25] Compliance reflects both the capacity and the distensibility of the organ (ie, the elastic properties of the gut wall), which are modified by the muscular activity. To measure compliance, the operating pressure of the barostat is increased while intraluminal volumes are measured. Ideally, the whole pressure/volume curve should be represented for each subject because the shape of the curve may be different

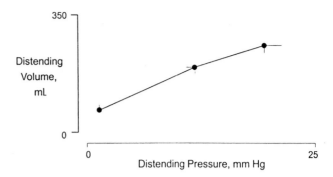

**FIGURE 11.31.** Intestinal compliance. Compliance was measured by increasing the pressure within a 36-cm-long intestinal bag, while measuring intrabag volume. Volume has been corrected using the compression factor. Adapted from Serra et al.[23]

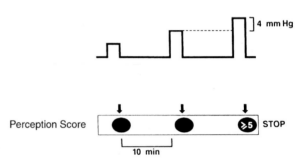

**FIGURE 11.32.** Sensitivity studies: methods. Intermittent phasic distentions can be applied at a regular interval (10 minute) in stepwise increments (4 mm Hg) up to the threshold for discomfort. After each distention, subjective perception is measured using a scale. Adapted from Azpiroz and Malagelada.[26]

in various conditions (Fig. 11.31).[23] Changes in the operating pressure require corrections in the recorded volume based on the compression factor. Indeed, by increasing the pressure, the air within the pump compresses and the wall of the air pump may deform so that the volume recorded by the barostat is larger than the real volume within the bag.[7]

The speed of the pressure change has to be adapted to the speed of the pump and the resistance to airflow through the connecting tube. The operating pressure has to be changed at a rate that can be followed by the barostat without overshooting. If the pressure is raised abruptly, the barostat will overpressurize the pump, and air will still be pressed into the bag after the desired pressure level has been reached and surpassed. The same phenomenon will apply to abrupt pressure reductions: the barostat will produce a vacuum in the pump, and air will be suctioned from the bag after the desired pressure set has been surpassed.

## SENSITIVITY STUDIES

The barostat operating at a low, constant pressure level is unperceived and does not modify the physiologic activity of the gut. However, intraluminal pressure increments may

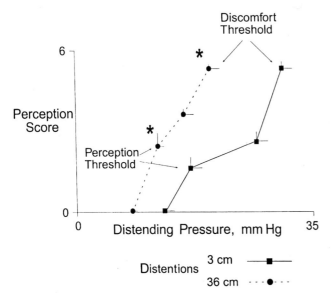

**FIGURE 11.33.** Stimulus-related perception of intestinal distention. Distention was performed by increasing the pressure either in a 3-cm-long intestinal bag or in a 36-cm-long bag. Perception was measured by a 0 to 6 scale. In the 3-cm segment, low intraluminal pressures did not induce perception; perception was related to the pressure from the threshold for perception up to the threshold for discomfort. Hence, perception depends on the intensity of the stimulus. However, perception also depends on the length stimulated, that is, on the number of receptors activated: distending pressures that were not perceived in the 3-cm segment, induced perception in the 36-cm segment, and distending pressures well tolerated in the short segment induced discomfort when applied in the long segment. Reproduced with permission from Serra J, Azpiroz F, Malagelada J-R. Modulation of gut perception in humans by spatial summation phenomena. J Physiol [Lond] 1998;506.2:579–87.

induce conscious perception and gut reflexes. Hence, the barostat can be used to produce gut stimulation and induce sensory and reflex responses.[19,26–28] Different stimulation paradigms can be used. Graded pressure increments can be applied either by phasic or stepwise pressure increments while measuring the intensity of perception by means of a scale (Fig. 11.32). With this simple method, stimulus response curves can be performed (Fig. 11.33). Alternatively, a tracking method can be used to determine pre-established perception levels, such as the threshold of first sensation and the threshold for discomfort.[29] This methodology can also be applied to study the relation between perception and visceral reflexes (Fig. 11.34). Indeed, both responses are mediated by different neural pathways and can be independently stimulated (Fig. 11.35).[19,26]

Initially, the barostat was thought to provide a better standardization of gut stimuli than fixed volume distentions. However, this is not really so. When gut compliance is similar, either fixed volume or barostat distentions produce standardized stimulation, but the stimuli are not comparable when the compliance is different. For instance, gastric distention at the same volumes results in lower intraluminal pressures and lower perception when the stomach is relaxed (Fig. 11.36).[18] On the contrary, using the barostat, the same pressure levels result in larger volumes and higher perception when the stomach is relaxed (Fig. 11.37).[18,24] Hence, neither volume (ie, elongation) nor intraluminal pressure is the factor that determines conscious perception. To try to solve this methodologic limitation, a computerized tensostat was developed, which is really an extension of the barostat concept.[24]

The tensostat is a computerized pump that, based on intraluminal pressure and volume, calculates the tension on the

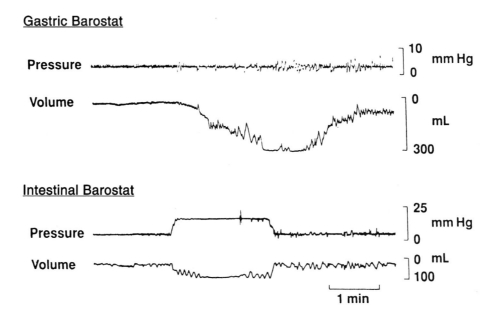

**FIGURE 11.34.** Enterogastric reflex elicited by the barostat. Duodenal distention was produced by increasing the pressure with the intestinal barostat, and the gastric relaxatory response was recorded by the gastric barostat as volume expansion at a constant pressure level. Reproduced with permission from Coffin B, Azpiroz F, Guarner F, Malagelada J-R. Selective gastric hypersensitivity and reflex hyporeactivity in functional dyspepsia. Gastroenterology 1994;107:1345–51.

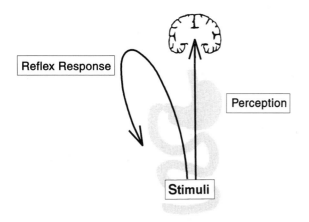

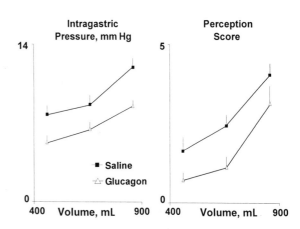

**FIGURE 11.35.** Responses to gut stimuli. Physiologic stimuli activate reflexes that regulate gut function without perception. Some stimuli may activate perception pathways and induce conscious sensations. However, reflexes and perception are mediated by independent mechanisms.

**FIGURE 11.36.** Gastric distention at fixed volume levels. Gastric distention was produced in healthy subjects both during baseline (intravenous saline administration) and during gastric relaxation induced by glucagon. At the same distending volumes, both intragastric pressure and perception scores were significantly smaller when the stomach was relaxed. Adapted from Notivol et al.[18]

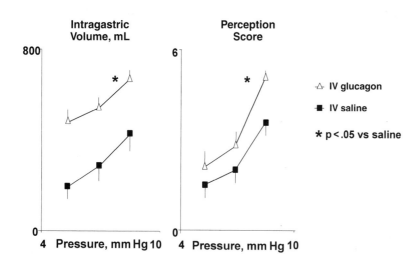

**FIGURE 11.37.** Gastric distention at fixed pressure levels. Using the barostat, fixed levels of intragastric pressure were tested both during baseline (intravenous saline) and during gastric relaxation (intravenous glucagon). At the same pressure levels, both intragastric volumes and perception scores were significantly higher when the stomach was relaxed. Adapted from Distrutti et al.[24]

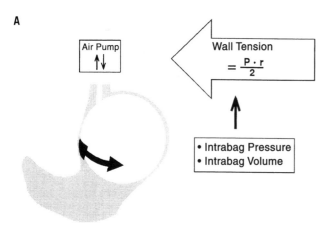

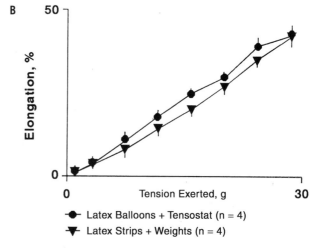

**FIGURE 11.38.** The tensostat. **A,** The tensostat is a computerized air pump that applies fixed tension levels on the gut wall. Based on intraluminal pressure and volume, the system calculates wall tension and drives the pump to maintain the desired tension level. Reproduced with permission from Distrutti E, Azpiroz F, Soldevilla A, Malagelada J-R. Gastric wall tension determines perception of gastric distension. Gastroenterology 1999;116:1035–42.

**B,** The tensostat was validated by comparing the elongation produced on a latex balloon by the tensostat to that produced by equivalent weights on 1-cm-wide latex strips. Reproduced with permission from Azpiroz F, Malagelada J-R, Distrutti E. Reply to letter to the editor: development of a tensostat for gastric perception studies. Gastroenterology 2000;118:A670.

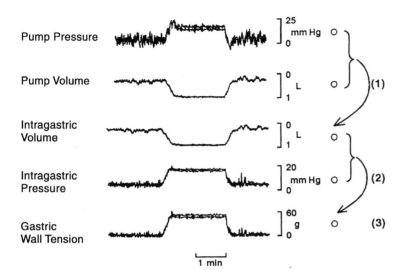

**FIGURE 11.39.** Operation of the tensostat. (1) Based on the pressure and the volume in the pump, the system calculates the real intragastric volume by applying the compression factor; (2) based on the corrected intragastric volume and the transmural pressure (intraluminal pressure minus intra-abdominal pressure calculated at the beginning of the experiment), the system calculates wall tension and (3) operates the pump to maintain the wall tension within ± 1 g of the preselected level. Reproduced with permission from Distrutti E, Azpiroz F, Soldevilla A, Malagelada J-R. Gastric wall tension determines perception of gastric distension. Gastroenterology 1999;116:1035–42.

gut wall by applying Laplace's law and maintains the preselected tension level (Figs. 11.38 and 11.39). The tensostat is based on the assumption that intraluminal air conforms to a regular shape, either spherical or cylindrical, which is obviously inexact. However, the studies performed serve as a bioassay to demonstrate the reliability of the system.[24] For instance, fixed tension levels applied by the tensostat produce similar perception whether the stomach is contracted or relaxed, despite the fact that intraluminal volumes are markedly different (Fig. 11.40). These data suggest that perception of gut distention depends on stimulation of tension receptors (Fig. 11.41). Hence, the advantage of the tensostat is that it allows standardization of gut stimuli and comparisons of perception independently of the size or the segment of the gut under study. The tensostat is a substantial methodologic advancement that is particularly useful for the evaluation of the effects on visceral perception of drugs that also modify gut compliance.[30]

## CLINICAL APPLICATIONS

The barostat has limited clinical applications, with very precise indications and restricted use in experienced laboratories. In clinical practice, the barostat may provide useful information on gastric tone, by measuring compliance and pharmacologic responses, and on gastric sensitivity, whereas the evaluation of reflexes may still be more experimental. The barostat is particularly useful in the evaluation of two gastrointestinal syndromes: functional dyspepsia and gastroparesis.

### Functional Dyspepsia

Patients with functional dyspepsia present upper abdominal symptoms in the absence of detectable abnormalities by conventional testing. In these patients, compliance is similar to healthy subjects, indicating that basal gastric tone is normal

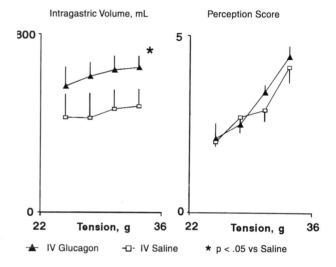

**FIGURE 11.40.** Gastric distention at fixed tension levels. Using the tensostat, fixed wall tension levels were applied both during baseline (intravenous saline) and during gastric relaxation (intravenous glucagon). The same tension levels produced significantly larger intragastric volumes when the stomach was relaxed. Perception was related to wall tension, and remained similar during baseline and during gastric relaxation, despite the larger intragastric volumes. Adapted from Distrutti et al.[24]

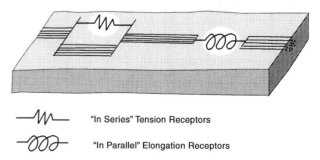

**FIGURE 11.41.** Putative mechanoreceptors in the gastric wall. Perception of gastric distention depends on stimulation of "in series" tension receptors. "In parallel" elongation receptors may be related to reflex pathways but do not seem involved in conscious perception.

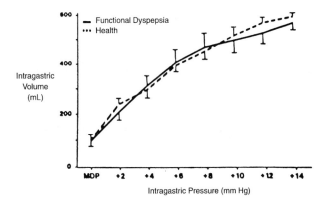

**FIGURE 11.42.** Gastric hypersensitivity in functional dyspepsia. Intragastric pressures that were unperceived in healthy subjects induced significant symptoms in patients with functional dyspepsia. MDP = minimal distending pressure. Reproduced with permission from Mearin F, Cucala M, Azpiroz F, Malagelada J-R. The origin of symptoms on the brain-gut axis in functional dyspepsia. Gastroenterology 1991;101:999–1006.

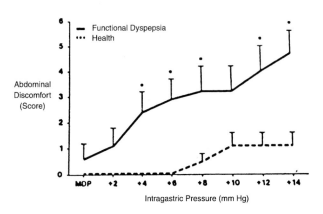

**FIGURE 11.43.** Gastric compliance in functional dyspepsia. Compliance was measured by increasing intragastric pressure in 2-mm Hg steps starting from the intra-abdominal pressure level (minimal distending pressure [MDP]) while recording intragastric volume. Compliance, that is, the volume–pressure relationship, was virtually identical in patients with functional dyspepsia and in healthy subjects. Reproduced with permission from Mearin F, Cucala M, Azpiroz F, Malagelada J-R. The origin of symptoms on the brain gut axis in functional dyspepsia. Gastroenterology 1991;101:999–1006.

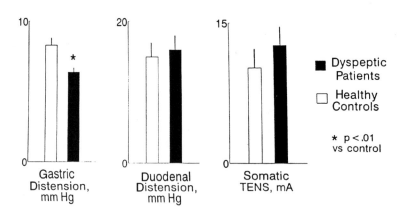

**FIGURE 11.44.** Visceral and somatic sensitivity in functional dyspepsia. Figure shows thresholds for discomfort to gastric distention, duodenal distention, and transcutaneous electrical nerve stimulation (TENS) applied on the hand. Patients with dyspepsia experienced discomfort at significantly lower intragastric pressures than healthy subjects, but perception of both duodenal and somatic stimuli was normal. Reproduced with permission from Coffin B, Azpiroz F, Guarner F, Malagelada J-R. Selective gastric hypersensitivity and reflex hyporeactivity in functional dyspepsia. Gastroenterology 1994;107:1345–51.

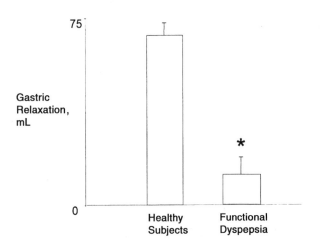

**FIGURE 11.45.** Enterogastric reflex induced by nutrients in functional dyspepsia. Duodenal nutrient infusion failed to induce a significant gastric relaxation in patients with functional dyspepsia (*$p < .05$ vs healthy subjects).

(Fig. 11.42).[17,28] Since gastric compliance is normal, gastric sensitivity in this group of patients can be evaluated by means of the barostat.

Using the barostat, it has been shown that patients with functional dyspepsia exhibit hypersensitivity of the stomach so that they perceive and tolerate significantly lower levels of intraluminal pressure and wall tension than healthy subjects (Fig. 11.43).[17,28] In a subgroup of patients with dysmotility-like dyspepsia, intestinal sensitivity has been shown to be normal (Fig. 11.44).[28] Furthermore, in these patients, somatic sensitivity is also normal, or a higher tolerance than healthy subjects is displayed.[17,28] This combination of visceral hypersensitivity and normal or even reduced somatic sensitivity is common to other functional gut syndromes, such as the irritable bowel.

It has also been shown that patients with functional dyspepsia have altered viscerovisceral reflexes that modulate gastric tone. The reflex gastric relaxation induced either by intestinal

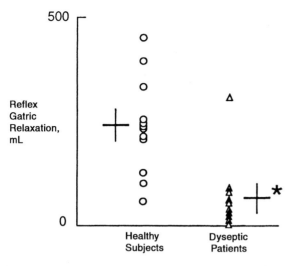

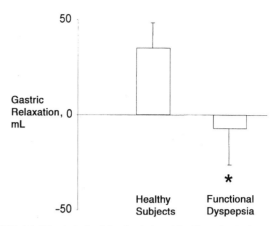

**FIGURE 11.47.** Antrofundal reflex induced by distention in functional dyspepsia. In healthy subjects, antral distention induces a relaxation of the proximal stomach, but this reflex is impaired in patients with functional dyspepsia (*$p < .05$ vs healthy controls). Adapted from Caldarella et al.[31]

**FIGURE 11.46.** Enterogastric reflex induced by distention in functional dyspepsia. Figure shows individual gastric relaxatory responses to duodenal distention in healthy subjects and dyspeptic patients. The gastric relaxatory response was significantly smaller in patients than in healthy controls (*$p < .05$). Reproduced with permission from Coffin B, Azpiroz F, Guarner F, Malagelada J-R. Selective gastric hypersensitivity and reflex hyporeactivity in functional dyspepsia. Gastroenterology 1994;107:1345–51.

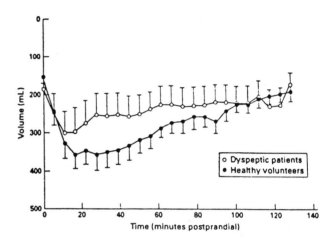

**FIGURE 11.49.** Gastric accommodation in functional dyspepsia. Gastric accommodation was measured as intragastric volume by the barostat before and at regular intervals after ingestion of a meal. Accommodation was significantly impaired in patients with dyspepsia as compared to healthy subjects ($p < .05$). Reproduced with permission from Salet GAM, Samson M, Roelofs JMM, et al. Responses to gastric distension in functional dyspepsia. Gut 1998;42:823–9.

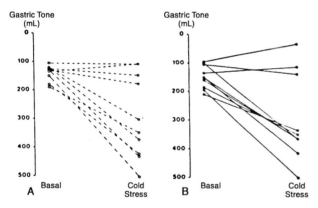

**FIGURE 11.48.** Somatovisceral reflex in functional dyspepsia. Hand immersion into iced water produces similar gastric relaxation in healthy subjects (**A**) and in patients with functional dyspepsia (**B**). Reproduced with permission from Mearin F, Cucala M, Azpiroz F, Malagelada J-R. The origin of symptoms on the brain-gut axis in functional dyspepsia. Gastroenterology 1991;101:999–1006.

## Gastroparesis

Gastroparesis is characterized by gastric retention caused by impaired emptying. The symptoms of these patients often cannot be distinguished from functional dyspepsia, and the diagnosis of gastroparesis is strictly based on a gastric emptying test. By definition, patients with gastroparesis have markedly delayed emptying, whereas patients with functional dyspepsia have normal gastric emptying or just exhibit a slight delay in emptying of solids but normal liquid emptying. In fact, the delayed solid emptying in dyspepsia may be related to impaired grinding of solids by the antrum and selective retention of solid particles by the pyloric sieve rather than to an alteration of the tonic propulsive force that produces empting.

nutrients or distention is impaired (Figs. 11.45 and 11.46).[28] Furthermore, the antrofundal reflex in response to gastric filling is altered, resulting in a defective gastric accommodation (Fig. 11.47).[31] By contrast, gastric responses to somatovisceral reflexes are normal (Fig. 11.48).[17] Impaired responses both to gastric filling and to intestinal nutrients contribute to an abnormal accommodation process (Fig. 11.49).[32,33] Dyspeptic symptoms are probably related to the combined reflex and sensory dysfunction in these patients (Fig. 11.50).

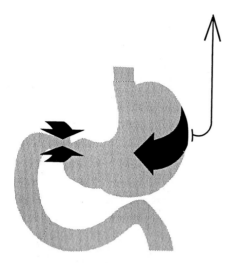

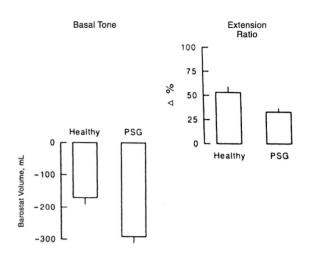

**FIGURE 11.50.** Putative mechanism of dyspeptic symptoms. Impaired accommodation to a meal in functional dyspepsia may not affect gastric emptying because final gastric outflow is regulated by antropyloric mechanisms. However, impaired relaxation after a meal produces an increment in gastric wall tension, which, particularly in these patients with hypersensitivity to distention, results in stimulation of sensory pathways and symptom perception.

**FIGURE 11.52.** Gastric response to distention in gastroparesis. At a low, constant intragastric pressure, basal gastric tone, that is, the volume measured by the barostat, was much larger in a group of patients with postsurgical gastroparesis (PSG) than in healthy subjects. By increasing the pressure, the extension ratio was significantly smaller in patients than in healthy subjects, indicating that the stomach behaves as a hypotonic, flaccid pouch.

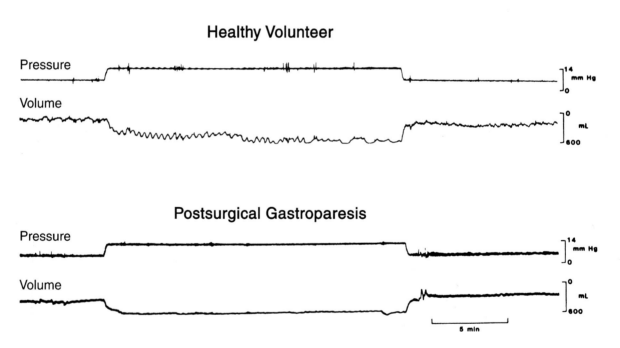

**FIGURE 11.51.** Examples of gastric response to distention. In a healthy subject, intragastric pressure increment by the barostat produced a contractile response. In a patient with surgical gastroparesis, the intragastric pressure increment did not produce a phasic response. Reproduced with permission from Azpiroz F, Malagelada J-R. Gastric tone measured by an electronic barostat in health and postsurgical gastroparesis. Gastroenterology 1987;92:934–43.

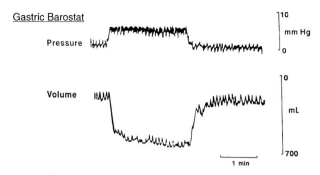

**FIGURE 11.53.** Visceral anesthesia. Example of unperceived gastric distention at a pressure level that produces marked gastric dilation in a patient with diabetic neuropathy and gastroparesis.

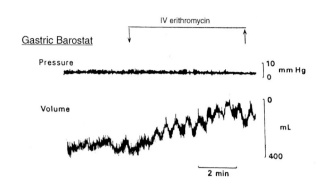

**FIGURE 11.54.** Therapeutic assay in gastroparesis. In a patient with gastroparesis and very low basal tone (large intragastric volume at a low pressure level), intravenous administration of erythromycin induces an increase in gastric tone (reduced baseline volume) with superimposed contractions (volume waves).

In patients with gastroparesis, the barostat demonstrates a flaccid stomach with low basal gastric tone and reduced distensibility (Figs. 11.51 and 11.52).[5] Since the stomach has very little basal tone, relaxatory drugs, such as glucagon, produce a small, if any, relaxation. Likewise, in the absence of basal tone, inhibitory reflexes cannot be reliably evaluated.

Gastric sensitivity in pure gastroparesis is normal. However, in some patients, the pathophysiologic mechanisms involved are various, and sensory abnormalities may also be present. For instance, in some patients with diabetic neuropathy, the most frequent cause of gastoparesis, sensory pathways may be affected and may exhibit impaired gastric perception or even complete anesthesia. Impaired sensitivity can be detected by a lack of perception to usually uncomfortable distention levels applied by the barostat or preferably by the tensostat (Fig. 11.53).

In patients with gastroparesis, the barostat may be used for a therapeutic assay, for instance, measuring the contractile response to intravenous administration of erythromycin (Fig. 11.54). A proper gastric response with vigorous contractions provides solid experimental base for a prokinetic trial.

## CONCLUSION

Over the years, the barostat has proven a useful tool to measure gut tone both for animal and human research studies (Table 11.1). However, the barostat has some limitations, which are

**TABLE 11.1.** Applications of the Barostat

| |
|---|
| Tone measurements |
|     Physiologic changes |
|     Reflex responses |
|     Pharmacologic effects |
| Compliance measurements |
| Visceral stimulation |
|     Sensitivity studies |
|     Induction of reflexes |

important to comprehend for reliable studies. The barostat can be used at a constant pressure set to measure variations in gut tone either physiologically, induced by reflexes, or pharmacologically. The barostat can also be used to manipulate intraluminal pressure and measure gut compliance and sensitivity. To date, the clinical applications of the barostat are still very limited and probably restricted to experienced groups.

## REFERENCES

1. Cannon WB. The movements of the stomach studied by means of the Roentgen rays. Am J Physiol 1898;1:359–82.
2. Szurszewski JH. Electrical basis for gastrointestinal motility. In: Johnson LR, editor. Physiology of the gastrointestinal tract. Vol 2. New York: Raven Press; 1981. p. 1435–66.
3. Azpiroz F, Malagelada J-R. Pressure activity patterns in the canine proximal stomach: response to distension. Am J Physiol 1984;247: G265–72.
4. Azpiroz F, Malagelada J-R. Physiologic variations in canine gastric tone measured by an electronic barostat. Am J Physiol 1985;248: G229–37.
5. Azpiroz F, Malagelada J-R. Gastric tone measured by an electronic barostat in health and postsurgical gastroparesis. Gastroenterology 1987;92:934–43.
6. Rouillon J-M, Azpiroz F, Malagelada J-R. Reflex changes in intestinal tone: relationship to perception. Am J Physiol 1991;261:G280–6.
7. Azpiroz F. Sensitivity of the stomach and the small bowel: human research and clinical relevance. In: Gebhart GF, editor. Progress in pain research and management. Vol 5: visceral pain. Seattle: IASP Press; 1995. p. 391–428.
8. Malagelada J-R, Azpiroz F. Determinants of gastric emptying and transit in the small intestine. In: Schultz SG, Wood JD, Rauner BB, editors. Handbook of physiology. Section 6: the gastrointestinal system. Vol 1: motility and circulation. 2nd ed. Bethesda (MD): American Physiology Society; 1989. p. 909–37.
9. Moragas G, Azpiroz F, Pavía J, Malagelada J-R. Relations among intragastric pressure, postcibal perception and gastric emptying. Am J Physiol 1993;264:G1112–7.
10. Cannon WB, Lieb CW. The receptive relaxation of the stomach. Am J Physiol 1911;29:267–73.
11. Villanova N, Azpiroz F, Malagelada J-R. Perception and gut reflexes induced by stimulation of gastrointestinal thermoreceptors in humans. J Physiol (Lond) 1997;502.1:215–22.
12. Azpiroz F, Malagelada J-R. Intestinal control of gastric tone. Am J Physiol 1985;249:G501–9.
13. Azpiroz F, Malagelada J-R. Perception and reflex relaxation of the stomach in response to gut distention. Gastroenterology 1990;98:1193–8.

14. Serra J, Azpiroz F, Malagelada J-R. Perception and reflex responses to intestinal distension are modified by simultaneous or previous stimulation. Gastroenterology 1995;109:1742–9.

15. Iovino P, Azpiroz F, Domingo E, Malagelada J-R. The sympathetic nervous system modulates perception and reflex responses to gut distension in humans. Gastroenterology 1995;108:680–6.

16. Villanova N, Azpiroz F, Malagelada J-R. Gastrogastric reflexes regulating gastric tone and their relationship to perception. Am J Physiol 1997;273:G464–9.

17. Mearin F, Cucala M, Azpiroz F, Malagelada J-R. The origin of symptoms on the brain gut axis in functional dyspepsia. Gastroenterology 1991;101:999–1006.

18. Notivol R, Coffin B, Azpiroz F, et al. Gastric tone determines the sensitivity of the stomach to distension. Gastroenterology 1995;108:330–6.

19. Rouillon J-M, Azpiroz F, Malagelada J-R. Sensorial and intestino-intestinal reflex pathways in the human jejunum. Gastroenterology 1991;101:1606–12.

20. Azpiroz F, Malagelada J-R. Importance of vagal input in maintaining gastric tone in the dog. J Physiol (Lond) 1987;384:511–24.

21. Azpiroz F, Malagelada J-R. Vagally mediated gastric relaxation induced by intestinal nutrients in the dog. Am J Physiol 1986;251:G727–35.

22. De Ponti F, Azpiroz F, Malagelada J-R. Reflex gastric relaxation in response to distention of the duodenum. Am J Physiol 1987;252:G595–601.

23. Serra J, Azpiroz F, Malagelada J-R. Modulation of gut perception in humans by spatial summation phenomena. J Physiol (Lond) 1998;506.2:579–87.

24. Distrutti E, Azpiroz F, Soldevilla A, Malagelada J-R. Gastric wall tension determines perception of gastric distension. Gastroenterology 1999;116:1035–42.

25. Kellow JE, Delvaux MM, Azpiroz F, et al. Principles of applied neurogastroenterology: physiology/motility-sensation. In: Drossman DA, Corazziari E, Talley NJ, et al, editors. Rome II: the functional gastrointestinal disorders. 2nd ed. McLean (VA): Degnon Associates; 2000. p. 91–156.

26. Azpiroz F, Malagelada J-R. Isobaric intestinal distention in humans: sensorial relay and reflex gastric relaxation. Am J Physiol 1990;258:G202–7.

27. Coffin B, Azpiroz F, Malagelada J-R. Somatic stimulation reduces perception of gut distension. Gastroenterology 1994;107:1636–42.

28. Coffin B, Azpiroz F, Guarner F, Malagelada J-R. Selective gastric hypersensitivity and reflex hyporeactivity in functional dyspepsia. Gastroenterology 1994;107:1345–51.

29. Whitehead WE, Delvaux M, and The Working Team. Standardization of tensostat procedures for testing smooth muscle tone and sensory thresholds in the gastrointestinal tract. Dig Dis Sci 1999;42:223–41.

30. Azpiroz F, Malagelada J-R, Distrutti E. Reply to letter to the editor: development of a tensostat for gastric perception studies. Gastroenterology 2000;118:642–3.

31. Caldarella MP, Azpiroz F, Malagelada J-R. The distal stomach is responsible for symptomatic gastric accommodation in functional dyspepsia [abstract]. Gastroenterology 2000;118:A670.

32. Salet GAM, Samsom M, Roelofs JMM, et al. Responses to gastric distension in functional dyspepsia. Gut 1998;42:823–9.

33. Tack J, Piessevaux H, Coulie B, et al. Role of impaired gastric accommodation to a meal in functional dyspepsia. Gastroenterology 1998;115:1346–52.

# CHAPTER 12

# Scintigraphy

*Alan H. Maurer, Henry P. Parkman, Linda C. Knight and Robert S. Fisher*

## GASTRIC EMPTYING

The advantages of radionuclide imaging for studying gastrointestinal tract function have remained the same since Griffith and colleagues first introduced the oral administration of radiolabeled $^{51}$Cr porridge to measure gastric emptying over 30 years ago.[1] In contrast to manometry, scintigraphy is noninvasive, does not disturb normal physiology, and permits quantification of bulk transit of solids and liquids. Compared with radiographic methods, scintigraphy results in low radiation exposure (see Table 7.2, Chapter 7), is easily quantified, and uses commonly ingested foods rather than non-nutrient substrates such as barium.

Once the solid or liquid phase of a meal is radiolabeled and appropriate corrections are made for attenuation and decay, the counts measured by a nuclear medicine camera are directly proportional to the volume of solid or liquid in the stomach. The retention of solids and liquids measured is therefore independent of any geometric assumptions used with other imaging modalities. Because of this ease of quantification and accuracy, scintigraphy has become the gold standard for measuring gastric emptying.

Recently, $^{13}$C- or $^{14}$C-labeled octanoic acid breath testing has been used to measure gastric emptying indirectly. Early studies have shown good correlation with gastric emptying scintigraphy.[2] At present, however, this technique is not widely available and does not permit imaging or regional assessment of gastric function.

Cannon was the first to observe that the fundus and antrum play separate roles in emptying liquids and solids.[3] He proposed that the fundus acts as a reservoir that undergoes receptive relaxation to receive food from the esophagus.[4] Normally, solid foods are temporarily stored in the fundus until slow, sustained contractions transfer the solids to the antrum. This early segregation of solids in the fundus is apparent in the initial images of a gastric emptying study (Fig. 12.1).

After solids reach the antrum, peristaltic contractions break down food particles by a process (trituration) in which large solid particles are mixed with gastric digestive juices and are ground into small particles of 1 to 2 mm, which are then able to pass through the pylorus.[5,6] The frequency of contractile activity of the antrum is controlled by a pacemaker located high on the greater curvature, at the boundary between the fundus and the antrum.

## INDICATIONS

Symptoms of gastric stasis include nausea, vomiting, abdominal fullness, pain, distention, early satiety, and weight loss. Gastric emptying studies are indicated to evaluate these symptoms and document emptying abnormalities after an anatomic cause has been excluded by either endoscopy, upper gastrointestinal series, or other imaging studies. Gastric emptying scintigraphy is also of value to objectively assess any response to treatment. In addition, with the development of

Tc-99m Solid Phase    In-111 Liquid Phase

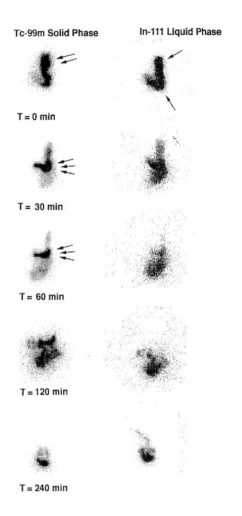

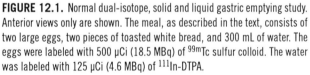

**Solid Phase**

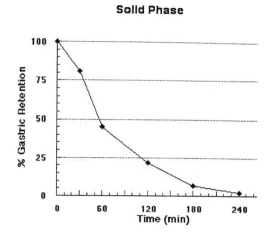

**Liquid Phase**

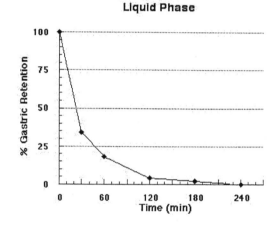

**FIGURE 12.1.** Normal dual-isotope, solid and liquid gastric emptying study. Anterior views only are shown. The meal, as described in the text, consists of two large eggs, two pieces of toasted white bread, and 300 mL of water. The eggs were labeled with 500 μCi (18.5 MBq) of $^{99m}$Tc sulfur colloid. The water was labeled with 125 μCi (4.6 MBq) of $^{111}$In-DTPA.

The images demonstrate early rapid distribution of liquids throughout both the proximal and distal stomach (*single arrow*) (t = 0 min). This is in contrast to the initial preferential localization of solids in the fundus (*double arrows*). With time, the solids move distally into the antrum (*triple arrows*),

where they are then ground to 1- to 2-mm particles before they begin to empty.

The solid emptying curve is normally sigmoidal in shape when plotted on rectilinear graph paper. However, as in this case, a normal emptying curve may show no significant lag phase. The lag phase may appear shortened if the subject has taken a relatively long time to eat the meal. In such cases, trituration and some emptying may have begun before the first images have been recorded. More complete chewing can also shorten the lag phase, especially for a soft meal such as eggs. There is therefore usually little clinical significance to a shortened or absent lag phase. The liquid emptying curve is monoexponential.

newer approaches to the treatment of gastroparesis, such as gastric pacing, scintigraphy will likely play an increasing role in analyzing regional gastric motor dysfunction.

## TECHNIQUE

### Patient Preparation

Gastric emptying scintigraphy is best performed in the morning after an overnight fast to avoid diurnal variations in emptying and residual food in the stomach. Premenopausal women should be studied in the early (ie, follicular) phase of the menstrual cycle to minimize hormonal effects on gastrointestinal

motility.[7] Any medication that affects gastric emptying should be discontinued for at least 2 to 3 days prior to the study (Table 12.1). Tobacco and alcohol should also be withheld.

### Instrumentation

With dual-isotope imaging, both solid and liquid radiopharmaceuticals can be measured simultaneously. The nuclear medicine gamma camera and collimator must be capable of imaging both indium 111 ($^{111}$In), with its higher-energy (247-keV) emission, and technetium 99m ($^{99m}$Tc), with its lower-energy (140-keV emission). As there is no need for high resolution or counting rates, imaging departments can use older cameras for gastric emptying studies and free up

**TABLE 12.1.** Medications That Delay Gastric Emptying*

Narcotic analgesics
Anticholinergics
Antidepressants including antispasmodics and tricyclic antidepressants
Calcium channel blockers
Gastric acid suppressants ($H_2$ receptor antagonists and proton pump inhibitors)
Somatostatin or octreotide (high dose)
Aluminum-containing antacids

Adapted from Parkman et al.[8]

**TABLE 12.2.** Stability of Several Radiolabeled Solids Tested In Vitro*

| Solid Meal | Percentage Bound in in Gastric Juice | Percentage Bound in 0.1 N HCl |
|---|---|---|
| $^{99m}$Tc-SC egg (whole) | 82 | 97 |
| $^{99m}$Tc-SC egg white (fat free) | >95 | 96 |
| $^{99m}$Tc egg (albuminum particles) | 65 | 95 |
| $^{99m}$Tc in vivo chicken liver | 98 | 94 |
| $^{99m}$Tc surface-labeled chicken liver | 84 | 90 |
| $^{99m}$Tc Chelex resin | 98 (24 h) | |
| $^{131}$I Fiber | 100 | 99 (48 h) |

Except where shown, all testing was at 3 to 4 hours.

* Adapted from Knight.[9]

$^{99m}$Tc-SC, technetium 99m sulfur colloid.

newer cameras for other uses. To perform quantification, the camera must be interfaced to a digital computer capable of standard region of interest analysis.

## RADIOPHARMACEUTICALS

For any test meal, the stability of binding of the radiolabel to the solid phase must be established to ensure that the radioisotope does not dissociate in gastric juice. Historically, in vivo labeling of chicken liver was the first method described for radiolabeling a solid food.[10] This is performed by injecting

$^{99m}$Tc sulfur colloid into the wing vein of a live chicken. The colloid is phagocytosed by the Kupffer's cells of the liver, resulting in an intracellular radiolabel that is the gold standard for stability to which all other solid food labels are compared.

Because of the impracticability of handling live chickens, several more convenient radiolabeled solid meals have been proposed. In the United States, the only radiopharmaceutical approved by the Food and Drug Administration for gastric emptying studies is $^{99m}$Tc sulfur colloid. When properly cooked with certain foods, the $^{99m}$Tc sulfur colloid does not dissociate from the solid phase of the meal and can be used to measure gastric emptying. Similar to the in vivo labeled chicken liver, there is minimal breakdown (Table 12.2).

For combined solid and liquid gastric emptying studies, the liquid phase can be imaged using $^{111}$In diethylenetriamine pentaacetic acid (DTPA), which is chemically inert. It is not absorbed from the gastrointestinal tract, nor does it bind to the solid phase of the meal. Because the 247-keV photon emission of $^{111}$In can easily be separated from the 140-keV photon emission of $^{99m}$Tc, dual-isotope imaging is possible (see Fig. 12.1). As oral $^{111}$In is not approved for routine clinical use in the United States, a broad license from a state or the federal Nuclear Regulatory Agency may be required for its use.

## THE TEST MEAL

The rate of gastric emptying is determined by the meal composition. Experimental studies in humans and animals have demonstrated that small intestinal receptors for glucose, lipids, amino acids, and osmolality feed back to inhibit the rate of gastric emptying.[11] Any test meal used for measuring gastric emptying must be standardized for volume, density, caloric content, and nutrients (protein, fat, and carbohydrate). Normal values for a variety of meals have been reported (Table 12.3).[12–16]

A simple and readily available test meal in common use, used for the examples in this chapter, consists of two scrambled whole large eggs served between two pieces of toasted

**TABLE 12.3.** Gastric Emptying Values for Various Meals*

| Solid Phase | Liquid Phase | Solid $T_{1/2}$ (min) (Mean ± 2 SD) | Solid 2, 3, 4 Hours (%) (Median 95th Percentile)* (Mean + 2 SD)** | $T_{1/2}$ Liquid (min) (Mean ± 2 SD) | Reference No. |
|---|---|---|---|---|---|
| Oatmeal | Milk | 44 ± 14.8 | | | 12 |
| Chelex resin | Water (100 mL) | | | | |
| Chicken liver | | | | | |
| 300 g | | 77 ± 10 | | | 13 |
| 900 g | | 146 ± 52 | | | |
| 1,692 g | | 277 ± 88 | | | |
| Chicken liver + ground beef | Water (150 mL) | 70 ± 14 | | 15 ± 4 | 14 |
| | 25% dextrose (150 mL) | 105 ± 26 | | 46 ± 14 | |
| Fat-free egg (EggBeater™) | Water (120 mL) | 83 (mean) | 2 h = 60%* | | 15 |
| | | | 4 h = 10% | | |
| Two-whole-egg sandwich | Water (300 mL) | 78 ± 22 | 2 h = 50%** | 28 ± 10 | 16 |
| | | | 3 h = 21%** | | |
| | | | 4 h = 10%** | | |

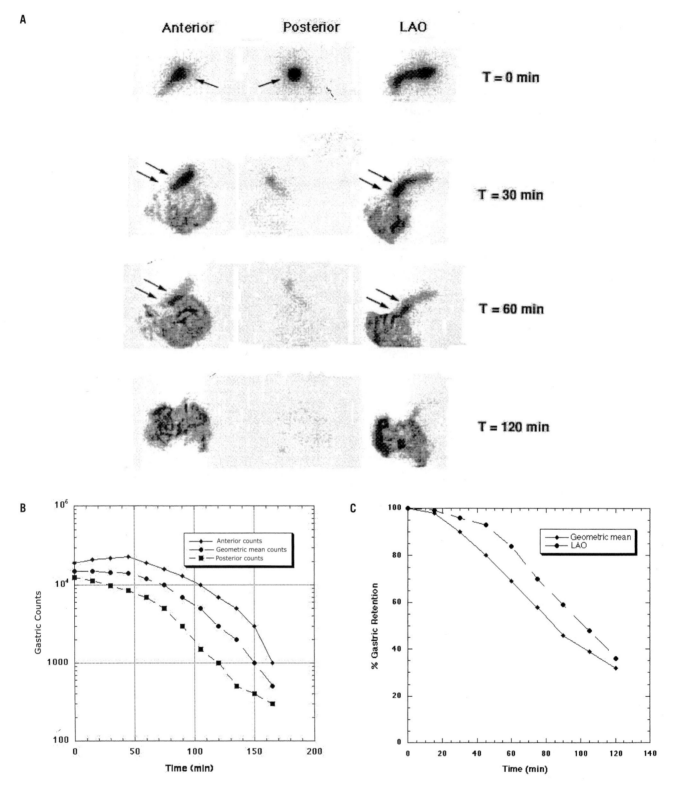

**FIGURE 12.2. A,** Comparison of solid-phase anterior, posterior, and left anterior oblique (LAO) images. Early (t = 0 min) anterior and posterior images show solids mostly localized in the fundus (*single arrows*). With time, the solids move from the fundus into the antrum (*double arrows*). The LAO view places the stomach in a plane parallel to the face of the nuclear medicine camera and minimizes the anterior-posterior differences in distance of the fundus and antrum from the camera. **B,** Anterior, posterior, and geometric-mean curves from **A**. The anterior counts appear to increase as activity moves closer to the camera. In contrast, the posterior counts decrease even before solids empty from the stomach as activity moves away from the camera. The geometric-mean corrected counts reflect the true volume of solids in the stomach and show the normal expected delay (lag phase) before the counts begin monoexponential emptying (see also Fig. 12.7). **C,** Left anterior oblique (LAO) versus geometric mean comparison. Compared with the geometric-mean curve, an LAO-only curve shows an increase in the lag phase as the LAO view does not completely correct for the fundal to antral depth changes.

white bread. It is served with 300 mL of water. This meal has 270 kcal with 23% protein, 40% fat, and 37% carbohydrate. The eggs are labeled with 500 μCi (18.5 MBq) of $^{99m}$Tc sulfur colloid. The water is labeled with 125 μCi (4.6 MBq) of $^{111}$In-DTPA. The patient is instructed to eat the meal within 10 minutes. The technologist performing the study should record the time taken to consume the meal and what portion of the meal, if any, was not consumed.

Recently, a multicenter study was performed with another standardized, low-fat meal showing excellent gastric emptying reproducibility.[15] The meal consists of fat-free egg substitute (EggBeater™) equivalent to the volume of two large eggs. It is served with two slices of bread, 30 g of strawberry jam, and 120 mL of water. The meal has a caloric value of 255 kcal with 24% protein, 2% fat, 2% fiber, and 72% carbohydrate. The radiolabel is stable in gastric juice (see Table 12.2). The gastric emptying half-time ($T_{1/2}$) measured with this meal is similar to the meal of two large whole eggs (see Table 12.3).

## ACQUISITION

The patient is usually imaged standing in front of the nuclear medicine camera. The study begins immediately after finishing the meal. This is typically recorded as time (t = 0). Lying in the supine positioning can significantly slow gastric emptying of solids: 20% emptying at 1 hour in a supine position versus 50% in an upright position.[17]

As solids move from the posteriorly located fundus to the more anteriorly located antrum, there will be an apparent increase in measured counts as the solids move closer to the camera when it is positioned in front of the patient. This increase in counts is attributable to the shorter distance of the solids from the camera, resulting in less attenuation from overlying soft tissue (Figs. 12.2A and 12.2B).

A method to correct for depth attenuation must therefore be applied when analyzing gastric emptying data. The attenuation method used determines what type of images (anterior, posterior, or left anterior oblique [LAO]) is acquired. A geometric-mean (anterior counts × posterior counts)$^{1/2}$ correction is most commonly used. Studies have shown that geometric-mean correction of gastric counts results in only a 3 to 4% variation for the depths typically encountered with gastric emptying studies.[18,19] Other methods for performing attenuation correction have been reported and include use of a lateral view, a peak-to-scatter ratio, and an LAO image.[20,21] A single LAO view is useful for patients who may not be able to stand and need to be imaged in a stretcher. The LAO method can cause some overestimation of the length of the lag phase and the gastric half-emptying time (Fig. 12.2C).[22]

Gastric emptying images are acquired using a minimum of 64 × 64 pixels in a byte mode matrix. For $^{99m}$Tc, the camera photopeak is set at 140 keV with a 20% window. For $^{111}$In, either the 172- or 247-keV photopeaks can be used alone or summed with a 20% window. For solid-phase-only studies

with $^{99m}$Tc, a general-purpose low-energy collimator is used. For dual-isotope studies, a medium-energy collimator must be used to collect the higher energies of $^{111}$In.

Until recently, gastric emptying studies were typically acquired for only up to 2 hours after meal ingestion. New studies have shown, however, that images should be acquired for up to 4 hours for greater sensitivity.[23] Some authors recommend that imaging should be done every 10 to 15 minutes if computerized mathematical curve fitting is to be performed.[16] Some recommend continuous imaging every 30 to 60 seconds for automated curve fitting and display of the images in a cine format. This may be helpful to look for esophageal reflux and overlap of small bowel with the gastric regions of interest.[7] Recently, Tougas and colleagues proposed that only four images (0, 60, 120, and 180 minutes) are needed to adequately characterize the solid-phase gastric emptying curve using a simplified, power exponential mathematical mode.[24]

In an effort to reduce cost and imaging time, we now acquire clinical studies immediately after ingestion of the meal (t = 0), at 30 minutes to look for rapid gastric emptying (dumping; Fig. 12.3), and then at 60, 120, 180, and 240 minutes. If there is no significant activity retained in the stomach at 2 hours, the study may be terminated before 4 hours. However, the study should not be terminated sooner if significant (>20%) activity remains in the stomach at 2 or 3 hours as some disorders of gastric emptying do not become apparent until 3 to 4 hours (Fig. 12.4).

## PROCESSING OF GASTRIC EMPTYING STUDIES

Computer regions of interest corresponding to the stomach are manually drawn to determine the gastric counts for both solids and liquids (Fig. 12.5). Care must be taken to recognize normal variations in the size and shape of the stomach and any other ancillary findings that may affect measurement of gastric emptying (Fig. 12.6).

Technetium 99m has a 6-hour half-life for radioactive decay and $^{111}$In has a 2.8-day half-life. The gastric counts must be corrected for this physical decay. After attenuation and decay correction, the percentage of activity remaining in the stomach is normalized by expressing it as a percentage of maximal gastric counts and is then plotted for all times.

Emptying of liquids is controlled by a sustained pressure gradient generated by the fundus. Liquids require no trituration and are normally distributed quickly throughout the stomach after ingestion. They empty monoexponentially (see Fig. 12.1). Thus, in contrast to solids, liquid emptying can be fully described by a simple $T_{1/2}$ value or the time to 50% emptying of gastric contents.[25]

A simple but clinically relevant approach to processing solid gastric emptying data is to determine a single $T_{1/2}$ emptying time or use a percentage of emptying measured at some time (2–4 hours) after ingestion of the meal. Tougas and colleagues reported that $T_{1/2}$ values are more normally distributed than the percentage of gastric activity measured at 2, 3, or 4 hours.

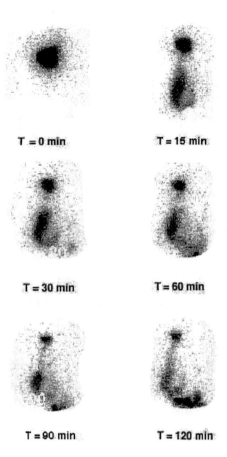

T = 0 min      T = 15 min

T = 30 min      T = 60 min

T = 90 min      T = 120 min

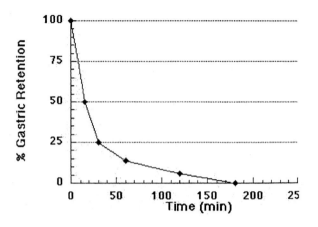

**FIGURE 12.3.** Rapid gastric emptying (solid phase, anterior only views shown). To detect rapid gastric emptying, images should be acquired early after the initial image. In this patient with a partial gastrectomy and symptoms of "dumping," there is filling of the gastric remnant and rapid emptying, with 75% emptied at 30 minutes. The normal emptying at 30 minutes for a standard two-egg meal is 20 ± 14% (mean ± 2 SD).

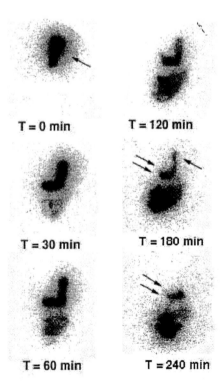

T = 0 min      T = 120 min

T = 30 min      T = 180 min

T = 60 min      T = 240 min

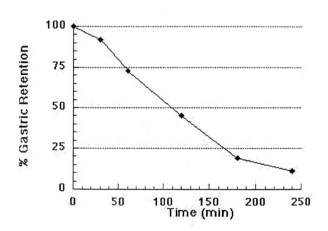

**FIGURE 12.4.** Normal early (up to 2 hours) gastric emptying but abnormal at 4 hours (solid phase, anterior only views shown). Some patients show borderline values, or even normal values for gastric emptying, at 2 hours (less than 50% retained for the two-whole-egg meal), as in this case. There is, however, abnormal gastric retention at 4 hours (12%). These patients typically show normal fundal filling and emptying (*single arrows*) but then demonstrate localized retention of solids in the antrum (*double arrows*).

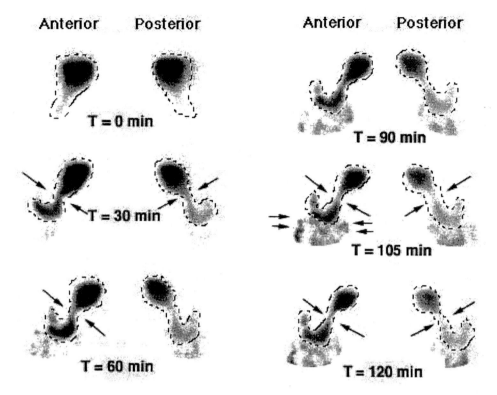

**FIGURE 12.5.** Computer regions of interest (ROIs) (only solid phase shown). The ROIs (*dotted lines*) are usually manually drawn to outline the stomach. Care is taken to avoid including activity from the small bowel (*double arrows*). A prominent and persistent contraction band (*single arrows*) separating the fundus and antrum is a common, normal finding.

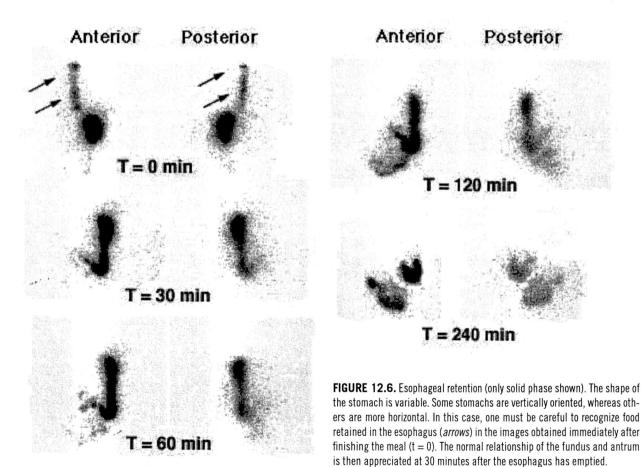

**FIGURE 12.6.** Esophageal retention (only solid phase shown). The shape of the stomach is variable. Some stomachs are vertically oriented, whereas others are more horizontal. In this case, one must be careful to recognize food retained in the esophagus (*arrows*) in the images obtained immediately after finishing the meal (t = 0). The normal relationship of the fundus and antrum is then appreciated at 30 minutes after the esophagus has emptied.

**Modified Power Exponential Curve Fit**

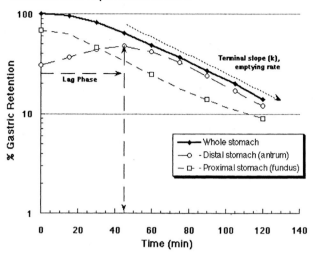

**FIGURE 12.7.** Normal antral and fundal solid-emptying curves with whole-stomach, modified, power exponential fit (geometric-mean corrected data shown). If separate analysis of the fundus and antrum is performed, the biphasic nature of gastric emptying and the relationship of the lag phase to antral function are more appreciated. During the first phase of gastric emptying, solids move from the fundus to the antrum. As the antrum fills, it begins to grind the solids. Once the solids have been broken down into small enough particles (1–2 mm), the antrum begins to empty (t = 45 min).

The peak in the antral filling curve corresponds to the end of the lag phase and the beginning of the second phase of gastric emptying. The monoexponential nature of the second portion of a solid emptying curve is best appreciated by plotting the data on a semilogarithmic graph, as shown here. The second portion of the whole-stomach curve appears linear (*small dotted line*) when using a modified power exponential curve fit since after the solids have been reduced to a size small enough to pass the pylorus, both solids and liquids empty at the same rate characterized by the slope (k). Adapted from Siegel et al.[16]

Given normally distributed data, the mean ± 2 SD is appropriate to determine the normal range for gastric emptying.[24] Single $T_{1/2}$ measures, although common in clinical practice, however, do not fully characterize the biphasic nature of solid-food gastric emptying.

The first phase of gastric emptying of solids includes the time for receptive relaxation and transient storage of solids in the fundus and the time required for grinding large particles to a size small enough to empty through the pylorus. This first phase is commonly referred to as the lag phase. In the second phase of gastric emptying of solids, the small particles that are suspended in the gastric liquid are emptied through the pylorus. During this phase, solids and liquids empty at the same rate (Fig. 12.7).[16]

There has been controversy over whether a lag phase for solid-food emptying exists. Moore and coworkers argued that the lag phase is an artifact created by failure to correct for attenuation.[19] Numerous studies, however, have since confirmed the existence of a lag phase.[26–28]

The best definition of the lag phase is one that incorporates all stages of gastric emptying. We define the lag phase as the time needed after solid food ingestion for the fundus to move solids into the antrum and then for the antrum to grind the solids into small particles so that the particles (suspended in the gastric liquid) can begin to empty.[29]

To characterize all phases of gastric emptying, it is best to fit the gastric emptying data to a mathematic function such as the power exponential first proposed by Elashoff and colleagues.[30] A modified power exponential function was later introduced by Siegel and colleagues. This function has been used successfully to characterize lag-phase differences owing to particle size and the physical composition of the meal.[16] Plotting the data on a semilogarithmic graph helps to demonstrate the biphasic nature of gastric emptying of solids (see Fig. 12.7). The modified, power exponential function is given by the following equation:

$$y(t) = 100 \times (1 - [1 - \exp(-kt)]^{\beta})$$

where y(t) is the percentage of gastric activity remaining at time t, k is the slope of the exponential fit to the terminal portion of the gastric emptying curve expressed in $min^{-1}$, and $\beta$ is the extrapolated y intercept of a linear fit to the terminal portion of the emptying curve. In this equation, the lag phase is given by (In$\beta$)/k. The end of the lag phase corresponds to the inflection point of the whole-stomach gastric emptying curve, where the second derivative equals zero. This corresponds to the time of peak activity in the antrum (see Fig. 12.7). Normal values for the two-whole-egg meal described earlier are (mean ± 2 SD) k = 0.0142 ± 0.0068 $min^{-1}$, lag phase (In $\beta$/k) = 31 ± 15 min, and $T_{1/2}$ = 77.6 ± 22.4 min.

Use of the modified, power exponential function for analyzing gastric emptying provides further insight into the function of both the fundus and antrum. Physically, the lag phase ends with peak filling of the antrum or when grinding is adequate such that the small suspended solids can begin to empty with the liquids. Urbain and colleagues showed that the lag phase increases with the density of the solid food and that once solids are triturated and suspended with the liquids, solids and liquids empty at the same rate, k (Fig. 12.8).[28]

## INTERPRETATION OF GASTRIC EMPTYING STUDIES

In addition to establishing normal values for a given test meal, studies have shown that results are affected by other factors such as gender[31] and the time of day at which the test is performed.[32] Interpretation of a gastric emptying study should always be based on comparison to a standardized meal and study protocol.

Performing liquid gastric emptying studies by themselves is of little clinical value because a delay in the gastric emptying of solids usually occurs before liquids.[33] Occasionally, a liquid or semisolid meal is useful without a solid phase in a patient who is unable to eat a solid meal because of severe nausea and vomiting.[34,35] In such cases, if liquid or semisolid

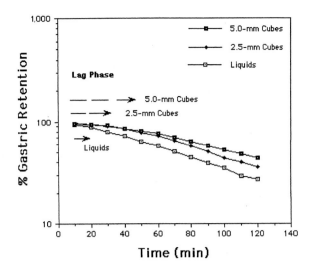

**FIGURE 12.8.** Effect of particle size on lag phase. To demonstrate the effect of particle size on the lag phase of gastric emptying, Urbain and colleagues administered isocaloric meals: (1) liquid (blenderized eggs), (2) 2.5-mm egg cubes, and (3) 5.0-mm egg cubes. The lag phase increased with solid particle size, but the terminal slope (rate of emptying) was the same. Adapted from Urbain et al.[28]

emptying is abnormal, significant gastroparesis for solids is also likely present.

We often perform dual-isotope, solid- and liquid-phase studies not because of the limited clinical information obtained about liquid gastric emptying but, more importantly,

to use the liquids to also record small bowel and colon transit.[36,37] As the symptoms of gastric and small bowel dysmotility may be similar, it is helpful to be able to assess both gastric and small bowel transit as part of a single study.

Since the emptying of [111]In-DTPA in water from the stomach is rapid, it serves as an excellent medium for recording small bowel transit (Fig. 12.9). We measure the percentage of administered liquids that have completed transit to the terminal ileum and/or cecum and ascending colon as an index of small bowel transit. Greater than 40% of the administered activity should pass through the small bowel by 6 hours in normal individuals. By recording additional images at 5 and 6 hours as part of a dual-isotope gastric emptying study, one can detect a small (11%) but significant occurrence of small bowel transit abnormalities in patients with dyspepsia.[32] Because of the long half-life of [111]In-DTPA, it can also be imaged at 24, 48, and 72 hours to record colon transit. The resulting whole-gut transit study is helpful when the patient's symptoms are not limited to upper gastrointestinal complaints.

One of the most common causes of delayed gastric emptying is insulin-dependent diabetes. This is usually related to autonomic neuropathy. The severity of gastric retention can range from mild to severe. Regionally within the stomach, the retention pattern most often seen is that of both fundal and antral retention (Fig. 12.10). Interestingly, studies on the role of gastric emptying and its relation to postprandial glucose control in non–insulin-dependent diabetics have shown no difference in solid emptying but accelerated gastric emptying of liquids.[38]

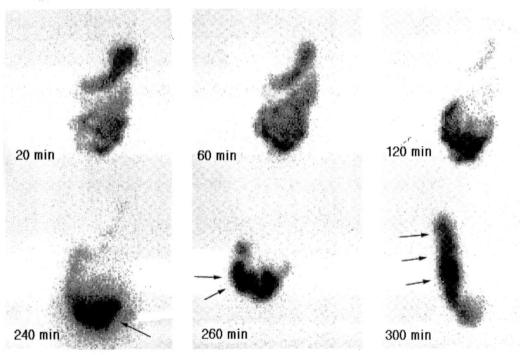

**FIGURE 12.9.** Normal small bowel transit (liquid phase, anterior only views shown). Sequential images of the liquid phase of a gastric emptying meal are shown. With time, an initially diffuse small bowel pattern begins to demonstrate accumulation of the activity in the terminal ileum, which acts as a temporary reservoir (*single arrow*) for intestinal chyme before it enters the cecum-ascending colon. This is followed by arrival of activity in the cecum-ascending colon area (*double arrows*). Following this, activity progresses to fill the ascending colon (*triple arrows*).

Severe gastric retention from surgical vagal nerve damage similar to what occurs in diabetic gastroparesis can be seen in patients with heart or lung transplantation (Fig. 12.11). This pattern of combined fundal and antral delayed emptying may also be seen with certain medications (see Table 12.1).

When there is severe gastric retention, it must not be assumed to be on the basis of gastroparesis. The interpretation of the gastric emptying study should always indicate to the referring physician that gastric outlet obstruction from an anatomic cause (tumor, ulcer) must be excluded.

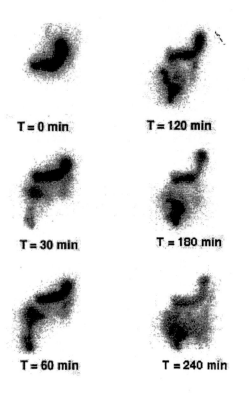

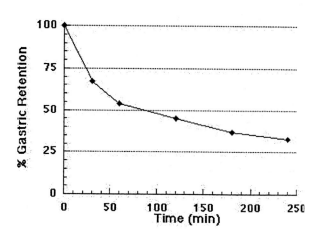

**FIGURE 12.10.** Diabetic gastroparesis (solid phase, anterior only views shown). This patient with insulin-dependent diabetes demonstrates retention in both the fundus and antrum. This diffuse retention pattern is typical of diabetic autonomic neuropathy. Of note, this patient shows an early borderline-normal 2-hour retention of 45% at 2 hours but clearly abnormally increased retention of 37% at 3 hours and 33% at 4 hours.

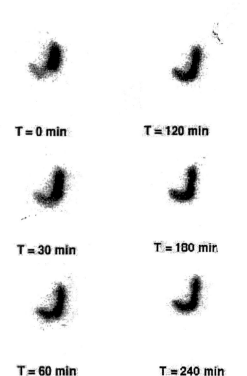

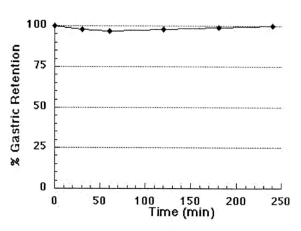

**FIGURE 12.11.** Post–cardiac transplantation gastroparesis (solid phase, anterior only views shown). This pattern of more severe retention in the fundus and antrum can be seen in patients with diabetes with more advanced gastroparesis than seen in Figure 12.10. In this case, the patient is post cardiac transplantation, and the etiology of the gastroparesis is likely related to direct vagal nerve damage. Anatomic outlet obstruction must always be excluded in such cases.

The determination of the percentage of gastric contents retained at a fixed time is a convenient measure for the whole stomach. The normal upper limits (mean + 2 SD) of retained gastric solids for our two-whole-egg meal are 50% at 2 hours, 21% at 3 hours, and 10% at 4 hours.[39] it is recognized, however, that there is often poor correlation of global measures of gastric emptying with symptoms, particularly in diabetics.[40] This has led investigators to examine the roles of the fundus and antrum in gastric emptying. Scintigraphy is unique in its ability to perform separate quantitation of fundal and antral emptying.[39]

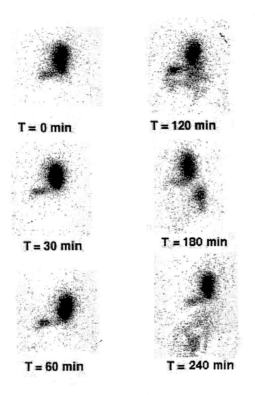

T = 0 min    T = 120 min

T = 30 min    T = 180 min

T = 60 min    T = 240 min

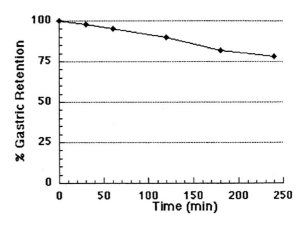

**FIGURE 12.12.** Localized fundal retention (solid phase, anterior only views shown). This patient with idiopathic gastroparesis shows persistent fundic retention (*arrows*) with failure of the solids to progress into the antrum. This is in contrast to the pattern seen in Figure 12.13, in which the fundus empties rapidly.

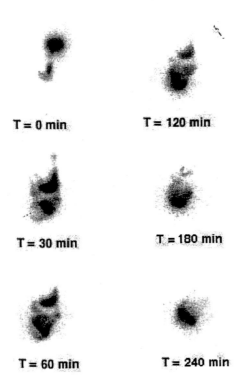

T = 0 min    T = 120 min

T = 30 min    T = 180 min

T = 60 min    T = 240 min

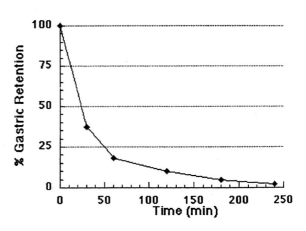

**FIGURE 12.13.** Loss of fundal accommodation (solid phase, anterior only views shown). This patient with symptoms of early satiety and abdominal pain has a gastric emptying study that does not demonstrate delayed gastric emptying. Rather, there is limited fundal accommodation with rapid movement of the solids from the fundus into the antrum. This loss of fundic accommodation may help explain the patient's symptoms.

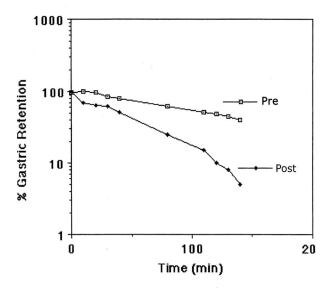

**FIGURE 12.14.** Gastric emptying studies before (Pre) and after (Post) therapy. These whole-stomach emptying curves show both a decrease in the lag phase and an increase in the rate of gastric emptying resulting from cisapride therapy in a patient with severe diabetic gastroparesis.

When reviewing gastric emptying studies, it is important to look at the scintigraphic images to assess the relative distribution of solids and liquids between the fundus and antrum.

Abnormalities of isolated fundal or antral dysmotility exist (Figs. 12.12 and 12.13). Troncon and colleagues examined whether the symptoms in a group of dysmotility-type dyspeptic patients could be the result of impaired fundal accommodation using a semisolid meal. They showed increased gastric contents in the distal stomach in dyspeptic patients (see Fig. 12.13).[41] This is consistent with ultrasonographic studies showing that dyspeptic patients tend to have larger postprandial antral volumes.[41,42]

Regional analysis of gastric emptying can also be helpful to evaluate the potential effect of drugs as treatment for gastroparesis. Gonlachanvit and colleagues have shown in patients with non–insulin-dependent diabetes that erythromycin speeds gastric emptying of solids and liquids primarily in the distal stomach, whereas morphine slows emptying in both the proximal and distal stomach.[43] In general, routine whole-stomach analysis is adequate to show objective evidence of a response to drug therapy (Fig. 12.14).

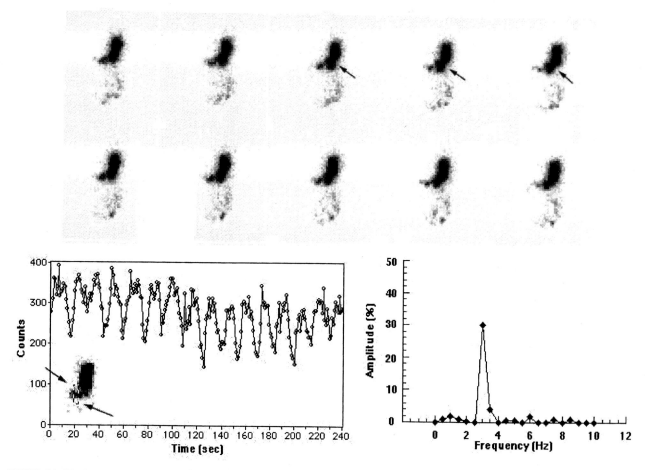

**FIGURE 12.15.** Scintigraphic analysis of antral contractions. To characterize the amplitude and frequency of antral contractions, images of the stomach are acquired rapidly at 1 second per frame. The upper two rows of images show a representative contraction wave as it sweeps across the antrum (*single arrows*). By placing a region of interest over the antrum (*double arrows, lower left insert*), a time activity curve of the counts in the region yields a recording of the antral contractions. These data are then analyzed by Fourier analysis to measure both the amplitude and frequency of antral contractions. In this example, the lower right insert shows a dominant normal antral frequency of 3 cycles per minute.

The existence and definition of the lag phase remain controversial. Although there is no consensus on the best definition of the lag phase, there are data supporting its clinical significance. The lag phase is a sensitive indicator of the efficacy of drugs used to treat diabetic gastroparesis.[44] Analysis of the lag phase has also been used to study the effects of ulcer surgery on gastric emptying. Mayer and colleagues found obliteration of the lag phase without an effect on trituration after truncal vagotomy and pyloroplasty.[45]

More advanced methods for analyzing the frequency and amplitude of antral contractions have been introduced (Fig. 12.15).[46,47] Normal antral contractions occur at a rate of three per minute. Measuring both the frequency and strength of antral contractions has further increased our understanding of gastric emptying. Differences in normal male and female gastric emptying have been shown to be attributable to the amplitude of antral contractions and not the frequency.[48] In diabetic gastroparesis, gastric emptying is delayed not only because of retention of food in the fundus but also decreased strength of antral contractions that occur at a higher frequency.[49]

## CONCLUSIONS

Today, advances in nuclear medicine imaging provide quantitative, physiologic analysis of the stomach and allow measurement of not only fundal and antral emptying of solids and liquids but also the frequency and amplitude of antral contractions. When combined solid- and liquid-phase meals are used, the study can be expanded to also provide information about small bowel and colon transit. For these reasons, scintigraphy will likely remain the gold standard for measuring gastric emptying and whole-gut transit.

### REFERENCES

1. Griffith GH, Owen GM, Kirkman S. Measurement of rate of gastric emptying using chromium-51. Lancet 1966;1:1244–5.
2. Choi MG, Camilleri M, Burton DD, et al. 13C octanoic acid breath test for gastric emptying of solids. Accuracy, reproducibility, and comparison with scintigraphy. Gastroenterology 1997;112:1155–62.
3. Cannon WB. The movements of the stomach studied by means of the Roentgen rays. Am J Physiol 1898;1:359–82.
4. Cannon WB. The receptive relaxation of the stomach. Am J Physiol 1911;29:267–73.
5. Meyer JH, Ohashi H, Jehn D, Thompson JB. Size of liver particles emptied from the human stomach. Gastroenterology 1981;80:1489–96.
6. Minami H, McCallum RW. The physiology and pathophysiology of gastric emptying in humans. Gastroenterology 1984;86:1592–610.
7. Donohoe KJ, Maurer AH, Ziessman HA, et al. Society of Nuclear Medicine procedure guideline for gastric emptying and motility. In: Donohoe KJ, editor. Society of Nuclear Medicine procedure guidelines manual. Reston (VA): Society of Nuclear Medicine; 1999. p. 37–40.
8. Parkman HP, Miller MA, Fisher RS. Role of nuclear medicine in evaluating patients with suspected gastrointestinal motility disorders. Semin Nucl Med 1995;25:289–305.
9. Knight LC. Radiopharmacy aspects of gastrointestinal imaging. In: Henkin RE, Boles MA, Dillehay GL, editors. Nuclear medicine. Vol 2. St. Louis; Mosby; 1996. p. 922–32.
10. Meyer JH. 99m Tc-tagged chicken liver as a marker of solid food in the human stomach. Am J Dig Dis 1976;21:296B.
11. Hunt JN, Stubbs DE. The volume and energy content of meals as determinants of gastric emptying. Am J Physiol 1975;245:209–25.
12. Wirth N, Swanson D, Shapiro B, et al. A conveniently prepared Tc-99m resin for semisolid gastric emptying studies. J Nucl Med 1983;24:511–4.
13. Christian PE Moore JG, Sorenson JA, et al. Effects of meal size and correction technique on gastric emptying time: studies with two tracers and opposed detectors. J Nucl Med 1980;21:883–5.
14. Collins PJ, Horowitz M, Cook DJ, et al. Gastric emptying in normal subjects—a reproducible technique using a single scintillation camera and computer system. Gut 1983;24:1117–25.
15. Tougas G, Eaker EY, Abell TL, et al. Assessment of gastric emptying using a low fat meal: establishment of international control values. Am J Gastroenterol 2000;95:1456–62.
16. Siegel JA, Urbain JL, Adler LP, et al. Biphasic nature of gastric emptying. Gut 1988;29:85–9.
17. Moore JG, Datz FL, Greenberg CE, Alazraki N. Effect of body posture on radionuclide measurements of gastric emptying. Dig Dis Sci 1988;33:1592–6.
18. Collins PJ, Horowitz M, Shearman DJC, Chatterton BE. Correction for tissue attenuation in radionuclide gastric emptying studies: a comparison of a lateral image method and a geometric mean method. Br J Radiol 1984;57:689–95.
19. Moore JG, Christina PE, Taylor AT, Alazraki N. Gastric emptying measurements: delayed and complex emptying patterns without appropriate correction. J Nucl Med 1985;27:1206–10.
20. Meyer JH, VanDeventer G, Graham LS, et al. Error and corrections with scintigraphic measurement of gastric emptying of solid foods. J Nucl Med 1983;24:197–203.
21. Fahey FH, Ziessman HA, Collen MJ, Eggli DF. Left anterior oblique projection an peak-to-scatter ratio for attenuation compensation of gastric emptying studies. J Nucl Med 1989;30:233–9.
22. Maurer AH, Knight LC, Vitti RA, et al. Geometric mean vs left anterior oblique attenuation correction: effect on half emptying time, lag phase, and rate of gastric emptying. J Nucl Med 1991;32:2176–80.
23. Guo JP, Fisher RS, Parkman HP, et al. Utility of four hour versus two hour gastric emptying studies. J Nucl Med 1999;40:190P.
24. Tougas G, Chen Y, Coates G, et al. Standardization of a simplified scintigraphic methodology for the assessment of gastric emptying in a multicenter setting. Am J Gastroenterol 2000;95:78–86.
25. Dugas MC, Schade RR, Lhotsky D, Theiel DV. Comparison of methods for analyzing gastric isotopic emptying. Am J Physiol 1982;243:G237–42.
26. Camilleri M, Malagelada JR, Brown ML, et al. Relation between antral motility and gastric emptying of solids and liquids in humans. Am J Physiol 1985;245:G580–5.
27. Collins PJ, Horowitz M, Chatterton BE. Proximal, distal and total stomach emptying of a digestible solid meal in normal subjects. Br J Radiol 1988;61:12–8.
28. Urbain JL, Siegel JA, Charkes ND, et al. The two-component stomach: effects of meal particle size on fundal and antral emptying. Eur J Nucl Med 1989;15:254–9.
29. Maurer AH, Knight LC, Krevsky B. Proper definitions for lag phase in gastric emptying of solid foods. J Nucl Med 1992;33:465–6.
30. Elashoff JD, Reedy TJ, Meyer JH. Analysis of gastric emptying data. Gastroenterology 1982;83:1306–12.
31. Datz FL, Christian PE, Moore J. Gender-related differences in gastric emptying. J Nucl Med 1987;28:1204–7.
32. Goo RH, Moore JG, Greenberg E, Alazraki NP. Circadian variation in gastric emptying of meals in humans. Gastroenterology 1987;93:515–8.
33. Loo FD, Palmer DW, Soergel KH, et al. Gastric emptying in patients with diabetes mellitus. Gastroenterology 1984;86:485–94.
34. Leb G, Lipp RW. Criteria for labeled meals for gastric emptying studies in nuclear medicine. Eur J Nucl Med 1993;20:185–6.

35. Lipp RW. Hammer HF, Schnedl W, et al. A simple scintigraphic method for continuous monitoring of gastric emptying. Eur J Nucl Med 1993;20:260–3.

36. Maurer AH, Krevsky B. Whole-gut transit scintigraphy in the evaluation of small-bowel and colon transit disorders. Semin Nucl Med 1995;25:326–38.

37. Bonapace ES, Maurer AH, Davidoff S, et al. Whole gut transit scintigraphy in the clinical evaluation of patients with upper and lower gastrointestinal symptoms. Am J Gastroenterol 2000;95:2838–47.

38. Frank JW, Saslow SB, Camilleri M, et al. Mechanism of accelerated gastric emptying of liquids and hyperglycemia in patients with type II diabetes mellitus. Gastroenterology 1995;109:755–65.

39. Parkman HP, Urbain JL, Knight LC, et al. Effect of gastric acid suppressants on human gastric motility. Gut 1998;42:245–50.

40. Horowitz M, Edelbroek M, Fraser R, et al. Disordered gastric motor function in diabetes mellitus. Recent insights into prevalence, pathophysiology, clinical relevance, and treatment. Scand J Gastroenterol 1991;26:673–84.

41. Troncon l, Bennet R, Ahluwalia N, Thompson DG. Abnormal intragastric distribution of food during gastric emptying in functional dyspepsia patients. Gut 1994;35:327–332.

42. Riucci R, Bontempo I, LaBella A, et al. Dyspeptic symptoms and gastric antrum distribution. An ultrasonographic study. Ital J Gastroenterol 1987;19:215–7.

43. Gonlachanvit S, Kantor SB, Knight LC, et al. Effects of erythromycin and morphine on regional gastric emptying in non-insulin dependent diabetes mellitus. 2000;12:481.

44. Horowitz M, Harding PE Chatterton BE, et al. Acute and chronic effects of domperidone on gastric emptying in diabetic autonomic neuropathy. Dig Dis Sci 1985;30:1–9.

45. Mayer EA, Thomson JB, Jehn D, et al. Gastric emptying and sieving of solid food and pancreatic and biliary secretions after solid meals in patients with nonresective ulcer surgery. Gastroenterology 1984;87:1264–71.

46. Urbain JL, Siegel Ja, Vancutsem E, et al. The isotope electrogastrogram: a new scintigraphic technique to visualize and noninvasively characterize gastric contractions. J Nucl Med 1990;31:775.

47. Akkerman LM, Jacobs F, Hong-Yoe O, et al. A noninvasive method to quantify antral contractile activity in man and dog (a preliminary report). In: Christensen J, editor. Gastrointestinal motility. New York: Raven Press; 1980. p. 195–202.

48. Knight LC, Parkman HP, Miller Ma, et al. Delayed gastric emptying in normal women is associated with decreased antral contractility. Am J Gastroenterol 1997;92:968–75.

49. Urbain JL, Vekemans MC, Bouillon R, et al. Characterization of gastric antral motility disturbances in diabetes using the scintigraphic technique. J Nucl Med 1993;34:576–81.

# CHAPTER 13

# Electrogastrography

*Kenneth L. Koch*

The stomach is a marvelous neuromuscular machine. It must accommodate the ingested foods we eat and then properly triturate and empty nutrient suspensions into the duodenum. The mixing and emptying activities of the stomach are paced by pacesetter potentials or slow waves.[1] The rhythmicity of the myoelectrical activity of the stomach is achieved by the interstitial cells of Cajal.[2,3]

During these physiologic mixing/emptying activities, the stomach produces many pleasurable sensations related to the satisfying epigastric fullness that accompanies the ingestion of a meal. On the other hand, when the neuromuscular apparatus of this sophisticated mixing chamber is dysfunctional, a variety of unpleasant and vague symptoms ranging from epigastric discomfort to nausea and vomiting are experienced.[4]

There are many analogies to cardiac physiology when the stomach is viewed as an electrocontractile mixing chamber and pump.[5] Thus, gastric electrocontractile abnormalities may be understood in terms of myoelectrical dysfunction that can influence the muscular function of the stomach. In this chapter, electrogastrography (EGG) is reviewed. The EGG reflects gastric myoelectrical events that produce normal stomach neuromuscular activities and gastric dysrhythmias that are associated with nausea and delayed gastric emptying.

## NORMAL GASTRIC MOTILITY: ELECTROMECHANICAL ACTIVITY

### Gastric Muscular and Electrical Regions

*Anatomy*

The anatomic and pacemaker regions of the stomach are described in Figure 13.1. The fundic area is considered the "proximal stomach," the area that relaxes to accommodate ingested food. The body and antrum are considered the "distal stomach," where the ingested solid foods are mixed and gently broken down by recurrent peristaltic waves.[6] When food particles are <1 mm in size, these nutrient suspensions are emptied into the duodenum by antral peristaltic contractions.[7]

*Pacemaker Region and Activity*

The pacemaker region is located on the greater curvature of the stomach, as shown in Figure 13.1. The 3 cycle per minute (cpm) pacesetter potentials or slow waves arise from the interstitial cells of Cajal located near the enteric neurons and the circular muscle layer (see Fig. 13.1).[2,3,7,8] The fundic muscle has no 3 cpm activity and is electrically "silent." The frequency of the pacesetter potentials is modulated by ongoing changes in vagal, splanchnic, and hormonal activity.[9] Pacesetter potentials migrate distally from the corpus toward the pylorus at a rate of 3 cpm with increasing velocity in the antrum.[10] The antrum is the site of most tachygastrias and tachyarrhythmias (3.75–10 cpm electrical waves).[11,12]

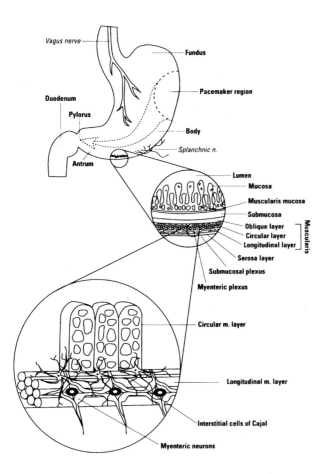

**FIGURE 13.1.** Gross and microscopic elements of the anatomy of the stomach. The proximal stomach is the fundus and the distal stomach is the body and antrum. The pyloric sphincter joins the antrum and the duodenum. Parasympathetic input to the stomach is supplied by the vagus nerve and the sympathetic nervous system innervates the stomach through the splanchnic nerves. On the greater curvature of the stomach between the fundus and the body is the general region of the pacemaker of the stomach. A telescoped and cross-sectional view of the antrum is shown in the circle in the middle of the figure. This view shows the gastric wall with the mucosal layer and the muscularis. The outermost muscle layer is the longitudinal layer; and running perpendicular to the longitudinal muscle layer is the circular muscle layer. There is also an oblique muscle layer in the stomach. Between the circular muscle and longitudinal muscle layers are neurons of the myenteric plexus and the enteric nervous system. The second telescoped view shown in the lower circle illustrates the anatomic proximities of the myenteric neurons and the interstitial cells of Cajal in the myenteric region between the circular and longitudinal muscle layers. The processes of the interstitial cells interdigitate with circular muscle fibers and the myenteric neurons. The interstitial cells in the myenteric plexus area are thought to be responsible for generation of slow waves or pacesetter potentials. The interstitial cells are also found in the submucosal layers, the deep musculatures plexus, and the intramuscular layers of the stomach.

## GASTRIC MYOELECTRICAL ACTIVITY AND ELECTROGASTROGRAPHY

### Basic Methods of Recording Gastric Myoelectrical Activity

The myoelectrical activity of the stomach may be measured from mucosal, serosal, or cutaneous electrodes (Fig. 13.2).[11–17] Each method has advantages and disadvantages. Electrodes may be sutured on the gastric serosa during invasive laparoscopic or operative procedures to record temporarily gastric myoelectrical activity. Mucosal electrodes yield direct myoelectrical recordings from the stomach, but the electrodes become dislodged during contractions that occur during fasting or after meals.

Figures 13.2 and 13.3 illustrate the electrical events that coordinate the gastric peristaltic waves that produce the emptying of nutrients. The key to normal peristaltic contractions is the proper aboral migration of the gastric pacesetter potentials from the pacemaker region to the distal antrum (see Fig. 13.2). The gastric slow wave itself produces a very tiny contraction in the circular muscle. Stronger contractions of the circular muscle that are needed for the work of gastric mixing/emptying require plateau and action potentials to bring the circular smooth muscle to contraction thresholds.[7,9] As measured with extracellular electrodes, a series of plateau or action potentials linked to the slow waves occur during depolarization of the circular muscle.[9] Thus, the electrical correlates of gastric peristaltic contractions are plateau and action potentials linked to the migrating pacesetter potentials (see Fig. 13.3).

The Ag-AgCl electrodes positioned on the epigastrium as shown in Figure 13.4 accurately record gastric myoelectrical activity and are termed EGGs. Electrogastrography refers to the method of recording gastric myoelectrical activity.[18,19] For the noninvasive cutaneous myoelectrical recordings, the skin is wiped with an alcohol swab before placement of the electrodes. Three to four electrodes are positioned on the epigastrium for clinical EGG recordings as shown in Figure 13.4. For example, electrodes 1 and 2 are referenced to electrode 3 to create one bipolar electrode: 1 to 2. Electrodes for gastric myoelectrical recordings are connected to amplifiers through couplers selected for the various myoelectrical frequencies to be analyzed. Filters are needed to create a frequency window from approximately 0.5 to 15 cpm, a range that encompasses normal EGG rhythms and gastric dysrhythmias. Methodologic details for recording EGGs have been published.[19]

### Normal EGG Frequency Ranges

The normal frequency ranges for EGGs encompass bradygastrias (approximately 0.5–2.5 cpm), the normal range (2.5–3.75 cpm), tachygastria (3.75–10.0 cpm), and the duodenal-respiratory range (10.0–15.0 cpm) (Fig. 13.5).[19,20] The respiration rate in some subjects occasionally is in the 10 to 15 cpm range, and the duodenal pacesetter potential ranges

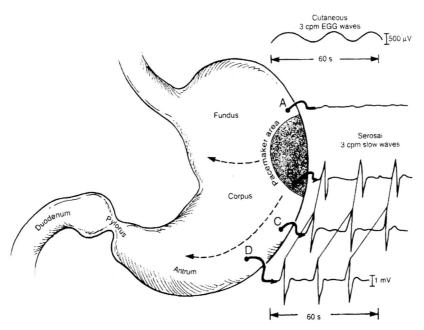

**FIGURE 13.2.** Gastric slow waves or pacesetter potentials are rhythmic depolarization and repolarization waves that begin in the pacemaker region. Slow waves migrate circumferentially as indicated by the horizontal arrow and, at the same time, migrate distally as shown by the arrow pointing to the antrum. In this figure, there are three electrodes on the gastric body and antrum and one electrode on the fundus. Note that a slow-wave sequence migrates from the pacemaker area into the antrum approximately every 20 seconds or 3 cycles per minute (cpm). The record-ing from the fundus, however, indicates no electrical rhythmicity. Also shown are cutaneous 3 cpm electrogastrogram (EGG) waves. The 3 cpm EGG waves represent the summation of electrical events from the stomach as measured from the cutaneous or surface electrodes. The surface record-ing of the stomach myoelectrical activity is an EGG. Reproduced with permission from Koch KL. The stomach. In: Schuster MM, editor. Atlas of gastrointestinal motility in health and disease. Baltimore: Williams and Wilkins; 1993. p. 158–76.

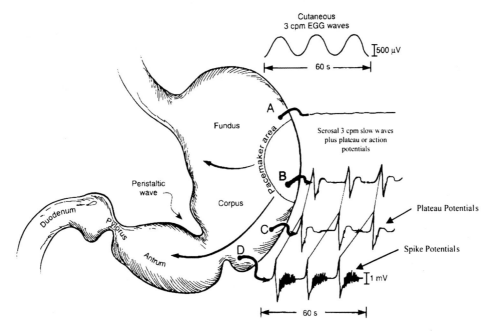

**FIGURE 13.3.** Slow waves linked to plateau potentials or spike potentials are the electrophysiologic basis for gastric peristalsis. The figure shows slow waves with a raised area after depolarization that represent plateau potentials (see electrode C). Contractions of the circular muscle occur during plateau potentials. The slow waves at electrode D show spike potentials associated with the slow waves. Circular muscle contraction also occurs during action potentials. Thus, the migrating slow waves linked to plateau or action poten-tials are the electrophysiologic basis for peristaltic contractions of the circu-lar muscle (peristaltic waves). A peristaltic wave is indicated by the *curved arrow*. The peristaltic wave is moving from the proximal corpus toward the pylorus and is shown by the indentation in the antrum. In their most regular form, gastric peristalses occur at a rate of 3 per minute. The cutaneous 3 cpm EGG waves are of greater amplitude when there is additional electrical activity of circular muscle depolarization/repolarization occurring at 3 cpm. An increase in the amplitude of 3 cpm EGG waves is correlated with increased antral contractions. In summary, plateau or spike potentials linked to slow waves are the electrophysiologic events that underlie recurrent gastric peristaltic waves that triturate and empty ingested meals.

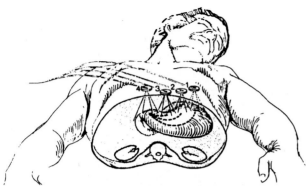

**FIGURE 13.4.** Placement of electrodes on the upper abdominal surface for recording electrogastrograms. These are recorded from silver-silver chloride electrodes placed in the epigastrium. The electrodes are placed in the mid-clavicular line 2 to 3 cm below the costal margin to avoid respiratory artifact. Electrodes 1, 2, and 3 are as referenced to electrode 4 to form bipolar electrode pairs. The bipolar electrode pairs record the electrical events that occur beneath the electrodes. By proper amplification and filtering of the signal, electrical waves between the frequency of 0.5 to 15 cpm are obtained and encompass the relevant frequencies from bradygastria (0.5–2.5 cpm), the normal range (2.5–3.75 cpm), tachygastria (3.75–10.0 cpm), and duodenal respiration frequencies (10.0–15.0 cpm).

from 12 to 14 cpm. Thus, it is important to know the respiratory rate before interpreting EGG frequencies in the 10 to 15 cpm range. Occasionally, the respiration rate is less than 10 cpm and may be confused with tachygastria (Fig. 13.6). Finally, deep breaths or coughs may create artifacts in the EGG signal, and it is extremely important that these minutes of EGG should be recognized as full of artifact and not subjected to computer analysis.[21]

## FASTING AND POSTPRANDIAL NEUROMUSCULAR ACTIVITY OF THE STOMACH AND EGG

The ultimate result of gastric myoelectrical and contractile work is the movement of liquids and solids from the stomach and into the small intestine, that is, gastric emptying. Gastric motility and emptying are measured by a variety of techniques ranging from pressure catheters to ultrasonography to scintigraphy to nuclear magnetic resonance methods. These topics are discussed in Chapters 10, 12, and 14. The myoelectrical patterns recorded by EGGs during fasting and postprandial periods are described below.

### Fasting Myoelectrical Activity

During prolonged fasting, such as an overnight fast, the stomach exhibits several stereotyped contractile patterns as described in Chapter 10. Phase 3 contractions are strong, rhythmic, antral contractions that occur at a rate of 3/min and continue for at least 2 to 3/min. Phase 3 contractions usually begin

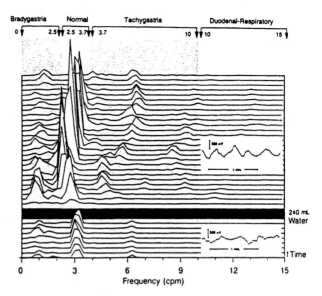

**FIGURE 13.5.** Electrogastrogram (EGG) recording before and after a healthy control subject ingests water. The EGG tracings are shown in the insets. The water load is indicated by the solid black line and 240-mL water. This figure also shows a series of peaks, the frequency analysis of the EGG signal, which is termed a running spectral analysis (RSA). Other figures in this chapter are presented in this same format. The x-axis from 0 to 15 represents the frequency in the EGG signal in cycles per minute (cpm). The y-axis indicates time. Each line in the RSA indicates the frequency peaks that occur in the 4-minute periods of EGG data. The next line indicates 1 new minute of EGG data added to the previous 3 minutes. Thus, there is a 75% overlap in each 4-minute period of EGG as analyzed in the EGG. A frequency analysis is performed for each of these 4-minute periods. The z-axis or third-dimension indicates the power at the various frequencies within the EGG signal. Power is the log of the microvolt$^2$ of any frequency that is present in the EGG signal. At the top of the figure, the normal frequency ranges are listed. In this figure, the baseline EGG tracing (*inset*) shows low-amplitude 3 cpm waves. After ingestion of water, the next EGG trace shows 3 cpm waves that have increased amplitude compared with the baseline recording. This is a normal EGG response to a water load. The RSA shows a series of peaks at the 3 cpm point during baseline before ingestion of water. The *black rectangle* indicates the 5-minute period of time during which water was ingested. The subjects ingested water until they felt full. After ingestion of water, there is a slight decrease in the EGG frequency to approximately 2.5 cpm, followed by a return to peaks at the 3 cpm frequency. The 3 cpm peaks are higher after ingestion of water compared with baseline peaks and indicate greater power (and amplitude) in the 3 cpm signal. This is a normal RSA pattern in a healthy subject after ingestion of water. Finally, it should be noted that there are a series of low-amplitude peaks from 5 to 6 cpm after ingestion of water. Very small peaks are also seen at 6 cpm at baseline. These peaks represent harmonics of the primary frequency, the 3 cpm signal. Six cpm waves are not seen in the actual EGG signal, but the 3 cpm waves are clearly noted. Thus, overall, this is a normal baseline EGG and a normal EGG response to ingestion of water. Reproduced with permission from Koch KL, Stern RM. Electrogastrography. In: Kumar D, Wingate D, editors. Illustrated guide to gastrointestinal motility. London: Churchill Livingstone; 1993. p. 290–307.

in the antrum and migrate into the duodenum and traverse the jejunum in 90 to 120 minutes.[22] The myoelectrical activities corresponding to Phases 1 to 3 of the interdigestive state have been recorded with strain gauges and serosal electrodes in dog.

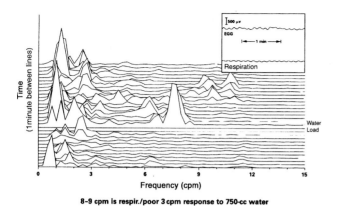

**8-9 cpm is respir./poor 3 cpm response to 750-cc water**

**FIGURE 13.6.** Electrogastrogram (EGG) signal with respiration artifact in a patient with chronic nausea. This figure shows the EGG rhythm strip and respiration rate (*inset*) and the running spectral analysis of the EGG at baseline and for 30 minutes after the water load test. The EGG recording and respiration recording in the inset show that the frequency of the EGG is approximately 8 cpm. Note that the respiration frequency in this patient is also 8 per minute. Thus, the 8 cpm waves in the EGG do not reflect a tachygastria but are, in fact, the respiration rate. The running spectral analysis shows almost no peaks in the normal 3 cpm range during baseline. After the patient ingested 750 mL of water during the water load, high peaks at approximately 8 cpm are seen for several minutes. At this same time, there are very few peaks in the normal 3 cpm range. As mentioned above, the 8 cpm peaks do not represent a tachygastria but are the respiration frequency. After the water load test and toward the end of the recording, some 3 cpm peaks are present.

Contractile activity during the interdigestive state is associated with high-power, low-frequency electrical waves.[23]

Gastric myoelectrical activity recorded with EGG during the interdigestive patterns was studied in humans.[24] The normal 3 cpm myoelectrical rhythm was most stable during Phase 1, or motor quiescence. A decrease in gastric frequency occurred during the transition from Phase 1 to 2, and the EGG frequency was very unstable during Phase 3. Only 44% of Phase 3 contractile complexes were reflected in the EGG signal as an increase in power at 3 cpm (Fig. 13.7).[24]

## Postprandial Gastric Myoelectrical Activity

Gastric neuromuscular responses after ingestion of a solid meal include fundic relaxation and corpus-antral contractions.[1,6,7] Details of these gastric smooth muscle responses to solid food are presented in Chapter 10.

### Postprandial Myoelectrical Activities in Response to Solid and Liquid Meals

As shown in Figure 13.8, a gastric peristaltic wave in the barium-filled stomach commences in the corpus and migrates distally to the pylorus. As the pacesetter potential linked with the depolarization and repolarization of the circular muscle migrates distally, a gastric peristalsis wave occurs, and several milliliters of gastric content are subsequently emptied into the duodenum.[15] These gastric peristaltic contractions occur three times a minute, the frequency of the gastric pacesetter potential.

### EGG Response to Water Load Test

The EGG recording with a water load test is a provocative and reproducible test for recording EGGs in patients with unexplained nausea or dyspepsia symptoms.[25] The water load provides a purely physical stimulus for gastric myoelectrical and contractile activity. The stomach must accommodate the water while the subject ingests water "until full" over a 5-minute period. The absence of calories in the test meal limits the effects of secretin, cholecystokinin, and other hormonal responses elicited by carbohydrate, fat, and protein on gastric electrical activity. The water load test also avoids stimulating colonic neuromuscular activity that accompanies ingestion of a caloric meal. The water load test provokes symptoms such as nausea and bloating and unmasks or increases gastric dysrhythmias and the failure of a normal 3 cpm response after the water load.

The EGG is recorded for 30 minutes after the water load is ingested, and the EGG pattern in response to the water load is analyzed. The patients' EGG results are compared with control values and an EGG diagnosis of normal or gastric dysrhythmia (bradygastria, tachygastria, poor 3 cpm response

### Migrating Myoelectrical Complex

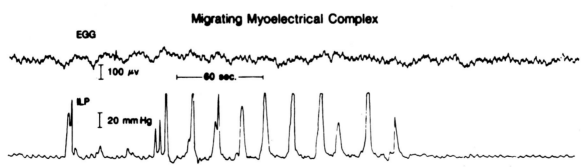

**FIGURE 13.7.** Electrogastrogram (EGG) recording during Phase 3 of the interdigestive motor complex. This figure shows an EGG recording in the upper tracing (EGG) and the simultaneously recorded intraluminal pressure (ILP) in the lower tracing (1). A burst of contractions at 3 per minute (Phase 3) is seen in the ILP recording obtained with a catheter in the antrum. During this time, there are 3 cpm myoelectrical waves seen in the EGG. When the Phase 3 contractions disappear, the EGG tracing shows waves with decreased amplitude and no distinct 3 cpm waves. Approximately 44% of the time, increases in amplitude of the 3 cpm EGG waves occur during Phase 3 contractions. Reproduced with permission from Koch KL. The stomach. In: Schuster MM, editor. Atlas of gastrointestinal motility in health and disease. Baltimore: Williams and Wilkins; 1993. p. 158–76.

or nonspecific dysrhythmia) can be made. Figures 13.5 and 13.9 show normal EGG responses to the water load in healthy subjects. A water load test elicited increased antral contraction and increased amplitude of myoelectrical signals in dogs.[17] Figure 13.10 shows the EGG signal analyzed and presented as a "gray-scale plot,"[26] and Figure 13.11 shows the EGG signal analyzed by adaptive filtering (see the figure legends for details).[27]

### Postprandial Myoelectrical Responses to Pain and Temperature

The amplitude of normal 3 cpm EGG activity decreases significantly in response to the cold pressor tests,[28] as shown in Figure 13.12. In response to the painful stimulation of cold caloric testing with 4°C water, gastric emptying is delayed, and antral hypomotility occurs.[29] The EGG signal, reflecting ongoing pacesetter potential activity, is also responsive to the

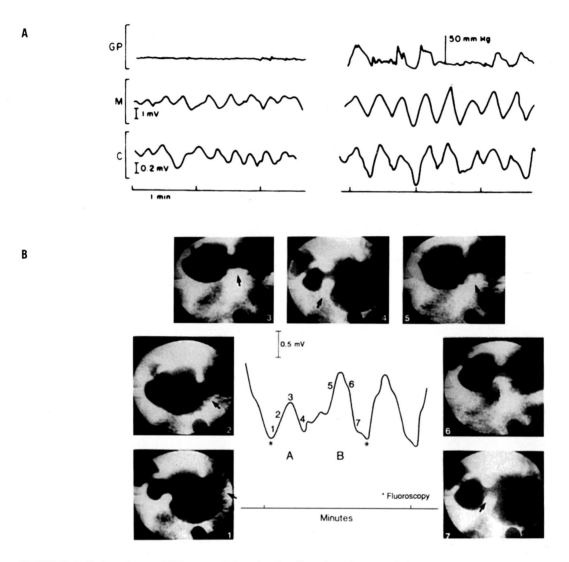

**FIGURE 13.8.** Electrogastrogram (EGG) response to ingestion of a milk meal (**A**) and EGG response to ingestion of a barium meal (**B**). **A** shows intragastric pressure (GP), EGG measured with a mucosal electrode (M), and EGG measured with a cutaneous electrode (C). The tracings on the left show the recordings during the fasting state and the tracings on the right show the pressure and EGG responses after ingestion of 240 mL of milk. Increased intraluminal pressure contractions and increased amplitude of EGG are seen in the panel on the right. Also, the cutaneous EGG and the mucosal EGG show similar frequencies at 3 cpm. **B** shows two gastric peristaltic sequences recorded during fluoroscopy of the barium-filled stomach. These two gastric peristaltic sequences correspond with the EGG waves labeled A and B. As EGG wave A was recorded (see numbers 1, 2, 3, and 4 located on the EGG wave), fluoroscopy of the barium-filled stomach resulted in pictures 1, 2, 3, and 4. As the EGG wave

A was recorded, a gastric peristaltic contraction (indicated by the *arrows* on the radiographs) traveled from mid-corpus (1), to the mid-antrum (2), to the distal antrum (3), and finally emptied barium into the duodenal bulb (4). Immediately thereafter, EGG wave B was recorded (see numbers 5, 6, and 7 on the EGG wave) with corresponding areas in the fluoroscopic pictures numbered 5, 6, and 7. Once again, the arrows on the fluoroscopic images indicate the migration of the antral peristaltic wave as it moved from mid-antrum (5) to the distal antrum (6 and 7) and emptied barium into the duodenal bulb. Note the similarities of pictures 4 and 7 showing the barium-filled duodenum. In the barium-filled stomach, each EGG wave reflected the electrical activity associated with a gastric peristaltic contraction. Reproduced with permission from Koch KL. The stomach. In: Schuster MM, editor. Atlas of gastrointestinal motility in health and disease. Baltimore: Williams and Wilkins; 1993. p. 158–76.

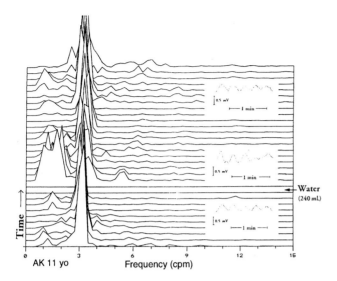

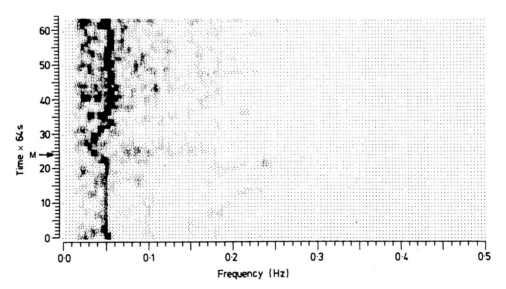

**FIGURE 13.9.** Electrogastrogram (EGG) response to a water load in a healthy subject. The baseline EGG rhythm strip shows a 3 cpm rhythm, and the normal rhythm is maintained after ingestion of 240 mL of water (see *insets*). Ingested water represents a physical volume to which the stomach must respond. The advantages of a water load are that there are no calories to stimulate secretin, cholecystokinin, or insulin release and cause additional effects on the stomach. Furthermore, because there are no calories, the water load test does not stimulate the gastrocolonic reflex and possibly affect the EGG signal with colonic neuromuscular activity. The running spectral analysis shows peaks at 3 cpm at baseline. After ingestion of water, there are transient rhythms at 1 and 2 cpm, but the 3 cpm rhythm is clearly maintained and represents a normal water load test in a healthy young subject.

**FIGURE 13.11.** The electrogastrogran (EGG) signal from a healthy subject plotted as running power spectra. The x-axis shows frequencies from 0 to 12 cpm. The lines on the y-axis represent discrete 2-minute periods of EGG signal that underwent spectral analysis. The z-axis indicates the power at the various frequencies in the EGG signal. The computer analysis shows many peaks in the 3 cpm range. In this technique, the percentage of all of the lines with the highest peak in the 2 to 4 cpm range is calculated. Reproduced with permission from Chen J, Stewart WR, McCallum RW. Adaptive spectral analysis of episodic rhythmic variations in gastric myoelectrical potentials. IEEE Trans Biomed Eng 1993;40:128–35.

**FIGURE 13.10.** Gray-scale plot of electrogastrogram (EGG) activity before and after a test meal (see *arrow* at M). This figure shows another way of displaying the frequencies in the EGG signal recorded from a healthy subject before and after ingestion of a yogurt meal. The x-axis indicates the EGG frequency in Hertz. The normal 3 cpm rhythm is 0.05 Hz. The y-axis shows time, with each dotted line indicating 256 seconds. The frequency analysis is performed on the 256 seconds, and the next line indicates an additional 64 seconds added to the previous 192 seconds. The power in the various frequencies is indicated by the darkness of the dots on the grid. The darker the area, the more power at that particular frequency. Thus, in this healthy subject, there is a clear dark line at 0.05 Hz (3 cpm), and after ingestion of the meal, there is a slight decrease in the frequency to approximately 0.04 Hz (2.4 cpm). Then the line becomes thicker and darker near 0.05 Hz. In addition, at baseline, a very faint gray line is seen at 0.1 Hz, which is 6 cpm and indicates a harmonic of the primary frequency of 0.05 Hz or 3 cpm. Reproduced with permission from Geldoff H, van der Schee EJ, van Blankenstein M, Gashuis JL. Electrogastrographic study of gastric myelectrical activity in patients with unexplained nausea and vomiting. Gut 1986;27:799–808.

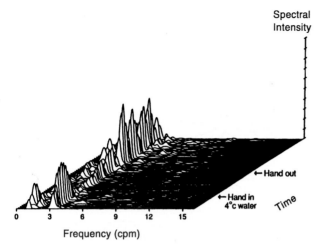

**FIGURE 13.12.** Effect of the cold pressor test on gastric myoelectrical activity. This figure shows a running spectral analysis of the EGG signal recorded from a healthy volunteer. During the baseline, there are regular peaks at the normal 3 cpm frequency. The cold pressor (hand in 4°C water) test is performed by having the subject plunge his/her hand into ice water (4°C). The figure shows that during the cold pressor test, there is a marked decrease in the height (power or spectral intensity) of the 3 cpm peaks. There are no tachygastrias or bradygastrias. The cold pressor test induces acute pain and increased sympathetic nervous system activity, a stimulus that markedly reduces the power or amplitude of the gastric myoelectrical activity. After the painful stimulus is removed (hand out), the 3 cpm peaks return to baseline power or intensity Reproduced with permission from Stern RM, Hu S, Koch KL. Effects of cold stress on gastric myoelectrical activity. J Gastrointest Motil 1991;3:225–8.

temperature of the ingested liquids. Cold temperature liquids suppressed the 3 cpm activity and produced immediate and temporary slower frequencies ("frequency dips"), whereas body temperature (37°C) liquids did not alter the EGG frequency immediately after ingestion of the liquid.[30]

### Sham Feedings and the EGG

In response to the cephalic vagal stimulation of sham feeding, EGG waves increase in amplitude at the 3 cpm frequency[31] and antral contractions increase (Fig. 13.13).[32] Furthermore, atropine blocks sham feeding–induced antral contractions, and patients with previous vagotomies failed to show an increase in 3 cpm electrical activity during sham feeding. These data indicate that activation of the cephalic vagal reflex increases the 3 cpm EGG signal via parasympathetic cholinergic pathways.[31]

### Duodenal Myoelectrical Activity

In normal subjects, the duodenal pacesetter potential frequencies from 12 to 14 cpm are not seen in the EGG recording, and only 5% of the total EGG power is within the duodenal-respiratory range of 10 to 15 cpm.[20] However, in patients with antrectomy and gastrojejunostomy anastomoses, the jejunal segment is near the abdominal surface. In these patients, the antrectomy has reduced the amount of stomach musculature and weakened the 3 cpm EGG signal, and duodenal or jejunal pacesetter potential can be detected.[33]

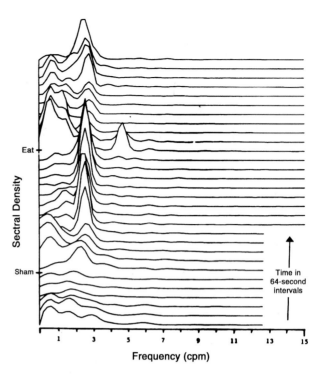

**FIGURE 13.13.** Effect of sham feeding on gastric myoelectrical activity. This figure shows a running spectral analysis of the electrogastrogram (EGG) signal recorded from a healthy subject. At baseline and before sham feeding, there are low-amplitude peaks in the 3 cpm range. The *arrow* indicates the point at which sham feeding occurs (Sham). Sham feeding was stimulated by chewing and spitting a hot dog on a roll over a 5-minute period. After sham feeding, there is an increase in the power at the 3 cpm frequency, indicated by the tall peaks at 3 cpm. This increase in EGG power at 3 cpm lasts approximately 10 minutes and then decreases to baseline levels. Thus, sham feeding stimulates parasympathetic activity and increases the EGG power at the normal 3 cpm EGG frequency in subjects who consider the experience neutral or positive. In subjects who found sham feeding to be a disgusting experience, the 3 cpm activity did not increase. Reproduced with permission from Stern RM, Crawford HE, Stewart WR, et al. Sham feeding. Cephalic-vagal influences on gastric myoelectrical activity. Dig Dis Sci 1989;34:521–7.

## GASTRIC MYOELECTRICAL DISORDERS: GASTRIC DYSRHYTHMIAS

### Gastric Dysrhythmias: Tachygastria and Bradygastria

Gastric dysrhythmias are abnormal frequencies of the gastric pacesetter activity that have been recorded in many clinical conditions. Gastric dysrhythmias originate in the body and antrum of the stomach as ectopic pacemakers.[11–14,34] Tachygastrias are abnormally fast rhythms ranging from 3.75 to 10 cpm (Fig. 13.14). Bradygastrias are abnormally slow rhythms ranging from flatline or arrhythmia patterns to high-amplitude, undulating waves in the 0.5 to 2.5 cpm range.[34] The normal pacemaker rhythm is generally not present when gastric dysrhythmias are active. However, in certain circumstances, several pacemaker areas may be active, and both the 3 cpm normal rhythm and gastric dysrhythmias may be recorded.

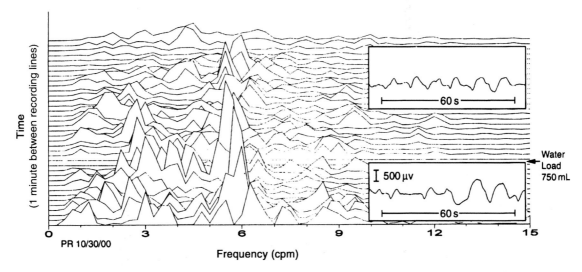

**FIGURE 13.14.** Tachygastria in a college student with chronic nausea 6 months after a viral illness. The EGG rhythm strips (*insets*) in this patient show a tachygastria at approximately 5 to 6 cpm during baseline and after the water load test. This is a regular tachygastria at 5 to 6 cpm. The running spectral analysis shows few peaks in the 3 cpm range at baseline, and most peaks are at 5 to 6 cpm. After ingestion of water, there is no increase in 3 cpm activity, and the tachygastria remains present at 5 to 6 cpm.

## Gastric Dysrhythmias in Various Disease States

### Nausea of Pregnancy

A spectrum of gastric dysrhythmias from bradygastrias to tachygastrias has been reported in patients with nausea of pregnancy (Fig. 13.15).[35] Electrogastrograms from these patients depict the spectrum of dysrhythmias that can be diagnosed by visual inspection of a high-quality EGG rhythm strip. See the figure legend for details.

### Diabetes Mellitus

In diabetic patients, the presence of a gastric dysrhythmia predicts delayed gastric emptying rates as determined by scintigraphic methods approximately 90 to 100% of the time.[3,36] Gastric dysrhythmias interfere with normal coordination and propagation of peristaltic waves, thereby decreasing the rate of gastric emptying.[36–38]

Figure 13.16 shows EGGs recorded from a patient with diabetic gastroparesis.[36] This bradygastria pattern resolved during treatment with domperidone. In six diabetic patients with gastroparesis treated with domperidone, gastric dysrhythmias converted to normal 3 cpm rhythms with an accompanying decrease in upper gastrointestinal symptoms. However, overall gastric emptying rates became normal in only one of six patients, suggesting gastric electrical and mechanical dissociation. Thus, the presence of gastric dysrhythmias, not the rate of gastric emptying, may be more relevant to epigastric symptoms such as nausea and early satiety.

### Idiopathic Gastroparesis

Figure 13.17 shows a bradygastria EGG pattern in a patient with idiopathic gastroparesis. Gastric dysrhythmias have been reported in patients with idiopathic gastroparesis,[20,39,40] in adults with functional dyspepsia and normal or delayed gastric

**A. Tachygastria**

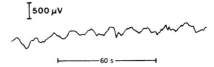

**B. Flatline**

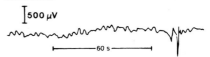

**C. Bradygastria**

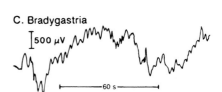

**D. Normal**

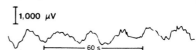

**FIGURE 13.15.** Gastric dysrhythmias in patients with first-trimester nausea of pregnancy. Rhythm strip A shows a 6 cpm tachygastria, whereas rhythm strip B is labeled in "flatline" because the electrogastrogram (EGG) has no discernible rhythm. The small waves are respiration signals at approximately 16 per minutes. This rhythm is also termed a low-amplitude bradygastria. The rhythm strip in C (bradygastria) is a high-amplitude 1 cpm wave. Rhythm strip D shows a normal 3 cpm rhythm recorded from a woman with no nausea on the morning of this EGG recording. On the other hand, the women with the gastric dysrhythmias reported nausea. Reproduced with permission from Koch KL. The stomach. In: Schuster MM, editor. Atlas of gastrointestinal motility in health and disease. Baltimore: Williams and Wilkins; 1993. p. 158–76.

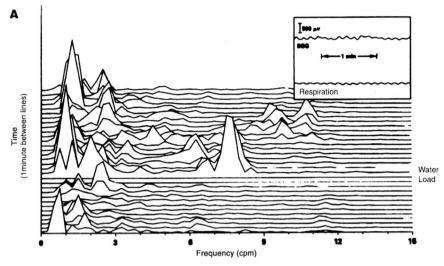

8–9 cpm is respir./poor 3 cpm response to 750-cc water

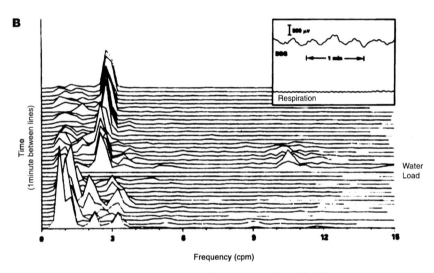

Regular 3 cpm activity after domperidone (20 mg PO quid)

**FIGURE 13.16.** Effect of domperidone on gastric myoelectrical activity in a patient with unexplained nausea. **A** shows an electrogastrographic (EGG) rhythm strip (*inset*) with no 3 cpm waves and mostly respiratory waves at 8 cpm. The running spectral analysis also shows very few 3 cpm peaks before and after the ingestion of water, although these are some of the 3 cpm peaks toward the end of the recording. This figure was also shown as Figure 13.8. **B** shows the EGG recording with water load test from the same patient after domperidone therapy. The inset now shows clear 3 cpm EGG waves in contrast to the respiratory waves. The running spectral analysis shows increased 3 cpm peaks at baseline compared with **A**. After ingestion of the water load, there are clear and increased 3 cpm peaks compared with **A**. This is a normal EGG response to a water load. The patient's nausea symptoms resolved with treatment with domperidone.

emptying rates,[41] and children with dyspepsia.[42] The bradygastria converted to a normal 3 cpm EGG pattern (an example of a pharmacologic "gastroversion") in a patient treated with cisapride. This patient's gastric emptying rate became normal during treatment with cisapride, indicating concordant electrical and mechanical activity. Metoclopramide (Reglan) also corrects gastric dysrhythmias (see below).

### Obstruction

Three cpm gastric electrical rhythms have been reported in patients with delayed gastric emptying caused by pyloric obstruction (Fig. 13.18). The EGG signals have persistent high-amplitude waves and lack the normal frequency variability recorded in healthy subjects (compare Fig. 13.18 with Fig. 13.9).[20]

### Ischemic Gastroparesis

Figure 13.19A shows a tachygastria in a patient with gastroparesis secondary to chronic mesenteric ischemia. After

mesenteric revascularization with bypass grafts of the obstructed celiac and superior mesenteric arteries, the patient had complete resolution of epigastric symptoms. The follow-up EGG recorded 6 months after revascularization (see Fig. 13.19B) shows the return of normal 3 cpm EGG signals. Delayed gastric emptying and gastric dysrhythmias resolve after mesenteric revascularization with bypass grafts for obstructions of the mesenteric arteries.[43,44]

### Dysmotility-Like Dyspepsia

From 35 to 58% of patients with dysmotility-like dyspepsia and negative endoscopic findings have gastric dysrhythmias.[40,45–47] Gastric dysrhythmias are pathophysiologic mechanisms associated with the vague symptoms of postprandial fullness, satiety, distention/discomfort, and nausea in dysmotility-like functional dyspepsia. The EGG with water load test identifies gastric dysrhythmias in approximately 60% of the patients with dysmotility-like functional dyspepsia (Fig. 13.20).[41] Some of these patients will also have gas-

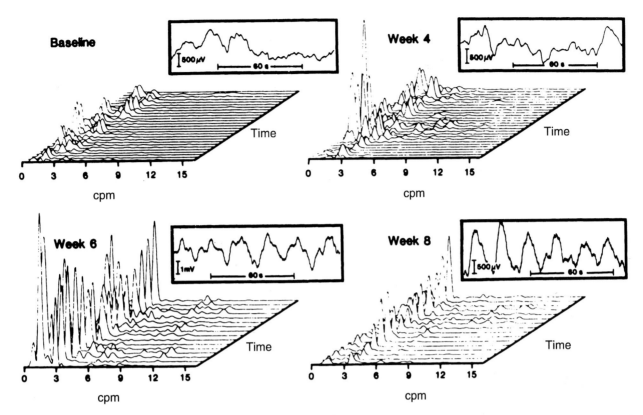

**FIGURE 13.17.** Effect of cisapride on bradygastria in a patient with unexplained nausea and vomiting. The *inset* shows a 1 to 2 cpm bradygastria at baseline before cisapride treatment. The running spectral analysis shows very few peaks at 3 cpm and the predominance of peaks in the 1 to 2 cpm bradygastria range. After treatment with cisapride, the electro- gastrogram (EGG) shows regular 3 cpm EGG waves at weeks 6 and 8. The running spectral analyses also show regular 3 cpm peaks in the normal 3 cpm range. Thus, the cisapride treatment converted the EGG rhythm to the normal 3 cpm pattern. The patient's nausea resolved during the treatment with cisapride.

troparesis (category 1), but most have a gastric dysrhythmia and normal gastric emptying (category 2). The presence of gastric dysrhythmias was associated with better symptom reduction during treatment with cisapride compared with patients who had normal EGG recordings.[47] Furthermore, correction of gastric dysrhythmias is associated with improvement in dyspepsia symptoms.[40,42,47]

On the other hand, approximately 40% of these dyspepsia patients have normal EGGs, suggesting visceral hypersensitivity (or nongastric causes of the symptoms) (category 3). Category 4 represents the combination of normal EGG pattern and delayed gastric emptying, a pattern associated with electromechanical dissociation or mechanical obstruction of the stomach.[20]

### Postsurgical EGG Patterns

The EGG pattern after gastric surgery may be very abnormal depending on the extent of the surgery. Patients with vagotomy, antrectomy, and Billroth I or II gastrojejunostomy may have tachygastrias or bradygastrias. Also, in patients who have had antrectomy and Billroth II contractions, the small bowel myoelectrical rhythm (eg, 12–14 cpm) may be the prominent signal in the EGG recording because the small bowel is closer to the surface.[33]

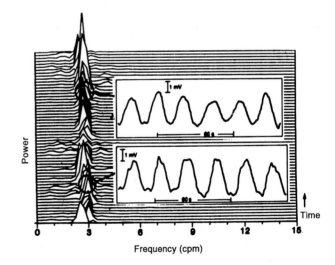

**FIGURE 13.18.** Electrogastrogram (EGG) pattern in a patient with pyloric stenosis and gastric outlet obstruction. The EGG *insets* show high-amplitude, very regular 3 cpm waves at two different time points during the 30-minute EGG recording. The running spectral analysis (RSA) shows the unvarying peaks at 3 cpm. The unvarying nature of the high-amplitude 3 cpm waves and peaks in the RSA is abnormal and suggests a possibility of mechanical obstruction in the antrum, pylorus, or duodenum. Reproduced with permission from Brzana RJ, Bingaman S, Koch KL. Gastric myoelectrical activity in patients with gastric outlet obstruction and idiopathic gastroparesis. Am J Gastroenterol 1998;93:1083–9.

**A**

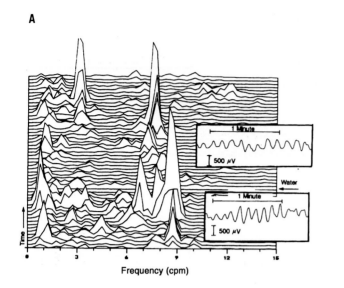

Frequency (cpm)

**B**

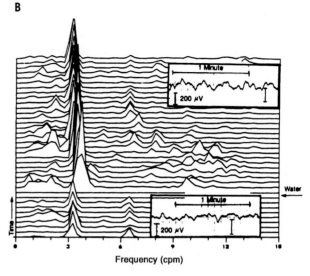

Frequency (cpm)

**FIGURE 13.19.** Gastric myoelectrical activity before and after mesenteric revascularization in a patient with ischemic gastroparesis. **A** shows electrogastrogram (EGG) rhythm strips (*inset*) showing a tachygastria pattern at approximately 8 cpm. The running spectral analysis also shows 8 to 9 cpm peaks and almost no 3 cpm peaks before or after ingestion of water. **B** shows the EGG recordings and running spectral analysis 6 months after mesenteric revascularization. The EGG signal now shows a 3 cpm rhythm, and the running spectral analysis shows many peaks in the 3 cpm range, indicating restoration of normal gastric myoelectrical activity. The patient had resolution of upper gastrointestinal symptoms and improved gastric emptying after the mesenteric revascularization.

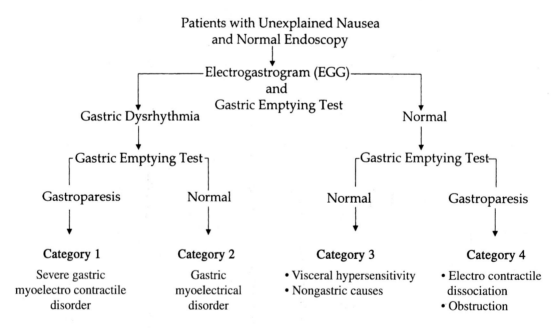

**FIGURE 13.20.** An algorithm for electrogastrogram (EGG) tests and gastric emptying tests to diagnose gastric neuromuscular disorders in patients with unexplained nausea and vomiting. This algorithm indicates a general approach to the patient with unexplained nausea and vomiting or functional dyspepsia. Careful history and physical examination should be performed. If physical examination and standard laboratory and diagnostic studies (endoscopy and ultrasonography) reveal no abnormalities, then the possibility of gastric neuromuscular dysfunction should be considered. An EGG will reveal whether there is a gastric dysrhythmia present versus normal gastric electrical activity. If a gastric dysrhythmia is diagnosed, then a gastric neuromuscular disorder is present. The patient with a gastric dysrhythmia may have delayed gastric emptying (category 1) or normal gastric emptying (category 2). Category 2 is a milder form of gastric neuromuscular disorder with gastric dysrhythmia only. On the other hand, if the EGG is normal, then there are several other diagnostic possibilities. The patient may have gastric visceral hypersensitivity or a nongastric cause of these symptoms (category 3). Nongastric causes include gastroesophageal reflux disease, irritable bowel syndrome, or central nervous system disorders. Appropriate tests may be needed to further follow up on these nongastric possibilities. If the gastric emptying test is delayed, then mechanical obstruction or electrocontractile dissociation should be considered.

A

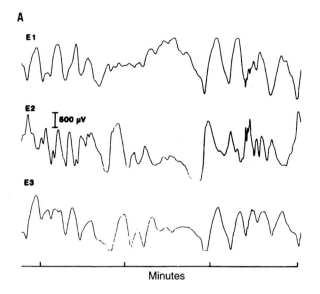

B

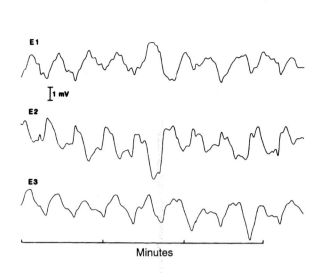

**FIGURE 13.21.** Effect of metoclopramide on gastric myoelectrical activity in a patient with idiopathic gastroparesis. The figures show three channels of electrogastrogram (EGG) recording (E1, E2, E3). **A** shows a tachygastria at 4 to 5 cpm. **B** shows the EGG signal from the same patient 20 minutes after ingestion of 20 mg of metoclopramide. The EGG rhythm has converted to normal 3 cpm activity and the patient's nausea disappeared, another example of a "gastroversion" and the pharmacologic correction of gastric dysrhythmia with improvement in nausea.

### Drugs That Eradicate Gastric Dysrhythmias

Drugs that improve the rate of gastric emptying (prokinetic agents) have also been shown to have antiarrhythmic properties in that gastric dysrhythmias are eradicated.[40,42,47] Since the precise mechanism of gastric dysrhythmias is unknown and ranges from sympathetic nervous system dominance to smooth muscle dysfunction to disorders of the enteric nervous systems and interstitial cells of Cajal, the exact site of the antiarrhythmic action of these drugs is unknown.

Metoclopramide is a gastroprokinetic drug with a variety of actions that include dopamine-2 antagonists, 5-hydroxytryptamine (5-HT$_3$) antagonists, and cholinomimetic (5-HT$_4$ agonist) properties. Metoclopramide decreases upper gastrointestinal symptoms, particularly nausea, in patients with gastroparesis and functional dyspepsia. Figure 13.21 shows an example of the antiarrhythmic effect of metoclopramide in a patient with a tachygastria (see legend for details).

Cisapride is a peripherally acting mixed 5-HT$_4$ agonist/5-HT$_3$ agonist that has effects on the fundus, corpus, and antrum of the stomach to promote an increased rate of gastric emptying. Cisapride improves gastric dysrhythmias in adults and children with functional dyspepsia and symptoms associated with gastroparesis.[40,47] Figure 13.17 shows the eradication of bradygastria during 8 weeks of treatment with cisapride (see legend for details).

Domperidone is a peripherally acting dopamine-2 antagonist that is approved in many countries around the world for nausea and functional dyspepsia symptoms. Domperidone improves upper gastrointestinal symptoms in patients with idiopathic and diabetic gastroparesis.[36,48] Figure 13.16 shows improvement in gastric myoelectrical rhythm over time in a diabetic patient treated with domperidone. The gastric dysrhythmia was eradicated, and a normal 3 cpm rhythm was produced.

### *Drugs That Evoke Gastric Dysrhythmias*

Many drugs produce adverse reactions in terms of nausea and vomiting. The mechanism of drug-induced nausea is unknown for most of these drugs and may be caused by central nervous system or peripheral gastrointestinal neuromuscular effects.

Glucagon induces gastric dysrhythmias and nausea.[49] Glucagon inhibits the smooth muscle of the gastrointestinal tract and may also inhibit inhibitory neurons, which leads to gastric dysrhythmias. Morphine sulfate commonly causes nausea when used for the relief of pain in the recovery room or other areas of the hospital. Figure 13.22 shows morphine-induced tachygastria in a healthy subject. The subject reported nausea during the development of the gastric dysrhythmia.[50] These findings indicate that some opioid pathways are relevant to the symptoms of nausea and to the mechanisms of gastric dysrhythmias. In this example, ondansetron treatment decreased nausea and restored the normal 3 cpm EGG rhythm (see figure legend).

Progesterone and estrogen are hormones that affect gastric myoelectrical activity.[51] The nausea of pregnancy and premenstrual upper gastrointestinal symptoms may be related to fluxes in progesterone and estrogen.[35] The effect of progesterone and estrogen medications was studied in healthy women who ingested standardized test meals. Those subjects with progesterone and estrogen treatment showed increased gastric dysrhythmias in the postprandial period.[51] The treatment of gastric dysrhythmias in the first trimester of pregnancy with protein-rich meals decreased nausea and gastric dysrhythmias.[52] Nicotine also induces gastric dysrhythmias.[53]

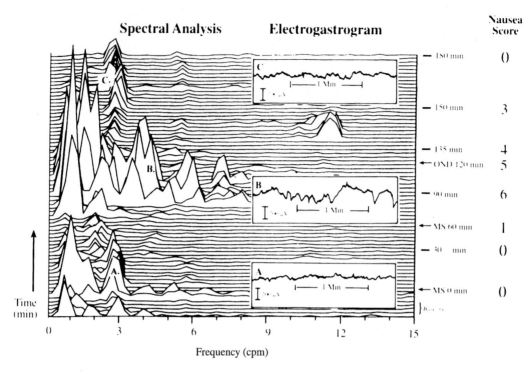

**Spectral Analysis**  **Electrogastrogram**  Nausea Score

**FIGURE 13.22.** Effect of morphine on gastric myoelectrical activity in a healthy subject. A variety of drugs cause nausea, and one of the common agents that induces nausea is morphine. Electrogastrogram (EGG) rhythm strips (*insets*) before (**A**) and after injection of morphine (**B, C**) are shown. **A** shows a low-amplitude 3 cpm rhythm immediately after morphine infusion (Ms 0 min). **B** indicates a tachyarrhythmia at the time of acute nausea (nausea score 6), and **C** shows restoration of 3 cpm EGG waves and peaks in the run-ning spectral analysis after treatment with intravenous ondansetron at 120 minutes (OND 120 min). The running spectral analysis shows 3 cpm peaks at **A** immediately after morphine infusion. At **B**, there are many peaks from 1 to 4 to 6 cpm, indicating the chaotic gastric dysrhythmias evoked by morphine. The peaks at **C** are regular 3 cpm peaks that are now normal after the ondansetron infusion. Gastric dysrhythmias have also been described after infusion of glucagon and administration of progesterone, estrogen, and nicotine.

### EGG Pattern in Children with Gastric Motility Disorders

Electrogastrography is of particular interest to pediatric gastroenterologists because of its noninvasive nature and ability to detect alterations in gastric myoelectrical activity. The recording of EGGs is feasible in neonates, newborns, and toddlers (Fig. 13.23).[54–56] However, movement artifact is a technical problem, and EGG recordings may not be interpretable because of these artifacts. However, recording the EGG in a quiet room, recording the EGG during the postprandial period, and using various techniques to keep the child contented can improve the quality and length of EGG recordings in children. Thus, EGG lends itself to studies of development of gastric rhythmicity in children, investigating unexplained nausea, vomiting, and other gastrointestinal symptoms in children.

Electrogastrograms have been recorded from neonates by several groups. Some developmental change over time has been described by most of the investigations.[55–56] The 3 cpm EGG rhythm is established at the time of normal gestational birth. In premature infants, there is more tachygastria activity present compared with normal adults.[54]

Electrogastrograms also contribute to the understanding of gastrointestinal neuromuscular disorders in children with unexplained nausea and vomiting or dysmotility-like dyspepsia. Combined with gastric emptying studies or antroduodenal motility studies, the EGG provides additional insights into neuromuscular abnormalities of the stomach. Gastric dysrhythmias are associated with dyspepsia symptoms; symptoms and dysrhythmias may resolve after treatment with cisapride.[42] In children with cyclic vomiting syndrome, a high incidence of gastric dysrhythmias has been recorded.[57]

### GASTRIC MYOELECTRICAL EVENTS DURING MOTION SICKNESS AND NAUSEA

The acute onset of nausea during vection-induced motion sickness in humans is preceded by several seconds to minutes by a shift from the normal 3 cpm gastric rhythm to abnormally fast, irregular myoelectrical activity, termed gastric tachyarrhythmias (Fig. 13.24).[58,59] Tachyarrhythmias include very fast frequencies in a 3.75 to 10.0 cpm range, as well as high-amplitude EGG waves in the bradygastria range. This chaotic myoelectrical activity from the stomach continues until the motion stimulus is stopped and homeostasis is re-established. During the recovery period, the gastric tachyarrhythmias dissipate, and 3 cpm gastric myo-

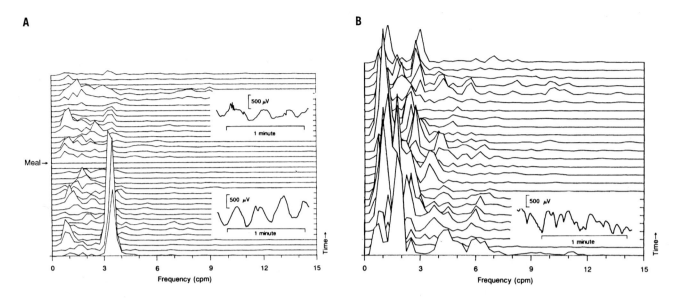

**FIGURE 13.23.** Gastric myoelectrical activity in neonates. **A** shows clear 3 cpm activity at baseline; after ingestion of a formula meal, there is decreased 3 cpm activity. **B** shows disordered gastric electrical activity with both tachygastria and bradygastria present in the EGG recording from a neonate. Reproduced with permission from Koch KL, Tran T, Bingaman S, Sperry N. Gastric myoelectrical activity in fasted and fed premature and term infants. J Gastrointest Motil 1993;5:41–7.

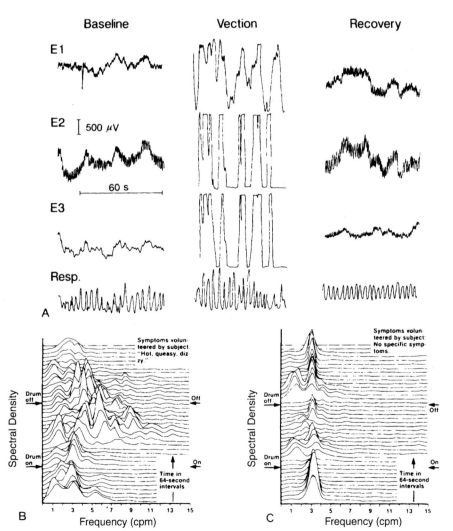

**FIGURE 13.24.** Gastric myoelectrical activity during vection-induced motion sickness. The EGG shows tachygastria during the nausea of motion sickness (**A**). The running spectral analysis shows disruption of the 3 cpm activity with abrupt and chaotic peaks in the tachygastria range during motion sickness symptoms (**B**). In contrast, the running spectral analysis (**C**) shows steady 3 cpm peaks in a subject with no motion sickness symptoms. Reprinted with permission from Koch KL. The stomach. In: Schuster MM, editor. Atlas of gastrointestinal motility in health and disease. Baltimore: Williams and Wilkins; 1993. p. 158–76.

electrical rhythm is re-established. The acute shift to gastric tachyarrhythmias during nausea is associated with activation of the sympathetic nervous system, the hypothalamic vaso-pressinergic system, and stress responses involving secretion of cortisol and β-endorphin.[60,61] In subjects with no motion sickness, the normal 3 cpm gastric electrical rhythm is maintained (see Fig. 13.24, B and C), and neither catecholamines, vasopressin, nor cortisol levels are increased.

## REFERENCES

1. Koch KL. The stomach. In: Schuster MM, editor. Atlas of gastro-intestinal motility in health and disease. Baltimore: Williams and Wilkins; 1993. p. 158–76.

2. Tuneberg L. Interstitial cells of Cajal: intestinal pacemaker cells? Adv Embryol Cell Biol 1982;71:1–130.

3. Sanders KM. A case for interstitial cells of Cajal as pacemakers and mediators of neural transmission in the gastrointestinal tract. Gastroenterology 1996;111:492–515.

4. Koch KL. Dyspepsia of unknown origin. Pathophysiology, diagnosis and treatment. Dig Dis 1997;15:316–29.

5. Koch KL. Review article: clinical approaches to unexplained nausea and vomiting. Adv Gastroenterol Hepatol Clin Nutr 1998;3:163–78.

6. Meyer JE. Motility of the stomach and gastroduodenal junction. In: Johnson LR, editor. Physiology of the gastrointestinal tract. New York: Raven Press; 1987. p. 393–410.

7. Lin HC, Hasler WL. Disorders of gastric emptying. In: Yamada T, editor. Textbook of gastroenterology. Philadelphia: JB Lippincott; 1995. p. 1318–46.

8. Smout AJPM, van der Schee EJ, Grashuis JL. What is measured in electrogastrography? Dig Dis Sci 1980;25:179–87.

9. Sarna S. In vivo myoelectrical activity: Methods, analysis, and interpretation. In: Schultz S, Wood JD, editors. Handbook of physiology: the gastrointestinal system. Baltimore: Waverly Press; 1989. p. 817–63.

10. Hinder RA, Kelly KA. Human gastric pacesetter potential: site of origin, spread and response to gastric transection and proximal gastric vagotomy. Am J Surg 1977;133:29–33.

11. You CH, Chey WY, Lee KY, et al. Gastric and small intestinal myoelectrical dysrhythmia associated with chronic intractable nausea and vomiting. Ann Intern Med 1981;95:449–53.

12. Bortolotti M, Sarti P, Barbara L, Brunelli F. Gastric myoelectrical activity in patients with chronic idiopathic gastroparesis. J Gastrointest Motil 1990;2:104–8.

13. Abell TL, Malagelada J-R. Glucagon-evoked gastric dysrhythmias in humans shown by an improved electrogastrographic technique. Gastroenterology 1985;88:1932–40.

14. Familoni BO, Bowes KL, Kingma YJ, Cote KR. Can transcutaneous recordings detect gastric electrical abnormalities? Gut 1991;32:141–6.

15. Koch KL, Stewart WR, Stern RM. Effect of barium meals on gastric electromechanical activity in man. A fluoroscopic-electrogastrographic study. Dig Dis Sci 1987;32:1217–22.

16. Hamilton JW, Bellahsene BE, Reicherlderfer M, et al. Human electrogastrograms. Comparison of surface and mucosal recordings. Dig Dis Sci 1986;31:33–9.

17. Lin Z, Chen JDZ, Schirmer BD, McCallum RW. Postprandial response of gastric slow waves: correlation of serosal recordings with the electrogastrogram. Dig Dis Sci 2000;45:645–51.

18. Stern RM, Koch KL. Electrogastrography: methodology, validation and applications. New York: Praeger; 1985.

19. Koch KL, Stern RM. Electrogastrography. In: Kumar D, Wingate D, editors. Illustrated guide to gastrointestinal motility. London: Churchill Livingstone; 1993. p. 290–307.

20. Brzana RJ, Bingaman S, Koch KL. Gastric myoelectrical activity in patients with gastric outlet obstruction and idiopathic gastroparesis. Am J Gastroenterol 1998;93:1083–9.

21. Verhagen MAMT, VanSchelven CJ, Samson M, Smout AJPM. Pitfalls in the analysis of electrogastrographic recordings. Gastroenterology 1999;117:453–60.

22. Labo G, Bortolotti M, Vezzadini P, et al. Interdigestive gastroduodenal motility and serum motilin levels in patients with idiopathic delay in gastric emptying. Gastroenterology 1986;90:20–6.

23. van der Schee EJ, Grashuis JL. Contraction-related, low-frequency components in canine électrogastrographic signals. Am J Physiol 1983;245:G470–5.

24. Geldof H, van der Schee EJ, Grashuis JL. Electrogastrographic characteristics of the interdigestive migrating complex in humans. Am J Physiol 1986;250:G165–71.

25. Koch KL, Hong S-P, Xu L. Reproducibility of gastric myoelectrical activity and the water load test in patients with dysmotility-like dyspepsia symptoms and in control subjects. J Clin Gastroenterol 2000;31:125–9.

26. Geldoff H, van der Schee EJ, van Blankenstein M, Grashuis JL. Electrogastrographic study of gastric myoelectrical activity in patients with unexplained nausea and vomiting. Gut 1986;27:799–808.

27. Chen J, Stewart WR, McCallum RW. Adaptive spectral analysis of episodic rhythmic variations in gastric myoelectrical potentials. IEEE Trans Biomed Eng 1993;40:128–35.

28. Stern RM, Hu S, Koch KL. Effects of cold stress on gastric myoelectrical activity. J Gastrointest Motil 1991;3:225–8.

29. Thompson DG, Richelson E, Malagelada J-R. Perturbation of upper gastrointestinal function in cold stress. Gut 1983;24:277–83.

30. ver Hagen MA, Luijk HT, Samson M, Smout AJMP. Effect of meal temperature on the frequency of gastric myoelectrical activity. Neurogastroenterol Motil 1998;10:175–81.

31. Stern RM, Crawford HE, Stewart WR, et al. Sham feeding. Cephalic-vagal influences on gastric myoelectrical activity. Dig Dis Sci 1989;34:521–7.

32. Katschinski M, Dahmen G, Reinshagen M, et al. Cephalic stimulation of gastrointestinal secretory and motor responses in humans. Gastroenterology 1992;103:383–91.

33. Schaap HM, Smout AJ, Akkermans LM. Myoelectric activity of the Billroth II gastric remnant. Gut 1990;31:984–8.

34. You CH, Lee KY, Chey WY, et al. Electrogastrographic study of patients with unexplained nausea, bloating and vomiting. Gastroenterology 1980;79:311–4.

35. Koch KL, Stern RM, Vasey M, et al. Gastric dysrhythmias and nausea of pregnancy. Dig Dis Sci 1990;35:961–8.

36. Koch KL, Stern RM, Stewart WR, et al. Gastric emptying and gastric myoelectrical activity in patients with symptomatic diabetic gastroparesis: effect of long-term domperidone treatment. Am J Gastroenterol 1989;84:1069–75.

37. Abell TL, Camilleri M, Hench VS, Malagelada J-R. Gastric electromechanical function and gastric emptying in diabetic gastroparesis. Eur J Gastroenterol Hepatol 1991;3:163–7.

38. Kim CH, Zinsmeister AR, Malagelada J-R. Effect of gastric dysrhythmias on postcibal motor activity of the stomach. Dig Dis Sci 1988;33:193–9.

39. Chen J, Schirmer BD, McCallum RW. Serosal and cutaneous recordings of gastric myoelectrical activity in patients with gastroparesis. Am J Physiol 1994;266:G90–8.

40. Rothstein RD, Alavi A, Reynolds J. Electrogastrography in patients with gastroparesis. Effect of long-term cisapride. Dig Dis Sci 1993;38:1518–24.

41. Koch KL, Medina M, Bingaman S, Stern RM. Gastric dysrhythmias and visceral sensations in patients with functional dyspepsia [abstract]. Gastroenterology 1992;102:A469.

42. Cucchiara S, Minella R, Riezzo G, et al. Reversal of gastric electrical dysrhythmias by cisapride in children with functional dyspepsia: report of three cases. Dig Dis Sci 1992;37:1336–40.

43. Liberski SM, Koch KL, Atnip RG, Stern RM. Ischemic gastroparesis: resolution of nausea, vomiting and gastroparesis after mesenteric artery revascularization. Gastroenterology 1990;99:252–7.

44. Balaban DH, Chen J, Lin Z, et al. Median arcuate ligament syndrome: possible cause of idiopathic gastroparesis. Am J Gastroenterol 1997;92:519–23.

45. Parkman HP, Miller MA, Trate D, et al. Electrogastrography in gastric emptying scintigraphy are complementary for assessment of dyspepsia. J Clin Gastroenterol 1997;24:214–9.

46. Lin Z, Eaker EY, Sarosiek I, McCallum RW. Gastric myoelectrical activity and gastric emptying in patients with functional dyspepsia. Am J Gastroenterol 1999;94:2384–9.

47. Bersherdas K, Leahy A, Mason I, et al. The effect of cisapride on dyspepsia symptoms and the electrogastrogram in patients with non-ulcer dyspepsia. Aliment Pharmacol Ther 1998;12:755–9.

48. Patterson DJ, Koch KL, Abell T, et al. Domperidone in diabetic gastroparesis: a placebo-controlled, double-blind, randomized study. Gastroenterology 1993;104:A564.

49. Abell TL, Malagelada J-R. Glucagon-evoked gastric dysrhythmias in humans shown by an improved electrogastrographic technique. Gastroenterology 1985;88:1932–40.

50. Koch KL, Bingaman S, Xu L, et al. Effect of ondansetron on morphine-induced nausea, gastric myoelectrical activity and plasma vasopressin levels in healthy humans. Gastroenterology 1996;110:A696.

51. Walsh JW, Hasler WL, Nugent CE. Progesterone and estrogen are potential mediators of gastric slow wave dysrhythmias in nausea of pregnancy. Am J Physiol 1996;270:G506–14.

52. Jednak MA, Shadigian EM, Kim MS, et al. Protein meals reduce nausea and gastric slow wave dysrhythmic activity in first trimester pregnancy. Am J Physiol 1999;277:G855–61.

53. Kohagen KR, Kim MS, McDonnell WM, et al. Nicotine effects on prostoglandin-dependent gastric slow wave rhythmicity in antro-motility in non-smokers and smokers. Gastroenterology 1996;110:3–11.

54. Koch KL, Tran T, Bingaman S, Sperry N. Gastric myoelectrical activity in fasted and fed premature and term infants. J Gastrointest Motil 1993;5:41–7.

55. Cucchiara S, Salvia G, Scarcella A, et al. Gestational maturation of electrical activity of the stomach. Dig Dis Sci 1999;44:2008–13.

56. Liang J, Co E, Zhang M, et al. Development of gastric slow waves in pre-term infants measured by electrogastrography. Am J Physiol 1998;274:G503–8.

57. Li B. Cyclic vomiting syndrome. Curr Treat Options Gastroenterol 2000;3:395–402.

58. Stern RM, Koch KL, Leibowitz HW, et al. Tachygastria and motion sickness. Aviat Space Environ Med 1985;56:1074–7.

59. Stern RM, Koch KL, Stewart WR, Lindblad IM. Spectral analysis of tachygastria recorded during motion sickness. Gastroenterology 1987;93:92–7.

60. Koch KL, Stern RM, Vasey MW, et al. Neuroendocrine and gastric myoelectrical responses to illusory-self motion in man. Am J Physiol 1990;258:E304–10.

61. Koch KL, Summy-Long, Bingaman S, et al. Vasopressin and oxytocin responses to illusory self-motion and nausea in man. J Clin Endocrinol Metab 1990;71:1269–75.

# CHAPTER 14

# Stable Isotope Breath Test and Gastric Emptying

*Doe-Young Kim and Michael Camilleri*

## REFERENCE METHOD AND VARIABILITY IN GASTRIC EMPTYING

Gastric scintigraphy (generally, technetium 99m [$^{99m}$Tc] and indium 111) is generally regarded as the reference method for the assessment of gastric emptying time. However, radioiso-

tope-based techniques have the inherent risk of radiation exposure for patients and personnel and require an expensive detection and data analysis system (a gamma camera). Breath tests have been developed to overcome those disadvantages. Breath tests measure the changes in the $^{13}$C-to-$^{12}$C ratio in expired air after administration of a stable isotope ($^{13}$C)-labeled test substance. The $^{13}$C-to-$^{12}$C ratio is measured by mass spectrometry or laser infrared spectroscopy, and gastric emptying is determined semiquantitatively from the kinetics of the breath $^{13}$CO$_2$ excretion. Breath tests are safely performed and noninvasive, substantially reduce the radiation burden, and appear promising for measuring gastric emptying of solids or liquids. When the stable isotope breath test was first introduced to measure gastric emptying, it required somewhat complicated mathematical analysis; subsequent studies have validated this approach, simplified the test by using fewer breath samples, developed office-based analysis methods for quantitation of breath $^{13}$CO$_2$, and simplified the mathematics to derive summaries of gastric emptying. Lately, the test has been applied to simulated diseases or actual disease states (eg, functional dyspepsia, diabetes, and dumping syndrome). In this chapter, the principles, technique (marker, analysis methods), and examples of the application of stable isotope breath tests are discussed.

In clinical practice, measurements of motility of the stomach and their interpretation are complicated by substantial day-to-day variability. The radioisotopic method is known to have a high degree of reproducibility within individuals; for example, in one study, the interindividual coefficient of variation was ~13%.[1] Reproducibility is better for solid than liquid test meals, and the test is also more reproducible in healthy subjects than in patients with gastric emptying disorders. Although the intrinsic variations discussed above cannot be reduced with the breath test, the latter has a number of advantages.

**TABLE 14.1.** Methods to Study Gastric Emptying

| | |
|---|---|
| Intubation techniques | Gastric aspiration |
| | Gastric dye dilution |
| | Duodenal dye dilution |
| Imaging techniques | Radiology |
| | Scintigraphy |
| | Ultrasonography |
| | Magnetic resonance imaging |
| Indirect techniques | Blood test |
| | Breath test |

Adapted from Vantrappen.[2]

## ADVANTAGES OF BREATH TESTS

Many techniques have been developed to study gastric emptying in humans, and they can be classified into intubation, imaging, and indirect techniques (Table 14.1).[2] Nonscintigraphic techniques have been developed to study gastric emptying, including applied potential tomography, acetaminophen (paracetamol) absorption test, or ultrasonography. These tests do not involve exposure to radiation. However, they are most effective in evaluating the gastric emptying of liquids.

The stable nonradioactive isotope breath test is an indirect method to measure gastric emptying of solids that produces results that are comparable with radioscintigraphy. Although lacking information about intragastric distribution of the different phases of the test meal, breath test measurements of gastric emptying offer several advantages over radioscintigraphy. First, in contrast to scintigraphy, which requires the patient and gamma camera to be located at the same site, the breath test does not require the sophisticated mass spectrometry equipment to be near at hand because the breath samples can be mailed to the analytic laboratory and can be stored for months without a change in isotopic enrichment of the breath samples. The other advantages of the breath test, which will be illustrated in this chapter, are as follows:

- It is noninvasive and easy to perform for the patients, even for elderly or disabled patients.
- No ionizing radiation is involved with $^{13}C$-labeled substrate as a marker of the test meal.
- Repeated gastric emptying studies are more acceptable, even in children and pregnant women.
- It has been validated, that is, it is sensitive to detecting pharmacologic effects on gastric motor activity and alterations in disease states.
- It can be applied to study patients away from gamma camera facilities, at the bedside, or in the community.

## PHYSIOLOGY OF GASTRIC EMPTYING

Gastric emptying is a complex physiologic process that is influenced by multiple factors: food particle size, consistency, osmolality, viscosity, and fiber, fat, or protein composition. Gastrointestinal hormone responses, diurnal variation, and intercurrent illness can also influence gastric emptying. Solid and liquid phases of a meal are delivered from the stomach at different rates. The proximal stomach controls the emptying of liquids, and the distal stomach, which includes the lower body and antrum, is thought to control that of solids by mixing, trituration, and propulsion. The functions of these regions are controlled and coordinated by intrinsic and extrinsic nerves and hormones.

Many studies have supported the concept of biphasic emptying for which the stomach requires a certain period of time (lag phase) to process solid foods before a subsequent equilibrium emptying phase. Once solids are reduced in size so that they are small enough to pass through the pylorus, both the liquids and solids are emptied at the same rate. Differences in lag phase can result from differences in (1) food particle size, (2) caloric content of the test meal, (3) type (eg, carbohydrate in liquid phase), (4) measurement methodology, and (5) disease states (eg, gastroparesis). The half emptying time ($t_{1/2}$) does not characterize either the lag period or reflect a measure of the actual rate of gastric emptying. However, it is a simple parameter that is useful in clinical practice.

## PRINCIPLES OF BREATH TESTS

The $^{13}C$-labeled substrate is emptied from the stomach, absorbed rapidly in the duodenum, metabolized in the liver, and excreted as breath $^{13}CO_2$. This test assumes that gastric emptying is the rate-limiting step in the ultimate delivery of $^{13}CO_2$ to the breath. The $^{13}CO_2$ enrichment of breath can be measured at regular intervals by isotope ratio mass spectrometry or laser infrared spectroscopy. This chapter discusses the substrates and techniques that have been used to measure gastric emptying of solids or liquids.

### Choice of Gastric Emptying Substrate

In most patients with gastroparesis, the gastric emptying of solids is delayed before there is an appreciable delay in the emptying of liquids. The majority of patients (55%) with delayed gastric emptying demonstrate delayed emptying of both liquids and solid food, but 45% show normal gastric emptying of liquids with delayed emptying of solid food.[3] Therefore, measuring gastric emptying of solids is more sensitive in the detection of delayed gastric emptying. On the other hand, after proximal gastric vagotomy, truncal vagotomy with pyloroplasty, or subtotal gastrectomy, the gastric emptying of liquids is often accelerated, whereas the emptying of solids is still normal or delayed. Therefore, the choice of substrate is determined by the clinical indication for the gastric emptying test, and, as with scintigraphy, the emptying of solids is most frequently evaluated in clinical practice and pharmacologic studies.

## GASTRIC EMPTYING OF SOLIDS: TECHNIQUES

### $^{13}$C-Labeled Test Substrate

An ideal substrate for a breath test to assess gastric emptying should mix thoroughly with the test meal, be stable in an acid environment, be easily absorbed on entering the duodenum, and be quickly metabolized on absorption.[4] The substrate should not be partitioned into the liquid phase. The same requirement is essential for the marker used for gastric scintigraphy.[5]

$^{13}$C-labeled substrates have been used for breath tests because $^{13}$C is stable and not radioactive. Substrates can be either synthetic products (eg, octanoic acid) or naturally occurring substances isolated from plant (eg, *Spirulina plantensis*) or animal materials. In fact, all carbon-containing products in food contain a certain amount of $^{13}$C. This natural abundance is generally in the order of 1.08% of all carbon atoms. However, the natural $^{13}$C abundance is not identical in all plant species; some plants produce carbohydrates with a higher $^{13}$C content. Naturally enriched carbohydrates include cornstarch, cane sugar, and pineapples, the so-called C4 plants. They are synthesized through the Hatch-Slack pathway[6] and have a $^{13}$C enrichment of 1.09%. This is different from other carbohydrates from most other plants—the C3 plants—that use the Calvin-Benson pathway[7] and have a $^{13}$C enrichment of 1.08%. These two pathways are photosynthetic processes by which carbon dioxide is converted to carbohydrate. C3 plants fix $CO_2$ into a three-carbon intermediate (C3) through the Calvin-Benson pathway, and C4 plants have a four-carbon intermediate in the Hatch-Slack pathway. Naturally labeled carbohydrates can be used as such in breath tests or fed to animals to produce other $^{13}$C-enriched materials (eg, $^{13}$C-labeled lactose from the milk of cows that were fed on cornstarch).[8] Other $^{13}$C-labeled test substrates can be obtained by having C3 plants (carbohydrate) or algae (carbohydrate, lipids) grow in atmospheric air artificially enriched with $^{13}CO_2$. *Spirulina* species are typical examples of such algae.

Octanoic acid and the proteinaceous algae, *Spirulina*, have been extensively used to measure the gastric emptying of solid meals, whereas acetate and glycine are used for liquid meals (Table 14.2).

### *Octanoic Acid*

Octanoic acid is an eight-carbon (medium-chain) fatty acid found in dietary fats, and $^{13}$C-octanoate is a synthetically labeled substance. Octanoic acid is readily solubilized in egg yolk[9] and is thus administered in an egg meal. It is fully retained in egg yolk during mixing and grinding in the acid environment of the stomach but is rapidly liberated in the duodenum. Being a medium-chain fatty acid, it is rapidly absorbed from the intestine (since it is not a triglyceride, lipolysis is not needed before absorption) and transported to the liver via the portal venous system. In the liver, it is rapidly and completely oxidized to $CO_2$ instead of being used in hepatic lipid synthesis.

### *Spirulina Platensis*

*Spirulina platensis* is an edible blue-green alga that is used as a health food and is comprised of 56 to 77% protein, 10 to 20% carbohydrate, and 9 to 14% lipid.[10] *Spirulina* is grown as a pure monoculture in a closed hydroponics chamber in a medium containing inorganic salts and is purged with pure $^{13}CO_2$. Resultant cells are uniformly labeled with $^{13}$C. The natural abundance level of $^{13}$C is increased from ~1 to 99%. When metabolized, the proteins, carbohydrates, and lipids of *Spirulina* give rise to respiratory $CO_2$ enriched in $^{13}$C. Because the contents of the algal cells are not freely diffusible, incorporation of labeled *S platensis* into a solid-phase meal occurs easily and represents the digestive state of the solid food matrix within which it is contained.

## Conduct of Study

The breath test should be performed after an overnight fast. Withholding food for 8 hours before and during the study reduces the baseline shifts in $^{13}$C abundance; unfortunately, fasting throughout this study can be difficult for infants or children.

### *Preparation of Test Meal*

The test meal used varies in different studies to date; however, there is a potential to develop standardized meals with a defined shelf life for future studies. In our laboratory, the test meal in the [$^{13}$C] substrate breath test consists of two egg whites and one yolk dosed with 100 mg of [$^{13}$C]octanoic

**TABLE 14.2.** $^{13}$C-Substrate in Literature for Measuring Gastric Emptying

| $^{13}$C-Substrate | Manufacturer | Meal Form | Commonly Used Dose (mg) | Test Meal |
|---|---|---|---|---|
| $^{13}$C-octanoic acid | 1) Isotec, Miamisburg, OH, 2) Aldrich Co, Milwaukee, WI 3) Eurisotop, Saint-Aubin, France 4) Promochem, Wesel, Germany | Solids Solids | 100 100 | Egg omelet (labeled in egg yolk) |
| $^{13}$C-*Spirulina platensis* | Meretek Diagnostics, Inc, Houston, TX | Solids | 200 | Egg meal, muffins, or biscuits |
| $^{13}$C-acetate | Cambridge Isotope Laboratories, Woburn, MA | Liquids | 150 | Oatmeal or any liquid meal |
| $^{13}$C-glycine | Isotec, Miamisburg, OH | Liquids | 100 | Water |

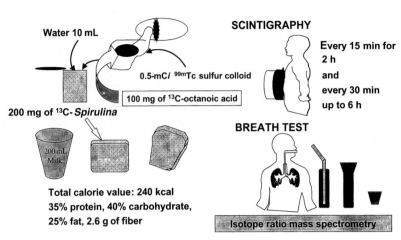

**FIGURE 14.1.** Simultaneous measurement of the retention of scintigraphic markers in the stomach and the excretion of labeled $CO_2$ in breath. The test meal consists of one egg white and one yolk dosed with 100 mg of $^{13}C$ octanoic acid or 200 mg of *Spirulina*. The egg white is mixed with 0.5-mCi technetium 99m ($^{99m}Tc$) sulfur colloid. Scintigraphic scanning with anterior and posterior cameras is performed with patients or volunteers standing. Imaging begins at the start of the test meal, and scans are obtained every 15 minutes for the first 2 hours and every 30 minutes up to 6 hours. Breath samples are taken at baseline before the meal and follow the same time schedule as the scintigraphic technique. Each breath sample is collected and stored in duplicate in glass containers using a straw to blow into the bottom of the tube. After restoppering the tubes, the $^{13}C$ breath content is determined in a centralized laboratory by isotope ratio mass spectrometry.

acid (Aldrich Co, Milwaukee, WI, or Isotec, Miamisburg, OH) or 200 mg of $^{13}C$ *S platensis* (Meretek Diagnostics, Inc, Houston, TX). The meal actually mimics that originally developed by the pioneering group at Leuven University, Belgium. In studies using simultaneous scintigraphy (Fig. 14.1), 0.5-mCi $^{99m}Tc$ sulfur colloid can be mixed with the egg whites, and the yolk and egg whites are cooked separately. The egg meal is placed on a slice of whole-wheat bread and given with a glass of skim milk for a total calorie value of 240 kcal and nutrient composition of 35% protein, 40% carbohydrate, 25% fat, and 2.6 g of fiber. In the future, $^{13}C$-labeled muffins (containing either $^{13}C$-octanoic acid or $^{13}C$-*Spirulina*) will be used, obviating the need to actually cook the meal before the test. The subject is encouraged to consume the entire test meal in less than 10 minutes for solid meals and 3 minutes for liquid meals.

### Breath Sampling

A breath test always starts with an air sample being taken for baseline $^{13}C$ enrichment in breath $CO_2$. During the test period, one or more breath samples are obtained at specific times to determine the change in breath $CO_2$ $^{13}C$ enrichment. Until recently, each breath sample was collected in a 3-L aluminum-coated plastic bag (Tecobag, Tesseraux Container, Bürstadt, Germany), and then a 25-mL aliquot of the breath sample was stored for subsequent $^{13}CO_2$ measurements. Nowadays, breath samples can be collected and stored in duplicate in glass containers (Vacutainer Tube; Becton Dickinson, Heidelberg, Germany) using a straw or a pipette to blow into the bottom of the tube, thereby "enriching" the air for subsequent sample analysis. As indicated below, breath sampling may be reduced to 2 or 3 hours with the test having the same accuracy as observed with scintigraphy. Breath sampling can be performed while the patient is reading or ambulatory. However, severe exercise should not be recommended throughout the breath test study because the exercise can influence the rate of absorption and the time needed for oxidation of $^{13}C$-substrate.

### Measurement of Labeled $CO_2$ in Exhaled Breath

$^{13}C$ can be detected by a number of techniques such as mass spectrometry, nuclear magnetic resonance spectroscopy, (NMRS), infrared spectroscopy, and laser resonance spectroscopy. For $^{13}CO_2$ analysis, isotope ratio mass spectrometry (IRMS) is the traditional technique; infrared and laser resonance spectroscopy are being developed as alternative techniques. With mass spectrometry, special equipment is required to measure $^{13}CO_2$ enrichment because a high level of accuracy is needed for the low level of enrichment (0.001–0.01%) generally obtained in breath tests. Isotope ratio mass spectrometry was originally developed for geologic applications in measuring the variation in natural $^{13}C$. The level of $^{13}C$ abundance in nature is not constant but is dependent on the origin of the carbon source; thus, it varies from around 1.06% for fossil fuels to 1.12% for carbonate stones. Similarly, the natural background of $^{13}C$ in breath $CO_2$ is 1.08 to 1.09% depending on the composition of C3 and C4 plant material ingested in the diet. The enrichment in $^{13}C$ during a breath test depends on the dose, $^{13}C$ enrichment of the substrate, and the degree of metabolic $^{13}CO_2$ production. Generally, the dose given results in a maximum absolute increase in $^{13}C$ abundance of breath $CO_2$ of about 0.005 to 0.05%.

Because the natural variations in the $^{13}C$ abundance are quite small, $^{13}C$ abundance is always measured against a defined standard. Thus, all values are either positive or negative differences from the standard according to the formula:

$$\delta^{13}C = \frac{^{13}C/^{12}C_u - ^{13}C_s/^{12}C_s}{^{13}C/^{12}C_s} \times 1,000‰$$

where u = unknown and s = standard.

$^{13}C$ abundance ($\delta^{13}C_{PDB}$) is expressed as per mil (‰) relative difference from the universal reference standard, usually the carbon from Pee Dee Belemnite (PDB) limestone (‰). $^{13}C$ enrichment is defined as the difference between the basal $^{13}C$ abundance before administration of substrate and

**TABLE 14.3.** Isotope Ratio Mass Spectrometry Instruments

| Manufacturer | Location | Instrument |
|---|---|---|
| Europa Scientific | Crewe, UK | ABCA |
| | | 20/20 |
| | | Tracermass |
| | | GEO |
| | | Orchid |
| Finnigan MAT | Bremen, Germany | MAT 250 |
| | | Delta S (/GC) |
| | | BreathMAT |
| VG Fisons (Micromass) | Manchester, UK | SIRA II |
| | | SIRA 10 |
| | | Optima |

Adapted from Stellaard and Geypens.[11]

the $^{13}$C abundance at a certain time point after administration and is expressed as $\Delta\delta^{13}C_{PDB}$ (‰). Biologic variation of baseline $\delta^{13}C_{PDB}$ values shows a variation (1 SD) in respiratory $CO_2$ of $\pm 0.5\%$.[11]

**INSTRUMENTS.** As mentioned, IRMS, infrared, or laser resonance techniques can be used to measure $^{13}CO_2$ enrichment in breath. Two types of IRMS equipment can be distinguished: one with a dual-inlet system in which each sample $CO_2$ and reference $CO_2$ is introduced directly and measured in sequence up to 10 times in a row. A second type is a continuous-flow system in which sample $CO_2$ and reference $CO_2$ are measured singly in one or in separate runs. This requires that $CO_2$ should be isolated or purified from breath by cryogenic trapping (on-line or off-line) or by gas chromatography. Instrument information (suppliers and commercial names of IRMS equipment) is listed in Table 14.3.

For sensitive and accurate measurement of the $^{13}CO_2$-to-$^{12}CO_2$ ratio in breath samples, IRMS is commonly used as the established standard method. However, studies indicate that infrared heterodyne radiometry and particularly infrared spectroscopy may prove to be valid, simpler, and easy-to-operate methods for analysis of breath samples under routine laboratory conditions. A newly designed nondispersive infrared spectrometer (NDIRS) (Wagner Analysentechnik, Worpswede, Germany, or IRIS, Iznita, Budapest, Hungary) for $^{13}CO_2$ measurements in breath samples has also become commercially available. So far, the principle of NDIRS has been used in a few limited studies for the detection of *Helicobacter pylori* infections by $^{13}$C urea breath tests. Schadewaldt and colleagues applied the NDIRS method to the $^{13}$C-octanoic acid breath test and compared results with the accurate standard IRMS.[12] Even though replicate results of NDIRS $^{13}CO_2$ measurement were somewhat less accurate than with the excellent IRMS analysis, they found a reasonable correlation between the two methods, suggesting that NDIRS may be applied in clinical laboratories.

**QUALITY OF REFERENCE COMPOUNDS AND CALCULATION OF $^{13}$C-RECOVERY.** Isotope ratios are measured by IRMS against a working standard that is calibrated against a certified PDB limestone

source. A conventional dual-inlet IRMS can determine differences in abundances with a precision of 0.1‰ or one part $^{13}$C in $10^6$ parts $CO_2$. At each point in time during the test, the breath $^{13}$C enrichment over baseline (DAB or DOB: delta above or over baseline) is determined. This result is then multiplied by the estimated $CO_2$ production rate per sampling period to determine $^{13}$C production. Usually, percentage dose recovered (PDR) is calculated from the following formula:

$$^{13}C \, (\% \text{ administered dose/hr})$$
$$= \frac{DOB}{^{13}C \text{ administered dose (mM)}} \times CO_2 \text{ production (mM/hr)} \times 100$$

where DOB is the percentage of $^{13}CO_2$ in total $CO_2$ in breath sample above natural background:

$$DOB = (\delta^{13}C_{PDB\,t=i} - \delta^{13}C_{PDB\,t=0}) \times R_{PDB} \times 10^{-3}$$

where $t$ = time, $R_{PDB}$ = 0.11273.

Total $CO_2$ production is assumed to be 300 mM/m² of body surface area (BSA)/hour (or 5 mM/m² BSA/min). Body surface area (m²) is calculated according to the classic weight-height formula of Haycock and colleagues (ie, BSA = weight [kg]$^{0.5378}$ × height [cm]$^{0.3964}$ × 0.024265).[13] Total $CO_2$ production can be further corrected for age and gender, as determined by Schofield.[14] The unit of $^{13}$C administered dose is changed to millimolar concentration using the following formula:

$$^{13}C \text{ administered dose (mM)} = \frac{\text{mg of substrate}}{\text{molar weight of } ^{13}C \text{ substrate}} \times P \times n/100$$

where P (%) is the purity of the substrate and n is the number of labeled carbon positions in the substrate. Subsequently, the cumulative PDR is computed, and this is frequently used as a final result of the breath test. $^{13}CO_2$ production over time is plotted graphically to construct a profile that is the reciprocal of the actual emptying process.

## Mathematical Analyses to Derive Gastric Emptying Parameters

Different mathematical analyses have been reported in the literature; we will describe them in chronologic order of development. The scope of this chapter precludes an exhaustive compilation of every detailed generation of the mathematical formula. However, before mentioning analysis methods, the following three parameters of gastric emptying need to be clarified:

### Half-Emptying Time

This is the time taken for half of the gastric contents passed to be emptied. In a study of 41 healthy volunteers evaluated by gastric scintigraphy, the normal range (10th to 90th percentile) for t½ in our laboratory was from 70 to 150 minutes.

## Lag Phase

This is a marker for the ability of the stomach to triturate solid food to a particle size that can be emptied through the pylorus. However, even for scintigraphy, there is no universally accepted method to calculate and express this variable. For convenience, it is defined as the time for 10% of the gastric solid contents to be emptied. The length of a lag phase depends on the meal volume, caloric density, food particle size, detection technique, and the presence of gastroparesis.[5] With liquid test meals, a lag phase is rarely observed unless the caloric density is high (eg, 25% of dextrose).

## Gastric Emptying Coefficient

This is an index of the global gastric emptying rate, which is derived from a formula described below.

Some studies (eg, $^{13}C$ - acetate or glycine breath test for liquid emptying) suggested time to peak $^{13}CO_2$ enrichment as a parameter. This parameter reflects the time of maximal gastric emptying rate.

## Nonlinear Regression Analysis

Two mathematical formulas were elaborated for the octanoic acid breath test by Ghoos et al.[15] The first formula fits well with the measured $^{13}CO_2$ recovery in breath, expressed as a percentage of excretion per hour of the given $^{13}C$ dose; the second formula is derived from the percentage of the cumulative $^{13}C$ dose curve excreted in breath. The first formula is expressed as:

$$y = at^b e^{-ct}$$

where y is the percentage of $^{13}C$ excretion in breath per hour, t is the time in hours, and a, b, and c are regression estimated constants.

The second formula is given by:

$$y = m(1 - e^{-kt})^\beta$$

where y is the percentage of cumulative $^{13}C$ excretion in breath, t is the time in hours, and m, k, and $\beta$ are regression estimated constants. In particular, m represents the total cumulative $^{13}C$ recovery when time is infinite and serves as a surrogate for the maximum gastric content at time = 0, that is, immediately after food ingestion.

This equation is derived from the empirical fact that the breath test curve representing the cumulative dose over time is inversely related but analogous to the scintigraphic curve of gastric emptying. Nonlinear regression analysis using commercial software programs such as the SAS NLIN program (SAS, Raleigh, NC) or Excel 4.0 macro program (Microsoft Corp., Redmond, WA) allows calculation of three main parameters of gastric emptying as measured by $^{13}C$ octanoic acid breath tests. These parameters are:

(1) $t_{1/2} = [(-1/k) \times \ln[1 - 2^{-(1/\beta)}]$ in minutes,

(2) $t_{lag} = (\ln\beta)/k$ in minutes, and

(3) gastric emptying coefficient (GEC) = ln(a), an index of the gastric emptying rate.

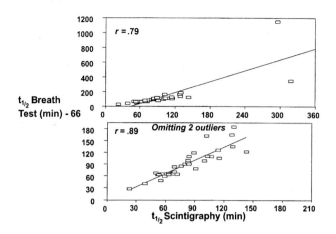

**FIGURE 14.2.** Correlation between half-emptying time ($t_{1/2b}$) determined by the breath test using a nonlinear regression analysis and $t_{1/2S}$ by scintigraphy. Note a correlation ($r = .79$) before (*upper figure*) and after ($r = .89$) two outliers were eliminated (*lower figure*). Note also that $t_{1/2}$ by breath test includes the subtraction of 66 (correction for intercept). Reproduced with permission from Ghoos YF, Maes BD, Geypens BJ, et al. Measurement of gastric emptying rate of solids by means of a carbon-labeled octanoic acid breath test. Gastroenterology 1993;104:1640–7.

The results presented using the original nonlinear method showed an excellent correlation between $t_{1/2}$ determined by the breath test and the scintigraphic $t_{1/2}$ time ($r = .89$) (Fig. 14.2).[15] This traditional analytic method is still being used in many institutions. However, this analysis showed that estimates of $t_{1/2}$ or $t_{lag}$ were markedly different between the breath test and simultaneous scintigraphy.[1,16,17]

**PITFALLS OF THE NONLINEAR MATHEMATICAL ANALYSIS.** In spite of the merits of the breath test, several pitfalls were identified. First, it is assumed that the $^{13}C$ breath test result depends on gastric emptying as the rate-limiting factor; however, postgastric processing such as absorption, metabolism, and excretion of $^{13}CO_2$ may vary in disease states affecting bowel mucosa, liver, or lungs (Fig. 14.3). Second, it is noteworthy that the breath test overestimated the $t_{1/2}$ measured by simultaneous scintigraphy by 66 minutes in Ghoos and colleagues'

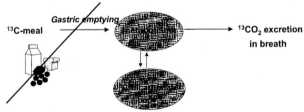

**FIGURE 14.3.** Pitfalls of breath tests for gastric emptying. $^{13}C$ can exit the bicarbonate pool and is subsequently released into the circulation at a rate that is unrelated to gastric emptying.

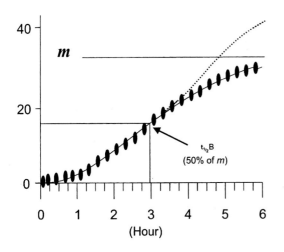

**FIGURE 14.4.** Pitfalls of $^{13}C$ breath test. One of the pitfalls of the breath test is the potential lack of steady-state excretion. Even after 6 hours, the cumulative $^{13}CO_2$ breath excretion was continuously increasing, thereby making estimation of *m* inaccurate.

method.[15] This correction factor was based on the intercept term on the linear regression of breath test versus scintigraphy. However, Choi and colleagues subsequently showed that the differences in t½ values obtained by the two methods varied widely from –33.1 to 169.6 (mean 48 minutes).

The reason for this difference is not known, but it is unlikely to be related to individual differences in absorption, metabolism, or excretion of octanoic acid since intraduodenal $^{14}C$-octanoic acid results in very rapid $^{14}CO_2$ appearance in breath.[18] Third, it has been demonstrated that the cumulative appearance of $^{13}CO_2$ in breath does not reach 100% or a steady state even after 6 hours from the time of $^{13}C$ meal ingestion (Fig. 14.4). This might be related to the "loss" or fixation of the administered isotope in the bicarbonate pool with subsequent release and appearance in breath. Thus, $^{13}CO_2$ continued to be excreted in breath long after gastric emptying was shown to be completed by simultaneous scintigraphy. These considerations led to refinements in the mathematical analyses used to calculate gastric emptying summaries.

### Deconvolution Analysis

Maes and colleagues developed a "separation" model to obtain a real-time gastric emptying curve.[18] By this model, the postgastric processing of octanoic acid could be mathematically separated from the $CO_2$ excretion curve after ingestion of a standard solid test meal. This approach to the analysis of breath test curve has two potential benefits. First, physiologically meaningful gastric emptying parameters can be calculated from breath test curves without correcting for postgastric processing of the label, which was based on the linear regression between radioscintigraphy and breath tests. Second, it allows for the evaluation of gastric emptying rates instead of measuring amounts of the emptied food as a function of time (flow curves).

**RATIONALE FOR THE SEPARATION MODEL.** To develop this mathematical model, three functions are introduced to describe three different processes:

1. The emptying rate of a labeled solid meal from mouth to pylorus is given by $M(t)$.

2. The rate of postgastric processing (absorption, metabolism, and excretion in breath) of the label is given by $D(t)$.
3. The global process of $CO_2$ excretion after ingestion of a labeled solid test meal is given by $T(t)$.

**$T(t) = M(t) + D(t)$.** The aim is to determine $M(t)$ given $T(t)$ and $D(t)$, both of which can be measured, and to describe the relation between the three functions. To achieve this aim, the following assumptions are required:

1. The meal is ingested at once, at time 0. For practical purposes, the time of ingestion is restricted to 10 minutes, and time 0 is taken as the time of completion of the ingestion of the meal. This is a reasonable assumption with solid meals, for which the lag time is almost invariably > 10 minutes.
2. $T(t)$, $D(t)$, and $M(t)$ are continuous functions not identical to zero and positive for each time $\geq 0$.
3. The rate of metabolism of the label [$D(t)$] is proportional to the rate of gastric emptying of the label $M(t)$. This implies that the kinetics of metabolism of the label are independent of the rate at which the label is emptied.

The formula for calculating t½ is discussed in detail in Maes and colleagues[18] and given by their references:

$$T_n = \sum_{i=1}^{n-1} D_{n-i} M_i \qquad (1)$$

$$T(t) = \int_0^t D(t - t_0) M(t_0) d_0 \qquad (2)$$

$$M_i = \frac{T_{i+1} - \sum_{j=1}^{i-1} D_{i+1-j} M_j}{D_1} \qquad (3)$$

If $T(t)$ and $D(t)$ are known, $M(t)$ can be separated from the total process $T(t)$ by decreasing the length of the time intervals.

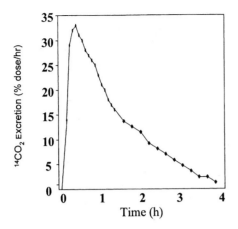

**FIGURE 14.5.** Dynamics of $^{14}CO_2$ appearance in breath after intraduodenal administration of 74 kBq of [$^{14}C$]octanoic acid in the second part of the duodenum in 20 healthy volunteers (mean ± SE). Reproduced with permission from Maes BD, Mys G, Geypens BJ, et al. Gastric emptying flow curves separated from carbon-labeled octanoic acid breath test results. Am J Physiol 1998;275:169–75.

To obtain the function of D($t$), Maes and colleagues positioned a flexible tube in the second part of the duodenum in 20 healthy volunteers. The dynamics of $^{14}CO_2$ appearance in breath were measured after intraduodenal administration of 74 kBq (2 µCi) of [$^{14}C$]octanoic acid. Figure 14.5 shows $^{14}CO_2$ excretion as a function of time in 20 healthy volunteers. $^{14}CO_2$ appeared in the breath almost immediately, with a peak excretion of 33.73% dose/h after 10.69 minutes, followed by an exponential decrease of $^{14}CO_2$ activity in the breath. The

half-excretion time of the curves was 67.5 minutes. The function T($t$) can be described as in the original Ghoos and colleagues' method.[15] Using these equations for T($t$) and D($t$), in Equation 3, the curve M($t$) is separated (Fig. 14.6). From the curve M($t$), gastric t½ and lag phase are obtained. Maes and colleagues reported an outstanding correlation between the gastric t½ ($r$ = .98) and lag phase ($r$ = .85) determined by scintigraphy and the breath test (Fig. 14.7).

### Linear Models

**GENERALIZED LINEAR REGRESSION MODEL.** To simplify the procedure for the $^{13}C$-octanoate breath tests, our group set out to identify the minimum number of breath samples, the optimal timing of samples, and the optimal total period of collection to predict accurately the information provided by simultaneous scintigraphic gastric emptying.[16] Reducing the number of breath samples analyzed will reduce costs for $^{13}CO_2$ measurement and increase the future application of the test in research and clinical practice.

Initially, a multiple linear regression analysis was used to identify, in 30 healthy subjects, the minimum set of breath samples that most accurately predicted the parameter estimates of the Ghoos and colleagues' nonlinear model using 24 breath samples obtained over 6 hours.[15] The following breath samples most accurately predicted ($r^2 > .95$) the 6-hour $^{13}CO_2$ cumulative curve's parameters ($\beta$, $\kappa$, and $m$): 35, 50, 95, 110, 140, 155, 215, 245, 260, 290, and 335 minutes. Breath samples at 50 minutes and beyond 4 hours (at 260, 290, and 335 minutes) after dosing had the highest weighting factors for predicting variable $m$. Although this approach gave more accurate estimates of scintigraphic t½, it was still cumbersome

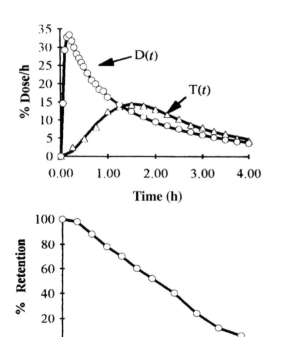

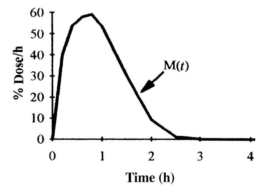

**FIGURE 14.6.** $^{14}CO_2$ excretion [T($t$)], postgastric processing [D($t$)], and gastric emptying [M($t$)] after ingestion of a [$^{14}C$]octanoic acid-labeled standard test meal in a subject with normal gastric emptying ($t_{½S}$ = 59 min) (% dose per hour as a function of time). Scintigraphic data are shown at *bottom* (% retention as a function of time). Reproduced with permission from Maes BD, Mys G, Geypens BJ, et al. Gastric emptying flow curves separated from carbon-labeled octanoic acid breath test results. Am J Physiol 1998;275:169–75.

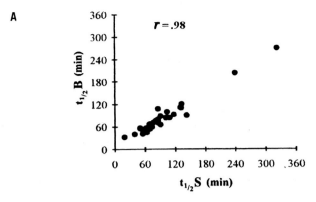 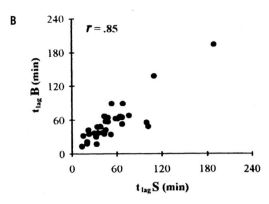

**FIGURE 14.7.** Scintigraphically determined gastric half-emptying time ($t_{\frac{1}{2}S}$) (**A**) and lag phase ($t_{lagS}$) (**B**) versus gastric half-emptying time and lag phase determined via breath test ($t_{\frac{1}{2}B}$ and $t_{lagB}$), using the separation model. Reproduced with permission from Maes BD, Mys G, Geypens BJ, et al. Gastric emptying flow curves separated from carbon-labeled octanoic acid breath test results. Am J Physiol 1998;275:169–75:

and required an impractical and prolonged long breath collection period. Hence, an improved model was developed, which, rather than predicting the 6-hour breath test results obtained by the Ghoos and colleagues' method, attempted to model the scintigraphic data.

**REDUCED "MAYO MODEL" AND INTERNAL CROSS-VALIDATION.** A preliminary analysis of the (reciprocally) transformed $t_{lag}$ and $t_{\frac{1}{2}}$ values using a simple stepwise multiple regression model provided candidate subsets of breath sample times to develop a reduced model using fewer time points (samples) in the generalized linear regression model. Since it is possible that evaluation of models to estimate $t_{lag}$ and $t_{\frac{1}{2}}$ may give an overly optimistic assessment when based on the same data, an internal cross-validation analysis was used to assess the results of the reduced models.[19] Thus, a "leave-one-out" approach was used to obtain the breath sample prediction of $t_{\frac{1}{2}}$ or $t_{lag}$ for each subject. In this analysis, each individual subject is left out of the calculations to estimate the regression parameters of the linear predictor for the regression model; then the predicted value for the subject omitted from the model (or left out) is computed using the regression model results based on the remaining subjects included in (or left in) the model. This is done repeatedly, with each subject, in turn, being left out and used as a (quasi) external validation observation.

Generalized linear regression models identified three time points as being significant predictors of $t_{lag}$ (75, 180 minutes) and $t_{\frac{1}{2}}$ (90, 180 minutes). Summaries of the mathematical models using data from three breath test samples (75, 90, 180 min) and of $t_{\frac{1}{2}}$ are:

$$T_{lag} = 1/LP_{lag}, \text{ where } LP_{lag} = 0.0250 + 0.0063 \times {}^{13}C_{75} - 0.0032 \times {}^{13}C_{180}$$

$$T_{\frac{1}{2}} = 1/LP_{\frac{1}{2}}, \text{ where } LP_{\frac{1}{2}} = 0.0097 + 0.0021 \times {}^{13}C_{90} - 0.0012 \times {}^{13}C_{180}$$

In these formulas, $t_{lag}$ and $t_{\frac{1}{2}}$ are really predicted values of

$t_{lag}$ and $t_{\frac{1}{2}}$ using breath test value concentrations in μM/min at the specific times of 75, 90, and 180 minutes; $LP_{lag}$ and $LP_{\frac{1}{2}}$ are the linear predictors (ie, weighted sums of breath test concentrations); and ${}^{13}Ci$ is the excreted quantity of ${}^{13}C$ (μM/min) for time $t_i = 75, 90,$ or 180 minutes.

The reduced model predicted $t_{lag}$ and $t_{\frac{1}{2}}$ values that were similar to scintigraphy and the standard deviation of differences in $t_{lag}$ and $t_{\frac{1}{2}}$ between the scintigraphy value, and the predicted value computed using the reduced model was only 10 minutes for both parameters (Figs. 14.8 and 14.9). Cross-validated predicted values also showed little change in the correlation coefficients.

### Stable Isotope Breath Test with a Standardized Off-the-Shelf Meal

Another study using a prepackaged, standard meal including a ${}^{13}C$ *Spirulina platensis* biscuit (Meretek Diagnostics, Inc) was performed in 27 healthy subjects.[19] After an overnight fast, participants ingested the standardized meal consisting of a 60-g rye roll (160 calories) and 120 mL of white grape juice (80 calories). The rye roll contained 200 mg of ${}^{13}C$ *S platensis*. Breath samples were collected at baseline (before meal) and at 75, 90, and 180 minutes, and gastric $t_{\frac{1}{2}}$ and $t_{lag}$ were estimated using the same mathematical formula as discussed for the reduced Mayo model. Data were compared with results from ${}^{13}C$ *S platensis* in our standard egg meal performed in the same individuals 5 to 9 months previously.

Figure 14.10 illustrates the distributions of $t_{lag}$ and $t_{\frac{1}{2}}$ estimates using the generalized linear regression model based on three breath ${}^{13}CO_2$ excretion data points for the ${}^{13}C$ *S platensis* egg meal and ${}^{13}C$ *S platensis* biscuit meal. Note the good agreement between results from the two meals (see Fig. 14.10); there were small differences in $t_{\frac{1}{2}}$ estimates within individuals (median 3 minutes, range –18 to 49) for the two meals, and these differences are consistent with the day-to-day variation in normal gastric emptying (median 12–15%) previously reported. These data suggest that the use of a standardized prepackaged meal may obviate the need to prepare the egg meal for these studies.

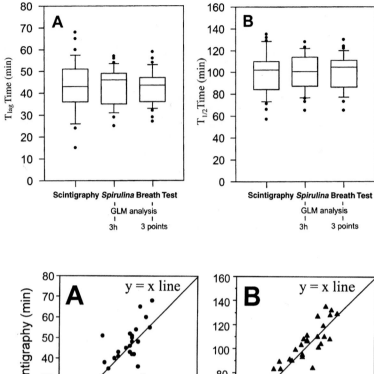

**FIGURE 14.8.** Comparison of gastric lag phase duration ($t_{lag}$) (**A**) and half-emptying times ($t_{\frac{1}{2}}$) (**B**) from scintigraphy and $^{13}C$ *S platensis* breath tests using the generalized linear regression models (GLM) in 30 healthy volunteers, shown as median values (*bars*), interquartile ranges (*boxes*), ranging from the 10th to the 90th percentile (*bar caps*), and actual data over the 10th to 90th percentiles (*dots*) for scintigraphy and breath tests. Note the excellent agreement between scintigraphy and GLMs. Reproduced with permission from Lee JS, Camilleri M, Zinsmeister AR, et al. A valid, accurate, office-based, nonradioactive test for gastric emptying of solids. Gut 2000;46:768–73.

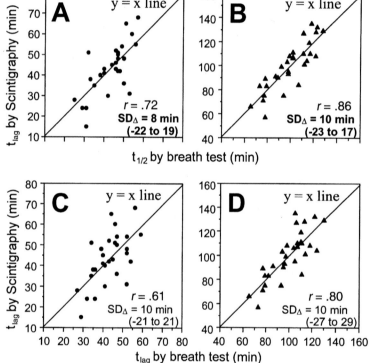

**FIGURE 14.9.** Comparison of lag phases ($t_{lag}$) and half-emptying times ($t_{\frac{1}{2}}$) between scintigraphy values and estimates from a generalized linear regression model based on breath test values. The *two upper figures* (**A** and **B**) are from the first 3 hours of data, and the *two lower figures* (**C** and **D**) are three sample data (baseline and 75 and 180 minutes for $t_{lag}$, baseline and 90 and 180 minutes for $t_{\frac{1}{2}}$). The y = x line is shown for comparison. The variation in differences between estimates by the two methods was expressed as $SD_{\bar{A}}$ and range. Note that standard deviations of differences in $t_{\frac{1}{2}}$ and $t_{lag}$ between scintigraphy and the "reduced model" were both only 10 minutes (**C** and **D**). Reproduced with permission from Lee JS, Camilleri M, Zinsmeister AR, et al. A valid, accurate, office-based, nonradioactive test for gastric emptying of solids. Gut 2000;46:768–73.

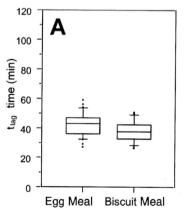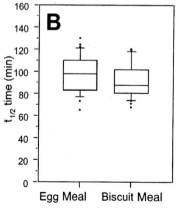

**FIGURE 14.10.** Distribution of $t_{lag}$ (**A**) and $t_{\frac{1}{2}}$ (**B**) using [$^{13}C$]*S platensis* breath test in an egg meal and in a biscuit meal in 27 healthy subjects, shown as median values (*bars*), interquartile ranges (*boxes*), ranging from the 10th to the 90th percentile (*bar caps*), and observed data over the 10th to the 90th percentiles (*dots*). Note the good agreement between the results from the two meals. Reproduced with permission from Lee JS, Camilleri M, Zinsmeister AR, et al. A valid, accurate, office-based, nonradioactive test for gastric emptying of solids. Gut 2000;46:768–73.

## Gastric Emptying in Symptomatic Diabetes Using the $^{13}$C Octanoic Acid Breath Test

A similar approach was used to optimize the $^{13}$C octanoic acid breath test.[17] We simultaneously measured gastric emptying of an egg meal (420 kcal) by scintigraphy and the $^{13}$C octanoic acid breath test in 22 symptomatic diabetic patients and 5 healthy controls. Review of simultaneous curves of gastric emptying by scintigraphy and the breath test showed that the cumulative excretion of $^{13}$CO$_2$ persisted even after 90% or more of the radiolabel had emptied from the stomach (Fig. 14.11). It is worth noting that the power exponential analysis fitted scintigraphic data points accurately. Despite 8 hours of breath sampling, the $t_{1/2}$ estimate using the conventional nonlinear method was markedly different from the scintigraphic value ($\Delta t_{1/2}$: median 113 minutes; range 19–282 minutes) (Fig. 14.12). The reduced models (Mayo model) for $t_{lag}$ and $t_{1/2}$ based on data from three samples (at baseline and 30 and 120 minutes for $t_{lag}$ or baseline and 30 and 150 minutes for $t_{1/2}$) and for $t_{1/2}$ were:

$$T_{lag} = 1/LP_{lag}$$

where $LP_{lag} = 0.001546 + 0.017694 \times {}^{13}C_{30} + 0.013779 \times {}^{13}C_{120}$

$$t_{1/2} = 1/LP_{1/2}$$

where $LP_{1/2} = 0.000853 + 0.006782 \times {}^{13}C_{30} + 0.004668 \times {}^{13}C_{150}$

In these formulas, $t_{lag}$ and $t_{1/2}$ are predicted $t_{lag}$ and $t_{1/2}$ using breath test concentrations in micromoles per minute at the specific time points ($^{13}C_{30}$, $^{13}C_{120}$, and $^{13}C_{150}$), $LP_{lag}$ and $LP_{1/2}$ are the linear predictors (ie, weighted sums of breath test concentrations), and is excreted quantity of $^{13}$C (μmol/min) for time $t_i$ = 30, 120, or 150 minutes.

## Application of Pharmacologic Perturbations in Gastric Emptying to Model Optimal Analyses of the Stable Isotope Breath Test.

We wished to validate a similar approach to measure the full range of gastric emptying that might be encountered clinically.[20] We assessed the accuracy of $^{13}$C *S platensis* breath test results relative to scintigraphy. Erythromycin (2.0 or 3.0 mg/kg) or atropine (0.01 or 0.02 mg/kg) was infused intravenously in healthy volunteers to accelerate or delay gastric emptying, respectively.

We applied the generalized linear regression models and cross-validated with the leave-one-out approach, as described above. The generalized linear regression models identified four breath samples or time points (45, 90, 105, 120 minutes) as being significant for accurately predicting $t_{1/2}$ measured by simultaneous scintigraphy. A summary of the mathematical model using data from these breath samples is:

$$t_{1/2} = 1/LP_{1/2}$$

where $LP_{1/2} = 0.0025 - 0.0039 \times {}^{13}C_{45} + 0.0088 \times {}^{13}C_{90} - 0.0063 \times {}^{13}C_{105} + 0.0024 \times {}^{13}C_{120}$

The breath test's sensitivity and specificity were both > 80% for the identification of accelerated or delayed emptying. Breath test and scintigraphic $t_{1/2}$ results were significantly correlated ($r = .88$, $p < .0001$). We concluded that the $^{13}$C *S platensis* breath test with breath samples at baseline and 45, 90, 105, and 120 minutes measures gastric emptying $t_{1/2}$ for solids with results that are comparable to scintigraphy under pharmacologic conditions that simulated dumping to severe gastroparesis.

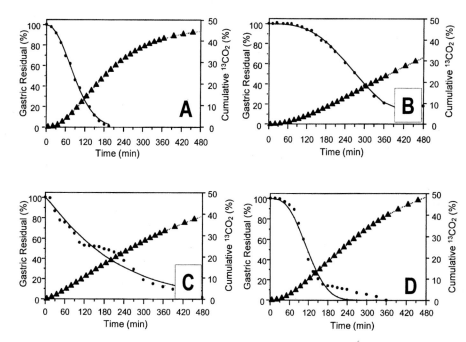

**FIGURE 14.11.** Curves of gastric emptying by simultaneous scintigraphy and the breath test in individual participants: a healthy volunteer (**A**), a diabetic patient with continuous but slow gastric emptying (**B**), a diabetic patient with intermittent but slow gastric emptying (**C**), and a diabetic patient with fast gastric emptying (**D**). The power exponential analysis closely fits the scintigraphic data points. Note that the cumulative excretion of $^{13}$CO$_2$ persisted even after 90% or more of the radiolabel had emptied from the stomach. This is even more apparent with curves that show intermittent emptying (**C**) or fast emptying (**D**). Reproduced with permission from Lee JS, Camilleri M, Zinsmeister AR, et al. Toward office-based measurement of gastric emptying in symptomatic diabetics using [$^{13}$C]octanoic acid breath test. Am J Gastroenterol 2000;95:2751–61.

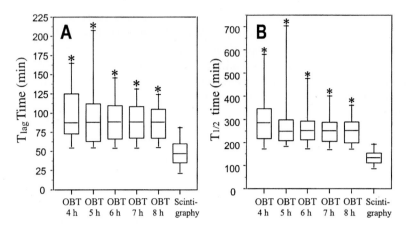

**FIGURE 14.12.** Gastric lag phase ($t_{lag}$) (**A**) and half-emptying times ($t_{1/2}$) (**B**) estimated by scintigraphy and $^{13}C$ octanoic acid breath test (OBT) in diabetic patients. Bar, median; box, interquartile range; bar cap, 5th to 95th percentile; *$p < .001$ compared to scintigraphy. Note that $t_{lag}$ and $t_{1/2}$ estimates are longer by the breath test using the uncorrected nonlinear model than with scintigraphy. Increasing the sampling time up to 8 hours reduces the variance but does not enhance the test's accuracy. Reproduced with permission from Lee JS, Camilleri M, Zinsmeister AR, et al. Toward office-based measurement of gastric emptying in symptomatic diabetics using [$^{13}C$]octanoic acid breath test. Am J Gastroenterol 2000;95:2751–61.

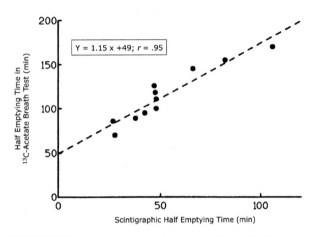

**FIGURE 14.13.** Correlation between the gastric half-emptying times in the $^{13}C$ acetate breath test and scintigraphy using a liquid test meal (225 kcal; n = 11). Note, however, that, despite the excellent correlation, the values by the breath test are "distant" from the line of identity and the intercept $t_{1/2}$ is 49 minutes. Reproduced with permission from Braden B, Adams S, Duan LP, et al. The $^{13}C$ acetate breath test accurately reflects gastric emptying of liquids in both liquid and semisolid test meals. Gastroenterology 1995;108:1048–55.

## GASTRIC EMPTYING OF LIQUIDS

### [$^{13}C$]Acetate Breath Test

Acetate can be used as a tracer molecule of the liquid phase in semisolid or liquid test meals. Acetate is a two-carbon volatile hydrophilic fatty acid that is not hydrolized in the stomach, is poorly absorbed in the stomach,[4] is readily absorbed in the small intestine, and is rapidly metabolized in humans. The time of maximum $^{13}CO_2$ excretion was the most convenient parameter of the $^{13}C$ acetate breath test used to characterize gastric emptying.[21]

#### *Preparation of Test Meal*
The test meal (oatmeal) is labeled with 150-mg sodium $^{13}C$ acetate (Cambridge Isotope Laboratories, Woburn, MA). For children, the acetate dose can be adjusted in accordance with $CO_2$ production linked to BSA: for example, 25 mg in neonates, 50 mg in infants, 100 mg in children, and 150 mg

in adolescents.[22] Subjects are requested to consume their test meal within 3 minutes.

#### *Technique*
Breath samples are collected before the meal, at 5-minute intervals during the first 2 hours and at 10-minute intervals thereafter during the next 4 hours for a total of 6 hours after ingestion of the $^{13}C$-labeled test meal. Breath samples are analyzed for isotopic enrichment by an isotope ratio mass spectrometer with an on-line gas chromatographic purification system.

Braden and colleagues reported that the $t_{1/2}$ for the $^{13}C$ acetate breath test closely correlated to those measured by scintigraphy both for semisolids ($r = .87$) and liquids ($r = .95$) (Fig. 14.13).[21] Despite the high correlation, the $t_{1/2}$ values by breath test are much higher than by scintigraphy, and further validation of this method is required. The time of maximum $^{13}CO_2$ exhalation also correlated with the $t_{1/2}$ obtained by scintigraphy ($r = .85$ for semisolids, $r = .94$ for liquids).

### Combined $^{13}C$-Glycine/$^{14}C$-Octanoic Acid Breath Test to Monitor Gastric Emptying Rates of Both Liquids and Solids

A dual-label breath test can be used with $^{13}C$-glycine for the liquid phase and $^{14}C$-octanoic acid for the solid phase to simultaneously measure gastric emptying of liquids and solids.[23] This test seems convenient for pharmacologic studies. Glycine was selected as a marker of the liquid phase because it is easily soluble in water. It is postulated that glycine is not absorbed in the stomach but is absorbed by active transport in the proximal intestine. Glycine is partly oxidized to $CO_2$ by different pathways. The test meal contained 150 mL of water, dosed with 100 mg of [1-$^{13}C$]-glycine (99% enrichment; Isotec, Miamisburg, OH), and there was a good to excellent correlation between the $t_{1/2}$ determined by the breath test and scintigraphy ($r = .91$ for liquids and $r = .92$ for solids).[23]

Estimation of $t_{1/2B}$ using this method involves a correction factor (minus 70 minutes) similar to the one used for solids,[15] based on the intercept value of the linear regression between

**TABLE 14.4.** Sensitivity and Specificity of the Breath Test Against Scintigraphy Reported in the Literature

| Literature (Year) | Breath Test | Subjects | Meals | Normal Value of $t_{1/2}$ by Scintigraphy* | Cutoff Value of $t_{1/2}$ by Breath Test | Sensitivity (%) | Specificity (%) |
|---|---|---|---|---|---|---|---|
| Ghoos et al[15] (1993) | $^{13}C$-octanoate | 16 healthy volunteers and 20 dyspeptic patients | Solid | $t_{1/2 S} < 75$ min | 80 min | 95 | 94 |
| Braden et al[21] (1995) | $^{13}C$-acetate | 20 healthy volunteers | Liquid | $t_{1/2 S} < 20$ min (mean + 2 SD) | 90 min | 80.0 | 77.8 |
| Ziegler et al[25] (1996) | $^{13}C$-octanoate | 34 diabetic patients | Solid | $t_{1/2 S} \leq 100$ min | 200 min | 75 | 86 ' |
| Delbende et al[26] (2000) | $^{13}C$-octanoate | 54 dyspeptic patients | Solid | $t_{1/2 S} \leq 109$ min (90th percentile of 34 healthy subjects) | 124 min | 67 | 80 |
| Viramontes et al[20] (2001) | $^{13}C$-Spirulina | 57 healthy volunteers (pharmacologically manipulated) | Solid | $70$ min $\leq t_{1/2 S} \leq 150$ min (10th and 90th percentiles of 42 healthy subjects) | 70 min (lower cutoff) 150 min (upper cutoff) | 86 | 80 |

*All were evaluated by simultaneous scintigraphy on the same subjects except Ziegler's report,[25] in which the breath test and scintigraphy were 2 days apart.

$t_{1/2 \text{breath test}}$ and $t_{1/2 \text{scintigraphy}}$. However, it is unclear whether some of the liquid marker may be partitioned with or adsorbed by the solid meal and "empty" more consistently more slowly in the presence of a solid meal,[24] and the consistency of the correction factor has not been confirmed in other laboratories. There is minimal exposure to radiation (less than 0.015 mGy) owing to $^{14}C$-octanoic acid, much less than the combined scintigraphic technique (0.78 mGy). Further research should be focused on gastric emptying tests using two different stable isotopes (eg, $^{13}C$, $^{15}N$) to avoid any radioactivity.

## Sensitivity, Specificity, and Reproducibility of Breath Tests

Gastric scintigraphy is generally regarded as the gold standard to assess the sensitivity and specificity of the breath test. However, it is likely that breath tests and scintigraphy do not measure exactly the same phenomena, and these may not be altered in exactly the same way in different pathologic conditions. Moreover, the accuracy of scintigraphy can be influenced by several factors such as count attenuation, downscatter, septal penetration, and imaging overlap.

Once delayed or accelerated gastric emptying (equivalent to disease) is defined by scintigraphic results, the sensitivity and specificity of the breath test can be obtained according to the cutoff values of the breath test, and receiver operating characteristic (ROC) curves can be constructed (x axis: false-positive fraction, y axis: true-positive fraction). Even though the trade-off between sensitivity and specificity is unavoidable (if the sensitivity is increased, the specificity is decreased, and vice versa), the most optimal cutoff value of the breath test (usually the left upper portion of the curve) can be estimated from a ROC curve.

Reported sensitivity and specificity of the breath test for detecting abnormal gastric emptying are summarized in Table 14.4.[20,21,25,26] Despite methodologic differences in the breath test performed at different centers, the sensitivity of the breath test ranged from 67 to 95% (median value of five studies 80%), and specificity ranged from 78 to 94% (median value of five studies 80%). Breath tests are well reproducible[1,15,16,21,22,26–28] and comparable to scintigraphy.[16,29] With breath tests, intraindividual variation is lower than interindividual variation, but this is also true for scintigraphy.[16] Reported coefficients of variation in the literature are described in Table 14.5 (solid meals) and Table 14.6 (liquid meals). Reproducibility is better using solid than liquid test meals and in healthy subjects than in nonulcer dyspepsia or diabetic patients.[21,28]

## Unsolved Problems in the Field of Application of Breath Tests

In spite of increasing reports about the use of breath tests to measure gastric emptying, there are still several problems to be solved. Further larger-scale validity studies are needed.

### Collection Period and Interval of Breath Sampling

To obtain the constant $m$ value in Ghoos and colleagues' mathematical model and to guarantee the discriminant value of the breath test, some researchers recommend breath sampling every 15 minutes for at least more than 4 or 5 hours.[15,18,21] It may be true that the more frequent and longer the collection period is, the more accurate the results will be. However, this may be cumbersome in some patients, rendering it difficult for office and epidemiologic studies. Moreover, Lee and colleagues have reported that even increasing the sampling time up to 8 hours did not enhance the breath test's accuracy (see Fig 14.12).[17]

**TABLE 14.5.** Coefficient of Variation of Gastric Half-Emptying Time of Solid Meals of the Breath Test and Scintigraphy Reported in the Literature

| Literature (Year) | Subjects | Breath Test | | Scintigraphy | |
|---|---|---|---|---|---|
| | | Intra (%) | Inter (%) | Intra (%) | Inter (%) |
| Ghoos et al[15] (1993) | 5 dyspeptic patients | 27 | — | — | — |
| Lartigue et al[29] (1994) | 12 healthy subjects | — | — | 19 | 20 |
| Lartigue et al[29] (1994) | 14 diabetic subjects | — | — | 29 | 76 |
| Choi et al[1] (1997) | 15 healthy volunteers | 12 | 20 | — | — |
| Duan et al[28] (1995) | 7 healthy subjects | 20 | — | — | — |
| Choi et al[16] (1998) | 30 (breath test) and 14 (scintigraphy) healthy volunteers | 15 | 23 | 14 | 44 |
| Delbende et al[26] (2000) | 18 healthy volunteers | 15 | 24 | — | — |

**TABLE 14.6.** Coefficient of Variation of Gastric Half-Emptying Time of Liquid Meals of the Breath Test and Scintigraphy Reported in the Literature

| Literature (Year) | Subjects | Breath Test | | Scintigraphy | |
|---|---|---|---|---|---|
| | | Intra (%) | Inter (%) | Intra (%) | Inter (%) |
| Lartigue et al[29] (1994) | 12 healthy subjects | — | — | 35 | 37 |
| Lartigue et al[29] (1994) | 12 healthy subjects | — | — | 67 | 84 |
| Branden et al[21] (1995) | 5 healthy subjects | 21.8 | — | — | — |
| Duan et al[28] (1995) | 5 healthy subjects | 5.58 | — | — | — |
| Barnett et al[27] (1999) | 28 healthy preterm infants | 23.9 | — | — | — |
| Gatti et al[22] (2000) | 30 healthy children and 30 patient children with gastroesophageal reflux | 5.34 | — | — | — |

### Intercept Term as a Correction Factor

Many articles report that the breath test overestimates $t_{1/2}$ by a certain amount of time compared to the scintigraphy $t_{1/2}$. Ghoos and colleagues reported that the breath test overestimated the scintigraphic $t_{1/2}$ by 66 minutes, and this intercept is similar among individuals.[15] Recently, Delbende and colleagues reported that this delay of the breath test over scintigraphy was 67 minutes.[26] Braden and colleagues reported that the delay was 49 minutes (liquid test) and 55 minutes (semisolid test meal) in the $^{13}$C-acetate breath test.[21] They speculated that low-molecular-weight acetate is absorbed and oxidized slightly more rapidly than [$^{13}$C]octanoate. However, Choi and colleagues reported that this intercept value varies among individuals, thereby resulting in differences in $t_{1/2}$ values obtained by the two methods (from −33.1 to 169.6 minutes).[1] Therefore, whether this time delay is constant among various disease groups and why this difference occurs are still unclear. This difference does not seem to be explained solely by the time required for postgastric processing (eg, absorption, metabolism, and excretion of $^{13}$C-substrate), because the peak excretion is observed around 10 minutes after intraduodenal instillation of *C-octanoate in healthy subjects (see Fig. 14.5).[18]

### Test Meals and Natural $^{13}$C Enrichment

Test meals and natural $^{13}$C enrichment vary between Europe and the United States. This factor should be considered since the breath test results are corrected for baseline $^{13}CO_2$ in breath.

### Application of Breath Tests

Since the breath test was introduced, it has been applied to measure gastric emptying of solids or liquids only in healthy subjects, the pediatric population,[22,27] and diseases such as nonulcer dyspepsia,[21,30] duodenal ulcer with *H pylori* infection,[31] diabetes,[17,25] hyperemesis gravidarum and nondyspeptic pregnancy,[32] Billroth II gastrojejunostomy,[33] and amyotrophic lateral sclerosis.[34] The breath test has also been applied to assess the effects of drugs. Thus, atropine,[20] octreotide,[35] propantheline,[36] and sumatriptan[37] delayed gastric emptying of solids in healthy subjects, whereas erythromycin[20,36] and cisapride[28] accelerated the gastric emptying rate of solids. Oral EM574, a new nonantibiotic motilide derived from erythromycin, also accelerated gastric emptying of solids,[38] and intragastric administration of 400 µg of capsaicin increased gastric emptying rate of liquids.[39]

### Limitation of Breath Tests

It should be borne in mind that the limitations of the breath test include the lack of information on the possible influence of impaired absorption or liver disease. In addition, the breath test does not provide information about intragastric meal distribution or concomitant small bowel and large bowel transit studies that are possible with scintigraphic techniques.

## Breath Test Application in the Pediatric Population

The breath test is more attractive for pediatric population studies and is preferable to gastric scintigraphy because it is easier. Gatti and colleagues reported that their results of the $^{13}$C-acetate breath test in the pediatric population closely correlated with those of scintigraphy.[22] Breath tests can be applied in premature infants, neonates, toddlers, children, and adolescents. The dose of $^{13}$C-substrate should be adjusted according to $CO_2$ production as predicted by BSA. The test meal for toddlers would need to be altered if they do not accept the adult test meal (scrambled eggs or pancakes). A test meal consisting of bread with $^{13}$C-octanoic acid containing chocolate spread has been suggested for this age group.[40]

## Cost Considerations

Whereas a gastric emptying study by scintigraphy may require dedication of a gamma camera for hours, the breath test can be performed for several patients simultaneously, thus rendering it more economic. The commercial rate for $^{13}$C measurement is approximately $15 per sample; restricting the number of samples for analysis thus helps reduce the overall costs of the test. Currently, expensive mass spectrometry is needed to measure breath $^{13}CO_2$. However, if less expensive methods such as NDIRS are used to measure $^{13}CO_2$ in the future, the test costs may be further reduced. These cost considerations justify efforts by investigators in this field to try to validate more cost-effective but accurate adaptations of the test.

## CONCLUSION

Breath tests are a promising, reliable, noninvasive way to measure gastric emptying. Efforts to improve, validate, and simplify the analytic methods have brought these tests to the threshold of clinical practice. Because test materials and breath samples can be easily and safely mailed to a central laboratory, tests can also be performed at home, in clinics, or in hospitals without facilities for mass spectrometry. Applications to larger groups of patients in clinical practice can be realistically envisaged in the near future.

### REFERENCES

1. Choi M-G, Camilleri M, Burton DD, et al. $^{13}$C-octanoic acid breath test for gastric emptying of solids: accuracy, reproducibility, and comparison with scintigraphy. Gastroenterology 1997;112:1155–62.
2. Vantrappen G. Methods to study gastric emptying. Dig Dis Sci 1994;39:91S–4S.
3. Pelot D, Dana ER, Berk JE. Comparative assessment of gastric emptying by barium burger and saline load tests. Am J Gastroenterol 1972;58:411–7.
4. Mossi S, Meyer-Wyss B, Beglinger C, et al. Gastric emptying of liquid meals measured noninvasively in humans with [$^{13}$C]acetate breath test. Dig Dis Sci 1994;39:107S–9S.
5. Siegel JA, Urbain J-L, Adler LP, et al. Biphasic nature of gastric emptying. Gut 1988;29:85–9.
6. Hatch MD, Slack CR. Photosynthesis by sugar-cane leaves: a new carboxylation reaction pathway of sugar formation. Biochem J 1966;101:103–11.
7. Quale J, Fuller A, Benson A, Calvin A. Enzymatic decarboxylation of ribulose diphosphate. J Am Chem Soc 1954;76:3610.
8. Swart GR, van den Berg JWO. $^{13}$C breath test in gastroenterological practice. Scand J Gastroenterol Suppl 1998;225:13-8.
9. Posati LP, Kinsella JE, Watt BK. Comprehensive evaluation of fatty acids in food. J Am Diet Assoc 1975;67:111–5.
10. Dillon JC, Phuc AP, Dubacq JP. Nutritional value of the alga *S. platensis*. World Rev Nutr Diet 1995;77:32–46.
11. Stellaard F, Geypens B. European interlaboratory comparison of breath $^{13}CO_2$ analysis. Gut 1998;43 Suppl 3:S2–6.
12. Schadewaldt PB, Schommartz B, Wienrich G, et al. Application of isotope-selective nondispersive infrared spectrometry (IRIS) for evaluation of [$^{13}$C]octanoic acid gastric-emptying breath tests: comparison with isotope ratio-mass spectrometry (IRMS). Clin Chem 1997;43:518–22.
13. Haycock G, Schwartz G, Wisotsky D. Geometric method for measuring body surface area: a height-weight formula validated in infants children and adults. J Pediatr 1978;93:62–6.
14. Schofield WN. Predicting basal metabolic rate, new standards and review of previous work. Hum Nutr Clin Nutr 1985;39 Suppl 1:5–41.
15. Ghoos YF, Maes BD, Geypens BJ, et al. Measurement of gastric emptying rate of solids by means of a carbon-labeled octanoic acid breath test. Gastroenterology 1993;104:1640–7.
16. Choi M-G, Camilleri M, Burton DD, et al. Reproducibility of $^{13}$C-octanoic acid breath test for gastric emptying of solids. Am J Gastroenterol 1998;93:92–8.
17. Lee JS, Camilleri M, Zinsmeister AR, et al. Toward office-based measurement of gastric emptying in symptomatic diabetics using [$^{13}$C]octanoic acid breath test. Am J Gastroenterol 2000;95:2751–61.
18. Maes BD, Mys G, Geypens BJ, et al. Gastric emptying flow curves separated from carbon-labeled octanoic acid breath test results. Am J Physiol 1998;275:169–75.
19. Lee JS, Camilleri M, Zinsmeister AR, et al. A valid, accurate, office-based, nonradioactive test for gastric emptying of solids. Gut 2000;46:768–73.
20. Viramontes BE, Kim D-Y, Camilleri M, et al. Validation of a stable isotope gastric emptying test for normal, accelerated or delayed gastric emptying. Neurogastroenterol Motil. [In press]
21. Braden B, Adams S, Duan LP, et al. The [$^{13}$C]acetate breath test accurately reflects gastric emptying of liquids in both liquid and semisolid test meals. Gastroenterology 1995;108:1048–55.
22. Gatti BC, di Abriola FF, Dall'Oglio L, et al. Is the $^{13}$C-acetate breath test a valid procedure to analyse gastric emptying in children? J Pediatr Surg 2000;35:62–5.
23. Maes BD, Ghoos YF, Geypens BJ, et al. Combined carbon-13-glycine/carbon-14-octanoic acid breath test to monitor gastric emptying rates of liquids and solids. J Nucl Med 1994;35:824–31.
24. Minami H, McCallum RW. The physiology and pathophysiology of gastric emptying in humans. Gastroenterology 1984;86:1592–610.
25. Ziegler D, Schadewaldt P, Mirza AP, et al. [$^{13}$C]Octanoic acid breath test for non-invasive assessment of gastric emptying in diabetic patients: validation and relationship to gastric symptoms and cardiovascular autonomic function. Diabetologia 1996;39:823–30.
26. Delbende B, Perri F, Courturier O, et al. $^{13}$C-octanoic acid breath test for gastric emptying measurement. Eur J Gastroenterol Hepatol 2000;12:85–91.
27. Barnett C, Snel A, Omari T, et al. Reproducibility of the $^{13}$C-octanoic acid breath test for assessment of gastric emptying in healthy preterm infants. J Pediatr Gastroenterol Nutr 1999;29:26–30.
28. Duan LP, Braden B, Caspary WF, Lembcke B. Influence of cisapride on gastric emptying of solids and liquids monitored by $^{13}$C breath tests. Dig Dis Sci 1995;40:2200–6.
29. Lartigue S, Bizais Y, des Varannes SB, et al. Inter- and intrasubject variability of solid and liquid gastric emptying parameters. A scintigraphic study in healthy subjects and diabetic patients. Dig Dis Sci 1994;39:109–15.

30. Maes BD, Ghoos YF, Hiele MI, Rutgeerts PJ. Gastric emptying rate of solids in patients with nonulcer dyspepsia. Dig Dis Sci 1997;42: 1158–62.

31. Perri F, Ghoos YF, Geypens BJ, et al. Gastric emptying and *Helicobacter pylori* infection in duodenal ulcer disease. Dig Dis Sci 1996;41: 462–8.

32. Maes BD, Spitz B, Ghoos YF, et al. Gastric emptying in hyperemesis gravidarum and non-dyspeptic pregnancy. Aliment Pharm Ther 1999;13:237–42.

33. Maes BD, Hiele MI, Geypens BJ, et al. Gastric emptying of the liquid, solid and oil phase of a meal in normal volunteers and patients with Billroth II gastrojejunostomy. Eur J Clin Invest 1998;28:197–204.·

34. Toepfer M, Folwaczny C, Lochmuller H, et al. Noninvasive (13)C-octanoic acid breath test shows delayed gastric emptying in patients with amyotrophic lateral sclerosis. Digestion 1999;60:567–71.

35. Maes BD, Goohs YF, Geypens BJ, et al. Influence of octreotide on the gastric emptying of solids and liquids in normal healthy subjects. Aliment Pharmacol Ther 1995;9:11–8.

36. Maes BD, Hiele MI, Geypens BJ, et al. Pharmacological modulation of gastric emptying rate of solids as measured by the carbon labelled octanoic acid breath test: influence of erythromycin and propantheline. Gut 1994;35:333–7.

37. Coulie B, Tack J, Maes B, et al. Sumatriptan, a selective 5-HT$_1$ receptor agonist, induces a lag phase for gastric emptying of liquids in humans. Am J Physiol 1997;272:G902–8.

38. Choi MG, Camilleri M, Burton DD, et al. Dose-related effects of N-demethyl-N-isopropyl-8,9-anhydroerythromycin A6,9-hemiacetal on gastric emptying of solids in healthy human volunteers. J Pharmacol Exp Ther 1998;285:37–40.

39. Debreceni A, Abdel-Salam OM, Figler M, et al. Capsaicin increases gastric emptying rate in healthy human subjects measured by [13]C-labeled octanoic acid breath test. J Physiol Paris 1999;93:455–60.

40. Galmiche JP, Delbende B, Perri F, Andrullin A. [13]C octanoic acid breath test. Gut 1998;43:S28–30.

CHAPTER 15

# Manometry

*John E. Kellow*

The motor functions of the small intestine include mixing food with digestive secretions, circulating chyme to ensure maximal mucosal contact, propelling contents in a net aboral direction, clearing residua or refluxate left over from the digestive process, and transporting secretions from the upper gut during fasting. These vital functions are accomplished by a combination of phasic and prolonged contractions, alterations in intestinal wall tone and other luminal properties, and alterations in compliance, the net result being luminal flow and transit through the intestine. Of these parameters, measurement of intraluminal pressure in the small intestine—manometry—adequately assesses the phasic and prolonged contractions only; assessments of small bowel myoelectrical activity via intraluminal catheters are not now undertaken for clinical purposes, whereas assessments of tone and compliance remain largely research tools.

Transit through the small intestine is considered in the following chapter; even though techniques for measurement of transit can be noninvasive, can assess both solid and liquid meal components, and can be quantified and performed with equipment currently available in many centers,

there is a very large variation in health, and alterations in transit in general provide little information regarding the underlying pathophysiology of gut motor disturbances. Thus, despite its invasive nature, manometry remains the most clinically relevant technique to assess the motor function of the small intestine.

## EVOLUTION OF HUMAN SMALL INTESTINAL MANOMETRY

Following Szurszewski's definitive characterization of the migrating motor complex (MMC) in dogs,[1] the systematic study of human small bowel motor physiology was initiated by Vantrappen and colleagues,[2] who described the periodic motor activity present in the small bowel during fasting. Over the next two decades, a large number of studies provided information on the spatial organization (ie, the relationship between occurrence of contractions at adjacent sites) and on the temporal organization (ie, the characteristics of contractions at a given site that change with time) of motor activity within the small bowel. Techniques used include ambulant radiotelemetry capsules tethered within the proximal small bowel[3] (now no longer employed in clinical practice); stationary water-perfused catheter systems using both short and longer (including overnight) recording periods; ambulant tube-mounted strain gauge catheter systems; and, most recently, a portable water-perfused micromanometric multichannel system. The description of human motor patterns is continuing to evolve, and, to date, recordings have been obtained from sites encompassing the entire small intestine (for periods of up to 24 hours), from sites limited to the duodenum and proximal jejunum (for periods of up to 72 hours), and in response to a wide variety of meal types and nutrients. In general, the smaller the caliber of the catheter system employed, the greater is the duration of recordings that can be comfortably and reliably obtained. However, the longer

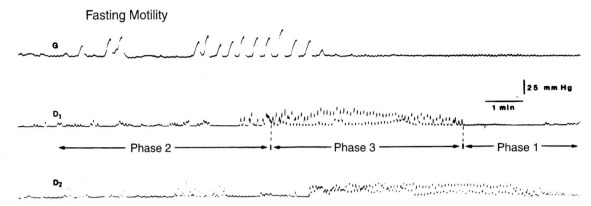

**FIGURE 15.1.** The three phases of the normal migrating motor complex (MMC), recorded diurnally in the fasting state using a stationary water-perfused catheter system. Recording side holes located in the gastric antrum (G) and the first and second parts of the duodenum (D$_1$ and D$_2$, respectively). In phase 3 of the MMC, also called the "activity front," a several-minute burst of rhythmic and regular contractions commences in the gastric antrum, progresses into the duodenum, and then migrates distally. In the small intestine, it is followed in time by phase 1, a period of motor quiescence, which, in turn, is followed after a variable interval by phase 2, a period of intermittent and apparently irregular phasic contractions. Pressure and time scales as shown.

the recording period and the greater the number of recording sensors, the greater is the technological sophistication required for data acquisition, display, and analysis.

## NORMAL PATTERNS OF HUMAN SMALL INTESTINAL MOTOR ACTIVITY

### Fasting Motor Patterns

The normal MMC, as recorded in the duodenum and jejunum during the waking state during fasting, has by convention three main phases (Figs. 15.1 to 15.4). Further description of the MMC component that occurs in the gastric antrum is provided in Chapter 10; this chapter will focus mainly on duodenojejunal, rather than gastroduodenal, manometric techniques. The manometric tracings in the following figures are depicted in a variety of formats to demonstrate some of the different types of recording and display systems that can be employed. Moreover, because of the complexity of small bowel pressure patterns, it is necessary to describe in some detail the normal patterns elucidated to date to maximize the validity of decisions regarding the presence of abnormal patterns in a particular patient.

Phase 3 of the MMC is, under normal circumstances, the most powerful propulsive sequence in the proximal small bowel; in direct contrast, during phase 1, the intestine appears relatively refractory to stimulation of contractile activity. The phase 2 component, in addition to phase 3, is important for propulsion, and the MMC has been termed "the intestinal housekeeper" because of its role in clearing the intestine of food residue during fasting. The phasic contractions during phase 3 are largely peristaltic, propagating over relatively short distances, but at a velocity considerably greater than the migration velocity of the overall phase 3 sequence itself. In late phase 3 in the duodenum—but not in the jejunum—some

retrograde contractions appear to be present, suggesting that the last portion of duodenal phase 3 subserves a "retroperistaltic" function.[4] The proportion of phase 2 contractions that are propagative remains controversial, owing to the technical limitations of obtaining multiple closely spaced sensors spanning a significant length of intestine.

Phases 1 and 3 of the MMC biorhythm are generated within the enteric nervous system, although modulation by the central nervous system (CNS) can occur; the normal intestinal microflora also appears to provide a stimulatory drive for the initiation and propagation of normal phase 3 activity.[5] Phase 2 motor activity, in contrast, depends more on central input as it is largely abolished during sleep and after vagotomy. Examples of recordings of proximal small bowel motility during sleep are shown in Figures 15.5 and 15.6. Appreciation of the regional variations and characteristics of fasting motor activity, and of the MMC, can best be obtained by recording simultaneously at multiple points along the small intestine, for prolonged periods (Figs. 15.7 to 15.16).[3,6–10]

### Postprandial Motor Patterns

Following ingestion of a meal or any type of nutrients, there is an immediate change in the contractile pattern of the small bowel to the so-called postprandial or "fed" pattern (Figs. 15.17 to 15.19).[11–13] These contractions—of variable frequency, amplitude, and propagation—enable the mixing of luminal contents and their subsequent aboral transport. The duration of this pattern relates, at least in part, to the time taken for digestible solids and liquids to empty from the stomach and to the caloric content of the meal; the pattern appears to be initiated by a vagal reflex and maintained by hormonal and paracrine effects. Fed pattern durations of about 180, 360, and 410 minutes occur in health after meals of 630, 1,260, and 2,520 kJ, respectively.[11] Fat produces a longer fed pattern than carbohydrate or protein, but the timing of the meal

**A**

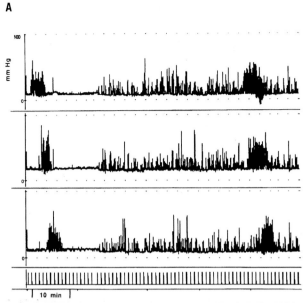

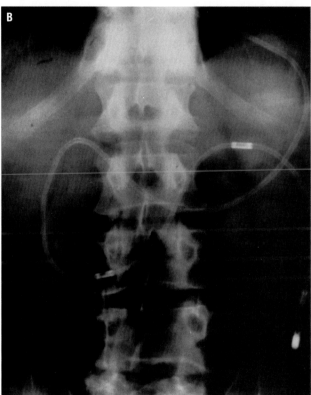

**FIGURE 15.2.** Manometric recording of computer-displayed fasting small intestinal motor activity (**A**) obtained using a triple-sensor strain gauge recording catheter positioned radiographically (**B**) with the sensors located in the third part of the duodenum (*top tracing*, **A**), at the duodenojejunal flexure (*middle tracing*), and in the proximal jejunum (*lower tracing*). From left, a phase 3 of the MMC is followed by phase 1 (motor quiescence) before phase 2 (irregular contractions) commences, culminating in a further phase 3. The precise cessation of phase 1 and commencement of phase 2 in the small bowel may not be apparent at times and can vary depending on the definition applied. Note that the individual contractions of the phase 3 of the MMC are not discernible on this display scale, the activity fronts appearing as dark blocks; note also that there is no apparent phase 1 component of the MMC following the second phase 3, a feature that can occur during diurnal recordings in some individuals.

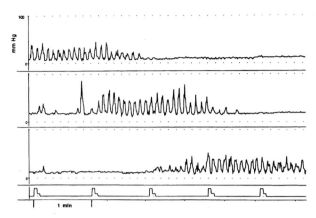

**FIGURE 15.3.** Portion of recording of fasting small intestinal motor activity from Figure 15.2A showing the first phase 3 in expanded scale. Note the sequential regular phasic contractions at each level of the proximal small bowel, with a maximal contraction rate of 12 cycles/minute in the middle tracing (duodenojejunal flexure).

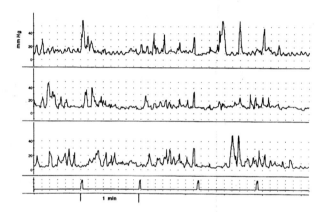

**FIGURE 15.4.** Portion of recording of fasting small intestinal motor activity from Figure 15.2A showing phase 2 activity in expanded scale. Note the irregular frequency of contractions and the irregular contractile amplitude. Some apparently propagated phasic contractions can be discerned.

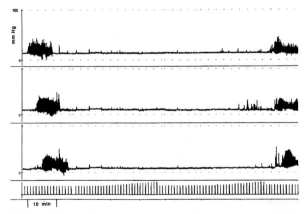

**FIGURE 15.5.** Recording of normal nocturnal (sleeping) small intestinal motor activity using a triple-sensor strain gauge recording catheter, positioned as in Figure 15.2 in the duodenum and proximal jejunum. Note the paucity of phase 2 activity between the first and second phase 3; it can be appreciated that recordings obtained during sleep thus expose more directly the phase 3 component of the MMC. Also, when compared to diurnal (awake) recordings, the propagation velocity of the phase 3 component is slower.

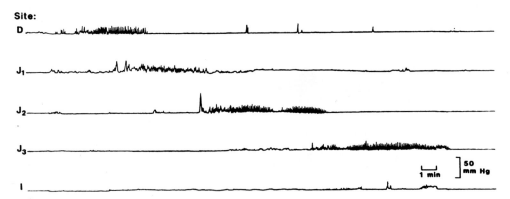

**FFIGURE 15.6.** Another example of manometric recording during sleep, on this occasion obtained with a stationary water-perfused catheter with side holes positioned in the duodenum (D), jejunum ($J_1$–$J_3$), and proximal ileum (I). Note the absence of phase 2 activity at all levels of the intestine; if a meal is ingested immediately prior to retiring, however, continuing phase 2 activity can be present during sleep. Note also the variable configuration of the phase 3 components, which commonly occurs in healthy subjects (even during sleep, and irrespective of the recording technique).

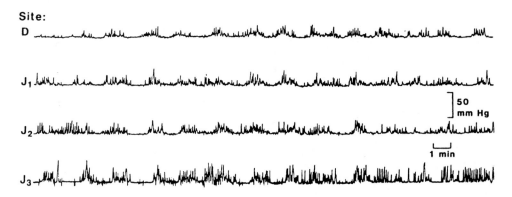

**FIGURE 15.7.** Water-perfused catheter recording from the distal duodenum (D) and three sites in the proximal jejunum ($J_1$–$J_3$) during diurnal phase 2 motor activity in a healthy subject. Clustering of contractions, with some sequences apparently propagated, is apparent from visual inspection of the tracings, in contrast to the irregular frequency of contractions usually observed. This pattern can be observed in some healthy individuals, especially in the latter stages of phase 2 activity, and usually intermittently. The control mechanism(s) or trigger for these "discrete clustered contractions" is not known but may be related to alterations in intestinal wall compliance. Reproduced with permission from Kellow JE, Borody TS, Phillips SF, et al. Human interdigestive motility: variations in patterns from esophagus to colon. Gastroenterology 1986;91:386–95.

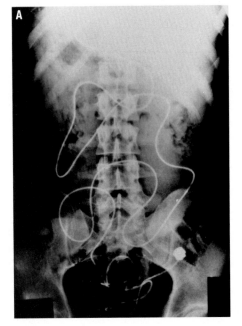

| Site | | cm from distal end |
|---|---|---|
| Esophagus | E | 185 |
| Body | B | 175 |
| Antrum | A | 165 |
| Duodenum | D | 150 |
| Jejunum { | $J_1$ | 125 |
| | $J_2$ | 100 |
| | $J_3$ | 75 |
| Ileum { | $I_1$ | 50 |
| | $I_2$ | 35 |
| | $I_3$ | 20 |
| | $I_4$ | 10 |
| Cecum | C | 0 |

**FIGURE 15.8.** Radiograph of a multilumen water-perfused catheter manometric assembly positioned in the upper gastrointestinal tract of a healthy adult (**A**); the tip of the assembly is situated in the cecum. The catheter has side holes positioned from the esophagus (E) to the cecum (C), as shown schematically in **B**. Figure 15.8B reproduced with permission from Kellow JE, Borody TS, Phillips SF, et al. Human interdigestive motility: variations in patterns from esophagus to colon. Gastroenterology 1986;91:386–95.

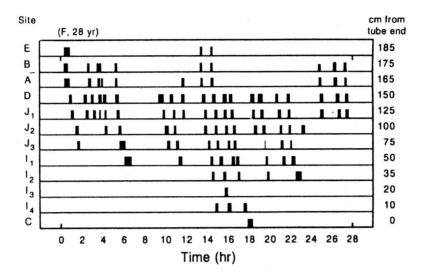

**FIGURE 15.9.** Example of "mapping" of migrating motor complex (MMC) along upper gastrointestinal tract during a prolonged period (greater than 24 hours) of fasting in a healthy female. Phase 3 components of the MMC are shown as dark blocks, and the position of water-perfused side hole sensors is as displayed in Figure 15.8. The variations in the MMC site of origin, extent of propagation, and periodicity can be readily discerned. Reproduced with permission from Kellow JE, Borody TS, Phillips SF, et al. Human interdigestive motility: variations in patterns from esophagus to colon. Gastroenterology 1986;91:386–95.

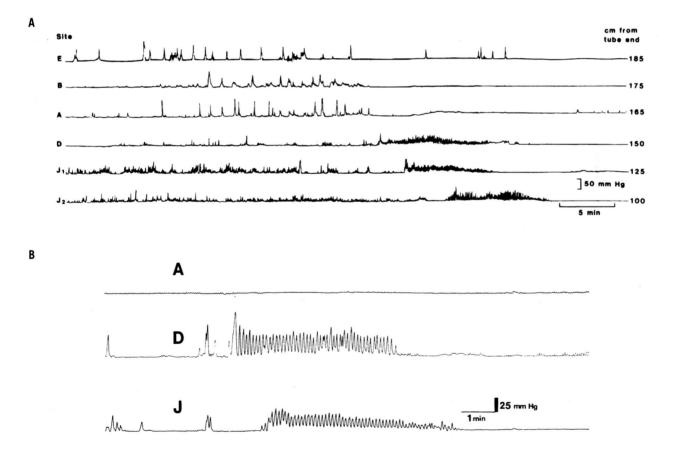

**FIGURE 15.10.** Portions of manometric recording obtained using the manometric catheter assembly displayed in Figure 15.8A/B. In **A**, note that phase 3 of the migrating motor complex (MMC) can be represented in the lower esophageal sphincter region (E), propagating through the gastric body (B) and antrum (A) and into the small intestine. The three phases of the MMC can be clearly identified in the duodenum (D) and proximal jejunum ($J_1$–$J_2$). In **B**, an expanded display of the manometric recording at a subsequent time point, and showing only three recording channels, note that the MMC can be seen to commence in the duodenum (D) without apparent gastric (A) representation. The MMC can also commence at more distal sites in the small intestine.

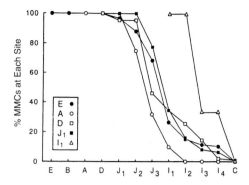

**FIGURE 15.11.** Relationship between the migrating motor complex (MMC) site of origin—for esophagus (E), gastric antrum (A), duodenum (D), proximal jejunum ($J_1$), and proximal ileum ($I_1$)—and the incidence (% of MMCs) at each subsequent intestinal locus, based on recordings of 24 hours duration in a group of healthy individuals. Recording side holes as per Figure 15.8. The distribution curves, representing the extent of propagation from each site of origin, are not significantly different, indicating that the site of MMC origin does not determine the extent of propagation.

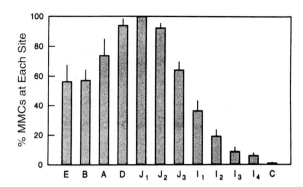

**FIGURE 15.12.** Incidence of migrating motor complexes (MMCs) in the human upper gastrointestinal tract, over a 24-hour period in a group of healthy individuals, where 100% has been assigned arbitrarily to the MMC incidence in the proximal jejunum. Recording side holes as per Figure 15.8. The greatest MMC incidence is in the proximal jejunum. Reproduced with permission from Kellow JE, Borody TS, Phillips SF, et al. Human interdigestive motility: variations in patterns from esophagus to colon. Gastroenterology 1986;91:386–95.

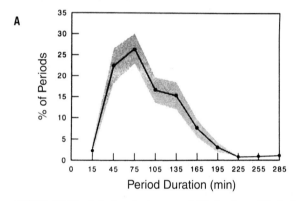

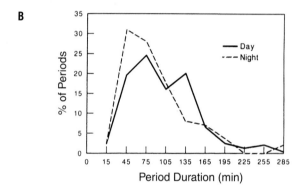

**FIGURE 15.13.** **A** displays the frequency distribution (mean %) of migrating motor complex (MMC) periods (cycle lengths) in the proximal jejunum over 24-hour recordings in health. Shaded area represents mean ± SEM. Each data point represents the midpoint of consecutive 30-minute time intervals. **B** represents the same data subdivided into daytime and nighttime (sleep) segments; note the shift to the left at night, with cycle lengths tending to be of shorter duration during this time. The MMC period can vary by several hours in the same individual, and the variance within subjects accounts for 90% of the total variance for the MMC periods.

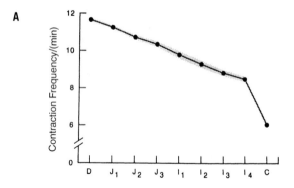

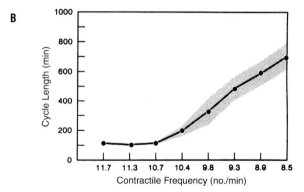

**FIGURE 15.14.** **A** displays the maximal frequency of contraction during phase 3 in a group of healthy subjects at various points along the small bowel (recording sites according to Fig. 15.8B). The frequency falls from about 12 cycles per minute in the duodenum and from 7 to 8 cycles per minute in the terminal ileum, reflecting the frequency gradient of the electrical slow wave in the small intestine. **B** shows the relationship between the average MMC cycle length (min) and the maximal contractile frequency (number of cycles/min) at different loci in the small intestine. Migrating motor complexes occur, on average, once each 300 minutes at a level at which the maximal contractile frequency is 10 cycles per minute, approximately equivalent to the midpoint of the small intestine. This relationship thus provides a useful functional definition of the site of recording within the small bowel. Shaded areas represent mean ± SEM. Figure 15.14B reproduced with permission from Kellow JE, Borody TS, Phillips SF, et al. Human interdigestive motility: variations in patterns from esophagus to colon. Gastroenterology 1986;91:386–95.

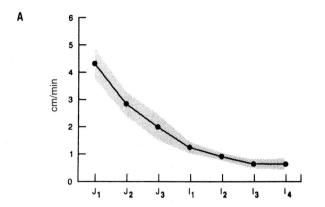 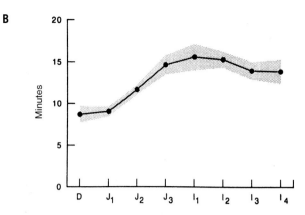

**FIGURE 15.15.** **A** shows the velocity of propagation of phase 3 of the migrating motor complex (MMC) along the small intestine. **B** shows the duration of phase 3 MMC along the small intestine. Note that the velocity slows considerably, and the duration increases (see also Fig. 15–6) as the MMC progresses distally. Phase 3 migration velocity is less variable within an individual than the other MMC characteristics. Shaded areas represent mean ± SEM and recording sites according to Figure 15.8B.

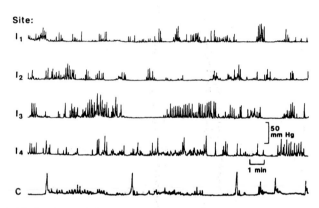 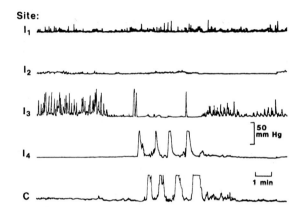

**FIGURE 15.16.** **A** shows a typical manometric recording from the ileum and cecum of a healthy fasting individual. In the ileum ($I_1$–$I_4$), short bursts of rhythmic phasic activity occur together with irregular contractions of varying amplitude and short periods of quiescence. The visual distinction between fasting and postprandial motor patterns is difficult as there are no apparent alterations in healthy ileal motor activity specific to the postprandial state. In the cecum (C), bursts of maximal contractile activity are interspersed with periods of irregular contractions and quiescence. In **B**, a group of high-amplitude prolonged contractions traverses the terminal ileum and cecum of a healthy subject. Such contractions occur infrequently during the day, in the fasting state or more often postprandially, and are highly propulsive, presumably clearing the remnants of a meal and any refluxed cecal material. They can be consciously perceived and have been reported to be directly associated with cramping abdominal discomfort in patients with irritable bowel syndrome. Reproduced with permission from Kellow JE, Borody TS, Phillips SF, et al. Human interdigestive motility: variations in patterns from esophagus to colon. Gastroenterology 1986;91:386–95.

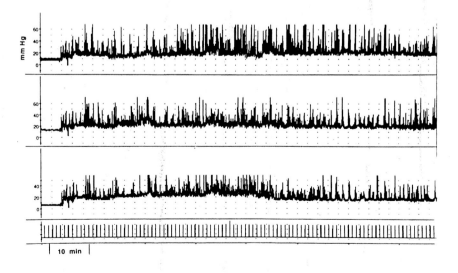

**FIGURE 15.17.** Manometric recording of postprandial small intestinal motor activity obtained in a healthy individual using a triple-sensor strain gauge recording catheter positioned as in Figure 15.2B and after ingestion of a 400-kcal (fat 44%, carbohydrate 47%, protein 12%) mixed meal. Note the continuous sequence of phasic contractions of varying frequency and amplitude, similar at each recording site, and with a greater intensity than phase 2 activity.

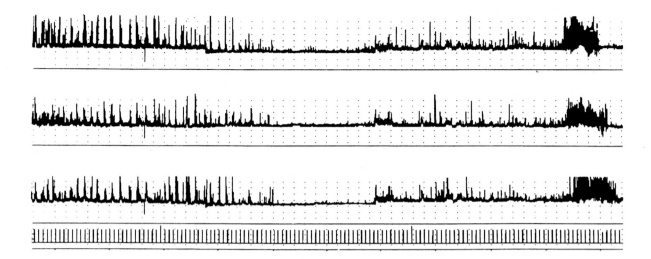

**FIGURE 15.18.** Continuation of the manometric recording of Figure 15.17, displaying the cessation of the postprandial pattern (after 300 minutes) and a brief period of motor quiescence, before the onset of phase 2 motor activity and a phase 3 component at the right of the tracing. In many recordings, it is difficult or not possible to visually distinguish between the cessation of the fed pattern and the resumption of fasting phase 2 activity, so by convention, the reappearance of a phase 3 is taken to represent the termination of the fed pattern. The return of the migrating motor complex postprandially can be jejunal rather than duodenal and can thus be undetected if only duodenal sensors are used to record postprandial activity. In this tracing, a pattern of discrete clustered contractions occurs in the late phase of the postprandial activity; such a pattern may occur postprandially in healthy subjects, particularly in elderly individuals. Scales for pressure and time as per Figure 15.17.

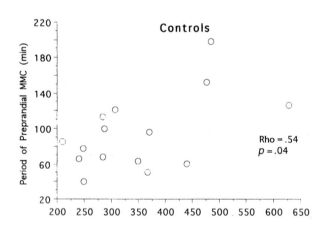

**FIGURE 15.19.** Relationship between postprandial (800-kcal meal) pattern duration (x-axis, min) and the period of the preprandial migrating motor complex (MMC) (min) in a group of healthy subjects (controls). The significant correlation suggests that the underlying enteric nervous system program that generates the cyclic MMC continues during the postprandial period, the latter representing only a temporary interruption to the phase 1 and 2 fasting patterns. These relationships require further study. Reproduced with permission from Evans PR, Bak Y-T, Shuter B, et al. Gastroparesis and small bowel dysmotility in irritable bowel syndrome. Dig Dis Sci 1997;42:2087–93.

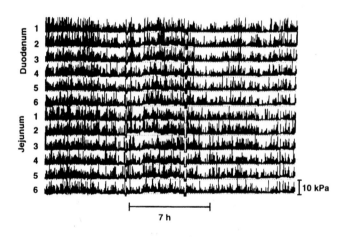

**FIGURE 15.20.** Manometric recordings from the small intestine of healthy subjects obtained over 20 hours using a portable water-perfused micromanometric system. Six side holes are located at 1-cm intervals in the mid-duodenum and six side holes also at 1-cm intervals in the proximal jejunum; the distance between the two groups of side holes is 25 cm. The protocol included lunch, dinner, and overnight sleep; the first two-thirds of the recording thus reveals largely postprandial activity and the latter one-third fasting activity. Reproduced with permission from Samsom M, Fraser R, Smout AJPM, et al. Characterization of small intestinal pressure waves in ambulant subjects recorded with a novel portable manometric system. Dig Dis Sci 1999;44:2157–64.

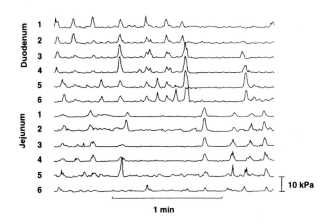

**FIGURE 15.21.** Expanded display of a 4-minute recording of postprandial jejunal and duodenal motor activity from recording in Figure 15.20 showing propagated pressure wave sequences spanning up to 5 cm. It appears that meal composition influences the number of isolated pressure waves and short-spanned pressure wave sequences but not the number of long-spanned pressure wave sequences. Reproduced with permission from Samsom M, Fraser R, Smout AJPM, et al. Characterization of small intestinal pressure waves in ambulant subjects recorded with a novel portable manometric system. Dig Dis Sci 1999;44:2157–64.

(breakfast, lunch, or dinner) does not appear to affect the contractile response of the intestine for the same nutrient load. Return of fasting (interdigestive) motor activity to the proximal small bowel often appears to occur, however, when nutrients are still present in the mid-distal small bowel. Usually, in a person consuming three meals a day, a least one phase 3 will occur between meals; if snacks are consumed between meals, then there may be no MMCs present during the day or even during the entire waking period. The possible functional significance of these variations in MMC occurrence during the waking hours has not been established. It has now become feasible to record small intestinal motor activity from multiple closely spaced water-perfused side holes for prolonged recording periods (up to 20 hours) using a portable low-compliance water pump.[14] With this technology, appreciation of the spatiotemporal organization of contractions, especially in the postprandial pattern, is possible (Figs. 15.20 and 15.21) and should lead to greater understanding of the functional significance of contractile patterns.

## CLINICAL APPLICATION OF SMALL BOWEL MANOMETRY

### Recording Techniques

#### Patient Preparation

Common to all techniques is the need for, among other aspects, fasting for at least 12 hours, cessation for 48 hours of medications that could affect motility, appropriate control of blood sugar level in diabetic patients, and a full explanation of the procedures.

### Manometric Technology

**CATHETER/TRANSDUCER OPTIONS.** Two types of catheters are generally used for clinical recordings: water-perfused and strain gauge.[15] A third type, using tube-mounted impedance sensors, is also available but is not routinely used in clinical practice.

The rationale for perfused tube (open-tip) manometry is that continuous intraluminal pressure recording will reveal phasic changes that approximate to the contractile activity of the intestinal segment under study. Intraluminal pressure is reflected by changes in pressure transmitted to an external strain gauge by a constant flow of water from a side hole in a catheter positioned in the bowel. The resistance to flow of the column of water depends on the nature of the contractions and the degree to which the side hole is occluded.

Standard equipment required for such recordings consists of a low-compliance, pneumohydraulic perfusion system linked to a multilumen catheter assembly and external strain gauge transducers. Pneumohydraulic perfusion is achieved by the use of degassed water contained in a reservoir that is maintained at a constant pressure (7.5–15 psi) by nitrogen gas or carbon dioxide; the latter pressure is reduced to atmospheric pressure before entering the manometric assembly by using capillary tubing, which provides a high resistance to flow. Thus, the perfusion rate also influences the compliance of the recording system. High-fidelity recordings of intraluminal pressure can be obtained with such a hydraulic capillary infusion system when catheter side holes with a diameter of, for example, 0.5 to 0.8 mm and perfusion rates of 0.1 to 0.3 mL/min are used. On sudden occlusion of the catheter side holes, the recording system should demonstrate a pressure rise of not less than 150 mm Hg/s. Micromanometric extrusions are available, as discussed earlier (see Fig. 15.20),[16] incorporating up to 20 recording side holes, with acceptable rise rates and suitable for transnasal intubation.

Perfused tube manometry has several advantages over other techniques to record intraluminal pressure. These include its relative simplicity, robust nature of the components, low running costs, versatility of the technique for studying different regions of the intestine, ability to readily incorporate a balloon for provocative testing, and ease of sterilization (especially for extruded plastic catheters). Disadvantages include the requirement for constant monitoring during the (stationary) recordings to ensure fidelity and the fact that the response is limited by hydraulic effects. The volume of water introduced into the lumen, when multiple side holes are employed, may also theoretically influence motor activity. Ambulant studies cannot be readily undertaken because of the requirement for an infusion pump, whereas prolonged stationary studies may be stressful in view of subject restriction.

The addition to a perfused tube catheter of a "sleeve" sensor can be used to assess motor activity in sphincteric regions (eg, the pylorus). Usually, a 4- to 6-cm membrane is positioned along the catheter assembly to span the study segment; pressure applied anywhere on the sleeve transmits the same pressure signal to the perfusion channel. Manometric side holes can also be included in the region of the sleeve to ensure that motor activity adjacent to the sphincter is detected separately from pressure activity recorded by the sleeve.

Commercially available strain gauge pressure transducer catheters for intraluminal use vary in coating material and flexibility; in general, they have a small external diameter (3–4 mm) and contain several sensors, typically three to six, and ideally a central lumen. When more than six sensors are included, an increase in the catheter diameter is required, thus reducing the tolerance of the subject to intubation for prolonged periods. For human recordings, catheter-mounted strain gauges are more sensitive in detecting intraluminal pressure changes than perfused tube manometry, but the differences are usually of such small magnitude to be of little practical importance (Fig. 15.22).[15] Peak amplitude can be more accurately determined with digital manometry provided that sampling frequency is sufficiently high.

There are a number of both practical and theoretical advantages to intraluminal strain gauge transducers. As well as their high fidelity, they are easy to insert transnasally and well tolerated. Prolonged recordings, including relatively comfortable sleep, are feasible, and with an isolation device and appropriate interfaces, the same catheter can provide both stationary and ambulant recordings. In addition, water perfusion is not required, and the catheters are easy to clean and sterilize. The disadvantages of these systems chiefly relate to the costs, both for the initial purchase and for repairs of defective transducers; the catheters are relatively fragile, especially if used for outpatient ambulant studies. Also, unlike perfused catheters, usually it is not feasible to have a range of strain gauge catheters, each with a different sensor configuration, for different clinical applications. One other important limitation is the minimum spacing of sensors (2.5–3 cm), which precludes more narrowly spaced sensors for antral manometry.

**OPTIMUM NUMBER AND LOCATION OF SENSORS.** With perfused tube manometry, many different arrangements of sensors and catheter lengths can be used to study different regions of the small bowel. Thus, sensors can be spaced widely to span the entire length of the small intestine or closely (1–2 cm) to record contractions from a localized segment or sphincteric region. For clinical purposes, recordings can usually be limited to the duodenum and proximal jejunum, with or without the gastric antrum. Two catheter designs that have been used extensively for short-term stationary recordings have side holes positioned at 0, 10, 20, 30, 40, 50, 60, 61, 62, 63, 64, and 65 cm from the distal end of a 175-cm tube and at 0, 10, 20, 30, 31, 32, 33, and 34 cm from the distal end of a 150-cm tube. These spacings provide for recordings across the antro-duodenal junction and at 10-cm intervals in the proximal small bowel. For recordings confined to the small bowel, a catheter with three sensors, where at least one, and preferably two, are positioned in the proximal jejunum—where MMCs

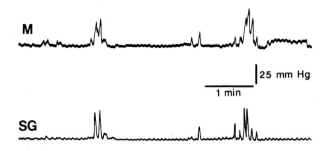

**FIGURE 15.22.** Simultaneous recordings of duodenal phase 2 activity from perfused tube manometric (M) and strain gauge manometric (SG) pressure sensors. Note tonic pressure change in manometric, but not strain gauge, recording. Reproduced with permission from Gill RC, Kellow JE, Browning C. The use of intraluminal strain gauges for recording ambulant small bowel motility. Am J Physiol 1990;258:61–5.

occur most frequently—represents the minimal requirement. Occasionally, it may be necessary to record from the ileum if this is felt to be the only site, or an important site, of a disease process. For recordings of intraluminal pressure from the terminal 30 to 50 cm of ileum, across the ileocecal sphincter, and from the proximal colon, a multilumen catheter with side holes located 0.5, 6.5, 8.0, 9.5, 11, 12.5, 17.5, 22.5, 37.5, and 52.5 cm from the distal tip can be used. With this catheter, when the terminal sensor is in the proximal colon, the closely spaced array of sensors usually straddles the ileocecal junction. If assessment of motor activity over the distal 100 cm of small bowel is required, an assembly with side holes located 0, 10, 20, 30, 40, 50, 75, 100, and 125 cm from the distal tip can be employed.

For ambulant small bowel monitoring, the most widely used strain gauge catheters have transducers positioned at 10- to 15-cm intervals from the distal tip. If three to six sensors are employed, the proximal sensor is positioned in the distal duodenum and the remaining sensors at and beyond the ligament of Treitz in the proximal jejunum. Prolonged ambulant recordings can also be obtained using longer catheters with sensors positioned in the distal jejunum and ileum.

### Placement of Catheters

The progress and final positioning of catheters is usually facilitated by image-intensification fluoroscopy. A freeze-frame facility enables radiation exposure to be limited. For tubes positioned in the proximal jejunum, for example, usually less than 5 seconds is required (0.2–0.4 mSv). Perfused tube catheters and strain gauge catheters can be positioned by using a steel-weighted tip at the end of the tube; an inflatable balloon tied or bonded over the tip allows for rapid transport of the catheter through the duodenum and beyond the ligament of Treitz once it has passed through the pylorus. In normal subjects, the catheter will reach the proximal jejunum usually within 1 hour and almost invariably within 2 hours; the terminal balloon is then deflated. For positioning of catheters in the ileum, manometric assemblies usually require up to 6 hours to be appropriately positioned. However, in patients with significant motility disorders of the upper gastrointestinal tract, passage through the pylorus can be difficult to achieve; in such cases, the catheter can be introduced into the stomach on the night before the study, hopefully to achieve passage through the pylorus during the night.

For perfused tube assemblies, another techique of placement involves use of a guidewire, over which a multilumen manometric assembly (incorporating a central channel) can be threaded and positioned in the proximal jejunum, under fluoroscopic control. The guidewire can be placed using a steerable catheter system or preliminary upper gastrointestinal endoscopy.

### Data Acquisition Devices

A variety of computer-based acquisition systems for stationary recordings are commercially available. These can accept a large number of primary input signals configurable by the user for recording from DC/transducers and can be set up for chart recorder modes. An analog to digital converter enables data to be stored on a commercially available portable solid-state recorder, which can be used for ambulant or stationary recordings. Currently available dataloggers for this techique are designed as lightweight, modular units with a power supply separated from the processing memory and interface circuitry, all mounted in a compact leather harness or shoulder bag. Typical specifications provide for sampling of several channels of pressure data for a period of up to 72 hours and a further channel for combined event and time information. To enable acquisition over such a period of time, a sampling rate of 2 Hz per channel is the minimum permissible for accurate recording of pressure events within the small bowel, allowing for at least 10 sampled points per contraction, which is adequate for clinical purposes in the current state of knowledge. Software residing on a host computer allows the datalogger to be controlled for calibration and data transfer and also for downloading recorded data to a chart recorder or similar program.

### Recording Protocols

The duration of recording required for clinical assessment depends on the type of disorder suspected and also on the available techniques for data analysis. One short-duration stationary protocol employs a 3-hour fasting recording period, followed by a 2-hour postprandial period, and a large amount of clinical data has been published using this protocol.[17] The variability of the patterns of small bowel motility suggests, however, that longer recording periods, which provide more information on all aspects of contractile activity, would be diagnostically superior to shorter recordings. This seems especially true for disorders where evaluation of the MMC propagation and incidence is required as a marker of enteric neural integrity.

Comparison of shorter (several hour) versus longer (24-hour) periods has received little attention, although there is some evidence that by prolonging a stationary fasting study to 6 hours, the same accuracy as an ambulant 24-hour study can be achieved in more than 90% of patients.[18] Certainly, prolonged monitoring of the motor response to food appears to offer no advantage over a short recording period. It should be noted, however, that a head-to-head comparison of the two types of recording periods using computer-aided analysis of all of the information available has not been undertaken. Moreover, in several patients in the above report, even though a short recording was considered to be abnormal, when small bowel motility was assessed using a long recording period, it was considered normal; this diagnostic change occurred in a greater number of patients than the reverse scenario. Data on the diagnostic usefulness of information provided during sleep recordings when compared to diurnal fasting recordings are also limited. Given the physiologic changes in motor patterns during sleep, however, it is reasonable to assume that such a period of assessment may be important in certain cases of disordered motility. Ambulant monitoring, particularly when performed on an outpatient basis with the subject continuing to conduct his or her usual daily activities, including sleeping at home, enables the incorporation of a potentially greater number of intrinsic and external modulatory influences on small bowel motility. These include different nutrient types, intestinal secretions, gas, fluctuating autonomic influences, enteric reflexes, and psychosocial issues. Ambulant monitoring also provides more potential to capture symptoms that may be intermittent or paroxysmal.

In terms of the postprandial pattern, for a short-duration stationary study, it is recommended that the test meal be of at least 400 kcal, which is known to provide a postprandial motor response of at least 2 hours; the meal is preferably a standard mixed, balanced solid/liquid meal, with 20 to 25% fat, 20 to 25% protein, and 50 to 55% carbohydrate, for which there are reasonable normative data available. Higher-fat meals can be used if motor or sensory hypersensitivity to fat is likely to be present based on the history; data for other provocative meals are not available for clinical use.

For ambulant and prolonged studies, several protocols can be used for clinical purposes. One protocol uses catheter insertion in the morning (7–9 am), a single 600-kcal meal given at 3 pm, thus providing a 6- to 7-hour fasting period, followed by a waking 8-hour postprandial period up until 11 pm. An 8-hour sleeping period is then recorded before the tube is removed the next morning. Over a period of ambulant recording of 48 hours, it has been shown that there is no appreciable change in the features of the MMC or of the postprandial pattern between the first and second 24-hour recording periods, and so unless further correlation of symptoms with specific motor patterns is desired, it is usually not necessary to prolong the recording period more than 24 hours. An alternative protocol employs at least one standard lower-energy meal (breakfast) and one standard higher-energy meal (dinner), with fasting in between, during the course of a 24-hour recording, and with a prior 8-hour overnight sleep period; the fed patterns following these two

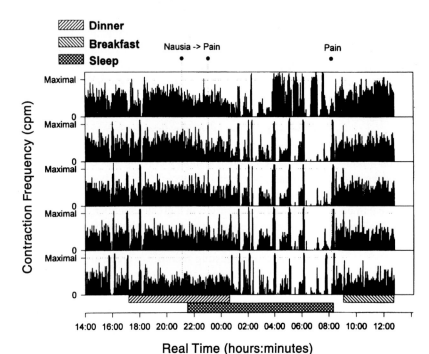

**FIGURE 15.23.** A frequency profile displaying five sites of contractile information, recorded using a five-sensor strain gauge catheter. Sensors are positioned in the duodenum (*upper two channels*), at the ligament of Treitz (*middle channel*), and in the proximal jejunum (*lower two channels*). The y-axis on each trace corresponds to the frequency of recognized contractions (number per minute) in successive time intervals, and beneath these traces is an indication of the timing of both meals and sleep periods. Note the increase in contraction frequency after meals, sustained for many hours before the return of the MMC activity, manifest by the phase 3 components apparent as discrete dark blocks. Reproduced with permission from Castillo FD, Benson MJ, Evans DF, et al. The intestinal datalogger: a tool for analysis of intestinal motor function. J Ambulatory Monitoring 1996;9:203–18.

standard meals can then be particularly evaluated and compared. A further protocol maintains the patient's usual routine of meals, as long as the evening meal is taken at least 3 hours before retiring. This type of meal protocol may be useful to provoke sensorimotor disturbances that are not demonstrable using a standard meal routine.

There are few published data on the use of provocative testing during clinical small bowel motility. Although meals of differing energy can be given, specific nutrients have not been well studied in man. Infusion or injection of various peptides such as cholecystokinin or somatostatin can be used, but the interpretation of the findings is difficult as normative data are lacking. Mechanical distention, using, for example, a small latex balloon, can be used to "evaluate" the peristaltic reflex, but the paucity of data in various disease states, including a lack of clinicopathologic correlation, has limited the use of this technique in clinical practice.

### Data Display and Analysis

Once the manometric data are downloaded from the datalogger, various graphic display programs can be used to display the overall nature of the contractile activity recorded (Fig. 15.23), and specific areas or regions of interest can be viewed selectively.[19] Qualitative and quantitative analysis can then be performed visually or by computer-assisted techniques. As discussed earlier, manometric nomenclature, although far from standardized, is based on specific pattern recognition, such as the characteristic phases of the MMC during fasting, and the postprandial pattern and various other types of contractile activity. Some relatively well-accepted qualitative definitions of small bowel motor activity are provided in Table 15.1. Based on these definitions, a set of criteria that can help define the presence of abnormal

proximal jejunal motor activity, when recorded for prolonged periods, can be generated (Table 15.2).[18] Most of these were developed based on short-term recording and can therefore be used in this context. A number of scoring systems, assigning arbitrary numeric scores to the alterations in Table 15.2, have been devised, but there is no internationally recognized system.

Computer analysis techniques, using various wave identification and recognition algorithms, artifact rejection techniques, and algorithms for detection of propagated activity, are beyond the scope of this chapter and are discussed in several reviews.[14,19,20] Such analyses, although not without their limitations, can produce an improved degree of objectivity in the analysis of pressure tracings and can provide quantitative analysis of a number of relevant parameters, which can then be compared individually to a normal range generated from the study of healthy subjects; an example is shown in Figure 15.24. There has been recent interest in the use of nonlinear mathematical models to improve the analysis, especially of the postprandial pattern, when compared to conventional computer-aided analysis[21]; further work is required before this can be applied clinically.

## Potential Clinical Indications

Based on the data presented in the previous sections, it can be seen that recording of small bowel motility can be used to test, in general terms,[22] the integrity of enteric neuromuscular function, the CNS pertubation of enteric neuromuscular function, and the enteric motor response to food. The role of small bowel motility in the clinical setting (Table 15.3) is therefore to define deviations, if any, from the normal patterns relative to these three areas and to categorize such

**TABLE 15.1.** Small Bowel Motor Parameters

| Parameter | Definition |
|---|---|
| Phase 3 (of the MMC) | A period with at least 2 min duration of uninterrupted regular phasic contractions at the maximum frequency for that locus, usually followed by quiescence[3] |
| Phase 3 periodicity | The time interval between the commencement of consecutive activity fronts[6] |
| Phase 3 propagation velocity | The distance between proximal and distal recording sensors divided by the time interval between the onset of phase 3 at the two sensors[7] |
| Phase 3 abnormality | Contractile irregularity or disruption, or simultaneous (>20 cm/min) or retrograde propagation[18] |
| Phase 2 (of the MMC) | A period of irregular and intermittent contractions with three or more contractions within 10 min[23] |
| Postprandial pattern | The period from the time of an evident increase in amplitude and/or frequency of contractions after commencement of a meal to the onset of the next phase 3[6] |
| DCCs | A period longer than 5 min with groups of clustered contractions with/without propagation, with at least 30 s of quiescence before and after each cluster[21] |
| Burst | A group of irregular uninterrupted contractions (10 contractions/min or more) longer than 2 min, with 50% or more of contractions higher than 20 mm Hg, without propagation[18] |
| SIPA | Sustained (>30 min), intense phasic pressure activity occurring in one or more segments with intestine while normal or decreased activity is being recorded simultaneously elsewhere[18] |
| Phase 3-like activity during postprandial pattern | Regular phasic contractions at the slow-wave frequency lasting longer than 1 min occurring 5 min or later after the intake of a meal, and if lasting longer than 2 min then not propagating through a number of channels or not obviously terminating the postprandial pattern[7] |

MMC, migrating motor complex; DCCs, discrete clustered contractions; SIPA, sustained incoordinated phasic activity.

**TABLE 15.2.** Criteria for Abnormal Proximal Jejunal Motor Activity

Migrating motor complex (MMC)
  No MMC per 24 h of recording
  More than three MMCs per 3 h of recording in awake state
  Phase 3 duration >10 min
  Phase 3 velocity <1 cm/min
  Simultaneous or retrograde phase 3
  Phase 2 duration > phase 1 duration during sleep
Postprandial pattern
  No establishment of fed pattern
  Duration <2 h after a 400-kcal (or greater) meal
Contraction amplitude
  <20 mm Hg (especially during phase 2 and/or 3 activity)
Presence of specific contractile patterns
  Bursts
  Sustained incoordinated phasic activity
  Multiple, simultaneous, prolonged (>8-sec) phasic contractions
  Postprandial discrete clustered contractions >30 min duration
  Postprandial phase 3-like activity

**TABLE 15.3.** Some Clinical Indications for Small Bowel Manometry

Suspected enteric/extrinsic neural morphologic abnormality
  Enteric and/or extrinsic neuropathy
    Primary: chronic idiopathic intestinal pseudo-obstruction/visceral neuropathy
    Secondary: diabetes mellitus, Parkinson's disease, post vagotomy
  Enteric myopathy
    Primary: chronic idiopathic intestinal pseudo-obstruction/hollow visceral myopathy
    Secondary: systemic sclerosis, amyloidosis
Suspected functional abnormality
  Mechanical obstruction of intestine
    Extrinsic
    Intrinsic
  Brain-gut dysregulation
    Gastroparesis/functional dyspepsia
    Functional constipation (severe idiopathic, esp. preoperatively)
    Functional diarrhea
    Functional abdominal pain
    ? Irritable bowel syndrome

deviations as either consistent with enteric neuropathy or myopathy,[18,24–29] consistent with a transient or reversible disorder of small bowel motor function owing to mechanical obstruction,[30–32] or consistent with disordered function in the absence of currently demonstrable histopathologic change.[9,21,33–40] Some prognostic information can also be obtained using this classification. Examples of these categorizations are provided in Figures 15.25 to 15.32. One further role for small bowel motility in the clinical setting is to evaluate the motor effects of pharmacologic agents, either those with therapeutic potential or those proposed as diagnostic agents. Such agents include prokinetic and antispasmodic drugs, visceral analgesics, opioids, and gastrointestinal peptides such as cholecystokinin and octreotide.[41] The choice

between stationary and ambulant recording techniques depends to some extent on the main aspect of small bowel motility to be explored, taking into account both the working diagnosis and the advantages and limitations of each technique, as outlined earlier (Table 15.4). It is important to note that, at present, data relating manometric findings to pathologic/histologic abnormalities in the small bowel are extremely limited and are based largely on extrapolations from the results of manometric recordings in well-defined systemic conditions (as in Table 15.3), where pathologic involvement of the intestine is known to occur. Moreover, because of the limited motor patterns that the gut can display, it is likely that different pathologic problems may provoke the same motor abnormality. The diagnostic sensitivi-

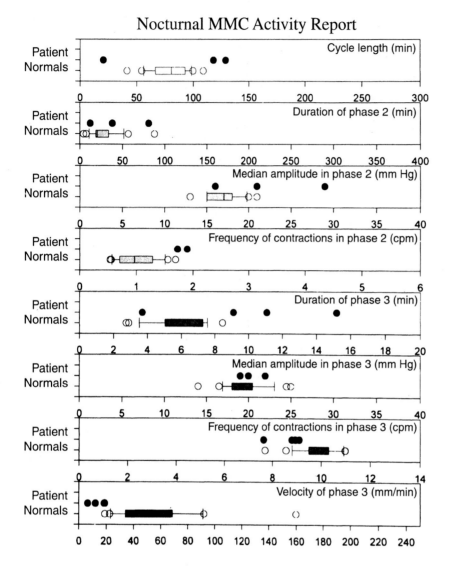

**FIGURE 15.24.** One published method of displaying individual patient data, where points corresponding to specific data from each recorded cycle of the migrating motor complex (MMC) in a single patient are plotted above a box and whisker representation of a range of normal data. Median values, interquartile range, 5th and 95th percentile values, and outliers are depicted for the normal values. Reproduced with permission from Castillo FD, Benson MJ, Evans DF, et al. The intestinal datalogger: a tool for analysis of intestinal motor function. J Ambulatory Monitoring 1996;9:203–18.

**TABLE 15.4.** Small Bowel Manometry Objectives Related to Available Recording Techniques

| | Recording Technique | | |
| | Short-Term Stationary* | Prolonged Ambulant | |
| Objective | | Diurnal | Nocturnal |
|---|---|---|---|
| Testing integrity of small bowel neuromuscular function (eg, enteric neuropathy, enteric myopathy) | ++ | ++ | +++ |
| Testing CNS pertubation of small bowel neuromuscular function (eg, extrinsic neuropathy, brain-gut dysregulation) | + | ++ | + |
| Testing small bowel motor response to food (eg, enteric/extrinsic neuropathy, enteric myopathy, mechanical obstruction) | +++[†] | ++[‡] | |

+ = technique provides limited data only, ++ = technique provides adequate data, +++ = technique provides detailed data.

*Prolonged stationary recordings feasible, including sleep, but patient required to remain in clinical facility; [†]technique also enables detailed evaluation of antropyloric motor activity after feeding; [‡]technique can be modified to provide limited evaluation of antropyloric motor activity after feeding.

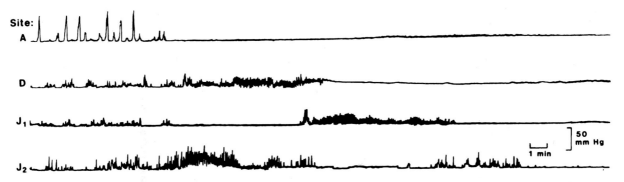

**FIGURE 15.25.** Water-perfused manometric recording of antral (A), duodenum (D), and proximal jejunal ($J_1$, $J_2$) motor activity during fasting in a patient with insulin-dependent diabetes mellitus. Note particularly the activity in channel $J_1$, consisting of a nonpropagated high-amplitude phase 3 component, followed by a poorly developed, although propagated from D and $J_1$, phase 3 component. These findings are suggestive of a neuropathic process affecting the small intestine.

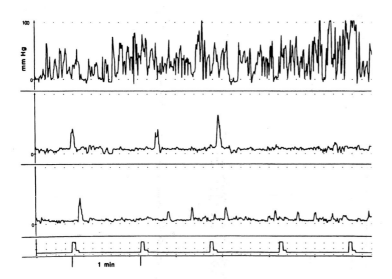

**FIGURE 15.26.** Expanded portion of a strain gauge ambulant recording of duodenal (*top tracing*) and proximal jejunal (*middle and distal tracings*) motor activity during fasting in a patient with unexplained gastrointestinal symptoms. Note the burst activity during phase 2, confined to the proximal recording site and suggestive of a neuropathic process affecting the small intestine.

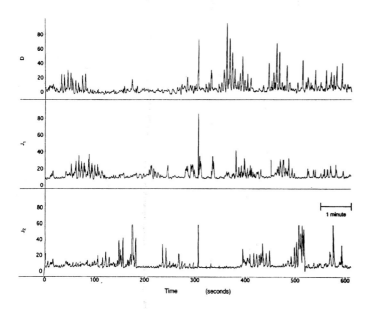

**FIGURE 15.27.** Strain gauge stationary recording of duodenal (D) and proximal jejunal ($J_1$, $J_2$) motor activity after a meal in a female patient with a history consistent with chronic idiopathic intestinal pseudo-obstruction. The fed pattern was established initially, but note the phase 3-like activity evident in this portion of the tracing and that occurred intermittently during this postprandial phase.

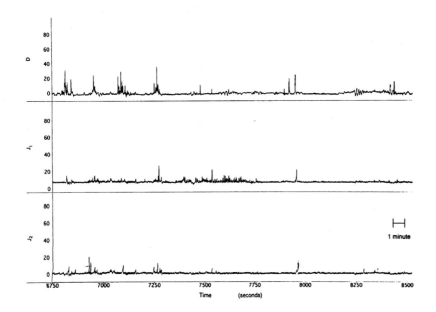

**FIGURE 15.28.** Strain gauge stationary recording of duodenal (D) and proximal jejunal ($J_1$, $J_2$) motor activity during fasting in a patient with scleroderma. Note the low-amplitude contractions especially during the phase 3 component in $J_1$, suggestive of a myopathic process affecting the small intestine.

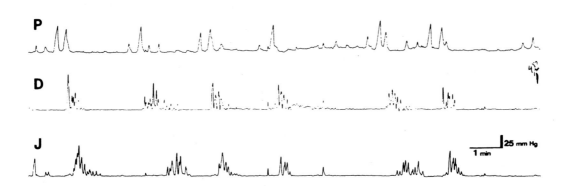

**FIGURE 15.29.** Portion of a perfused tube stationary manometric recording from the pylorus (P), duodenum (D), and proximal jejunum (J) during the postprandial state in a male patient with recurrent episodes of abdominal pain, who was subsequently shown at laparotomy to have an adhesive band obstruction in the mid-jejunum. Note the occurrence of repetitive clusters of phasic and tonic contractions of relatively high amplitude and occurring every 2 to 3 minutes.

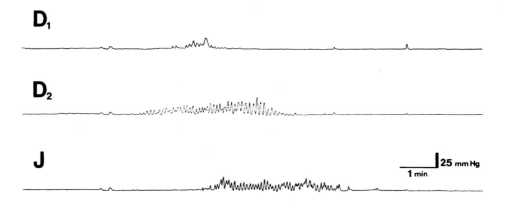

**FIGURE 15.30.** Phase 3 of the migrating motor complex recorded from the duodenum and jejunum during sleep using perfused catheter manometry in a patient with severe functional constipation. Note the low contractile amplitude, which can be present in such patients, indicating a possible myopathic process affecting the small intestine.

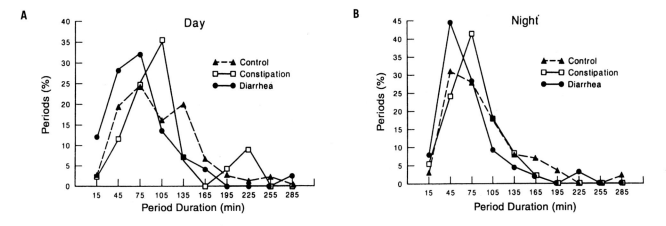

**FIGURE 15.31.** Frequency distribution (mean percent) of migrating motor complex (MMC) periods (cycle lengths) in the proximal jejunum of a group of healthy subjects (controls) and subgroups of patients with irritable bowel syndrome, predominant constipation, and predominant diarrhea **(A)** during daytime fasting and **(B)** during sleep at night. Each data point represents the midpoint of consecutive 30-minute time intervals. Note the tendency for shorter periods in the diarrhea-predominant group and for longer periods in the constipation-predominant group, during daytime only. The significance of such changes in MMC cycle lengths during periods of fasting is not known but may indicate altered central nervous system modulation.

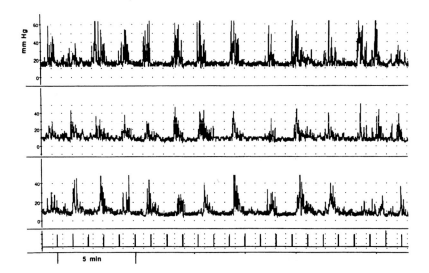

**FIGURE 15.32.** Portion of an ambulant strain gauge fasting recording from the duodenum (*upper tracing*) and jejunum (*middle and distal tracings*) in a patient with irritable bowel syndrome. Note the prominent clustered contractions present during phase 2 activity. These may occur more frequently, and in particular be of longer duration during the day, than in healthy subjects, but the significance is not known.

ty and the specificity of the alterations in motility, such as those in Table 15.2, in specific diseases have not been established, and the results of the manometric study need to be considered, particularly taking into account the other clinical information available, such as concurrent medical conditions, previous surgery, family history, medications, the physical examination, and the results of investigations involving radiology and blood testing.

## CONCLUSION

At present, small bowel manometry has a limited but important place in the array of diagnostic investigations in clinical gastroenterology. Expansion of this role, and more widespread use, will depend on continuing techno-

logical developments (manometric and computer technology), standardization of techniques and protocols internationally to obtain more definitive normal databases and determine the significance of subtle deviations from normal, and further elucidation of histopathologic and pathophysiologic correlations, including CNS/enteric nervous system interactions.

### *Acknowledgments*
The author wishes to thank Professors S.F. Phillips and D.L. Wingate for their support and encouragement and the following past and present colleagues in the Gastrointestinal Investigation Unit at the Royal North Shore Hospital in Sydney for their help, including the preparation of figures: Drs. P. Evans, Y-T Bak, Y-K Chan, E. Bennett, X-Y Gui, R. Hansen, and A. Malcolm.

**REFERENCES**

1. Szurszewski JH. A migrating motor complex of the canine small intestine. Am J Physiol 1969;217:1757–63.
2. Vantrappen G, Janssens J, Hellemans J, et al. The interdigestive motor complex of normal subjects and patients with bacterial overgrowth of the small intestine. J Clin Invest 1977;59:1158–66.
3. Thompson DG, Wingate DL, Archer L, et al. Normal patterns of human upper small bowel activity recorded by prolonged radiotelemetry. Gut 1980;21:500–6.
4. Bjornsson ES, Abrahamsson H. MMC-related duodenojejunal antegrade and retrograde peristalsis in humans. Neurogastroenterol Motil 1994;6:303–9.
5. Husebye E, Hellstrom PM, Midvedt T. The intestinal microflora stimulates myoelectric activity of rat small intestine by promoting cyclic initiation and aboral propagation of the migrating myoelectric complex. Dig Dis Sci 1994;39:946–56.
6. Kellow JE, Borody TS, Phillips SF, et al. Human interdigestive motility: variations in patterns from esophagus to colon. Gastroenterology 1986;91:386–95.
7. Husebye E, Skar V, Aalen, OO, et al. Digital ambulatory manometry of the small intestine in healthy adults. Dig Dis Sci 1990;35:1057–65.
8. Kumar D, Wingate DL, Ruckebusch Y. Circadian variation in the propagation velocity of the migrating motor complex. Gastroenterology 1986;91:926–30.
9. Kellow JE, Gill RC, Wingate DL. Prolonged ambulant recordings of small bowel motility demonstrate abnormalities in the irritable bowel syndrome. Gastroenterology 1990;98:1208–18.
10. Lindberg G, Iwarzon M, Stal P, et al. Digital ambulatory monitoring of small bowel motility. Scand J Gastroenterol 1990;35:1057–65.
11. Ouyang A, Sunshine AG, Reynolds JC. Caloric content of a meal affects duration but not contractile pattern of duodenal motility in man. Dig Dis Sci 1989;34:528–36.
12. Soffer EE, Adrian TE. Effect of meal compositon and sham feeding on duodenojejunal motility in humans. Dig Dis Sci 1992;37:1009–14.
13. Evans PR, Bak Y-T, Shuter B, et al. Gastroparesis and small bowel dysmotility in irritable bowel syndrome. Dig Dis Sci 1997;42:2087–93.
14. Samsom M, Fraser R, Smout AJPM, et al. Characterization of small intestinal pressure waves in ambulant subjects recorded with a novel portable manometric system. Dig Dis Sci 1999;44:2157–64.
15. Gill RC, Kellow JE, Browning C. The use of intraluminal strain gauges for recording ambulant small bowel motility. Am J Physiol 1990;258:610–5.
16. Omari T, Bakewell M, Fraser R. Intraluminal micromanometry: an evaluation of the dynamic performance of micro-extrusions and sleeve sensors. Neurogastroenterol Motil 1996;8:241–5.
17. Malagelada J-R, Camilleri M, Stanghellini V. Manometric diagnosis of gastrointestinal motility disorders. New York: Thieme Medical; 1986.
18. Soffer EE. Thongsawat S. Small bowel manometry: short or long recording sessions? Dig Dis Sci 1997;42:872–7.
19. Castillo FD, Benson MJ, Evans DF, et al. The intestinal datalogger: a tool for analysis of intestinal motor function. J Ambulatory Monitoring 1996;9:203–18.
20. Benson MJ, Castillo FD, Wingate DL, et al. The computer as referee in the analysis of human small bowel motility. Am J Physiol 1993;264:G645–54.
21. Michoux N, Lalaude O, Maheu B, et al. Postprandial duodenojejunal motility in health and idiopathic severe gastroparesis: from conventional analysis to nonlinear dynamic analysis. Neurogastroenterol Motil 2000;12:75–85.
22. Husebye E. The patterns of small bowel motility: physiology and implications in organic disease and functional disorders. Neurogastroenterol Motil 1999;11:141–61.
23. Remington M, Malagelada J-R, Zinsmeister A, et al. Abnormalities in gastrointestinal motor activity in patients with short bowels: effect of a synthetic opiate. Gastroenterology 1983;85:625–36.
24. Stanghellini V, Camilleri M, Malagelada J-R. Chronic idiopathic intestinal pseudo-obstruction: clinical and intestinal manometric findings. Gut 1987;28:5–12.
25. Rees WD, Leigh RJ, Christofides ND, et al. Interdigestive motor activity in patients with systemic sclerosis. Gastroenterology 1982;83:575–80.
26. Camilleri M, Malagelada J-R. Abnormal intestinal motility in diabetics with the gastroparesis syndrome. Eur J Clin Invest 1984;14:420–7.
27. Greydanus MP, Camilleri M. Abnormal postcibal antral and small bowel motility due to neuropathy or myopathy in systemic sclerosis. Gastroenterology 1989;96:110–5.
28. Camilleri M, Carbone LD, Schuffler MD. Familiar enteric neuropathy with pseudo-obstruction. Dig Dis Sci 1991;36:1168–71.
29. Samsom M, Jebbink RJ, Akkermans LM, et al. Abnormalities of antroduodenal motility in type 1 diabetes. Diabetes Care 1996;19:21–7.
30. Summers RW, Anuras S, Green J. Jejunal manometry patterns in health, partial intestinal obstruction, and pseudo-obstruction. Gastroenterology 1983;85:1290–300.
31. Camilleri M. Jejunal manometry in distal subacute mechanical obstruction: significance of prolonged simultaneous contractions. Gut 1989;30:468–75.
32. Frank JW, Sarr MG, Camilleri M. Use of gastroduodenal manometry to differentiate mechanical and functional intestinal obstruction: an analysis of clinical outcome. Am J Gastroenterol 1994;89:339–44.
33. Kellow JE, Phillips SF. Altered small bowel motility in irritable bowel syndrome is correlated with symptoms. Gastroenterology 1987;92:1885–93.
34. Kellow JE, Eckersley GM, Jones M. Enteric and central contribution to intestinal dysmotility in irritable bowel syndrome. Dig Dis Sci 1992;37:168–74.
35. Gorard DA, Libby GW, Farthing MJ. Ambulatory small intestinal motility in "diarrhea" predominant irritable bowel syndrome. Gut 1994;35:203–10.
36. Jebbink RJ, Van Berge-Henegouwen GP, Akkermans LM, et al. Antroduodenal manometry: 24-hour ambulatory monitoring versus short-term stationary manometry in patients with functional dyspepsia. Eur J Gastroenterol Hepatol 1995;7:109–16.
37. Schmidt T, Hackelsberger N, Widmer R, et al. Ambulatory 24-hour jejunal motility in diarrhea-predominant irritable bowel syndrome. Scand J Gastroenterol 1996;31:581–9.
38. Small PK, Loudon MA, Hau CM, et al. Large-scale ambulatory study of postprandial jejunal motility in irritable bowel syndrome. Scand J Gastroenterol 1997;32:39–47.
39. Wackerbauer R, Schmidt T, Widmer R, et al. Discrimination of irritable bowel syndrome by non-linear analysis of 24-hour jejunal motility. Neurogastroenterol Motil 1998;10:331–7.
40. Glia A, Lindberg G. Antroduodenal manometry findings in patients with slow-transit constipation. Scand J Gastroenterol 1998;33:55–62.
41. Haruma K, Wiste JA, Camilleri M. Effect of octreotide on gastrointestinal pressure profiles in health and in functional and organic gastrointestinal disorders. Gut 1994;35:1064–9.

# CHAPTER 16

# Scintigraphy

*Charlene M. Prather*

Scintigraphic small bowel transit measurements are typically obtained in conjunction with gastric emptying or colonic transit studies. Quantification of small bowel transit is most commonly used in the research setting to assess transit changes in response to pharmacologic manipulations. Measurement of small bowel transit may also be used clinically in the assessment of a variety of functional gastrointestinal symptoms including abdominal discomfort, bloating, and diarrhea.

Directly measuring small bowel transit has proved difficult owing to several technical challenges. The small bowel cannot be accessed noninvasively. Small bowel transit begins following emptying from the stomach. For this reason, small intestinal transit is often assessed indirectly using orocecal transit measurements, which include gastric emptying and small intestinal transit. Clinically, small bowel transit is usually assessed noninvasively by lactulose hydrogen breath testing (see Chapter 24). Lactulose hydrogen breath testing provides a measure of fasting orocecal transit time but has a few limitations. Lactulose itself can accelerate small bowel transit.[1] In addition, it is unclear how the findings of small bowel transit performed during the fasting period reflect what occurs in the fed state. An additional limitation occurs in the presence of bacteria in the upper gastrointestinal tract that metabolize the sugar, causing an artificial peak in breath hydrogen that can masquerade as rapid transit.[2] The move to using a nonabsorbable, nonmetabolized scintigraphic marker into a solid or liquid meal has been advantageous in the measurement of small bowel transit.

Several methods have been described for detecting small bowel transit. Malagelada and colleagues studied the transit of solids and liquids through the small intestine using [131]iodine-labeled fiber and [99m]technetium diethylenetriamine pentaacetic acid (DTPA)–labeled water.[3] The use of [111]indium- or [99m]technetium-labeled resin beads has also been described.[4,5] More recently, [111]indium DTPA added to water has been proposed as a simpler technique for the determination of small intestinal (and also colonic) transit.[6] For reasons of convenience, expense, radiation exposure, and isotope half-life, [99m]technetium is the isotope most commonly used for the purpose of measuring small intestine transit. This is usually performed in conjunction with measuring gastric emptying. The choice of measuring small intestinal transit of solid or liquids is a matter of preference. Solids and liquids travel through the small intestine at similar rates.[3] Thus, labeling of either the solid or liquid phase is a reasonable strategy for measuring small intestine transit.

## TECHNIQUES

Small bowel transit is performed as an extension of the usual scintigraphic gastric emptying or colonic transit study.[5,6] A variety of techniques are proposed in the literature. The techniques described here are among the most straightforward and easily reproduced.

### Liquid Small Bowel Transit

To limit the influence of gastric emptying on the small bowel transit time, the isotope is given in a liquid formulation, such as water.[6] The isotope-labeled water empties from the stomach rapidly, except in profound gastric emptying delay.[6] The patient or study subject is given 300 mL of water mixed with 125 µCi of [111]indium DTPA. Using a large-field-of-view camera with a medium-energy collimator, anterior and posterior images are obtained immediately and every 30 minutes for up to 360 minutes. Longer imaging times may be needed

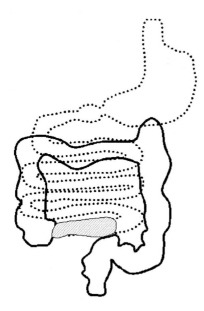

**FIGURE 16.1.** Region of the terminal ileum (*shaded area*). This is the location of relative stasis that occurs prior to emptying into the cecum. This is also the site where isotope may be identified on a scintigraphic scan for small bowel transit.

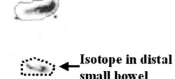

← **Isotope in distal small bowel**

**FIGURE 16.2.** Gastric emptying and small bowel transit scan of a patient with scleroderma. The scan was obtained at 4 hours and showed 50% retention in the stomach (*solid line*), which was prolonged. Small bowel transit is normal with 23% of the isotope residing in the distal ileum (*dotted line*).

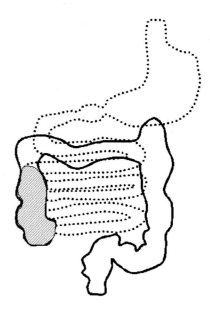

**FIGURE 16.3.** Region of the cecum and ascending colon (*shaded area*). This is the region of interest that may be identified in order to evaluate small bowel transit.

in the case of slow transit, waiting until the isotope has accumulated in the terminal ileum or cecum. To assist in later image interpretation, the addition of an external marker attached to the iliac crest may be helpful. The images are analyzed using a standard computer-based region of interest program. The ileum serves as a reservoir of relative stasis that can usually be readily identified on the scans. Regions are drawn around the distal ileum (Figs. 16.1 and 16.2). A geometric mean is taken of the anterior and posterior counts, and correction is also made for radioisotope decay.[7] Small bowel activity may be calculated by subtracting any remaining gastric counts from the total abdominal counts. The percentage of arrival of small bowel activity residing in the terminal ileum, cecum, and ascending colon at 6 hours provides a measure of small bowel transit.[6,8] Using this technique, normal small bowel transit time has been described as greater than 40% accumulation in these regions.[6] It is highly likely that significant variations in normal small bowel transit measurement occur from laboratory to laboratory because of the inter-

pretation of what constitutes a region. Determination of normal values in an individual laboratory will allow greater quality assurance in the performance of these studies.

### Solid Small Bowel Transit

Scintigraphic gastric emptying is performed more commonly than scintigraphic measurement of colonic transit. The radiolabeled meal can be followed to its arrival in the colon, providing a measure of small intestine transit. This has been described using the resin bead method of measuring gastric emptying.[5,9] The region of interest identified is the cecum and ascending colon (Figs. 16.3 to 16.5). The normal value for colonic filling at 6 hours is quite broad at 11 to 70%.[9] Normal values for small bowel transit used in conjunction with the more recently described gastric emptying technique of labeling an egg meal with $^{99m}$technetium are anticipated.[10]

Scintigraphic small bowel transit has the advantage of studying intestinal transit in the fed state without disturbing the physiologic events involved in the transit process. Some limitations exist with this technique as well. The identification of the terminal ileum or cecum may be difficult in some patients. The cecum may also overlap with the small intestine, obscuring this landmark.[11] This limitation can be overcome by analyzing time activity curves for the ascending colon and hepatic flexure.[11] Several approaches have been described for the analysis of small bowel transit using scintigraphy.[3,12,13] The ideal technique is the one that can be most reliably and readily reproduced in the individual laboratory. Among the simplest techniques, subtracting the 10% time for gastric emptying from the 10% colonic filling time or the time for 10% colonic filling may be the most practical.[8,12]

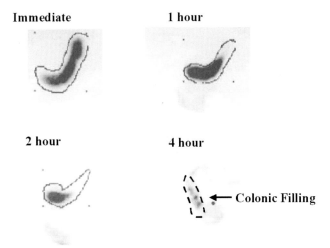

**Immediate**  **1 hour**

**2 hour**  **4 hour**

← Colonic Filling

**FIGURE 16.4.** Gastric emptying and small bowel transit study performed in a patient with abdominal bloating and discomfort. Gastric emptying is fairly rapid, with 50% retention at 1 hour, 5% retention at 2 hours, and 2% retention at 4 hours (*solid outline*). At 4 hours, filling of the colon can be seen, with 80% of the isotope residing in the colon (see Fig. 16.5). This represents rapid small bowel transit.

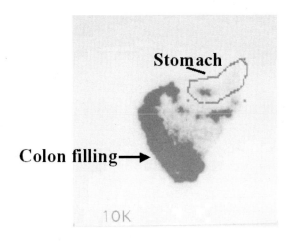

**Stomach**

**Colon filling** →

10K

**FIGURE 16.5.** The 4-hour image in Figure 16.4 after having been contrast-adjusted to show the degree of colonic filling. The cecum, the ascending colon, and the transverse colon can be readily identified. A small amount of residual radioactivity can be noted in the stomach.

Scintigraphic small bowel transit provides physiologic, quantitative information of small bowel transit. Although some centers use small bowel transit studies clinically, it is predominantly used in research studies to identify changes in response to pharmacologic manipulation. It is difficult to suggest the best scintigraphic method for measuring small bowel transit. The easiest method to adopt is likely the extension of the normal gastric emptying study with measurement of colon uptake at 4 or 6 hours. The methodologies for these techniques have been simplified, making them generally applicable for both the clinical and research laboratories. Scintigraphic small intestinal transit quantification provides

separation of normal from rapid or delayed transit.[5] This may allow more reliable targeting of therapy for patients who present with similar gastrointestinal complaints but exhibit abnormalities of transit localized to different regions of the gastrointestinal tract.

## REFERENCES

1. Miller MA, Parkman HP, Urbain JL, et al. Comparison of scintigraphy and lactulose breath hydrogen test for assessment of orocecal transit: lactulose accelerates small bowel transit. Dig Dis Sci 1997;42:10–8.
2. Rhodes JM, Middleton P, Jewell DP. The lactulose hydrogen breath test as a diagnostic test for small-bowel bacterial overgrowth. Scand J Gastroenterol 1979;14:333–6.
3. Malagelada JR, Robertson JS, Brown ML, et al. Intestinal transit of solid and liquid components of a meal in health. Gastroenterology 1984;87:1255–63.
4. Camilleri M, Colemont LJ, Phillips SF, et al. Human gastric emptying and colonic filling of solids characterized by a new method. Am J Physiol 1989;257:G284–90.
5. Charles F, Camilleri M, Phillips SF, et al. Scintigraphy of the whole gut: clinical evaluation of transit disorders. Mayo Clin Proc 1995;70:113–8.
6. Bonapace ES, Maurer AH, Davidoff S, et al. Whole gut transit scintigraphy in the clinical evaluation of patients with upper and lower gastrointestinal symptoms. Am J Gastroenterol 2000;95:2838–47.
7. Hardy JG, Perkins AC. Validity of the geometric mean correction in the quantification of whole bowel transit. Nucl Med Commun 1985;6:217–24.
8. Maurer AH, Krevsky B. Whole-gut transit scintigraphy in the evaluation of small-bowel and colon transit disorders. Semin Nucl Med 1995;25:326–38.
9. Camilleri M, Zinsmeister AR. Towards a relatively inexpensive, non-invasive, accurate test for colonic motility disorders. Gastroenterology 1992;103:36–42.
10. Tougas G, Chen Y, Coates G, et al. Standardization of a simplified scintigraphic methodology for the assessment of gastric emptying in a multicenter setting. Am J Gastroenterol 2000;95:78–86.
11. Caride VJ, Prokop EK, Troncale FJ, et al. Scintigraphic determination of small intestinal transit time: comparison with the hydrogen breath technique. Gastroenterology 1984;86:714–20.
12. Greydanus MP, Camilleri M, Colemont LJ, et al. Ileocolonic transfer of solid chyme in small intestinal neuropathies and myopathies. Gastroenterology 1990;99:158–64.
13. Read NW, Miles CA, Fisher D, et al. Transit of a meal through the stomach, small intestine, and colon in normal subjects and its role in the pathogenesis of diarrhea. Gastroenterology 1980;79:1276–82.

CHAPTER 17

# Manometry

*Gabrio Bassotti and Michael D. Crowell*

Among the hollow viscera of the human body, the colon is the least known and understood concerning its motor functions.[1] This is somewhat disappointing in that functional motor abnormalities of the large bowel (such as idiopathic constipation) are relatively frequent in the general population and may affect up to 20% of subjects.[2] Techniques have been developed (especially manometric ones) that allow recording of human colonic motility in relatively physiologic conditions for extended periods of time (24 hours or more) and obtaining information on large bowel normal motility.[3]

The main functions of the human colon are absorption (water, some electrolytes, bacterial metabolites, short-chain fatty acids), net distal propulsion of contents, and storage of fecal matter until defecation is (socially) convenient.[4] Because of the anatomic conformation, the proximal portions of the large bowel are not easy to reach, and many (if not most) data in humans have been obtained from the distal (sigmoid, rectum) portions of the viscus.[1] However, it must be stressed that these segments may not be fully representative of overall colonic motor behavior, and this is supported by the fact that proximal and distal segments of the viscus seem to display different physiologic properties.[5]

## ASSESSMENT OF COLONIC MOTILITY

Owing to the fact that, in contrast to upper gastrointestinal tract segments, the human colon moves its content in hours or days, instead of seconds or minutes, prolonged observation periods (up to 24 hours, or more) are needed.[6] Given the complexity of colonic motor activity and its anatomic conformation, it is therefore not surprising that an "ideal" technique for measuring this activity is lacking. Only pancolonic manometry has to date been used to evaluate colonic motor function over the entire length (pancolonic recordings) or over limited segments (segmental recordings) of the colon. A major difference between the two methods is that pancolonic recordings require colonoscopy for probe placement because of the length of the viscus (Fig. 17.1). Pancolonic manometry provides the most information on overall colonic motor activity and has been used as both research and diagnostic tools over recent years. The equipment used to record colonic motility is substantially similar between the pancolonic and segmental methods except for the length of the recording assembly. Both perfused and solid-state techniques have been employed for recording pancolonic and segmental activity. Once the probe has been inserted, recording is carried out for 24 hours or more to assess the wide variability of colonic motor events (see below). During the recordings, one or two meals are usually given to evaluate the response of the colon to a meal in a physiologic way: the standard protocol in our laboratory is to give two 1,000-kcal meals (lunch, dinner) and a 450-kcal continental breakfast during the study.[7]

## ANALYSIS OF THE TRACINGS

Colonic motility tracings are usually analyzed according to a general protocol involving calculation of a Motility Index (MI) in one or more segments, both basally and after physi-

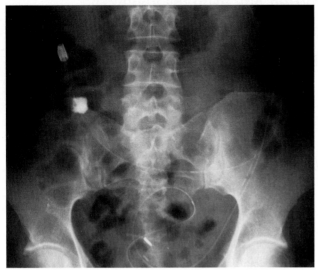

**FIGURE 17.1.** Colonoscopically positioned manometric probe in the large bowel.

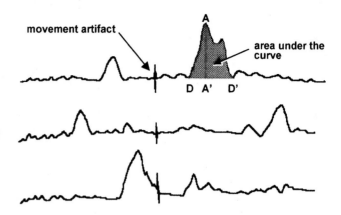

**FIGURE 17.2.** The drawing shows how a Motility Index may be calculated (manually or by computer assistance) by taking into account, for each wave, amplitude (A-A', usually expressed in mm Hg) and duration (D-D', usually expressed in seconds). An area under the curve (*gray area*) may thus be calculated, assuming a triangular shape for each wave. Movement artifacts are easily distinguished by contraction waves because of their spike-like appearance.

ologic stimuli (meals). Specific motor events (in particular mass movements) are then calculated separately. The MI may be calculated in several ways: one of the more common (also often employed in our laboratory) when making calculations is by visual analysis of appropriate wave forms and summary calculations perfomed by hand. This technique for data reduction assumes that pressure waves are triangular in shape and estimates the product of their mean amplitude multiplied by the sum of their duration for a given time period. Contractile amplitude is calculated by subtracting the mean resting colonic pressure, taken at baseline, from the peak pressure wave. Movement artifacts are easily recognized as rapid fluctuations occurring simultaneously at all recording sites (Fig. 17.2).

More recently, computerized programs have become available that allow such calculations in a more efficient (and, perhaps, reliable) fashion. Computerized scoring also allows the investigator to better recognize specific motor patterns that may occur infrequently in the colon[8]: these programs also allow for automatic calculation of the area under the curve (see Fig. 17.2). However, notwithstanding the use of an automated system, most authors still employ visual analysis to evaluate colonic motility tracings, especially for specific events (eg, mass movements), since reliable computerized systems are lacking.

## NORMAL COLONIC MOTILITY PATTERNS

Human colonic motor activity may be substantially divided in three broad categories: (1) individual contractions, (2) organized groups of phasic contractions, and (3) special propulsive contractions.[9] The first two categories represent the so-called segmental activity and the third is the propagated activity. However, to date, no standard classification

of contractile colonic events exists; hence, the same phenomenon has been defined differently by different investigators. For this reason, we have recently proposed a simple classification of these events in humans, a classification that takes into account data from myoelectrical studies and that is basically in agreement with previous radiologic descriptions (Tables 17.1 and 17.2).[10]

### Segmental Activity

These motor events represent the majority of overall daily motor activity of the human colon. Contractile amplitude generally fall, within a range of 5 to 50 mm Hg, although single waves of higher amplitude may be seen sporadically. Segmental activity may appear as single, isolated contractions (Fig. 17.3) or as small groups (bursts) of contractile waves (Fig. 17.4). The contractile patterns are usually arrhythmic, but a rhythmic frequency may occasionally be recorded (<6% of the overall daily contractile activity), especially in the sigmoid colon, where a 3 cpm frequency seems to predominate (Tables 17.3 and 17.4).[11] The regular pattern of 3 cpm has also been frequently recorded at the level of the rectosigmoid junction (Fig. 17.5), and it has

**TABLE 17.1.** Human Colonic Contractile Patterns

| |
|---|
| Segmental activity |
|     Single contractions |
|     Groups (bursts) of contractions |
|         Rhythmic |
|         Arrhythmic |
| Propagated activity |
|     Low-amplitude propagated contractions |
|     High-amplitude propagated contractions |

Adapted from Bassotti et al.[5]

**TABLE 17.2.** Contractile Events of the Human Colon and Their Putative Myoelectrical Equivalent

| Contractile Event | Other Definitions | Putative Electrical Equivalent |
|---|---|---|
| Segmental contractions | | |
|   Single | Type 1, 2, and 3 waves (Adler et al, 1941[12]; Code et al, 1952[13]) Short-duration contractions (Sarna et al, 1982[14]) | Electrical response activity (Sarna et al, 1975[15]); contractile electrical complex (Sarna et al, 1975[15]) |
|   Groups (bursts) | Long-duration contractions (Sarna et al, 1982[14]) | Continuous electrical response activity (Sarna et al, 1975[15]); short spike bursts (Fioramonti et al, 1980[16]) |
| Propagated contractions | | |
|   Low-amplitude propagated contractions | | ?Migrating long spike bursts (Fioramonti et al, 1980[16]) |
|   High-amplitude propagated contractions | Large bowel peristalsis (Hardcastle and Mann, 1968[17]); mass movements (Holdstock et al, 1970[18]); giant migrating contractions (Karaus and Sarna, 1987[19]); colonic propagating sequence (Bampton et al, 2000[20]) | Migrating long spike bursts (Fioramonti et al, 1980[16]) |

Adapted from Sarna.[9]

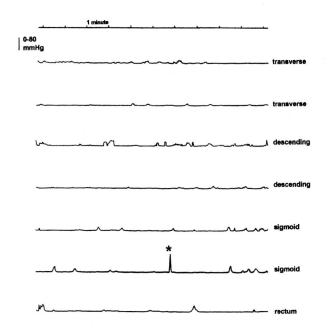

**FIGURE 17.3.** Colonic manometric tracing showing segmental activity represented by low-amplitude, isolated waves. Sporadic, higher-amplitude single contractions (*) may occasionally be observed. Recording points are spaced 12 cm apart.

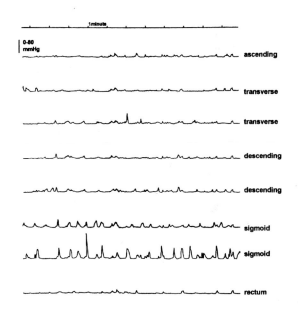

**FIGURE 17.4.** Manometric tracing obtained in the same subject of Figure 17.3, at a different time. It may be noted that, especially in the sigmoid colon, contractile activity is arranged in groups (bursts) of waves, mostly arrhythmic.

**TABLE 17.3.** 24-Hour Contractile Frequency Patterns in the Human Colon

| Cycles/min | % |
|---|---|
| 2 | 5.5 |
| 3 | 80.0 |
| 4 | 8.5 |
| 5 | 3.9 |
| 7–8 | 1.9 |

Adapted from Bassotti et al.[10]

**TABLE 17.4.** Percentage of Time Occupied by Rhythmic Contractile Patterns (in toto) Over 24 Hours in Single Colonic Segments

| | % |
|---|---|
| Ascending | 0.9 |
| Transverse | 12.4 |
| Descending | 37.5 |
| Sigmoid | 49.2 |

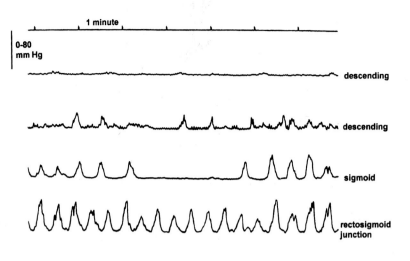

**FIGURE 17.5.** Regular colonic contractile activity in the 3 cpm range, evident at the sigmoid and rectosigmoid recording points (spaced 12 cm apart). Note how in the rectosigmoid area, this kind of activity is continuous (sometimes for long periods of time) and may represent a sort of functional sphincter, acting as a barrier toward the incoming flux of contents.

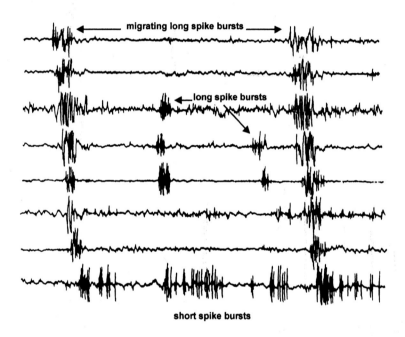

**FIGURE 17.6.** Colonic myoelectrical tracing showing the electrical equivalent of segmental contractions (short spike bursts) and propagated contractions (long spike bursts). Adapted from Fioramonti J. [Compared study of large bowel motor functions. PhD thesis.] Toulouse: Université Paul Sabatier; 1981.

been suggested to form a type of functional sphincter.[21] However, it is important to note that the percentage of time occupied by a rhythmic activity in the rectosigmoid only approaches 50% (see Table 17.4). Therefore, one should not overestimate the true incidence of regular contractile activity in colon. Segmental contractions slow colonic transit, allowing mucosal absorption that is enhanced by anatomical haustrations in the proximal segments. Combined manometric-scintigraphic recordings showed that boluses injected at the splenic flexure level may spread in both oral and aboral directions, depending on the frequency and pressure gradients between the site of the injection and that at adjacent segments.[22,23] These data support previous radiologic observations showing that segmental contractions can propel colonic contents in either direction, although generally over rather short distances.[24] Segmental contractions, in fact, may generate forward progression of contents, provided that an aborally directed pressure gradient occurs.[25]

## Propagated Activity

Contractile patterns represent a minority, albeit an important one, of the overall colonic motility. Based on contractile amplitude (which may have different pathophysiologic implications), we have arbitrarily divided propagated waves into two groups: low-amplitude propagated contractions (LAPCs) and high-amplitude propagated contractions (HAPCs). Both contractile patterns are thought to be the manometric equivalent of long spike bursts observed during myoelectric recordings, whereas segmental contractions are thought to be the equivalent of short spike bursts (Fig. 17.6).[26]

The LAPCs, which have been poorly characterized in humans, are propagated waves with amplitude ranging from 5 to 40 mm Hg (Fig. 17.7), with a daily frequency and distribution similar to that described below for higher contractions. The scarce data available on LAPCs suggest that

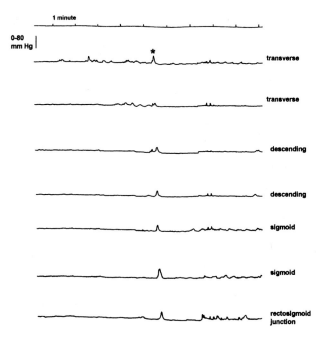

**FIGURE 17.7.** Representative manometric tracing showing a low-amplitude propagated contraction (*) running oroaborally across the colon. These waves are more frequently observed after meals and after morning awakening. Adapted from Bassotti et al.[27]

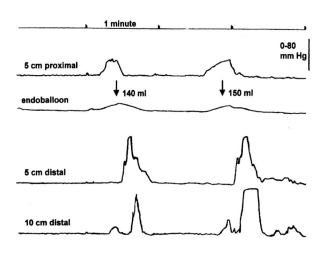

**FIGURE 17.8.** Colonic propagated contractions evoked by endoballoon distention of 140 and 150 mL of air. Colonic distention may elicit this kind of activity in more than 50% of subjects tested, suggesting that endoluminal stimuli play a role in the genesis of propulsive activity. Adapted from Bassotti et al.[29]

they occur approximately 60 times per day per subject, and the frequency increases after meals.[27] There is some evidence that LAPCs are involved in the transport of colonic contents. Supporting evidence has been reported for fluid transport,[28] during balloon distention of the viscus (Fig. 17.8),[29] and with the passage of flatus (see below).[30]

At the beginning of the century, radiologic observations in humans demonstrated an infrequent, intense propagating activity capable of shifting a discrete amount of colonic contents over a long tract of the viscus (Fig. 17.9).[31,32] This activity was subsequently confirmed and labelled as mass movements.[33] Subsequently, manometric studies have confirmed a direct relationship between "mass movements" and the HAPCs.[34] More recently, we and others have investigated and characterized these events in healthy humans through pancolonic manometry[7,35,36] and showed that (1) HAPCs represent an infrequent event in humans, appearing on average 6 times/day/subject; (2) the average amplitude of HAPCs is about 100 mm Hg, which makes them easily identifiable from the background contractions on manometric recordings (Fig. 17.10); (3) HAPC parameters are relatively constant when recorded from different colonic segments (Table 17.5) and when recorded from stationary and ambulatory techniques (Table 17.6); (4) most HAPCs propagate oroaborally; in a few subjects, about 25% of HAPCs may be observed propagating in a retrograde fashion, usually in the distal sigmoid colon, and are associated with forward-propagated events; (5) HAPCs may be associated with abdominal sensations, such as borborygmus and defecatory stimulus,

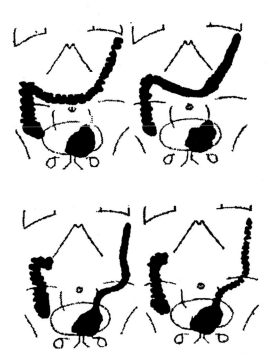

**FIGURE 17.9.** Drawing from radiologic observations of colonic "peristalsis" (subsequently defined mass movements) in man at the very beginning of the last century. It is worth noting that such an activity was observed only twice in over 1,000 radiologic examinations. Adapted from Holzknecht.[32]

and may precede defecation (see below); (6) repeated studies in the same healthy subjects have shown that HAPCs are a consistently present physiologic phenomenon[37]; (7) the diurnal and nocturnal patterns of HAPCs are directly related to physiologic events (see below).

## DAILY DISTRIBUTION OF COLONIC MOTOR EVENTS

It is well established that the human colon displays both circadian and diurnal patterns of motility (Fig. 17.11),[38] paralleled by similar changes in muscle tone. These motor patterns are influenced by specific physiologic events and by central nervous system centers. For instance, sleep exerts a strong inhibitory influence on both segmental and propagated activity (Fig. 17.12).[39] Maximal contractile activity is consistently recorded during waking hours and is directly associated with specific physiologic events (see below), whereas during the nocturnal period (and especially during the sleep), the colon is less active and often exhibits total quiescence. These observations imply that the human colon possesses a circadian pattern of motility. Diurnally, it is evident that both segmental and propulsive motor activity dramatically increase following meals and with morning awakening.

In contrast to the upper gut and the colon of some animal species (ie, the dog), the human colon does not exhibit reg-

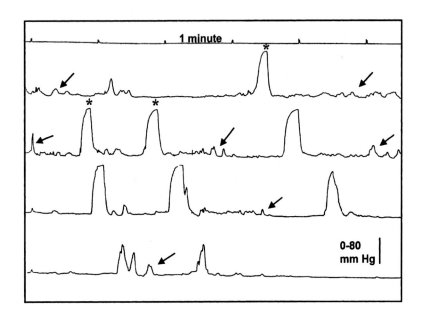

**FIGURE 17.10.** Recording of high-amplitude propagated contractions (HAPCs) in the human colon. Because of their amplitude, HAPCs (*) are easily differentiated from the more common segmental contractions, some of which are marked by arrows. Note that the HAPCs invariably propagated oroaborally. Recording points, spaced 12 cm apart, are from the proximal transverse (proximal tracing) to the mid-descending colon (distal tracing). Adapted from Bassotti and Gaburri.[35]

**TABLE 17.5.** HAPC Parameters in Single Colonic Segments

|  | Amplitude (mm Hg) | Duration (s) | Propagation Velocity (cm/s) |
|---|---|---|---|
| Ascending | 114.7 ± 6 | 15.9 ± 0.9 | 1.8 ± 0.1 |
| Transverse | 109.5 ± 6 | 14.6 ± 0.8 | 1.1 ± 0.1 |
| Descending | 117.6 ± 7 | 13.9 ± 0.7 | 1.0 ± 0.1 |
| Sigmoid | 95.3 ± 5 | 13.0 ± 0.7 | 0.8 ± 0.1 |

Values are presented as mean ± SEM.
HAPC, high-amplitude propagating contraction.
Adapted from Holzknecht.[32]

**TABLE 17.6.** Comparison of HAPC Parameters Obtained from Stationary and Ambulatory Recording Techniques

| Recording Method | HAPC/24 h | Amplitude (mm Hg) | Duration (s) | Propagation Velocity (cm/s) |
|---|---|---|---|---|
| Stationary | 6.0 ± 8.1 | 115.5 ± 6.5 | 14.5 ± 0.81 | 1.11 ± 0.10 |
| Ambulatory | 6.9 ± 1.5 | 150.5 ± 11.4* | 11.2 ± 0.88* | 1.24 ± 0.13 |

Values are presented as mean ± SEM.
*p < .05.
HAPC, high-amplitude propagating contraction.
Adapted from Crowell et al.[7]

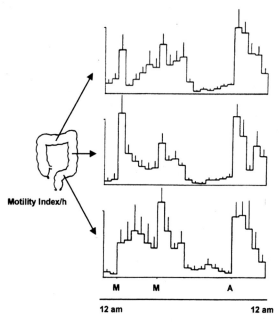

**FIGURE 17.11.** Twenty-four-hour trend of motor activity in different colonic segments (transverse, descending, and sigmoid). Note the Motility Index increase after meals (M) and awakening in the morning (A). Note also the sharp decrease of motility during the night. Adapted from Narducci et al.[38]

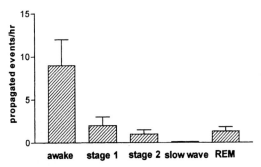

**FIGURE 17.12.** Occurrence of colonic propagated events during the night in the various stages of sleep. Awake defines periods of nocturnal wakefulness interspersed among periods of stable sleep. It is worth noting that propagated events are almost absent during slow-wave sleep. Adapted from Furukawa et al.[39]

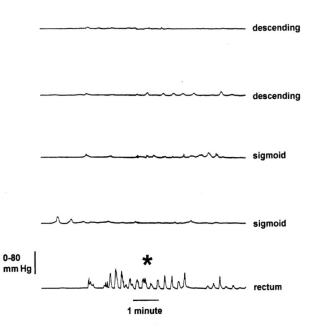

**FIGURE 17.13.** Rectal motor complex (*). Note that this type of activity appears in the rectum, displays an harmonic frequency (about 3 cpm), and is independent from other colonic segments. Adapted from Bassotti et al.[10]

ular cyclic motor patterns. However, in the rectum (and possibly in the distal sigmoid), a periodic phenomenon has been described: the rectal motor complex (RMC). The RMC consists of rectal contractions with a frequency of 2 to 3/min, with duration >3 minutes and wave amplitude >5 mm Hg (Fig. 17.13).[40] The RMC occurs independently from the migrating motor complexes in the small bowel, is not linked to motor activity of other colonic segments, and is accompanied by a rise in anal canal pressure, and its probable function is to avoid rectal stasis and preserve fecal continence, especially during sleep.

## SPECIFIC PHYSIOLOGIC EVENTS

### Colonic Motor Response to Eating

The gastrocolic and reproducible physiologic responses of the large bowel consist of a prompt (within 1–3 minutes) activation of the viscus following ingestion of a meal.[41]

This response lasts up to 3 hours in healthy subjects and is chiefly represented by segmental contractions (Fig. 17.14), although LAPCs and HAPCs also increase after meals. Postprandial motility is influenced by both the caloric content of the meal composition: fat and carbohydrates stimulate,[42] although to a different extent (Fig. 17.15), and amino acids and protein inhibit large bowel motor activity.[43] Moreover, different colonic segments respond differently with respect to a meal: the proximal segment ones display a prompt but less sustained response, suggesting a mixing and storage function, whereas the distal colon segments act more as a

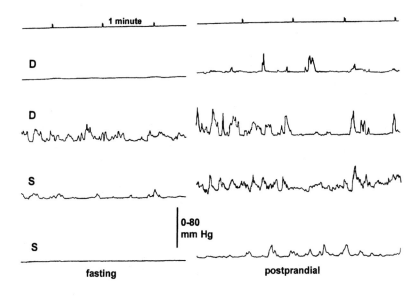

**FIGURE 17.14.** Motor response to eating (*right side of the figure*) recorded in the descending (D) and sigmoid (S) colon. Note the motor increase in all segments in the postprandial tracing, represented mainly by segmental, relatively low-amplitude contractions.

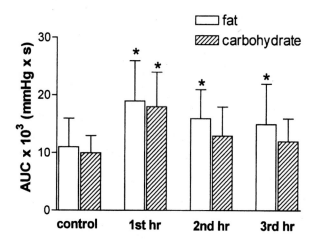

**FIGURE 17.15.** Effects of fat and carbohydrate meals on the area under the curve (AUC) in healthy volunteers. Note that both meals are able to stimulate colonic motor activity, although the effects of carbohydrate are shorter with respect to fat meals. *$p < .05$ versus control (fasting). Adapted from Rao et al.[42]

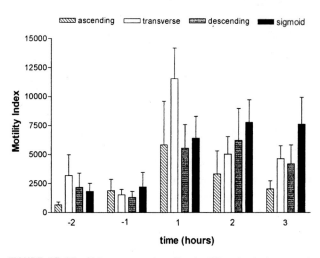

**FIGURE 17.16.** Motor response to eating in different colonic segments. Note the strong increase of the Motility Index after a 1,000-kcal standard meal, an increase that is significantly different from basal (fasting) values up to the third postprandial hour. Also note the different behavior among segments: the proximal ones (ascending and transverse) display a strong immediate response with a subsequent sharp decrease, whereas the distal ones (descending and sigmoid) have a lesser but more stable magnitude in the time course. Adapted from Bassotti et al.[44]

conduit to propel fecal matter to the rectum (Fig. 17.16).[44] In addition to the direct effects of gastric stimulation, the smell, sight, and/or taste of food may also influence colonic motor activity.[45]

## Defecation

This act is a private one and scarcely susceptible to study by physiologic means. The defecation process is two phased: the first phase is involuntary, in which colonic contents are transported toward the rectum, and the second phase is voluntary, with behavioral mechanisms that include increased intra-abdominal pressure, pelvic floor relaxation and descent, and subsequent straightening of the anorectal angle. Increased intrarectal distention and pressure leads to relaxation of the internal anal sphincter by reflex. Stools are then expelled during the subsequent, voluntary relaxation of the external anal sphincters. The majority of data on the defecatory process have been gathered indirectly using short-term recordings of anorectal motility. However, in recent years, 24-hour motility recordings from the colon have shown that defecation is often preceded (as early as 1 hour before stool expulsion) by an increase of HAPCs.[20] Additionally, coordinated motor patterns have been identified between upper colonic segments and the anorectal area, suggesting a direct link between HAPCs and relaxation of the anal sphincters after the propulsive wave sweeps contents from above (Fig. 17.17).

## Flatus

The few studies available suggest that gas transport may be mediated by LAPC, with a mechanism similar to that observed for defecation and that in some way resembles that

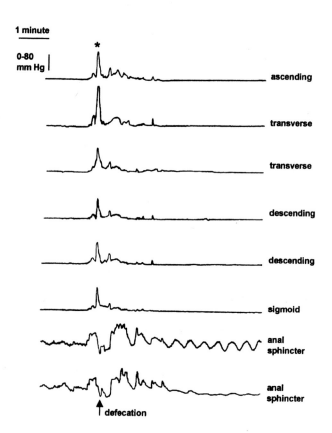

**FIGURE 17.17.** Manometrically recorded defecation. Note the high-amplitude propagated contraction (*) traveling oroaborally across the colon and the concomitant relaxation of the proximal and distal portions of the anal sphincter (*arrow*), which allows fecal contents to be expelled. Adapted from Bassotti et al.[10]

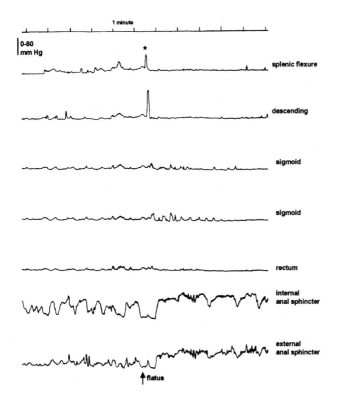

**FIGURE 17.18.** Motility events recorded during flatus emission (*arrow*). This is preceded by an oroaboral propagated contraction (*), the amplitude of which progressively decreases in the more distal colonic segments. Note the concomitant relaxation of both the internal and external parts of the anal sphincter. Adapted from Bassotti et al.[30]

**TABLE 17.7.** HAPC Parameters in Controls and Patients with Severe Idiopathic Constipation

|  | Controls | Patients |
|---|---|---|
| No./24 hours | 6.1 ± 0.9 | 2.7 ± 0.7* |
| Amplitude (mm Hg) | 110.4 ± 6.4 | 60 ± 14.2** |
| Duration (s) | 14.2 ± 0.8 | 6 ± 1.5** |
| Propagation velocity (cm/s) | 1.0 ± 0.3 | 0.74 ± 0.2 |

Values are presented as mean ± SEM.
*$p < .02$; **$p < .05$
HAPC, high-amplitude propagating contraction.
Adapted from Bassotti et al.[44]

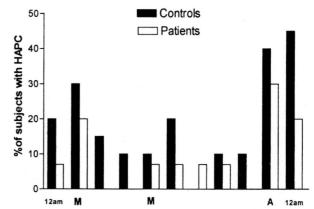

**FIGURE 17.19.** Hourly percentage of high-amplitude propagated contractions (HAPCs) displayed during 24-hour recordings of colonic motility in healthy volunteers and chronically constipated patients: the latter group had an overall significantly ($p < .05$) reduced number of events during the recording session. M, meals; A, awakening in the morning. Adapted from Bassotti et al.[46]

observed during swallowing. In fact, the coordinated motor pattern displays oroaboral LAPC associated with early relaxation of the anal sphincter (Fig. 17.18).

## COLONIC MOTILITY IN DISEASE STATES

It should be stressed that colonic manometry to date has not been established as a reliable, clinical diagnostic tool, although under specific conditions it may represent a useful adjunct for making therapeutic decisions. In spite of the lack of current acceptance as a diagnostic tool, colonic manometry is extremely valuable for understanding not only the physiology of colonic function but also the pathophysiology of colonic dysfunction.

### Chronic Constipation

Colonic manometry has been most employed clinically as an adjunct test in patients with slow transit constipation in which a surgical option is being contemplated. Studies involving relatively homogeneous groups of chronically constipated patients have yielded significant findings. First,

chronically constipated patients display, on average, a significantly reduced number of HAPCs (that also are of lesser amplitude and shorter duration), suggesting that colonic propulsive activity is impaired (Table 17.7 and Fig. 17.19).[46,47] Second, the colonic motor response to eating (ie, the gastrocolic response) in constipated patients is severely blunted or absent in all colonic segments, indicating a total dysfunction of the viscus in response to a physiologic stimulus.[48,49] In extreme cases, such as true colonic inertia, only a few contractions may be recorded from the colon during any 24-hour period.

Altered characteristics of the RMC may prove in the future to be useful for clinical diagnostics. Decreased and/or disorganized RMC patterns have been reported in patients with severe constipation and may represent abnormal neuromuscular control in the distal bowel.[50] Direct challenge of the colonic neuromuscular apparatus may provide clinically useful information. Intraluminal instillation of bisacodyl during colonic manometry has been suggested as a physiopharmacologic test to functionally assess residual propulsive activity of the large bowel in severely constipated patients.[51] Studies have demonstrated that chronically constipated patients with colons judged to be "dead" were able

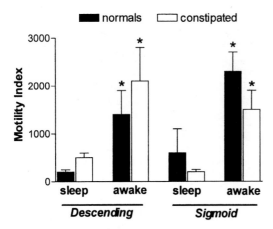

**FIGURE 17.20.** Effect of sudden awakening from sleep on descending and sigmoid colon Motility Index in healthy volunteers and in patients with chronic constipation. *$p < .05$ vs sleep. Adapted from Bassotti et al.[52]

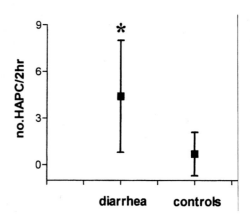

**FIGURE 17.21.** Postprandial number of high-amplitude propagated contractions (HAPCs) in patients with diarrhea and in healthy volunteers. *$p < .05$. Adapted from Choi et al.[58]

to respond to the bisacodyl challenge test, thus suggesting that residual propulsive activity was still present and a more aggressive medical treatment was needed to avoid surgery. By means of colonic manometry, it has also been possible to demonstrate that severely constipated patients have an intact motor response to sudden awakening (Fig. 17.20),[52] suggesting that the brain-gut control of some fundamental mechanisms governing colonic motility is preserved and that the motor abnormalities described in such patients may be caused by an intrinsic dysfunction of the viscus.

### Irritable Bowel Syndrome

The IBS is one of the most controversial areas among functional gastrointestinal syndromes. Although a colonic "dysmotility" has been frequently implicated as being responsible for associated gastrointestinal symptoms, a consistent motor abnormality has not been demonstrated. Although several colorectal motor abnormalities have been described in patients with irritable bowel syndrome (IBS), most are in response to direct stimulation and include an exaggerated response to eating[53,54] and emotional arousal.[55] It should be stressed, however, that these studies were mostly carried out in the distal rectosigmoid area. Unfortunately, studies throughout the colon focusing on spontaneous colonic motility are very scarce. We have recently reported a study on colonic motility in patients with IBS (constipation and alternating bowel habit subtypes) that showed (1) there were no differences with respect to controls concerning HAPC number and the Motility Index over 24 hours (MI/24 hours); however, IBS patients with constipation had a lower daily MI; (2) HAPCs and the MI were significantly reduced during sleep in both patients and controls; (3) HAPCs were significantly more frequent before as compared to after defecation; (4) HAPCs were significantly more frequent after compared to before meals.[56] These results seem to suggest that colonic motility plays a secondary role in the pathogenesis of IBS.

**TABLE 17.8.** Postprandial Propagated Contractions in Healthy Subjects and Patients with Functional Diarrhea

|  | Healthy Subjects | Patients |
|---|---|---|
| No. of contractions | 1.75 ± 3.0 (1–3) | 5.42 ± 0.8 (2–8)* |
| Onset after eating (min) | 59.20 ± 5.7 (37–82) | 23.1 ± 6.8 (4–52)* |
| Propagation velocity (cm/s) | 0.94 ± 0.2 (0.4–4.1) | 2.61 ± 0.4 (0.5–10)** |

Values are presented as means ± SD (range).
*$p < .003$; **$p < .004$.
Adapted from Niederau et al.[54]

### Chronic Diarrheal Diseases

Few studies have dealt with colonic manometry in subjects complaining of chronic diarrheal diseases. One combined manometric/scintigraphic study in subjects with functional diarrhea suggested that the overall amount of segmental contractions is reduced and that of propagated contractions are increased, especially in the postprandial period (Table 17.8).[57] A manometric/tonometric study showed that patients with diarrhea due to functional disorders or dysautonomia had no different MI with respect to controls but displayed a higher number of postprandial HAPCs (Fig. 17.21).[58]

A manometric/scintigraphic study in patients with ulcerative colitis showed that these patients have decreased colonic contractile activity overall, without significant pressure gradients among different segments, and an increased number of LAPCs that were associated with rapid movement of the scintigraphic tracer into the sigmoid colon.[59]

**REFERENCES**

1. Bassotti G, Crowell MD, Whitehead WE. Contractile activity of the human colon: lessons from 24 hour studies. Gut 1993;34:129–33.
2. Drossman DA. Idiopathic constipation: definition, epidemiology and behavioural aspects. In: Kamm MA, Lennard-Jones JE, editors. Constipation. Petersfield (UK): Wrightson Biomedical Publishing; 1994. p. 11–7.
3. Bassotti G. Manometry: why, when, and how? In: Ewe K, editor. Constipation and ano-rectal insufficiency. Falk Symposium no. 95. Dordrecht: Kluwer Academic Publishers; 1997. p. 68–74.

4. Bassotti G. Physiology of colonic motility. In: Barbara L, Corinaldesi R, Gizzi G, et al, editors. Chronic constipation. London: WB Saunders; 1996. p. 38–50.

5. Bassotti G, Germani U, Morelli A. Human colonic motility: physiological aspects. Int J Colorect Dis 1995;10:173–80.

6. O'Brien MD, Phillips SF. Colonic motility in health and disease. Gastroenterol Clin N Am 1996;25:147–62.

7. Crowell MD, Bassotti G, Cheskin LJ, et al. Method for prolonged ambulatory monitoring of high-amplitude propagated contractions from colon. Am J Physiol 1991;261:G263–8.

8. Parker R, Whitehead WE, Schuster MM. Pattern-recognition program for analysis of colon myoelectric and pressure data. Dig Dis Sci 1987;32:953–61.

9. Sarna SK. Physiology and pathophysiology of colonic motor activity. Part I. Dig Dis Sci 1991;36:827–62.

10. Bassotti G, Iantorno G, Fiorella S, et al. Colonic motility in man: features in normal subjects and in patients with chronic idiopathic constipation. Am J Gastroenterol 1999;94:1760–70.

11. Bassotti G, Bucaneve G, Pelli MA, Morelli A. Contractile frequency patterns of the human colon. J Gastrointest Motil 1989;2:73–8.

12. Adler HF, Atkinson AJ, Ivy AC. A study of motility of the human colon. An explanation of dyssynergia of the colon, or the "unstable colon." Am J Dig Dis 1941;8:197–202.

13. Code CF, Hightower NC, Morlock CG. Motility of the alimentary canal in man. Review of recent studies. Am J Med 1952;13:328–51.

14. Sarna SK, Latimer P, Campbell D, et al. Electrical and contractile activities of the human rectosigmoid. Gut 1982;23:698–705.

15. Sarna SK. Gastrointestinal electrical activity. Terminology. Gastroenterology 1975;68:1631–35.

16. Fioramonti J, Bueno L, Frexinos J. Sonde endoluminale pour l'éxploration électromyographique de la motricité colique chez l'homme. Gastroenterol Clin Biol. 1980;4:546–50.

17. Hardcastle JD, Mann CV. Study of large bowel peristalsis. Gut 1968;9:412–20.

18. Holdstock DJ, Misiewicz JJ, Smith T, et al. Propulsion (mass movements) in the human colon and in relationship to meals and somatic activity. Gut 1970;11:91–99.

19. Karaus M, Sarna SK. Giant migrating contractions during defecation in the dog colon. Gastroenterology 1987;92:925–33.

20. Bampton PA, Dinning PG, Kennedy ML, et al. Spatial and temporal organization of pressure patterns throughout the unprepared colon during spontaneous defecation. Am J Gastroenterol 2000;95:1027–35.

21. Chowdhury AR, Dinoso VP, Lorber SH. Characterisation of a hyperactive segment at the rectosigmoid junction. Gastroenterology 1976;71:584–8.

22. Moreno-Osset E, Bazzocchi G, Lo S, et al. Association between posprandial changes in colonic intraluminal pressure and transit. Gastroenterology 1989;96:1265–73.

23. Cook IJ, Furukawa Y, Panagopoulos V, et al. Relationships between spatial patterns of colonic pressure and individual movement of content. Am J Physiol 2000;278:G329–41.

24. Barclay AE. Direct x-ray cinematography with a preliminary note on the nature of nonpropulsive movements of the large intestine. Br J Radiol 1935;8:652–8.

25. Garcia-Olmo D, Garcia-Picazo D, Lopez-Fando J. Correlation between pressure changes and solid transport in the human left colon. Int J Colorect Dis 1994;9:87–91.

26. Frexinos J, Bueno L, Fioramonti J. Diurnal changes in myoelectric spiking activity of the human colon. Gastroenterology 1985;88:1104–10.

27 Bassotti G, Clementi M, Antonelli E, Tonini M. Low-amplitude propagated contractile waves: a relevant propulsive mechanism of the human colon. Dig Liver Dis 2001;33:36–40.

28. Chauve A, Devroede G, Bastin E. Intraluminal pressures during perfusion of the human colon in situ. Gastroenterology 1976;70:336–40.

29. Bassotti G, Gaburri M, Imbimbo BP, et al. Distension-stimulated propagated contractions in human colon. Dig Dis Sci 1994;39:1955–60.

30. Bassotti G, Germani U, Morelli A. Flatus-related colorectal and anal motor events. Dig Dis Sci 1996;41:335–8.

31. Hertz AF. The passage of food along the human alimentary canal. Guys' Hosp Rep 1907;61:389–427.

32. Holzknecht G. Die normale Peristaltik des Colon. Münch Med Wochenschr 1909;56:2401–3.

33. Holdstock DJ, Misiewicz JJ, Smith T, Rowlands EN. Propulsion (mass movements) in the human colon and in relationship to meals and somatic activity. Gut 1970;11:91–9.

34. Torsoli A, Ramorino ML, Ammaturo MV, et al. Mass movements and intracolonic pressures. Am J Dig Dis 1971;16:693–6.

35. Bassotti G, Gaburri M. Manometric investigation of high-amplitude propagated contractile activity of the human colon. Am J Physiol 1988;255:G660–4.

36. Lémann M, Flourié B, Picon L, et al. Motor activity recorded in the unprepared colon of healthy humans. Gut 1995;37:649–53.

37. Bassotti G, Betti C, Fusaro C, et al. Colonic high-amplitude propagated contractions (mass movements): repeated 24-h studies in healthy volunteers. J Gastrointest Motil 1992;4:187–91.

38. Narducci F, Bassotti G, Gaburri M, Morelli A. Twenty four hour manometric recording of colonic motor activity in healthy man. Gut 1987;28:17–25.

39. Furukawa Y, Cook IJ, Panagopoulos V, et al. Relationship between sleep patterns and human colonic motor patterns. Gastroenterology 1994;107:1372–91.

40. Orkin BA, Hanson RB, Kelly KA. Intermittent rectal motor activity: a rectal motor complex? J Gastrointest Motil 1989;1:5–8.

41. Bassotti G, Imbimbo BP, Gaburri M, et al. Transverse and sigmoid colon motility in healthy humans: effects of eating and of cimetropium bromide. Digestion 1987;3:163–9.

42. Rao SSC, Kavelock R, Beaty J, et al. Effects of fat and carbohydrate meals on colonic motor response. Gut 2000;46:205–11.

43. Battle WM, Cohen S, Snape WJ. Inhibition of post-prandial colonic motility after ingestion of an amino acid mixture. Dig Dis Sci 1980;25:647–52.

44. Bassotti G, Betti C, Imbimbo BP, et al. Colonic motor response to eating: a manometric investigation in proximal and distal portions of the viscus in man. Am J Gastroenterol 1989;84:118–22.

45. Rogers J, Raimundo AH, Misiewicz JJ. Cephalic phase of colonic pressure response to food. Gut 1993;34:537–43.

46. Bassotti G, Gaburri M, Imbimbo BP, et al. Colonic mass movements in idiopathic chronic constipation. Gut 1988;29:1173–9.

47. Bassotti G, Chiarioni G, Vantini I, et al. Anorectal manometric abnormalities and colonic propulsive impairment in patients with chronic idiopathic constipation. Dig Dis Sci 1994;39:1558–64.

48. Bazzocchi G, Ellis J, Villanueva-Meyer, et al. Post-prandial colonic transit and motor activity in chronic constipation. Gastroenterology 1990;98:686–93.

49. Bassotti G, Imbimbo BP, Betti C, et al. Impaired colon motor response to eating in patients with slow transit constipation. Am J Gastroenterol 1992;87:504–8.

50. Waldron DJ, Kumar D, Hallan RI, et al. Evidence for motor neuropathy and reduced filling of the rectum in chronic intractable constipation. Gut 1990;31:1284–8.

51. Bassotti G, Chiarioni G, Germani U, et al. Endoluminal instillation of bisacodyl in patients with severe (slow transit type) constipation is useful to test residual colonic propulsive activity. Digestion 1999;60:69–73.

52. Bassotti G, Germani U, Fiorella S, et al. Intact colonic motor response to sudden awakening from sleep in patients with chronic idiopathic (slow-transit) constipation. Dis Colon Rectum 1998;41:1550–6.

53. Sullivan MA, Cohen S, Snape WJ. Colonic myoelectrical activity in irritable bowel syndrome. Effect of eating and anticholinergics. N Engl J Med 1978;298:878–83.

54. Niederau C, Farber S, Karaus M. Cholecystokinin's role in regulation of colonic motility in health and in irritable bowel syndrome. Gastroenterology 1992;102:1889–98.

55. Welgan P, Meshkinpour H, Beeler M. The effect of anger on colon motor and myoelectric activity in irritable bowel syndrome. Gastroenterology 1988;94:1150–6.

56. Bassotti G, Crowell MD, Cheskin LJ, et al. Physiological correlates of colonic motility in patients with irritable bowel syndrome. Z Gastroenterol 1998;36:811–7.

57. Bazzocchi G, Ellis J, Villanueva-Meyer J, et al. Effect of eating on colonic motility and transit in patients with functional diarrhea.

58. Choi MG, Camilleri M, O'Brien MD, et al. A pilot study of motility and tone of the left colon in patients with diarrhea due to functional disorders and dysautonomia. Am J Gastroenterol 1997; 92:297–302.

59. Reddy SN, Bazzocchi G, Chan S, et al. Colonic motility and transit in health and ulcerative colitis. Gastroenterology 1991;101:1289–97.

Simultaneous scintigraphic and manometric evaluations. Gastroenterology 1991;101:1298–306.

# Barostat Measurements

*Michel M. Delvaux*

The barostat was initially designed by Azpiroz and Malagelada to evaluate the tone of a hollow organ, and the first studies were performed on the dog stomach to evaluate relaxation of the fundus.[1] Over the last decade, the barostat has been used in many studies to measure changes in the tone of hollow organs: to maintain the pressure constant in a bag placed in the organ, the barostat inflates or deflates the bag. The movements of air are thought to reflect changes in the tone of the organ.

On the other hand, a lot of attention has been paid over the last decade to visceral sensitivity and particularly to the hypersensitivity that characterizes many of the patients suffering from functional digestive disorders.[2] Following the initial report by Ritchie,[2] the barostat has been used by many investigators as a distending device to evaluate visceral sensitivity. Luminal distention is one of the most common methods to elicit visceral sensations. Although a barostat is not needed to perform distention studies, it has made those easier to design and has allowed more complete results to be obtained.

Colonic motility had mainly been studied with manometry or electromyography until the last decade.[3] From these studies, various types of colonic contractions were identified: segmental localized contractions dividing the lumen and its content into haustra to promote mixing of the digesta; propulsive contractions preceded by the disappearance of the haustral pattern, migrating distally along the colon and usually named "mass movements"; and antiperistalsis, which is the main motor activity of the proximal colon. These methods allowed the description of physiologic and pathologic motility patterns but failed to evaluate colonic relaxation and tone. The barostat has provided the means to approach these questions as it did for other digestive organs.

The purpose of this chapter is to review the technical aspects of the use of a barostat to evaluate colonic tone and explore visceral sensitivity with distention tests and to describe the current knowledge about physiologic and pathologic colonic tone and sensitivity.

## TECHNICAL DESCRIPTION OF THE BAROSTAT

The barostat consists of a pumping device controlled by a computer that maintains the pressure in the bag connected to the inflation line constant (Fig. 18.1). To achieve this, the barostat aspirates or inflates air in the bag, and the changes in bag volume reflect changes in the tone of the gut. The pumping device may either be a bellows or a syringe.[1,4]

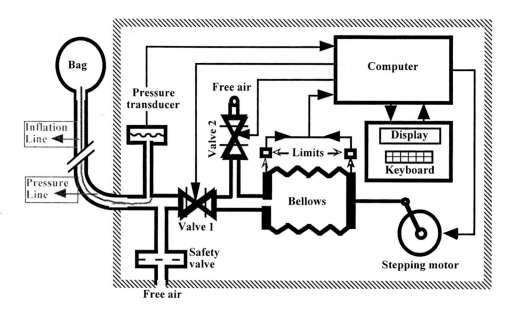

**FIGURE 18.1.** Scheme of a barostat using a bellows as a pumping device and showing the air circuit within the barostat. It is important to note that the probe attached to the barostat must ideally have distinct lines for inflation of air within the bag and measurement of the intrabag pressure. A safety valve triggered by a mechanical button allows the investigator to deflate the bag very rapidly in case of emergency.

Both have advantages and disadvantages (see Chapter 11). However, we must point out that some calculations must be performed by the system to compensate for artifacts in pressure and volume measurements. A careful calibration of the system is also mandatory. Some technical issues have recently been addressed by a group of experts in the field regarding the use of a barostat for tone and distention studies.[5]

## Tone Recording

By maintaining a low but constant pressure in the bag placed in the colon, the barostat deflates the bag and adapts it closely to the wall of the colon. Colonic bags are usually of cylindrical shape and must be large enough so that, at any time, the bag remains fully compliant to changes imposed by the barostat and does not interfere with the measurements. To achieve this goal, it is recommended to use thin polyethylene bags rather than latex balloons that heavily interfere with the response of the barostat to tone changes (Fig. 18.2). The size of the barostat bag must be adapted to the organ to be studied. For the colon, the maximal volume of the bag should not exceed 700 mL, with a maximal diameter of 10 cm and a length of about 10 cm, to not interfere with the physiologic behavior of the organ during measurements. For the rectum, spherical bags can be used with a maximal volume of 600 mL, the diameter when completely inflated being about 12 cm. Bags of such size are expected to not interfere with measurements as, in most conditions, volumes used for either tone or distention studies will not exceed the 90% of their maximal capacity and, as shown in Figure 18.2, will remain infinitely compliant.

For performing tone studies, the bag is placed in the organ and then inflated slowly with a moderate volume of 200 mL of air to unfold it. After the subject has recovered from anesthesia (if applied) and expelled excessive air from the colon (in case of colonoscopy), sessions designed to record gut tone should start with an equilibration period during which the pressure is maintained constant at the operating pressure (see below) and the volume of the bag continuously monitored until it reaches a stable baseline value. In most published reports, the time required for baseline stabilization has not exceeded 15 to 20 minutes,[6-8] except under special conditions. After this equilibration period, the proper experiment would be started.

The operating pressure is the constant pressure that will be maintained in the bag for the duration of the study. This pressure is usually established as the pressure that allows one to detect events that raise intra-abdominal pressure (eg, respiratory movements, strain, or cough).[6-8] In this case, the operating pressure should be reported, at least as a mean value for each experimental group. However, other investigators have used a standard operating pressure fixed a priori in every subject studied,[9] which is sufficiently high to keep the bag from being completely collapsed in any subject. Usual pressures are in the range of 10 to 12 mm Hg, whatever the method used for establishing them. Although a clear demonstration has not been provided that bags inflated at 10 to 12 mm Hg pressure do or do not interfere with physiologic gut motility, some studies have suggested a possible influence.[10]

Owing to significant differences in digestive motility and tone between fed and fasting states,[6,11-13] reports on barostat studies should clearly specify whether subjects were

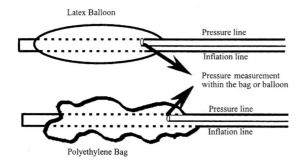

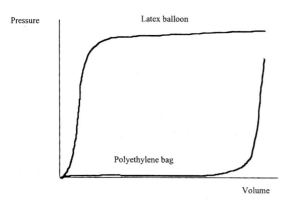

**FIGURE 18.2.** Schematic representation of a polyethylene bag and a latex balloon that can be used for distention studies. Note the separation between the pressure and the inflation lines. The shape and size of the bag or balloon have to be fixed depending on the organ studied (see Table 18.1). The chart shows theoretical compliance curves of the polyethylene bag and latex balloon when they are inflated in air. The polyethylene bag is infinitely compliant until the volume of air inflated is up to 90% of the maximal capacity of the bag. On the contrary, latex balloons are poorly compliant, and the pressure increases rapidly within them.

fasted at the time of recording. Usually, the recording session should start with the subject fasted. This baseline record should last up to 1 hour. Some authors have suggested that glucagon be administered to abolish muscle tone as a way of documenting the sensitivity of the recording system.[7] However, prolonged side effects cannot be totally ruled out even though the duration of action of glucagon is short. When a complete evaluation of tone is intended, and unless the goal of the experiment specifically prohibits such an approach, the study should include a recording of tone in both the fasting and fed states.[6,7,11-13] In some conditions, where the effect of a definite event or that of a drug is being investigated, the recording should continue at least until the baseline value is reached again.

Another major point to keep in mind when starting barostat studies for recording colonic or rectal tone is the position of the subject. There have been many reports demonstrating the importance of the subject's position during tone recording sessions.[7,11] The general guideline is to keep the balloon as close to the upper surface of the body as possible. When colonic tone was studied, a 30-degree semisupine

position was used by several authors.[6,7] When rectal tone was studied,[11] a prone position was used. The position of the subject is certainly of importance in all barostat studies because the weight of adipose tissue overlying the organ and the tone of the abdominal wall directly influence barostat recordings. Consequently, within a study, body position should be carefully standardized in all subjects.

## Distention Studies

The advantages of using a barostat as a distending device are multiple. The size of the bellows or the syringe may be adapted to the organ to distend; thus, it is possible to obtain very fast inflation of the bag, which provokes a rapid stretch of the gut wall. Because of the computer-driven inflation system, the barostat allows one to perform various types of distending protocols and to inflate the bag several times in a reproducible way. Speed of inflation, duration of the inflation, and pressure or volume limit are electronically controlled; thus, repeatability of distentions is ensured. The main advantage of the barostat is that it measures precisely both the volume and the pressure when a distention is performed. Whenever the fixed parameter defining the distention step is the pressure (isobaric distentions) or the volume (isovolumic distentions), the other parameter is measured at the same time. This is important for studying compliance of the gut wall to distention.

When studying tone, an important point is whether a balloon or a bag should be used for barostat studies. Latex balloons made from condoms have been widely used.[2,14,15] These balloons frequently have an ovoid or cylindrical form and are characterized by a rapid increase in internal pressure for small volume changes that reflect their elastic properties (see Fig. 18,2). When the pressure increases above the elastance threshold, they become plastic and may accommodate large volumes with little increase in pressure.[16] By contrast, polyethylene bags display an infinite compliance at low pressure until the volume of air within the bag is equal to the volume of the bag itself. Thereafter, any further increase in volume will induce a rapid increase in internal pressure.[6,7,11] In distention studies, the bag or the balloon must not interfere with the measurements of volume (or pressure when thresholds are defined by the volume) needed to reach a given pressure level and not modify the pressure-volume relationship (compliance). For this reason, it has been recommended that a bag be used instead of a balloon.[5]

The bag must be oversized, based on the organ to be distended. The volume capacity of the bag must be greater than the largest volume of air to be injected. At volumes greater than 90% of its maximal capacity, the bag will interfere with pressure and volume measurements. Moreover, the diameter of the bag must be larger than the maximal diameter of the gut segment being tested. The form of the bag should also be adapted to the organ. For studies in the rectum,[11] it is advisable to use bags that, when inflated, conform to a spherical shape. For tubular regions of the gastrointestinal tract, such

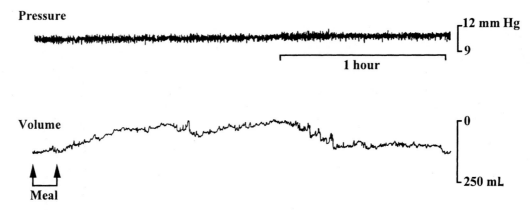

**FIGURE 18.3.** Colonic response to eating showing an increase in colonic tone recorded with a barostat bag placed in the left colon. The 1,000-calorie meal induces a sustained increase in tone, marked by a decrease of the barostat bag volume down to nearly zero during at least 2 hours. Notice the very fast onset of the response after the meal. Record obtained in a healthy male volunteer.

as the colon,[6] cylindrical bags with a fixed length should be used (ie, the bag should be attached to the probe at both ends to avoid any appreciable change in length during inflation).

## STUDIES OF COLONIC TONE

### Colonic Tone in Physiologic Conditions

Colonic muscle maintains a continuous tone, which may vary in physiologic conditions, such as the postprandial period. When a barostat bag is placed in the left colon in humans, the volume at operating pressure ranges between 50 and 150 mL.[6,7,11] During the fasting state, balloon volumes are generally constant; small fluctuations in volume are not accompanied by phasic contractile activity.[7]

After a meal, the volume of a barostat bag placed in the left colon consistently decreases. The decrease in bag volume, which corresponds to an enhanced colonic tone, occurs 5 to 20 minutes after the beginning of the meal and lasts up to 3 hours (Fig. 18.3).[6,7] In the study by Steadman et al,[7] filling the stomach with water failed to enhance colonic tone. During nocturnal sleep, colonic tone seems to be decreased as the bag volume may increase up to 60% above the baseline diurnal volume. In this study, colonic tone increased again after awakening. Like colonic tone, rectal tone increases after a meal.[11]

Variations in colonic tone recorded in physiologic conditions correlate with those of contractile phasic activity that is recorded by manometry or electromyography. However, the components of phasic contractile activity that are responsible for tone changes in the colon are not known. Using atropine, which inhibits both the phasic and tonic activities of the colon, it was suggested that tone might be related to the occurrence of stationary contractions seen as short spike bursts of action potentials in the left colon,[17] but this observation has not been confirmed by further studies. In another study,[7] atropine inhibited both the baseline and

the postprandial tonic activities of the colon, but no correlation was made with manometric recordings.

Colonic tone, however, seems not to change in a similar way along the whole colon. In a study performed in healthy volunteers, the postprandial increase in tone was more pronounced in the transverse than in the sigmoid colon.[18] By contrast, the phasic contractile activity was significantly stronger in the sigmoid than in the colon in the postprandial state. Interestingly, this study also showed that the fasting volume of the colon was significantly correlated with the magnitude of the tonic response to a meal. Regional differences in colonic tone have been further studied in healthy volunteers.[19] This study showed that the postprandial tonic response of the colon was much more marked in the distal than in the proximal colon (cecum and ascending colon). In some subjects, a postprandial relaxation of the proximal colon could even be observed.

Physiologic stimuli of the tonic-colonic response to eating are not entirely understood. As shown by Steadman et al,[7] the energy content of the meal is important as well as the volume in determining the tonic-colonic response to eating. Cholecystokinin seems not to play a major role as it relaxed both the proximal and distal colon in healthy volunteers but had divergent effects, stimulating phasic contractile activity in the distal colon and inhibiting it in the proximal colon.[20] Relaxation of the proximal colon could be understood as an adaptive response to the arrival of chyme in the ileocecal region. However, in a study performed in dogs, it was shown that tone increases in response to a meal in the proximal colon.[12] Tone is also enhanced when nutrients or even saline is perfused in the distal ileum, indicating that the late response to food is at least partly attributable to stimulation by intraluminal content in the dog. Mediators of the tonic-colonic response to eating are not known precisely. In a study in healthy volunteers, ondansetron, a 5-hydroxy-tryptamine (5-$HT_3$) antagonist, was able to inhibit the tonic response, as well as the phasic contractile activity of the colon to a high-energy meal, indicating that a serotonin-dependent pathway is involved.[13] A recent study did not show any significant difference in the intensity of the tonic-colonic response to a meal between males and females.[21]

### Colonic Tone in Diseases

The responsibility of changes in colonic tone in the pathophysiology of digestive diseases has not yet been clearly established. Studies that have evaluated the role of abnormal tonic motility of the colon are very few. Most of the attention has been paid to irritable bowel syndrome since these patients have been studied frequently in distention studies for evaluation of visceral perception. Studies comparing patients with IBS and healthy controls have up to now failed to demonstrate specific abnormalities of colonic tonic motility. Patients with IBS, whatever their bowel disturbances, show similar tonic motility of the colon as healthy subjects.[6,22] Tonic response to a meal seems to be preserved.

A clear demonstration of an abnormal tonic motility of the colon has been obtained only in patients with carcinoid diarrhea, who show a baseline hypertony and an exaggerated tonic response of the colon to a meal.[23] This enhanced postprandial response of the colon was inhibited by the 5-HT$_3$ antagonist ondansetron, which returned the response to values observed in healthy subjects.[24] On the other hand, in a group of patients with functional diarrhea or diarrhea associated with dysautonomia, the colonic response to eating was found to be reduced as compared with controls, and there was no significant change in baseline volume of the barostat bag.[25] The limited information available does not allow any conclusion regarding the changes of colonic tone that might be involved in the pathogenesis of diarrhea.

Likewise, no significant change could be shown in patients with chronic constipation. Comparing healthy controls and patients with slow transit time constipation, normal transit time constipation, or outlet obstruction, O'Brien and colleagues did not find any significant change in the tonic motility patterns of the left colon at baseline or in the postprandial period.[26] These authors concluded that barostat studies did not help in the management of patients with chronic constipation. This observation is in agreement with other reports from studies of patients with IBS and constipation, which did not show any significant change in baseline volume of the barostat bag or in the intensity and duration of colonic tonic response to a meal from controls.[6]

Colonic tone is also influenced by central nervous system lesions. Studying two patients with spinal cord injury, Bruninga and Camilleri showed that baseline barostat bag volumes were similar to those recorded in healthy subjects, whereas the postprandial increase in tone characterizing the colonic response to eating was markedly impaired in patients.[27] On the contrary, local injury to the colonic wall (ie, the creation of a surgical anastomosis) leads to an increase in tone that is marked on the first 3 days after the surgical procedure,[28] indicating that postoperative hypertony of the colon might be at least partly involved in postoperative ileus. In this study, hypertony was associated with an increase in phasic contractile activity of the colon.

## DESIGN OF STUDIES FOR EVALUATING COLONIC SENSITIVITY

Over the last decade, the considerable interest that has been raised for studies on visceral perception has also included the evaluation of colonic perception. In this chapter, we revise the design of such studies to help investigators in designing their studies and then summarize the current knowledge about hypersensitivity to distention, which has been recognized as a frequent characteristic of patients with IBS.[3]

### Technical Parameters Influencing Sensitivity Studies

The distention protocol may considerably affect the results of visceral perception studies. The pressure or volume defining a sensory threshold and subsequently the concept of hyperreactivity or hypersensitivity to distention will be influenced by the method of distention.[5]

When the barostat is used to perform luminal distention of a digestive segment, the first parameter to fix is whether the level of distention will be defined according to the pressure level reached in the bag (isobaric distentions) or to the volume of air present in the bag (isovolumic distentions). Some problems may arise with volume-scaled stimuli. Volume is not linearly related to balloon diameter or pressure because (1) air is being inflated into a bag of approximately cylindrical shape in most cases, (2) air is compressible, (3) small variations in bag shape and dimensions may affect the measurements and dimensions of the bag and thus affect the pressure-volume relationship, and (4) the volume is, to some extent, influenced by the anatomy of the subject. Therefore, balloon or bag pressure is more reproducible between laboratories and between subjects because the pressure scale compensates for the different factors possibly influencing the volume of the bag: bag shape, gut wall compliance, contractile activity, and subject's anatomy. Thus, it is recommended to define sensory thresholds by the distending pressure. Bias described here may interfere more with measurements performed in the rectum.

Various distention protocols have been proposed. They are mainly based on the use of two different types of stimuli: the continuous, progressive, and cumulative distention (ramp distention) and the intermittent, rapid, time-limited distention inducing an abrupt stretch of the gut wall (phasic distention). Using these different protocols (Fig. 18.4), some authors have reported variations in subject's responses elicited by luminal distention. Comparing ramp distention to phasic distention, Mayer and coworkers found that hypersensitivity to rectal distention characterizing patients with IBS was triggered only by phasic distention.[29] In another study reporting results obtained with two types of distention (rapid phasic

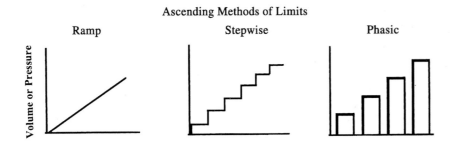

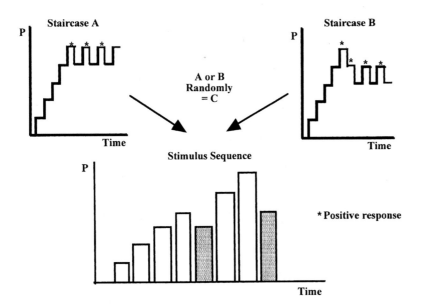

**FIGURE 18.4.** Schematic representation of the most common distention protocols. The advantages and disadvantages of these protocols are discussed in Table 18.1.

distention and cumulative stepwise distention), the pain threshold elicited by rapid phasic distention was significantly lower than the one elicited by stepwise distention.[6] This observation may suggest that different afferent nerve pathways are triggered by the various types of distention, but a role for distinct mechanoreceptors or for multisensitive nociceptors within the gut wall has not been ruled out.[30]

Although ramp or phasic distention may be used in distention studies depending on the question to be addressed, it is important to know that some sensory test protocols (eg, double random staircase or signal detection) can be done only with phasic distentions. As a general recommendation, when phasic stimuli are used, the duration of distention steps has to be at least 60 seconds and the interval between steps also equal to or higher than 60 seconds. In case of phasic distentions, the subject's sensations will not be recorded immediately after the onset of the pressure in the balloon since the time required for wall adaptation may be 3 to 5 seconds and reflex contractions may occur during 10 to 20 seconds after onset of inflation.[31]

Sensory thresholds are higher for rapid inflation than for slow inflation rates,[32] and the differences between patients with IBS and healthy controls are greater for rapid than for slow distention.[29] Rates up to 40 mL/s are able to efficient-

ly compensate for changes in balloon pressure associated with coughing or other movement artifacts. Whatever rate of inflation is chosen, it should be constant for all distention steps in one experiment. This will have the effect that distentions at higher pressure levels require longer to reach the target pressure (or volume), but this is preferable to inflating at different rates to fix the duration of inflation.

## Protocols of Distention for Evaluation of Colonic Sensitivity

The response of the subject to distention of the rectum or the colon may be influenced by his past experience and psychological factors such as the fear of pain, which are collectively called response bias. Therefore, some distending protocols were designed to eliminate these biases.

Ascending limits protocols are based on the progressive increase in intensity of the distending stimulus, using either ramp, stepwise, or phasic distention, until the subject reports pain or another sensation of interest (see Fig. 18.4). The assumption underlying the "ascending method of limits" is that pain is qualitatively different from other sensations produced by distention and that there is a discrete threshold at which pain is first experienced. This method is believed

**TABLE 18.1.** Advantages and Disadvantages of the Various Distention Protocols

| Method | Definition | Advantages | Disadvantages |
|---|---|---|---|
| Ascending method of limits | Each distention larger than last until subject reports pain | Simple, few trials | Vulnerable to psychological bias; stimuli are predictable; only one judgment depicts thresholds |
| Random sequence | Random series; subject rates each distention | Less psychological bias; sequence is unpredictable; relatively few trials | Impossible to use because some distentions would be too painful; must use pseudorandom sequence, approximating ascending limit method |
| Tracking technique | After each pain report, next distention is randomly same or lower; after each report of no pain, next distention is randomly same or higher | Sequence is unpredictable; threshold is based on multiple judgments | Requires large number of distentions (up to 45 trials) |
| Double random staircase | In staircase A, distention decreases after every pain report and increases after report of no pain; staircase B works in the same way; computer randomly alternates A and B | Sequence is unpredictable; threshold is based on multiple judgments | Requires large number of distentions (up to 30 trials) but fewer than tracking |

to be maximally sensitive to psychological biases, especially the fear of pain, because stimuli are predictable to the subject. In addition, the patients' learning history may influence where on the continuum of stimulus intensity they report pain. Therefore, the thresholds recorded using this method seem less reliable, and it should not be recommended. However, in our point of view, the ascending limits method has some advantages, including its simplicity and the smaller number of presentations of the stimulus, and it has recently been proven reproducible in carefully controlled double-blind studies.[33,34]

Various protocols have been designed to circumvent the problem of response biases. They are based on the presentation of multiple stimuli to the subject using a random order or jumping randomly from one technique of tracking the response of the subject to another one. This latter method is called the "double random staircase." One may even make the sequence of stimuli unpredictable to the investigator when the computer program determines this sequence, based on the response of the subject, without any intervention of the investigator. We must emphasize that, independently of the protocol used, the trial must start with an ascending limits method phase to detect the pressure (or volume) threshold at which the subject will report pain or discomfort. This is mandatory to detect the pain threshold and avoid inflation of the bag at pressures higher than during the second part of the trial. Then multiple stimuli are presented around this threshold pressure to assess the reliability of the subject's response. Finally, the threshold pressure is defined as the mean intensity of the thresholds eliciting the sensation of interest.

Signal detection uses two stimuli of rather similar intensity so that most of the subjects cannot distinguish between them without making mistakes. The stimuli are presented numerous times in random order (up to 200 in some studies on somatic perception). The number of times the stimuli have

qualified as painful or nonpainful are counted.[35] One practical problem with these protocols is that it is difficult to fix the distention pressure to be used during the test. If the same distending pressure is used for all of the subjects, some will report only nonpainful sensations, whereas some others will report only painful ones. Therefore, a search for pain threshold by an ascending limits protocol is needed beforehand.

One could summarize the problem of choice of a distending protocol with the following statements:
- Multiple distentions at each pressure or volume step yield more reliable estimates of sensory thresholds. However, practical considerations may limit the number of trials that can be presented.
- For measuring the threshold for urgency, discomfort, or pain, the ascending method of limits is frequently used but is more vulnerable to psychological influence on sensory reports.

The advantages and disadvantages of the various distention protocols are summarized in Table 18.1.

### Evaluation of Compliance

Compliance is the capacity of a hollow organ to adapt to the imposed distention. It is defined as the ratio dV/dP, which characterizes the derived function of the pressure-volume curve and is expressed in mL/mm Hg$^{-1}$ when isobaric distentions are performed (Fig. 18.5). To evaluate compliance, one needs to measure the volume of the distending bag at each pressure step, build the pressure-volume curve, and calculate the slope of this curve, which represents the compliance. The shape of the pressure-volume relationship may be considerably different, depending on the studied organ. It is usually linear in the range of the intermediate pressure steps but may show inflection points at lower or higher pressure steps.[6,15,34,36]

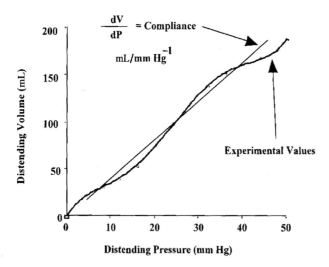

**FIGURE 18.5.** Theoretical pressure-volume curve observed when the colon is distended by a polyethylene bag. The first derived function of the curve dV/dP is a straight line. The compliance corresponds to the slope of this line and is expressed in mL/mm Hg$^{-1}$.

Compliance is influenced by many factors, including the tone of the organ, contractile activity, and surrounding anatomy. It may also be influenced by the elastic properties of the distending device (barostat + probe and bag). As already mentioned, polyethylene bags and latex balloons behave quite differently when inflated in air. Latex balloons are poorly compliant and dramatically influence the compliance measurements, so that when latex balloons are used, the compliance of the system must be carefully evaluated in air before performing distention studies and then subtracted from the compliance measured during distention sessions. On the contrary, polyethylene bags are extremely compliant if they are oversized as compared to the range of volumes to be used during distention studies, so that the maximal distending volume never exceeds 80% of the maximal capacity of the bag.

Evaluation of compliance is important when one compares the sensitivity of an organ in different experimental conditions (eg, in fasted versus fed state or on placebo or a drug that is thought to modify sensory thresholds). Changes in compliance may then explain variations of volumes observed during isobaric distentions.[37] Changes in compliance may also interfere with the results of studies comparing thresholds detected by isovolumic distentions under various conditions. The slopes of pressure-volume curves need to be carefully compared in such cases to rule out changes in compliance before concluding a change in sensory thresholds.

On the other hand, the absence of changes in compliance while pressure thresholds are significantly different between various experimental conditions or between various groups of subjects indicates that these changes are related to modifications of sensory pathways and not to changes in elastic properties of the wall of the organ.

## COLONIC AND RECTAL DISTENTION TESTS IN THE IRRITABLE BOWEL SYNDROME

Over the last decade, studies on colonic sensitivity have widely used distention tests to evaluate the changes in perception of painful and nonpainful sensations in patients with IBS. These studies have established the role of visceral hypersensitivity as one of the pathophysiologic characteristics of the condition. Hypersensitivity of the gut to distention was suggested 27 years ago by Ritchie, who showed that patients with IBS experienced pain at lower distending volumes during rectal distention than controls.[2]

### Pathophysiology of Visceral Hypersensitivity in Patients with IBS

In another study, pain thresholds elicited by rectal distention were much lower in patients with functional diarrhea than in constipated patients, suggesting an influence of colonic transit on visceral perception.[30] Colonic hypersensitivity has also been observed in patients with constipation-prone IBS,[6,15,29,34] and the lowered pain threshold observed in these patients could be normalized up to the distending pressure required to induce pain in controls by octreotide.[39]

As in the colon, visceral hypersensitivity has been observed when distending the jejunum in patients with IBS as compared to controls.[40] It has recently been shown by Francis and colleagues that in patients with IBS, hypersensitivity to distention was a diffuse disorder involving the esophagus, various segments of the small intestine, the colon, and the rectum.[41] The pathophysiology of visceral hypersensitivity in patients with IBS remains controversial. Some authors have claimed that it could be related to a default in relaxation of the colonic wall resulting in an increase in parietal tension when a contraction occurs and in a subsequent stimulation of parietal mechanoreceptors. However, Whitehead and colleagues have simultaneously recorded colonic phasic activity by manometry and distended the colon by a balloon and have shown that abdominal pain was induced by distention in the absence of any alteration of colonic motility.[15] This observation was confirmed by studies performed with the barostat, which concluded that colonic compliance (ie, the elastic properties of the colon) was not different in patients with IBS and in controls.[6,16] These results suggest that the primary disorder responsible for the visceral hypersensitivity in patients with functional bowel disorders could be located on visceral afferents. However, the exact level of this abnormality has not yet been defined. Recently, it was suggested that patients with diarrhea-predominant IBS would show a lower compliance to distention than controls and patients with constipation-prone IBS.[42] However, this observation made at the rectal level must be interpreted cautiously as patients with diarrhea may have interference of continence feelings with painful sensations that might interfere with the measurements during distention studies.

Experimental data have been published supporting the involvement of peripheral afferents in the pathophysiology of visceral hypersensitivity in IBS. As already said, octreotide restores sensory thresholds to colonic distention in patients with IBS without modifying colonic compliance[39,44] and decreases the intensity of cortical and spinal evoked potentials.[46] Comparison between electrical stimulation of jejunal afferents and mechanical distention of the jejunum to induce an intestino-intestinal reflex in patients with IBS and healthy volunteers has shown that only thresholds of pain perception triggered by mechanical distention were lower in IBS than in controls, whereas perception of electrical stimulation was rather similar in both groups.[46] This observation suggests that the primary disorder could be located at the level of parietal mechanoreceptors themselves. On the other hand, comparing patients with IBS, controls, and patients with a section of the lumbar spinal cord, Lembo and colleagues have assumed that the primary disorder explaining visceral hypersensitivity in patients with IBS might be located at the level of splanchnic lumbar afferents.[29]

Finally, attention has also been paid to the role of the central nervous system (CNS) in visceral hyperalgesia observed in patients with IBS. The initial reports used models of stress to demonstrate the influence of the CNS. Indeed, healthy subjects submitted to a stress, either physical or psychological, showed hypersensitivity to rectal distention,[47] and this effect lasted at least 2 hours after the end of the stress itself. More recently, Mönnikes and colleagues showed that the effect of stress on perception of rectal distention was different in healthy volunteers and patients with IBS.[48] Whereas healthy volunteers were distracted by application of a psychological stress and reported pain at higher pressure than during baseline distention, patients with IBS did not show any difference under stress and baseline conditions and were always more sensitive to distention than healthy controls. This observation suggests that patients with IBS might be hypervigilant to abdominal sensations. Such hypervigilance has been further suggested by studies made with the new brain imaging techniques.[49] In this study, the cortical areas stimulated by the perception of painful rectal distention were different in patients with IBS and controls, but one of the main observations was that this difference correlated with an anticipation phenomenon in patients with IBS that might partly explain the observation of lowered thresholds. However, studies on brain imaging are too recent to draw firm conclusions about the regions of the cortex that are stimulated by rectal or colonic distention, and recent reports have brought contradictory results.[50]

## Factors Influencing the Perception of Rectal and Colonic Distention

Sensory thresholds measured during distention studies are influenced by several factors, inside and outside of the colon, that need to be carefully controlled during any study.

These factors may sometimes explain the differences observed between studies.

Elastic properties of the colonic wall certainly have an influence on the perception of distention, but their actual role in hypersensitivity is not understood. In conditions that modify the tone of the colonic wall, thresholds have been different, both in healthy subjects and in patients with IBS. When the tone is enhanced by the response to a meal, sensory thresholds have been found higher than at baseline.[51] By contrast, relaxation of the rectal wall with glucagon has not been shown to alter the sensory thresholds elicited by luminal distention.[52]

Subjects' characteristics also influence the results of distention studies. Sensory thresholds, perception and pain, increase with age in healthy subjects.[53] The influence of gender on sensory thresholds has been discussed for several years. Previous reports have suggested that women were more sensitive than men to rectal distention.[54] However, in a recent study, no difference was seen between males and females in the perception of rectal distention.[55] Differences owing to gender, however, have recently been confirmed by a study including rectal distention tests and brain imaging.[50] The results of these studies must be carefully analyzed as anatomic differences between genders may affect the results of studies using volume-scaled stimuli. As described above, the activity of the central nervous system influences the perception of rectal distention. Stress and arousal may have different effects.[56] More important is the link that has been shown between the intensity of IBS-related symptoms and the sensory thresholds measured during distention studies. In a study of about 25 patients with IBS undergoing rectal distention at 6-week intervals, the sensory thresholds were elevated when symptoms improved.[36] This observation shows that hypersensitivity to rectal distention is not permanent in patients with IBS; thus, it is currently impossible to propose distention tests in clinical practice for the diagnosis of IBS.

## Pharmacologic Modulation of Colonic Sensory Thresholds

The advances in knowledge about the functioning of digestive afferents have allowed the identification of many neurotransmitters involved in the processing of information along these nerve pathways.[57] On the other hand, the possibility of performing distention studies with a good reproducibility of sensory thresholds has led some investigators to evaluate the effect of drugs on visceral sensitivity. Somatostatin has been studied in many trials, which have shown that it was able to increase sensory thresholds during rectal[46,58] and colonic[39] distention. Moreover, somatostatin decreases the intensity of evoked potentials triggered by electrical stimulation of the rectal wall.[45] This observation suggests that somatostatin could act directly on peripheral afferent pathways.

The second class of compounds that has been evaluated over the last decade is the group of 5-HT$_3$ antagonists. The 5-HT$_3$ receptors are one of the best known examples of recep-

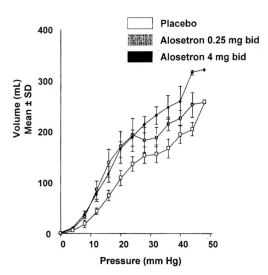

**FIGURE 18.6.** Effect of alosetron on colonic compliance evaluated as the slope of the pressure-volume relationship established from measurements performed during phasic distention of the left colon, with a barostat, in patients with IBS. Reproduced with permission from Delvaux M, Louvel D, Mamet JP, et al. Effect of alosetron on responses to colonic distension in patients with irritable bowel syndrome. Aliment Pharmacol Ther 1998;12:849–55.

**TABLE 18.2.** Substances Proven Effective in Altering Sensory Thresholds

Results of human studies
    Somatostatin (octreotide)
    5-HT$_3$ antagonists: granisetron, alosetron, cilansetron
    Kappa-opioid agonist: fedotozine
    Oxytocin
    Dopamine-2 antagonists: levosulpiride
    β3-Adrenergic agonist (SR 58611)
    Antidepressants: amitriptyline
    Spasmolytics: trimebutine
Indications from animal studies
    Cholecystokinin antagonists (?)
    5-HT$_4$ agonists
    Antagonists of tachykinin receptors: NK1, NK2
    Bradykinin (under special conditions?)

5-HT, 5-hydroxytryptamine.

tors involved in the activation of peripheral afferents for the processing of information originating from both somatic[59] and digestive afferents.[60,61] In the same way, 5-HT$_3$ receptors are involved in visceral reflexes triggered by rectocolonic distention in animals with chemically induced experimental colitis.[60] In humans, granisetron increases the thresholds of visceral perception induced by rectal distention in patients with IBS.[37] Alosetron, another 5-HT$_3$ antagonist, has also been shown to influence perception of colonic distention in patients with IBS.[62] However, the effect of alosetron did not modify the pressure thresholds elicited by distention of the left colon but the volume of the barostat bag at thresholds, indicating a modification of colonic compliance induced by the drug (Fig. 18.6). Alosetron has been shown effective in treating female patients with diarrhea-predominant IBS, the main result being expressed as a global improvement, including diarrhea and abdominal pain.[63] However, alosetron has recently been withdrawn from the American market because of side effects resulting in colonic obstruction owing to slowing in transit and several cases of ischemic colitis.

Recently, we have also shown that fedotozine, which acts peripherally as an agonist of kappa-opioid receptors, was able to inhibit the hypersensitivity of patients with IBS to colonic distention.[34] Fedotozine has also been shown to improve the abdominal symptoms of patients with IBS.[64] Moreover, in animals, fedotozine was shown to affect viscero-visceral reflexes, indicating that it could act on afferent pathways.[65] On the other hand, fedotozine does not alter the compliance of the colonic wall.[34]

Among the other drugs acting on sensory thresholds, we have shown that oxytocin acts on sensory thresholds in a cut-off manner, independent of the dose.[66] Recently, we have obtained experimental evidence that the effect of oxytocin is not mediated through a release of enkephalins since it is not inhibited by naloxone.[66] Other compounds are expected to act on perception of colonic distention in patients with IBS, but the results of ongoing experiments have not been published so far. Table 18.2 summarizes the classes of compounds that might be of interest in this indication.

## CONCLUSION

The barostat has been widely used over the last 5 years to explore the sensitivity of the gut to luminal distention. The results of these studies have brought new insights in the pathophysiology of functional bowel disorders and have demonstrated the importance of visceral perception disturbances in these patients. The knowledge has also been increased about visceral afferents and their implication in perception disorders.

Drug trials based on the evaluation of sensory thresholds are now published and in the future will provide an interesting approach to test the potential therapeutic effect of drugs designed to treat functional bowel disorders. However, at the moment, distention tests lack the specificity to discriminate between functional patients and normals or patients with organic diseases. Therefore, the results of drug trials based on the evaluation of effects on sensory thresholds must presently be considered as indicative but not predictive of the clinical action of the drug. Multicenter trials will answer these questions in the future.

Finally, we would like to stress the dramatic influence of the technical conditions of distention studies on their results. As stated here, we need standardization of the experimental procedures to enable comparisons between different studies. At the least, the reports of these studies should include a clear description of methods and procedures and provide technical specifications of distending devices, probes, and bags or balloons. The Working Party Report by a group of investigators with expertise in the use of the barostat is intended to provide the users of barostats with recommendations to accurately address these technical issues.[5]

## REFERENCES

1. Azpiroz F, Malagelada J-R. Physiological variations in canine gastric tone measured by an electronic barostat. Am J Physiol 1985;248:G229–37.

2. Ritchie J. Pain from distension of the pelvic colon by inflating a balloon in the irritable colon syndrome. Gut 1973;14:125–32.

3. Frexinos J, Delvaux M. Normal colonic motility. In: Wingate DL, Kumar D, editors. Illustrated guide of motility. Edinburgh: Churchill Livingstone; 1994. p. 427–48.

4. Hachet T, Caussette M. A multifunction programmable computerized barostat. Gastroenterol Clin Biol 1993;17:347–51.

5. Whitehead WE, Delvaux M. Standardization of barostat procedures for testing smooth muscle tone and sensory thresholds in the gastrointestinal tract. Dig Dis Sci 1997;42:223–41.

6. Bradette M, Delvaux M, Staumont G, et al. Evaluation of colonic sensory thresholds in IBS patients using a barostat: definition of optimal conditions and comparison with healthy subjects. Dig Dis Sci 1994;39:449–57.

7. Steadman CJ, Phillips SF, Camilleri M, et al. Variation of muscle tone in the human colon. Gastroenterology 1991;101:373–81.

8. Von der Ohe MR, Hanson RB, Camilleri M. Comparison of simultaneous recordings of human colonic contractions by manometry and a barostat. Neurogastroenterol Motil 1994;6:231–22.

9. Whitehead WE, Crowell MD, Davidoff A, et al. Is sexual abuse associated with lower thresholds for pain due to balloon distention of the rectum [abstract]? Gastroenterology 1993;106:A588.

10. Toma TP, Phillips SF, Sarr MG. Does a barostat bag stimulate colonic motility in the dog [abstract]? Gastroenterology 1994;106:A579.

11. Bell AM, Pemberton JH, Hanson RB, Zinsmeister AR. Variations in muscle tone of the human rectum: recordings with an electromechanical barostat. Am J Physiol 1991;260:G17–25.

12. Basilisco G, Phillips SF, Cullen JJ, Chiravuri M. Tonic responses of canine proximal colon: effects of eating, nutrients and simulated diarrhea. Am J Physiol 1995;268:G95–101.

13. Von der Ohe MR, Hanson RB, Camilleri M. Serotoninergic mediation of post-prandial colonic tone and phasic responses in humans. Gut 1994;35:536–41.

14. Kullman G, Fielding JF. Rectal distensibility in the irritable bowel syndrome. Ir Med J 1981;74:140–2.

15. Whitehead WE, Holtkotter B, Enck P, et al. Tolerance for recto-sigmoid distention in irritable bowel syndrome. Gastroenterology 1990;98:1187–92.

16. Toma TP, Zighelboim J, Phillips SF, Talley NJ. Methods for studying intestinal sensitivity and compliance: in vitro studies of balloons and a barostat. Neurogastroenterol Motil 1996;8:19–28.

17. Delvaux M, Staumont G, Louvel D, et al. Effect of atropine on colonic tone and myoelectrical activity in patients with irritable bowel syndrome [abstract]. Hellen J Gastroenterol 1992;5:62.

18. Ford MJ, Camilleri M, Wiste JA, Hanson RB. Differences in colonic tone and phasic response to a meal in the transverse and sigmoid human colon. Gut 1995;37:264–9.

19. Jouet P, Coffin B, Lemann M, et al. Tonic and phasic motor activity in the proximal and distal colon of healthy volunteers. Am J Physiol 1998;274:G459–64.

20. Coffin B, Fossati S, Flourie B, et al. Regional effects of cholecystokinin octapeptide on colonic phasic and tonic motility in healthy humans. Am J Physiol 1999;276:G767–72.

21. Soffer EE, Kongara K, Achkar JP, Gannon J. Colonic motor function in humans is not affected by gender. Dig Dis Sci 2000;45:1281–4.

22. Vassallo MJ, Camilleri M, Phillips SF, et al. Colonic tone and motility in patients with irritable bowel syndrome. Mayo Clin Proc 1992;67:725–31.

23. Von der Ohe M, Camilleri M, Kvools LK, Thomforde GM. Motor dysfunction of the small bowel and colon in patients with the carcinoid syndrome and diarrhea. N Engl J Med 1993;329:1073–8.

24. Von der Ohe M, Camilleri M, Kvools LK. A 5-HT3 antagonist corrects the postprandial colonic hypertonic response in carcinoid diarrhea. Gastroenterology 1994;106:1184–9.

25. Choi MG, Camilleri M, O'Brien MD, et al. A pilot study of motility and tone of the left colon in patients with diarrhea due to functional disorders and dysautonomia. Am J Gastroenterol 1997;92:297–302.

26. O'Brien MD, Camilleri M, Von der Ohe M, et al. Motility and tone of the left colon in constipation: a role in clinical practice? Am J Gastroenterol 1996;91:2532–8.

27. Bruninga K, Camilleri M. Colonic motility and tone after spinal cord and cauda equina injury. Am J Gastroenterol 1997;92:891–4.

28. Huge A, Kreis ME, Zittel TT, et al. Postoperative colonic motility and tone in patients after colorectal surgery. Dis Colon Rectum 2000;43:932–9.

29. Lembo T, Munakata J, Mertz H, et al. Evidence for the hypersensitivity of lumbar splanchnic afferents in irritable bowel syndrome. Gastroenterology 1994;107:1686–96.

30. Jaenig W, Koltzenburg M. On the function of spinal primary afferent fibers supplying colon and urinary bladder. J Autonom Nerv Syst 1990;30:589–96.

31. Whitehead WE, Engel BT, Schuster MM. Irritable bowel syndrome. Physiological and psychological differences beween diarrhea-predominant and constipation-predominant patients. Dig Dis Sci 1980;25:404–13.

32. Sun WM, Read NW, Prior A, et al. The sensory and motor responses to rectal distention vary according to the rate and pattern of balloon inflation. Gastroenterology 1990;99:1008–13.

33. Delvaux M, Louvel D, Lagier E, et al. Reproducibility of sensory thresholds triggered by rectal distension in healthy volunteers [abstract]. Gastroenterology 1995;108:A590.

34. Delvaux M, Louvel D, Lagier E, et al. The kappa agonist Fedotozine relieves hypersensitivity to colonic distension in patients with irritable bowel syndrome (IBS). Gastroenterology 1999;116:38–45.

35. Bradley LA, Scarinci IC, Richter JE. Pain threshold levels and coping strategies among patients who have chest pain and normal coronary artries. Med Clin North Am 1991;75:1189–202.

36. Mertz H, Naliboff B, Munakata J, et al. Altered rectal perception is a biological marker of patients with irritable bowel syndrome. Gastroenterology 1995;109:40–52.

37. Prior A, Read NW. Reduction of rectal sensitivity and postprandial motility by granisetron, a 5-HT3 receptor antagonist, in patients with irritable bowel syndrome [abstract]. Gut 1990;31:A1174.

38. Prior A, Maxton DG, Whorwell PJ. Anorectal manometry in irritable bowel syndrome: differences between diarrhoea and constipation predominant subjects. Gut 1990;31:458–62.

39. Bradette M, Staumont G, Delvaux M, et al. Somatostatin analogue increases thresholds of discomfort and pain perception to colonic distension in irritable bowel syndrome patients. Dig Dis Sci 1994;39:1171–8.

40. Accarino AM, Azpiroz F, Malagelada J-R. Symptomatic responses to stimulation of sensory pathways in the jejunum. Am J Physiol 1992;263:G673–7.

41. Francis CY, Houghton LA, Whorwell PJ, et al. Enhanced sensitivity of the whole gut in patients with irritable bowel syndrome [abstract]. Gastroenterology 1995;108:A601.

42. Lee OY, Naliboff BD, Olivas T, et al. Differences in rectal mechanoelastic properties according to predominant bowel habit in IBS patients [abstract]. Gastroenterology 2000;118:A667.

43. Latimer P, Campbell D, Latimer M, et al. Irritable bowel syndrome: a test of the colonic hyperalgesia hypothesis. J Behav Med 1979;2: 285–95.

46. Hasler W, Soudah H, Owyang C. A somatostatin analogue inhibits afferent pathways mediating perception of rectal distension. Gastroenterology 1993;104:1390–7.

45. Chey WD, Beydoun A, Roberts DJ, et al. Octreotide reduces perception of rectal electrical stimulation by spinal afferent pathway inhibition. Am J Physiol 1995;269:G821–6.

46. Accarino AM, Azpiroz F, Malagelada J-R. Selective dysfunction of mechanosensitive intestinal afferents in irritable bowel syndrome. Gastroenterology 1995;108:636–43.

47. Erckenbrecht J. Noise and intestinal motor alterations. In: Buéno L, Collins S, Junien JL, editors. Stress and digestive motility. London: John Libbey Eurotext; 1989. p. 93–6.

48. Mönnikes H, Heymann-Mönnikes I, Arnold R. Patients with irritable bowel syndrome have alterations in the CNS-modulation of visceral afferent perception [abstract]. Gut 1995;37:A168.

49. Silverman DH, Munakata JA, Ennes H, et al. Regional cerebral activity in normal and pathological perception of visceral pain. Gastroenterology 1997;112:64–72.

50. Berman S, Munakata J, Naliboff BD, et al. Gender differences in regional brain response to visceral pressure in IBS patients. Eur J Pain 2000;4:157–72.

51. Lagier E, Delvaux M, Metivier S, et al. Colonic tone influences thresholds of sensory perception to luminal distension in IBS patients [abstract]. Gastroenterology 1996;110:A700.

52. Siproudhis L, Bellissant E, Juguet F, et al. Octreotide acts on anorectal physiology: a dynamic study in healthy subjects. Clin Pharmacol Ther 1998;64:424–32.

53. Lagier E, Delvaux M, Vellas B, et al. Influence of age on rectal tone and sensitivity to distension in healthy subjects. Neurogastroenterol Motil 1999;11:101–8.

54. Blanc C, Maillot C, Delvaux M, et al. Influence of gender and menstrual cycle on visceral perception in healthy volunteers [abstract]. Gastroenterology 1999;116:A724.

55. Soffer EE, Kongara K, Achkar JP, Gannon J. Colonic motor function in humans is not affected by gender. Dig Dis Sci 2000;45:1281–4.

56. Ford MJ, Camilleri M, Zinsmeister AR, Hanson RB. Psychosensory modulation of colonic sensation in the human transverse and sigmoid colon. Gastroenterology 1995;109:1772–80.

57. Bueno L, Fioramonti J, Delvaux M, Frexinos J. Mediators and pharmacology of visceral sensitivity: from basic to clinical investigations. Gastroenterology 1997;112:1714–43.

58. Plourde V, Lembo T, Shui Z, et al. Effects of the somatostatin analog, octreotide on rectal afferent nerves in humans. Am J Physiol 1993;265:G742–5.

59. Meller ST, Lewis SJ, Brody MJ, Gebhart GF. The peripheral nociceptive actions of intravenous administered 5-HT in the rat requires dual activation of both $5\text{-HT}_2$ and $5\text{-HT}_3$ receptor subtypes. Brain Res 1992;561:61–8.

60. Morteau O, Eeckhout C, Buéno L. Effect of the $5\text{-HT}_3$ antagonists (granisetron and KC9946) on viscerosensitive response to colorectal distension before and during experimental colitis in awake rats. Fundam Clin Pharmacol 1994;8:553–62.

61. Moss H, Sanger GJ. Antagonism by BRL43694 of pseudoaffective reflexes evoked by duodenal distension [abstract]. Br J Pharmacol 1987;92:531P.

62. Delvaux M, Louvel D, Mamet JP, et al. Effect of alosetron on responses to colonic distension in patients with irritable bowel syndrome. Aliment Pharmacol Ther 1998;12:849–55.

63. Camilleri M, Northcutt AR, Kong S, et al. Efficacy and safety of alosetron in women with irritable bowel syndrome: a randomised, placebo-controlled trial. Lancet 2000;355:1035–40.

64. Dapoigny M, Abitbol JL, Fraitag B. Efficacy of peipheral kappa agonist fedotozine versus placebo in treatment of irritable bowel syndrome. A multicenter dose-response study. Dig Dis Sci 1995;40:2244–8.

65. Gué M, Junien JL, Buéno L. The kappa-agonist fedotozine modulates colonic distension-induced inhibition of gastric motility and emptying in dogs. Gastroenterology 1994;107:1327–34.

66. Louvel D, Delvaux M, Fioramonti J, et al. Oxytocin increases thresholds of colonic visceral perception in IBS patients. Gut 1996;39:741–7.

# CHAPTER 19

# Radiopaque Markers and Transit

*Ghislain Devroede*

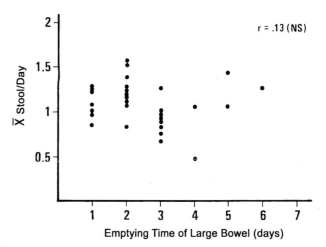

**FIGURE 19.1.** Relationship between whole gut transit time and stool frequency. There is no correlation between per day stool frequency and total emptying of large bowel, here defined as number of days between the appearance of the first marker and the disappearance of the last marker. The same goes for the correlation between stool frequency and mean transit time of one marker. NS, not significant.

## ASSESSING COLORECTAL TRANSIT TIME

Recent epidemiologic studies have confirmed the old observation that stool frequency correlates poorly with colorectal transit time.[1] From a simple theoretical point of view, this is hardly surprising since colorectal transit times are a reflection of what happens as feces is propelled along the large bowel as a consequence of diverse motor elements at work in the bowel wall. Propulsion results in stool output, and stool output is the product of stool frequency and stool weight. It is easy to understand that defecating once (stool frequency) a stool, weighing 200 g, 400 cm long, expelled from the splenic flexure down[2-4] results from different physiologic mechanisms than defecating also once (stool frequency) a stool, weighing 50 g, 5 cm long, expelled from the ampullary part

of the rectum,[5] after considerable straining efforts and sometimes against a pelvic floor that does not relax, as occurs in anismus.[6] Most likely, total and segmental colorectal times will be faster in the former case.[7] Thus, one expects colorectal transit time not to correlate with stool frequency (Fig. 19.1) but with stool output. Yet stool frequency is still the basis used by many clinicians to make a diagnosis of constipation, and it is highly unreliable.[7,8]

### Correlation with Stool Output

Colorectal transit times reflect stool output. But collecting, freezing, and weighing stool is a messy ordeal and has not gained wide clinical popularity. Dietary fiber increases stool

**FIGURE 19.2.** Self-reported disturbed bowel habits in the United States. Self-reported constipation occurs more often in women than in men and in blacks than in whites. It increases with age.[12]

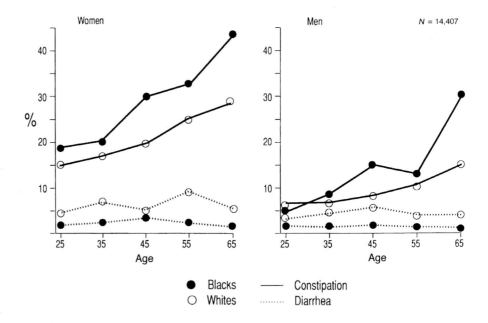

### Correlation with Subjective Complaints

Is it better to rely on patients' complaints? If the gold standard is the sign (stool frequency or colorectal transit times), there is no correlation between the prevalence of self-reported constipation and that of stool frequency. For instance, self-reported constipation increases with age (Fig. 19.2), but stool frequency remains constant (Fig. 19.3).[12] Constipation is neither a disease nor a sign. As a symptom, it may be indicative of many diseases, and the differential diagnosis covers as wide a spectrum as for abdominal pain. A symptom is a subjective appreciation that is highly variable from patient to patient. Dismissing the symptom as unimportant as compared with the sign and dismissing the emotions as marginally relevant are bound to lead to an oversimplified approach to constipation.

Another example is the prevalence of laxative ingestion. The more severe the constipation, the more frequent is its intake, but many people ingest some even if they do not report constipation, do not experience infrequent defecation, and do not pass hard stools.[12,13] The percentage of laxative consumers in a general population increases with age,[13,14] even at equal severity of the problem.[15] Worse, there is no relationship between laxative intake and observed stool frequency, gastrointestinal transit time, or segmental colorectal transit time.[13] Thus laxative consumption is largely part of a culture and a poor indication of pathophysiologic derangement.[7] Not surprisingly, a very recent study provided con-

clusive evidence from a community-based epidemiologic evaluation that self-reports are virtually worthless in terms of reflecting reality.

For all of these reasons, measurement of colorectal transit times should be the gold standard of evaluation in the approach to constipated patients. It has the merit of placing the complaint of constipation in perspective with the functional derangement. There are patients who claim they do not defecate, but markers are seen clearly to disappear (by defecation) from plain films of their abdomen.[16–18] This denial of fecal expulsion makes these patients belong to the group with factitious disorders. If the consequence of their denial is negligible, except for the physician's frustration and puzzled questioning, this is merely a case of pseudologia fantastica, but if surgery is performed, this is clearly automutilation, and the falsely constipated patient belongs to the group of patients with Munchausen syndrome.[18] The in-depth analysis of the later patients[19] suggests that they have a psychotic personality structure, and this should be known before embarking on treatment.

### Significance of History of Sexual Abuse

Sexual abuse is found in the past history of every other woman with functional gastrointestinal disorder,[21] particularly those with lower gastrointestinal disorders[22] who complain of constipation among other symptoms. The medical consequences of sexual abuse are horrendous: women abused by their fathers in their childhood undergo on average eight operations throughout their life, see 19 consultants on average, gastroenterologists and surgeons included, have charts 10 cm thick on average, and go for 18 years before the abuse is detected.[23] This is important to know because 75% of the operations were, in retrospect (on the basis of reviewing operative and pathologic reports), completely unnecessary, and this includes surgery for constipation. Many constipated

**FIGURE 19.3.** Self-reported stool frequency in the United States. Although constipation increases with age, stool frequency remains constant with increasing age.[12]

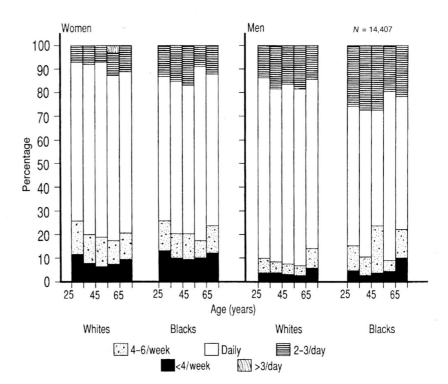

patients go from one operation to another. The value of these procedures is limited and has not been compared to the natural history or less invasive approaches such as psychotherapy.[7] Not uncommonly, patients succeeded in blackmailing a surgeon, through suicidal threats, into performing an operation that is unnecessary because colorectal transit times were perfectly normal.[18] Thus, colorectal transit time measurements are mandatory before treating a patient who claims to remain constipated after having tried a high-fiber diet.

## AVAILABLE TECHNIQUES AND THEIR LIMITATIONS

Ideally, the measurement of colorectal transit time should be done in a physiologic way. It should not be invasive and should reflect faithfully what occurs to digestive contents as they proceed along the gastrointestinal tract. The technique should be practical, simple, reproducible, and reliable, not only in a specialized tertiary setting but also in community facilities. It should obtain easy acceptance by patients, their treating physicians, and specialists who may be involved, such as radiologists or nuclear medicine physicians. Available techniques include radiographs of the abdomen,[16,24–33] colonic scintigraphy,[34–40] or a biomagnetic method.[41] Most experience has been accumulated with the radiopaque markers technique, which, although not perfect, constitutes at present the best available way to evaluate colorectal transit times.

Following ingested markers from day to day on plain films of the abdomen permits one to sort out constipated patients from healthy controls. Thus, markers are retained longer in constipated patients than they are in healthy controls.[16,24,25] Normal subjects expel the first marker within 3 days and 80%

of them within 5 days.[16,24] This can be shown by taking radiographs of the abdomen or of the stools, but the latter method is less convenient in a clinical setting. A plain film taken 3 days after ingestion of 20 markers allows one to make a reliable diagnosis of constipation in 100% of cases, giving the test a powerful discriminant value. Constipated subjects on that day retain 18 or more markers. Table 19.1 shows that it is on that day that the greatest difference on average is found as compared with healthy controls or controls who claim that stress does not modify their bowel habits or trigger abdominal pain.

### Principles Regarding Measurements

The measurement of colorectal transit times is based on the same principles governing calculations from dye dilution curves in cardiovascular evaluation of blood flow. Thus, injection ought to be quasi-instantaneous, and what happens proximally will influence distal events. Because of this principle, there is no perfect technique at present. For instance, ingested radiopaque markers take a while before they reach the cecum and do not all arrive at once. Fortunately, transit time from the mouth to the cecum occurs in a matter of hours, whereas transit from the cecum until expulsion through the anus is longer. It is this relative difference in a rate of transit that permits the use of ingested radiopaque markers.

Segmental gastrointestinal transit time is more difficult to evaluate for the same reason. If the traffic of markers through the ascending colon is slow, they will enter the left colon and rectosigmoid area with some delay, and this by itself may account for "delayed" left colorectal transit, even if there is no abnormality whatsoever at this site. Segmental interdependence is thus an essential element to consider.

**TABLE 19.1** Markers in the Abdomen in Healthy Subjects and Constipated Patients (Mean ± SD)*

| | Days after Ingestion of 20 Markers | | | | | |
|---|---|---|---|---|---|---|
| | 1 | 2 | 3 | 4 | 5 | 6 |
| Stress-free controls | 12.9 ± 6.4 | 4.0 ± 4.3 | 0.4 ± 1.2 | 0.0 ± 0.0 | 0.0 ± 0.0 | 0.0 ± 0.0 |
| Healthy controls | 15.3 ± 6.2 | 8.0 ± 7.8 | 3.7 ± 6.3 | 1.7 ± 4.2 | 0.4 ± 1.9 | 0.3 ± 1.4 |
| Constipated patients with delayed transit | 19.8 ± 0.7 | 19.1 ± 2.1 | 18.2 ± 2.7 | 12.3 ± 7.9 | 9.8 ± 7.3 | 7.5 ± 7.6 |
| Constipated patients with normal transit | 16.0 ± 5.8 | 8.3 ± 7.2 | 1.7 ± 2.0 | 0.5 ± 0.9 | 0.2 ± 0.5 | 0.0 ± 0.2 |
| | *t* Value between Constipated Patients with Delayed Transit and | | | | | |
| Stress-free controls | 6.01 | 17.80 | 34.10 | 8.85 | 7.60 | 5.60 |
| Controls | 4.10 | 7.86 | 11.99 | 6.74 | 7.03 | 5.31 |
| | *t* and *p* Values between Constipated Patients with Delayed Transit and | | | | | |
| Stress-free controls | 1.84 NS | 2.58 $p < .02$ | 2.77 $p < .01$ | 2.79 $p < .01$ | 2.01 $p < .05$ | 1.00 NS |
| Controls | 0.41 NS | 0.16 NS | 1.65 NS | 1.52 NS | 0.52 NS | 0.81 NS |

*Data from Bouchoucha et al.[31]

$p < .001$ for all significant values.

NS, not significant.

These are not merely theoretical considerations because a number of studies have shown that some patients who complain of constipation may have perfectly normal overall colorectal transit times yet have segmental delays.[28,42–44] Bony structures serve to segregate three segments of large bowel: right colon, left colon, and rectosigmoid area. The spinal processes and imaginary lines from the fifth lumbar vertebra to the pelvic outlet serve as landmarks. A large cecum sometimes overlaps the rectal area. Markers are considered to be still in the cecum if a clear bowel outline of the cecum is visible and no markers have gone through the left colon.

### Formulas for Calculations

Mean transit time ($\Delta t$) of the markers is calculated in the following ways:

$$\overline{\Delta t} = \frac{1}{N} \sum_{i=1}^{N} \Delta t_i \qquad (1)$$

where $\Delta t_i$ is the transit time of a given marker through the studied site and $N$ is the total number of markers.

If $n$ is the number of markers present in the studied site at a given time, one may demonstrate that:

$$\sum_{i=1}^{N} \Delta t_i \approx \int_{0}^{\infty} n \, dt \qquad (2)$$

Plain films of the abdomen are taken at time $t_1, t_2 \ldots t_j$ (at 24-hour intervals in this study). On these films, one can see $n_1, n_2 \ldots n_j$ markers until $n_j = 0$ at time $t_j$. Thus, the integral in Equation 2 can be replaced by an approximation:

$$n_1 \left[ \frac{t_1 + t_2}{2} - \frac{t_0 + t_1}{2} \right] + n_2 \left[ \frac{t_2 + t_3}{2} - \frac{t_1 + t_2}{2} \right] \qquad (3)$$
$$\cdots + n_j \left[ \frac{t_j + t_{(j+1)}}{2} - \frac{t_{(j-1)} + t}{2} \right]$$

where $t$ is the time elapsed from ingestion of markers to the time when the film is taken to $t_0 = 0$.

From this, a working formula can be deduced and is shown graphically in Figure 19.4.

$$\overline{\Delta t} = \frac{1}{N} \sum_{i=1}^{N} n_i \left[ \frac{t_{(i+1)} + t_{(i-1)}}{2} \right] \qquad (4)$$

For example, if 20 markers are ingested, films are taken every 24 hours, and on successive films, 16, 8, 6, 2, and 0 markers are found in the ascending colon:

$$\text{means transit time} = \frac{1}{20}[(16 \times 24)] + (8 \times 24) + (6 \times 24)$$
$$+ (2 \times 24)] = 38.4 \text{ hours}$$

Thus, when intervals ($T$) are constant, Equation 4 can further be simplified into:

$$\overline{\Delta t} = \frac{1}{N} \sum_{i=1}^{j} n_i T = \frac{T}{N} \sum_{i=1}^{j} n_i \qquad (5)$$

This working formula is independent of the number of swallowed markers and the time interval between plain films of the abdomen. It is important to know in a daily clinical setting because occasionally not all markers are ingested or a film of the transit series is skipped. Some authors have erroneously studied clearances using the percentage of disappearing markers as an index of segmental transit time and

**FIGURE 19.4.** Measuring colorectal transit time is based on the principles of a dye dilution curve. Columns of markers counted at times $t_1$, $t_2$, $t_3$, ... $t_j$ can be transformed into a triangle. The mean transit time of one marker will reflect half of the area under this triangle.

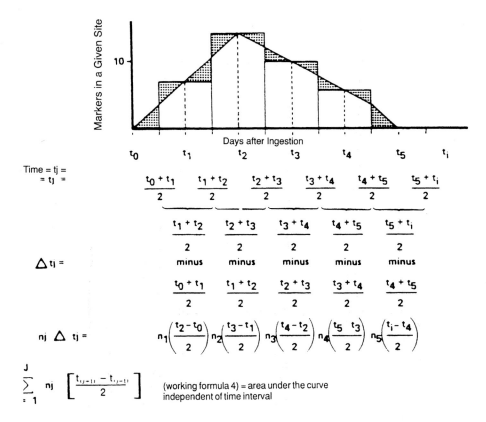

instead of the actual number of markers.[45] Percentage is both relative and dependent on proximal events. The technique described above measures the mean transit time of one radiopaque marker. It can be further simplified by using a standard number of markers and a standard set of hours between films. For instance, if 20 markers are ingested, and films are taken every 24 hours, Equation 5 becomes:

$$TT = 24 \times \sum n_i / 20 = 1.2 \times \Delta n_i \qquad (6)$$

where $n_i$ is the number of markers on day $i$ in the studied zone and $TT$ is the mean transit time (Equation 6) of a single marker in a given site. It can be even further simplified by giving 24 rather than 20 markers. This eliminates the need to multiply Equation 6, that is by 1.2 in 24/24 = 1. Thus, markers are counted in successive films, and the addition provides the mean transit time. Markers (Sitzmarks, Konsyl Pharmaceutical Inc., Fort Worth, TX) are now commercially available.

### Validity Testing

The validity of using radiopaque markers to study gut transit times has been tested. A comparison has been made between the transit time of these pellets and that of a simultaneously administered dose of chromium-51-labeled sodium chromate. A dose of 3 to 6 μCi of the isotope in 5 to 10 mL of the solution was given. The results showed that transit times to appearance of the first markers are similar, but that, in several patients, later pellets take less time to traverse the large bowel

than the corresponding proportion of sodium chromate (Fig. 19.5). Ileostomy research indicates that at least part of the more rapid transit of markers is in the upper gut.[24] A comparison has also been made between transit of rates of pellets and that of simultaneously administered gelatin capsules of powdered carmine, the comparison being limited to transit times for the first and last red color as there is no simple method available for measuring carmine in the stool. In 25 of 30 comparisons,

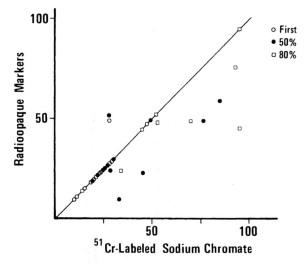

**FIGURE 19.5.** Whole gut transit time (hours). The correlation between the transit of radiopaque markers and that of chromium-51-labeled radium chromate is good but far from perfect, particularly for the latest pellets.[24]

the times of the first marker and the first appearance of the carmine were the same, and in 16 occasions, they were the same for 100% of markers and the last visible carmine.[24]

These studies provide evidence for a gross but imperfect similarity between passage of radiopaque marker pellets and that of radioactive chromium or powdered carmine. Factors to consider are the nature of the pellets themselves and the gastrointestinal segment that they traverse. Transit through the esophagus, stomach, and small bowel is delayed in patients with constipation[46] and in those with irritable bowel syndrome,[47] some of whom have mainly constipation, and this is corrected by treatment.[46,48] Thus, rapid transit of radiopaque markers as compared with chromium 51 in the upper gastrointestinal tract is likely to induce errors to evaluate differences between constipated patients and controls in a zone in which transit is rather fast. In the large bowel, the transit time of radiopaque markers is also faster than that obtained by scintigraphy.[38,39] Plastic pellets have a laxative action,[49] which may explain this.

## Single Ingestion-Multiple Films versus Multiple Ingestions-Single Film

Recent studies have focused on a practical goal: reducing the amount of radiation exposure. The basic principle has been to increase the frequency of marker ingestion and concomitantly decrease the frequency of radiographs taken with the use of multiple films[27–30] or a single film.[31–33] These studies (even if they compare well with that using daily films[26]) are open to a number of criticisms. After only 3 days of ingestion, steady-state conditions of marker intake and output may not have been reached.[27–30] In those studies, which used a prolonged period of ingestion of markers in the hope of reaching the necessary steady-state conditions,[31–33] segmental transit times were not always calculated,[33] and an empirical approximation was used to determine the number of days of ingestion; this may not be valid in all groups of patients. The use of different types of markers to evaluate retrograde movement is based on the major assumption that the transit time of a single radiopaque marker is reproducible from day to day.[27–30] Because defecation frequency is not as autonomous as colorectal function, the correlation between the multiple marker and the multiple film techniques decreases as one progresses along the bowel, and for the same reason is better in constipation, when subjects defecate less often, than in health (Fig. 19.6). When a single film is taken, it is impossible to evaluate the change in distribution of markers on a day-to-day basis. This may be pertinent since reflux of markers from distal to more proximal colon is associated with differences in personality and psychophysiologic relationships[50] and probably with retrograde movement of propagating electrical activity in the large bowel.[43] Finally, in the single[29,30] or triple[27,28] film-multiple marker ingestion techniques, the dispersion of data is noticeable, and its significance has not been explored.

For these reasons, a technique has been devised that is more flexible and can be adapted to individual needs.[31] Patients ingest radiopaque markers at 9 am on 6 consecutive days. An abdominal x-ray film is taken the day after the last ingestion of the markers (Fig. 19.7). Segmental and total colonic transit time is calculated (Equation 6) as follows:

$$TT = 24 \times n/10 = 2.4 \times n$$

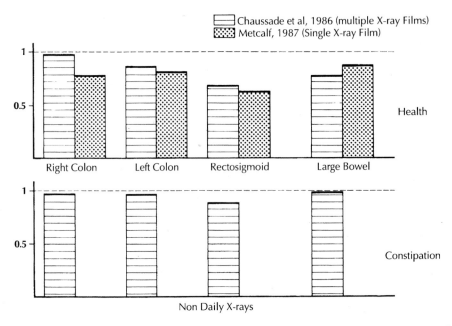

**FIGURE 19.6.** Alternate ways to measure colonic transit time (correlations). The correlation between the single ingestion of markers-multiple films technique[27] and that of multiple ingestions-single film[29] is better in constipation and better proximally in the large bowel, presumably because of the subjective and random effect of defecation.

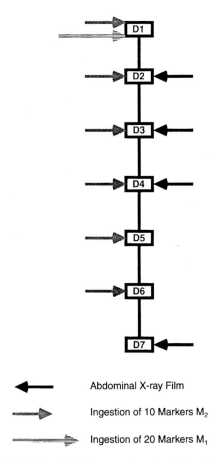

**FIGURE 19.7.** Two methods for measuring colorectal transit time. In the first one, 20 markers $M_1$ are ingested once (*large arrow*), and a plain film of the abdomen is then taken on days 2, 3, and 4, when markers had disappeared from the abdomen, and the test was thus stopped. In the second method, 10 markers $M_2$ are ingested every day for 6 days. A single film is taken the next day (D7).[31]

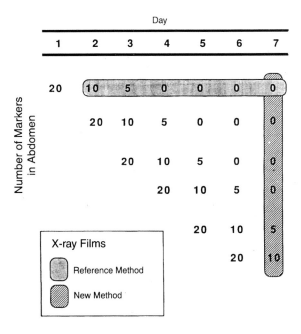

**FIGURE 19.8.** This illustrates Figure 19.7. *Reference method* calls for a single ingestion of radiopaque markers-multiple films technique. *New method* calls for a multiple ingestion-single film technique.[31]

The principle of the equivalence between the two methods of measurement is indicated in Fig. 19.8.

This study permits one to draw a number of conclusions. In the subjects who have simultaneously both types of studies (single film-multiple marker ingestions versus multiple films-single marker ingestion), there is a very good correlation between the two techniques. Correlation is .70 for right and left colon, .66 for the rectosigmoid area, and .69 for total colonic transit time (all significant at $p < .001$) (Fig. 19.9).

On films taken on successive days, markers can be seen to decrease in number, and a model of this decrease can be drawn. Parameters characteristic of the decreasing curves of markers appear in Table 19.2. Curves shown in Fig. 19.10 are calculated, rather than measured, from these parameters. Greatest variations are in the $T$ parameter, ranging from 1.55 in stress-free subjects to 8.22 in patients with colonic inertia. The spread in variance in the colonic inertia group is much greater than in the other groups and demonstrates more heterogeneity.

In patients who have asynchronous measurements, transit times are similar at first and second examinations. This is important to know because the natural history of constipa-

tion has hardly been explored; thus, we need a reproducible technique to measure transit. The correlation coefficients vary according to site and, although very significant, are far from one.

The number of markers to be counted on the single film may become considerable. If five markers are ingested every day, using the same formula, ingestion of markers may be reduced to 3 weeks ($2 \times 10.7$) in colonic inertia and 2 weeks in hindgut dysfunction ($2 \times 60.0$) and outlet obstruction ($2 \times 7.2$). These transit times, up to now, could not be calculated and used for statistical analysis because all that could be said was that they actually exceeded a given measured value.[53,54] This is easy to understand: a comparison of the various available methods used to measure colorectal transit times is in order. The technique of single ingestion of a bolus of markers[26] measures the mean transit time of a single marker. In contrast, all techniques using multiple ingestions of markers with single film provide data on a mean

**TABLE 19.2.** Model of Decrease in Number of Markers (Parameters)*

| Groups | $k$ (Mean $\pm$ 2 SD) | $T$ (days) (Mean $\pm$ SD) |
|---|---|---|
| Stress-free controls | 1.89 ± 0.43 | 1.55 ± 0.12 |
| Healthy controls | 2.09 ± 0.65 | 2.06 ± 0.20[†] |
| Constipation with normal transit | 2.11 ± 0.56 | 2.08 ± 0.18[†] |
| Colonic inertia | 1.78 ± 1.37 | 8.22 ± 3.68[†] |
| Hindgut dysfunction | 2.61 ± 1.06 | 5.02 ± 0.57[†] |
| Outlet obstruction | 3.58 ± 1.45 | 6.33 ± 0.59[†] |

*Adapted from Bouchoucha et al.[31]

[†]$p < .05$ as compared to stress-free controls.

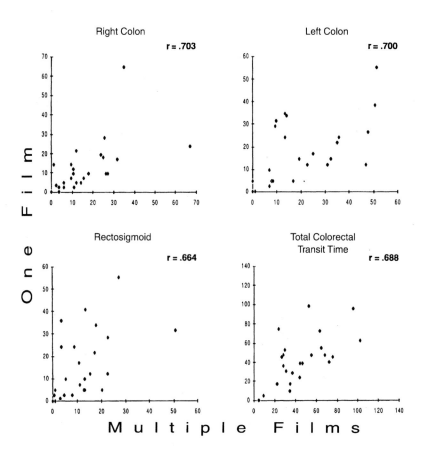

**FIGURE 19.9.** Good correlation between the two techniques (single film-multiple marker ingestion and multiple film-single marker ingestion) in three segments of colon and in total colonic transit times.

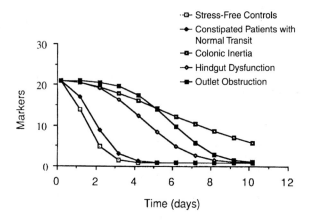

**FIGURE 19.10.** Calculated curve of daily elimination of marker under differing conditions.

transit time, made of successive mean transit times of a single marker already shown to vary from day to day.[29,51] It is not surprising that the correlation coefficient is only 0.7, and this explains less than 50% of the variance of the measured values ($0.7 \times 0.7$). This is rather constant and does not vary much from site to site, being maximum in the right colon and minimum in the rectosigmoid segment. This results from the imprecision of the measurement, which is amplified when a 3-day study is performed.[27–30] Correlation with the daily ingestion of markers is independent of the site of measure-

ment, with more prolonged ingestion of markers, 6 days,[31] which minimizes the influence of time of defecation, a voluntary act. Ingestion of pellets for only 3 days maximizes the importance of day 3, which is the more discriminant day.[31]

The technique of multiple daily films permits one to detect situations for which patients deny defecation by comparing a diary, in which no stool is reported, with clear evidence on the film of that day of a decrease in the number of markers. Similar information can be obtained with the technique using multiple ingestions of markers and a single film: if patients claim they did not defecate at all, all ingested markers should be present on the abdominal x-ray film. However, if patients claim they defecated only once, for instance, and the x-ray film confirms that some of the ingested markers have been defecated, it is impossible to know with the film technique if they actually defecated more than once.

This chapter does not deal with colonic scintigraphy (which is covered in Chapter 20, "Scintigraphy"). Differences between the results obtained from radiopaque markers technique and from colonic scintigraphy are relevant to discuss, however. Transit of radiopaque markers appears to be faster than that of radiopaque material as evaluated by colonic scintigraphy. It must be remembered that if particle sizes are important,[49] methods to obtain dye dilution curves are also important. Thus, when a nondigestible capsule enters the cecum,[37] or when indium 111 is incorporated into a coated capsule that disperses into the ileocecal region,[38,39] we have the same situation as in old methods using radiopaque mark-

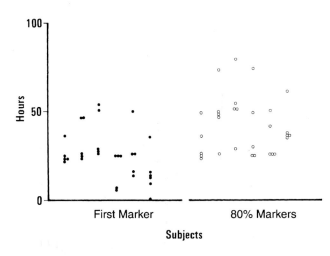

**FIGURE 19.11.** Transit times of radiopaque markers in whole gut replicate studies. Although reproducible,[31] there is a rather large variation coefficient to radiopaque marker studies of large bowel transit time.[24]

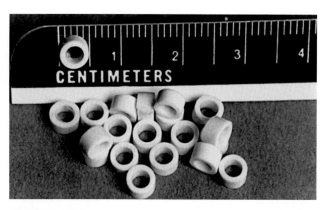

**FIGURE 19.12.** Radiopaque markers for the study of colorectal transit time.

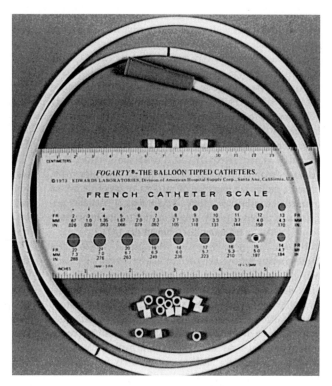

**FIGURE 19.13.** Markers can be cut from radiopaque Levine tubing (15 French).

ers, when they were simply counted from day to day on plain films of the abdomen.[16,24,25] The considerations given above about the measurement of segmental colonic transit time[26] apply to colonic scintigraphy. It is not clear at this stage of our knowledge how this will be dealt with.

## TECHNIQUES IN CLINICAL SETTINGS

### Techniques and Examples

Measurement of colonic transit time with radiopaque markers is a simple and reproducible technique that can be performed in any radiology department. There are two contraindications to such studies: pregnancy, because radiation may be harmful to the fetus, and bowel obstruction, because the results are invalidated by the obstruction.

Patients with complaints of constipation or diarrhea should first undergo a general history and physical examination to rule out obvious etiologies. Most patients will require radiographic or endoscopic evaluation of the gastrointestinal tract. Additional tests such as anorectal manometry, balloon and saline defecation, external sphincter electromyography, and defecography will usually be required in addition to the transit studies for a complete evaluation in patients with constipation. Patients with diarrhea will usually require studies to rule out malabsorption syndromes or infectious etiologies. The details of this evaluation have been covered elsewhere.[7] Radiopaque marker techniques should not be performed unless a "diagnosis" of chronic idiopathic constipation has been arrived at, of course by exclusion.

Although markers are commercially available (site markers), they may also simply be cut from radiopaque tubes. The advantage of preparing markers, other than decreased expense, is that multiple distinguishable shapes can be fashioned, which allows one to gauge factors such as the vari-

ability in day-to-day transit and patient compliance. Some authors believe this is essential,[30] but the author has never done this in practice or in a research situation. Markers (Fig. 19.12) can be cut in circular (2 × 6 mm) or semicylindrical shapes (6 × 6 mm) from 16F radiopaque Levine tubes (Tomac 19947-9616 K10R, American Hospital Supply, Evanston, IL), or cylindrical shapes (1 × 6 mm) can be cut from radiopaque pediatric tubing. If neither of these is readily available, alternate radiopaque markers can be constructed from Levine or Salem sump tubes (Fig. 19.13), although the degree of radiopacity will need to be checked. Markers of the size described can be placed in gelatin capsules. Separate norms need to be calculated for each of these techniques.

All contrast material from previous studies should be cleared from the colon prior to the onset of the test, and no

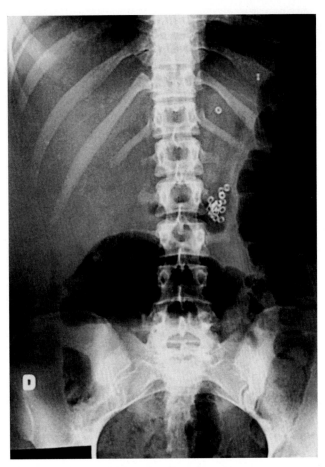

**FIGURE 19.14.** This patient just swallowed 20 radiopaque markers, 2 of which are in the fundus of the stomach. Note the gaseous outline of the colon, which is clearly distinct. This film is not essential and can be omitted but is needed to make sure that the patient did swallow the markers (some are noncompliant and pretend they did) and that the patient received and swallowed 20 markers, so that the mathematics to calculate transit times does not need to be changed (see text).

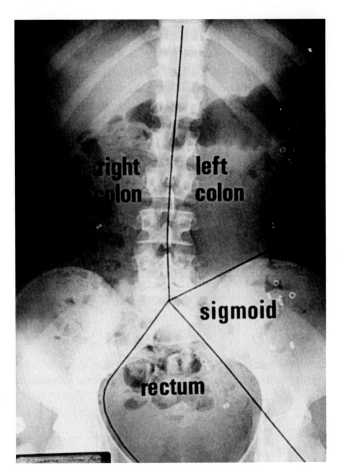

**FIGURE 19.15.** How to attribute markers to a given large bowel segment. In fact, most authors now combine the left colon and sigmoid zone, as in Table 19.3. A simple way is just to check for the spinal column and the pelvic rim.

contrast studies should be scheduled for the duration of the test. Patients should be instructed to consume their usual diet, continue usual activities, and omit the use of laxatives, enemas, or other medications known to affect gastrointestinal motility. Patients should be on supplemental fiber or a high-residue diet for the duration of the study. Patients should swallow 20 markers in one bolus in the morning, and films should be taken subsequently (Fig. 19.14).

Stools may be examined radiographically or, to distinguish between the different types of constipation, the progression of markers along the colon may be followed by daily radiographs of the abdomen. Most normal subjects will have passed all markers within 4 to 5 days following ingestion, whereas patients with severe constipation may not have passed all of the markers by 10 days after the study onset. Abdominal x-ray films should include the diaphragms and the pubis to ensure that all markers in the colon are visualized. Films are taken until all markers are expelled or for a maximum of 7 days after ingestion.

To calculate segmental transit times, markers are counted in the right colon, left colon, and rectosigmoid area by using the bony landmarks of the spine and pelvic contours (Fig. 19.15). Occasionally, a large cecum overlaps the pelvis, or a transverse colon is sagging into the abdomen; this can be recognized either by gaseous shadows or by barium enema in the same patient on another day. A simple formula can be obtained if the patient swallows 20 markers and a film is obtained every 24 hours: markers are counted in the segment of colon each day until distal total progression; these numbers are added and the sum is multiplied by 1.2.

To minimize radiation, markers may be ingested repetitively, after which a single x-ray film of the abdomen is taken following a variable length of time. It should be clearly understood, however, that this technique does not measure the mean transit time of a single marker, as the previous technique does, but the mean of mean transit times, presuming that they do not change from day to day (which they do). Moreover, the technique requires the establishment of steady-state conditions, and these require longer periods of ingestion as the severity of constipation increases. It is possible to obtain reliable measurements of colorectal transit times in

**TABLE 19.3.** Number of Markers Present

| Film | Right Colon | Left Colon | Rectosigmoid | Colon |
|------|-------------|------------|--------------|-------|
| 1st | 10 | 6 | 4 | 20 |
| 2nd | 2 | 4 | 6 | 12 |
| 3rd | 1 | 2 | 2 | 5 |
| 4th | 0 | 0 | 1 | 1 |
| 5th | 0 | 0 | 0 | 0 |
|  | 13 | 12 | 13 | 38 |

Mean right colon transit    $= 1.2 \times 13 = 15.6$ hours
Mean left colon transit     $= 1.2 \times 12 = 14.4$ hours
Mean rectosigmoid transit   $= 1.2 \times 13 = 15.6$ hours
Mean colonic transit        $= 1.2 \times 38 = 45.6$ hours

**TABLE 19.4.** Number of Markers Present

| Film | Right Colon | Left Colon | Rectosigmoid | Colon |
|------|-------------|------------|--------------|-------|
| 4th | 10 | 12 | 12 | 34 |
| 7th | 0 | 0 | 1 | 1 |
|  | 10 | 12 | 13 | 35 |

Right colon transit $= 1.2 \times 10 = 12$ hours
Left colon transit  $= 1.2 \times 12 = 14.4$ hours
Rectosigmoid        $= 1.2 \times 13 = 15.6$ hours
Colon               $= 1.2 \times 35 = 42$ hours

severe constipation, but markers should be ingested at least for 1 week in patients with normal transit constipation, 2 weeks in those with left colon dysfunction, and 4 weeks in those with colonic inertia. Of course, if a subject swallows 20 markers a day for 3 weeks, it will become close to impossible to count all of these markers on a plain film of the abdomen: if there was no defecation in this period of time,

420 markers should be present. The formula described is very flexible and allows adaptation: 5 markers may be given once a week for 1 month, and the multiplying number becomes

$$7 \times 24 = 168 \text{ (hours between films)}$$

5    5 (bolus) $= 33.6$ n markers (maximum in a month would be $5 \times 4 = 20$ in abdomen)

If total colonic transit times are calculated, all markers in the colon are tabulated for each abdominal film and used in the calculations. In calculating segmental transit times, the number of markers in a particular segment of the colon in each film is tabulated and substituted in the formula (Table 19.3).

If a multiple marker technique is used, the same formula can be used as long as 20 of each kind of marker are given, and markers are given at 24-hour intervals.

Again, in this situation, the total number of markers in each segment is used in the formula regardless of type (Table 19.4).

In the situation of diarrhea evacuation, the simplified formula may be modified to allow for the difference in time interval between abdominal x-ray films or administration of markers.

### Normograms

Normal values in adults have been obtained. Although acceptable for gross motor abnormalities and severe constipation, using them may be misleading for subjects complaining of minor constipation. Transit times of controls are shorter if they claim they do not have abdominal pain or changes in bowel habits when placed in stressful conditions: the longest transit time through the large bowel is only 43 hours instead of 93. Available data are found in Table 19.5.

Using radiopaque marker studies permits one to detect situations in which patients lie or misrepresent their complaint.

**TABLE 19.5.** Maximum "Normal" Transit Time though the Large Bowel (Mean + 2 SD, in Hours)*

| Adults | Chaussade et al, 1986[27] | Chaussade et al, 1990[62] | Metcalf, 1990[30] | Arhan et al, 1981[26] | Hinds et al, 1989[61] | Bouchoucha, 1992[31] | Bouchoucha et al, 1992[31†] |
|--------|------|------|------|------|------|------|------|
| Markers Technique | | | Multiple Ingestion | | | Single Ingestion | |
| Right colon | 24 | 24 | 32 | 38 | 24 | 37 | 20 |
| Left colon | 30 | 31 | 39 | 37 | 32 | 26 | 14‡ |
| Rectosigmoid | 44 | 33 | 36 | 34 | 45 | 41 | 25 |
| Colon and rectum (total) | 67 | 67 | 68 | 93 | 76 | 88 | 43‡ |

| Children | Arhan et al, 1981[26] (Single Ingestion) | Bautista et al, 1991[63] (Multiple Ingestion) |
|----------|------|------|
| Right colon | 18 | 18 |
| Left colon | 20 | 18 |
| Rectosigmoid | 34 | 19 |
| Colon and rectum (total) | 62 | 50 |

*Except for data from Arhan et al's study, which are not calculated from a Gaussian curve but are the maximal experimental values.

†Stress-free controls.

‡$p < .01$, as compared with other controls.

In such an event, it is best to use the discovery of misrepresentation as encouragement and relate the information back to the patient as evidence of improvement. Transit studies may also be used to evaluate segmental colonic transit time to detect specific areas of the bowel that are not functioning properly; the results of these studies may be abnormal even though patients have more than three stools per week. During follow-up, marker studies serve the purpose of providing objective data reflecting the clinical course.

Markers can also be counted in stools. This approach is useful to evaluate mouth-to-anus transit time but cannot be used to detect segmental abnormalities along the gastrointestinal tract. The first marker should be excreted by the end of the third day after ingestion and 80% within 5 days.

## CLINICAL RESULTS

Mechanisms of constipation can be approached in two different ways: following the progress of feces along the large bowel or evaluating bowel wall muscular activity and tone. The first method provides an estimate of the end results induced by abnormalities demonstrated by the second method.

### Types of Constipation

On the basis of radiopaque marker studies, patients with constipation may be divided into three different groups. In the first, there is delay in the colon.[16,24,25,55,56] Various labels have been used for this. Slow transit constipation refers to a situation in which markers are retained too long in the colon and/or rectum in the presence of a barium enema, which does not indicate the presence of megacolon and/or megarectum. In colonic inertia, there is slow transit of radiopaque markers in the ascending colon (Fig. 19.16), whether this is caused by sluggish bowel wall activity or distal functional or organic obstruction producing retropulsion of markers (Fig. 19.17); in the latter situation, a proposal has been made to call this constipation by colonic delay to distinguish hyper- from hypomotile situations.

Relatively few patients have a delayed transit in the ascending colon.[25,28,42,56,67] The incidence is 15% of the entire cohort complaining of constipation or 16 to 41% of those found to have delayed colorectal transit—this, of course, depending on the level of care (physicians in tertiary centers see more severely constipated patients). Right colonic stasis is very seldom limited to that site and is practically always associated with overall colorectal delayed transit.[28,57]

In the second situation, feces pass normally along the colon but are stored too long in the rectum.[16,53,58,59] Patients with hindgut dysfunction have normal right colon transit and distal delay. Thirty-three percent of patients with less than two stools per week have such a pattern, with half having delay in the left colon and rectosigmoid area and another half having outlet obstruction.[42] It is not clear whether these two groups of patients should be pooled together and classified

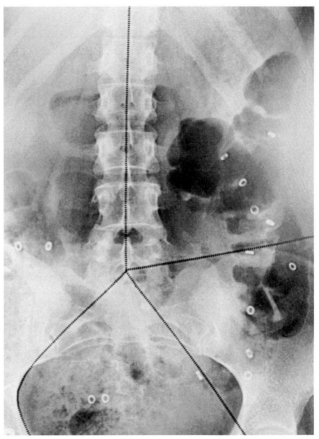

**FIGURE 19.16.**  One week after ingestion, this patient still had markers in the ascending colon. An extra film, taken for other reasons 1 week later, shows that 14 days after ingestion there are still three markers in the ascending colon.

under the broader term of distal constipation. Some patients with delayed transit in the ascending colon have clear evidence of reflux from left to right colon,[55] and, in some, the delay is not reproducible.[50] One explanation is that distal spasm slows down transit through the ascending colon, and these patients probably belong to the group of subjects constipated by hindgut dysfunction. Isolated stasis in the left colon occurs in 15% of a constipated cohort, or 36% of those found to have delayed overall large bowel transit.[28]

Some patients have normal colonic function but rectal stasis (Figs. 19.18 and 19.19); they suffer from outlet obstruction.[25,53,54] This is also relatively rare and occurs in only 13% of a constipated cohort but in 31% of those found to have delayed overall large bowel transit.[28]

In the third situation, the transit time of the radiopaque markers is normal. Twenty-nine percent of patients with less than two stools per week and 50% of those with less than three stools per week have "normal" transit in the large bowel.[42,43] This indicates the influence of diagnostic criteria used by clinicians. Patients with "normal" transit may have isolated delayed segmental transit in the descending colon, and some may have "normal" segmental transit times with overall delayed transit.[28,42,43] Only one-third of patients with "nor-

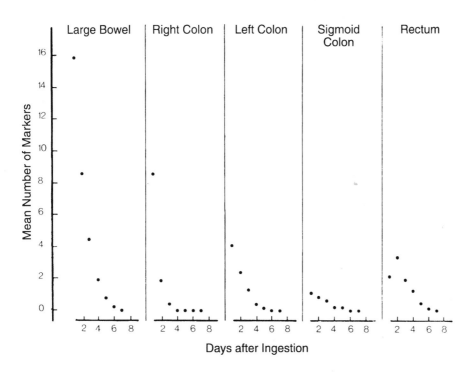

**FIGURE 19.17.** Transit of radiopaque markers through the large intestine. Although this figure represents average data, it is a helpful way to show an exponential decrease in the number of markers at a given site. Once a peak number is reached on successive days, normally, the number decreases. However, in some patients there is retropulsion of markers.

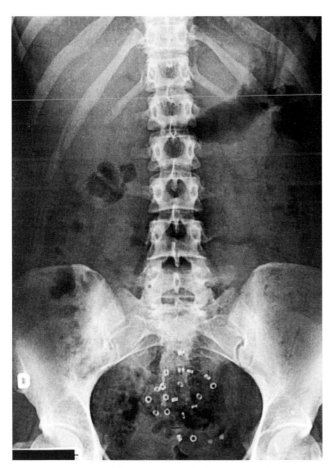

**FIGURE 19.18.** In this patient, all 20 ingested markers, 6 days after ingestion, have now been sitting in the rectum for 3 days in a row. Colon transit time is normal in the right and left colon. The patient has a megarectum.[53] In this situation, one can speak of outlet obstruction.

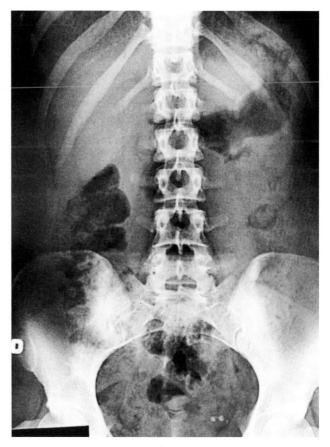

**FIGURE 19.19.** Same patient as in Figure 19.18. Between the taking of these two films, the patient defecated a very large stool and plugged the toilet bowl. Note the two phleboliths in the left part of the pelvis, also visible in Figure 19.18, which should not be confused with radiopaque markers, which have all been defecated at once.

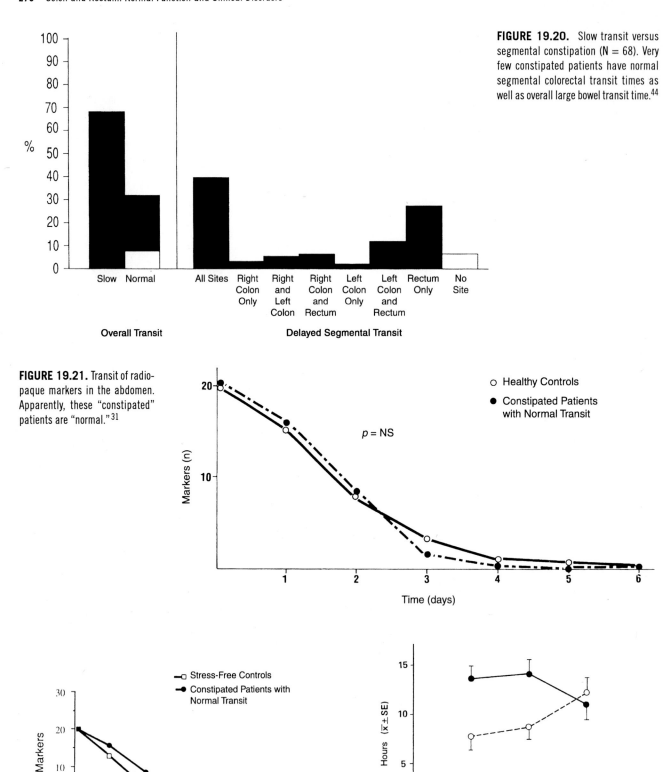

**FIGURE 19.20.** Slow transit versus segmental constipation (N = 68). Very few constipated patients have normal segmental colorectal transit times as well as overall large bowel transit time.[44]

**FIGURE 19.21.** Transit of radiopaque markers in the abdomen. Apparently, these "constipated" patients are "normal."[31]

**FIGURE 19.22.** Although the "constipated" patients charted in Figure 19.21 appear "normal" when compared to controls who claim that stress does not modify their bowel habits and does not trigger abdominal pain, their colonic transit is slightly delayed. There is an excess number of markers 2 ($p < .05$), 3 ($p < .01$), 4 ($p < .01$), and 5 days ($p < .05$) after ingestion.[31]

**FIGURE 19.23.** Segmental transit time through the human colon. Feces spend more time in the colon than in the rectum in adults (*solid circles*); the reverse is true in children (*open circles*). Overall, for the large bowel there is no difference.[26] In this study, the notion of stress and normal function was not investigated.

mal" colorectal transit also have "normal" segmental transit time,[44] (Fig. 19.20), and in only 4 of 61 patients were both anorectal manometry and studies of colorectal transit times "normal."[57] Subjects who are immune to stress have faster transit times[31]: several constipated patients with "normal" transit times (Fig. 19.21), in fact, have "delayed" transit when compared to this type of control (Fig. 19.22).[31] Thus, great care should be used before dismissing a patient as being "normal."

The complaint of constipation is confirmed by the physiopathologic finding of a delayed transit more often in women than in men.[28,31] Moreover, there are no differences in times of colorectal transit between men and women who are immune to stress.[31] This, and the joint analysis of colonic transit time with clinical signs, suggests that data collected during patient interview have little usefulness in distinguishing the different subsets of transit disturbance. For instance, the use of digital pressure to assist defecation, although relevant to an assessment of the severity of constipation, does not differentiate right colonic from rectosigmoid stasis.[28] However, low stool frequency and abdominal distention occur more frequently and abdominal distention occur more frequently when colorectal transit time is prolonged.

## Effects of Age, Exercise, and Alcohol

Age is an important variable. Although overall large bowel transit time does not differ in adults and children, the relative transit time in the colon is greater in adults (Fig. 19.23).[26] More recent data in children cast some doubts that rectal stasis is common at a younger age (see Table 19.3). However, occasionally, during in-depth psychoanalysis,[7] a patient may revert from an "adult" pattern to a "childlike" pattern. Whether this is regressive infantilization or cure from a stressful pattern is not known (Fig. 19.24). The reader is referred to a full review of the subject of constipation,[7] including mechanisms of constipation that are related to the classification described above. Patient selection (Fig. 19.25) and natural history (Fig. 19.26) are important variables to know to understand and interpret transit studies.

Apart from idiopathic constipation, little has been done in terms of understanding colorectal motility and transit time. Football players, who engage in strenuous physical activity as compared with much more sedentary students, do not have faster colorectal transit times. However, right colon transit is considerably slower, left colon and rectum transit

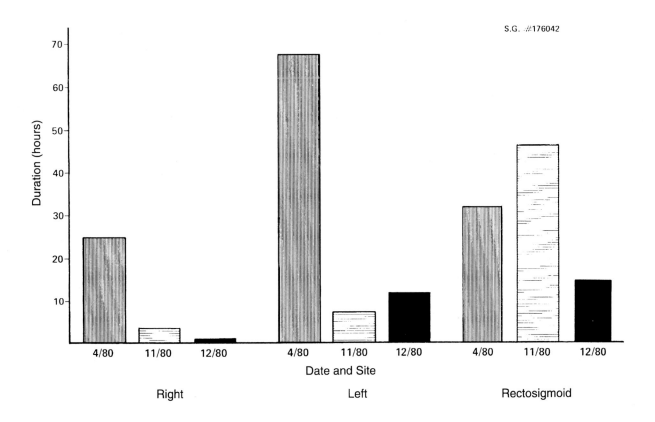

**FFIGURE 19.24.** Segmental colonic transit time. Successive transit studies were obtained as quality control of therapy in this 24-year-old women, a victim of incest who initially defecated once a week for 20 years. Without medication, there is clear acceleration of the transit time. In April, transit in the left colon is markedly delayed. By December, the patient had cathartic experiences about what she lived sexually and emotionally in her family. Transit has become very fast in the ascending colon and normal in the left. Rectal transit is normal, and this is where the feces stay longer. The patient thus has reverted to a "childlike" or "infantile" pattern of colorectal motility; however, she remained asymptomatic for 12 years.

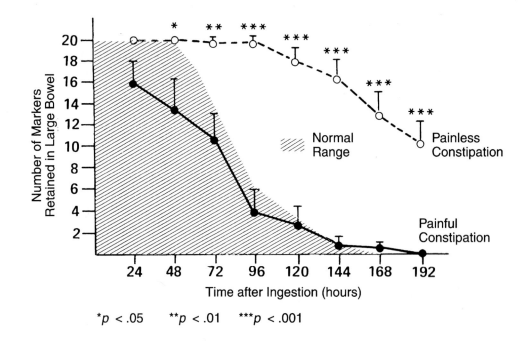

**FIGURE 19.25.** Transit of radiopaque markers in chronic idiopathic constipation. Patients with painless constipation have slower transit than those with painful constipation. (See Devroede[7] for a full discussion.) It is essential to know the selection criteria of patients before making an interpretation of transit studies with radiopaque markers.

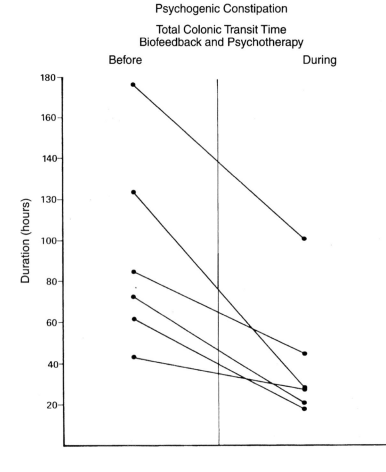

**FIGURE 19.26.** During biofeedback therapy for anismus combined with psychotherapy there may be physical evidence of improvement obtained with radiopaque marker transit studies.

being somewhat prolonged and making up the delay so that there is no overall difference.[60] Alcoholic patients often complain of chronic diarrhea. Its origin is multifactorial, but withdrawal of alcohol profoundly modifies colorectal transit. Thus, using radiopaque markers, it was demonstrated that, after withdrawal, large bowel transit becomes slower but only because of rectosigmoid transit, which becomes three times as long; colonic transit is unaffected.[61] In summary, techniques using radiopaque markers have proved of great value to study the mechanisms of constipation and can help one to choose among the modalities of treatment. They are simple, reliable, and reproducible. They should be the gold standard against which newer techniques should be checked, keeping in mind the considerations, limitations, clinical findings, and pitfalls exemplified in this chapter.

## REFERENCES

1. Devroede G. Dietary fiber, bowel habits, and colonic function. Am J Clin Nutr 1978;10 Suppl 31:157–60.
2. Hertz F, Newton A. The normal movements of the colon in man. J Physiol 1913;47:57–65.
3. Halls J. Bowel content shift during normal defecation. Proc R Soc Med 1965;58:859–60.
4. Ritchie JA. Colonic motor activity and bowel function. Part I. Normal movement of contents. Gut 1968;9:442–56.
5. Lesaffer LPA. Digital subtraction defecography. In: Smith LE, editor. Practical guide to anorectal testing. New York/Tokyo: Igaku-Shoin; 1990. p. 127–34.
6. Preston DM, Lennard-Jones JE. Anismus in chronic constipation. Dig Dis Sci 1985;30:413–8.
7. Devroede G. Constipation. In: Sleisenger M, Fordtran J, editors. Gastrointestinal disease: pathophysiology, diagnosis, management, 5th ed. Philadelphia: WB Saunders Co.; 1993.
8. Whitehead WE, Chaussade S, Corazziari E, Kumar D. Report of an international workshop on management of constipation. Gastroenterol Int 1991;4:99–113.
9. Davies GJ, Crowder M, Dickerson JWT. Dietary fibre intake of individuals with different eating patterns. J Hum Nutr Appl 1985;39:139–48.
10. Tucker DM, Sandstead HH, Logan GM Jr, et al. Dietary fiber and personality factors as determinants of stool output. Gastroenterology 1981;81:879–83.
11. Cummings JH. Constipation, dietary fiber and the control of large bowel function. Postgrad Med J 1984;60:811–9.
12. Everhart JE, Go VL, Johannes RS, et al. A longitudinal survey of self-reported bowel habits in the United States. Dig Dis Sci 1989;34:1153–62.
13. Corazziari E, Materia E, Baurano G, et al. Laxative consumption in chronic nonorganic constipation. J Clin Gastroenterol 1987;9:427–30.
14. Dent OF, Goulston KJ, Zubrzycki J, Chapuis PH. Bowel symptoms in an apparently well population. Dis Colon Rectum 1986;29:243–7.
15. Milne JS, Williamson J. Bowel habits in older people. Gerontol Clin 1972;14:56–60.
16. Hinton JM, Lennard-Jones JE. Constipation: definition and classification. Postgrad Med J 1968;44:720–3.
17. Preston DM, Pfeffer JM, Lennard-Jones JE. Psychiatric assessment of patients with severe constipation [abstract]. Gut 1984;25:582.
18. Devroede G. Obstipation: what is the appropriate therapeutic approach? In: Barkin JS, Rogers AI, editors. Difficult decisions in digestive diseases. Chicago: Year Book; 1989. p. 458–84.
19. Cremora-Barbaro A. The Munchausen syndrome and its symbolic significance: an in depth case analysis. Br J Psychiatry 1987;151:76–9.
20. Drossman DA, Li Z, Andruzzi E, et al. U.S. household survey of functional gastrointestinal disorders. Prevalence sociodemography and health impact. Dig Dis Sci 1993;38:1569–80.
21. Drossman DA, Leserman J, Nachman G, et al. Sexual and physical abuse in women with functional or organic gastrointestinal disorders. Ann Intern Med 1990;113:828–33.
22. Leroi AM, Bernier C, Watier A, et al. Prevalence of sexual abuse among patients with functional disorders of the lower gastrointestinal tract. Int J Colorectal Dis 1995;10:200–6.
23. Arnold RP, Rogers D, Cook DAG. Medical problems of adults who were sexually abused in childhood. BMJ 1990;300:705–8.
24. Hinton JM, Lennard-Jones JE, Young AC. A new method for studying gut transit times using radiopaque markers. Gut 1969;10:842–7.
25. Martelli H, Devroede G, Arhan P, Duguay C. Mechanisms of idiopathic constipation: outlet obstruction. Gastroenterology 1978; 75:623–31.
26. Arhan P, Devroede G, Jehannin B, et al. Segmental colonic transit time. Dis Colon Rectum 1981;24:625–9.
27. Chaussade S, Roches H, Khyari A, et al. Mesure du temps de transit colique (TTC): description et validation d'une nouvelle technique. Gastroentérol Clin Biol 1986;10:385–9.
28. Chaussade S, Khyari A, Roche H, et al. Determination of total and segmental colonic transit time in constipated patients. Results in 91 patients with a new simplified method. Dig Dis Sci 1989;34:1168–72.
29. Metcalf AM, Phillips SF, Zimsmeister AR, et al. Simplified assessment of segmental colonic transit time. Gastroenterology 1987;92:40–7.
30. Metcalf A. Transit time. In: Smith LE, editor. Practical guide to anorectal testing. New York/Tokyo: Igaku-Shoin; 1990. p. 17–22.
31. Bouchoucha M, Devroede G, Arhan P, et al. What is the meaning of colorectal transit time measurement? Dis Colon Rectum 1992;35: 773–82.
32. Abrahamsson H, Antov S, Bosacus I. Gastrointestinal and colonic segmental transit time evaluated by a single abdominal x ray in healthy subjects and constipated patients. Scand J Gastroenterol 1988;23 Suppl 152:72–80.
33. Fortherby KJ, Hunter JP. Idiopathic slow transit constipation: whole gut transit times, measured by a new simplified method, are not shortened by opioid antagonist. Aliment Pharmacol Ther 1987;1:331–8.
34. Krevsky B, Maurer AH, Fisher RS. Patterns of colonic transit in chronic idiopathic constipation. Am J Gastroenterol 1989;84:127–32.
35. Kamm MA, Lennard-Jones JE, Thompson DG, et al. Dynamic scanning defines a colonic defect in severe idiopathic constipation. Gut 1988;29:1085–92.
36. Bazzocchi J, Ellis J, Villanueva-Meyer J, et al. Postprandial colonic transit and motor activity in chronic constipation. Gastroenterology 1990;98:686–93.
37. Stubbs JB, Valenzuela GA, Stubbs CC, et al. A noninvasive scintigraphic assessment of the colonic transit of nondigestible solids in man. J Nutr Med 1991;32:1375–81.
38. Proano M, Camilleri M, Phillips SF, et al. Transit of solids through the human colon: regional quantification in the unprepared bowel. Am J Physiol 1990;258:G856–62.
39. Stivland T, Camilleri M, Vassallo M, et al. Scintigraphic measurement of regional gut transit in idiopathic constipation. Gastroenterology 1991;101:107–15.
40. McLean RG, Smart RC, Gaston-Parry D, et al. Colon transit scintigraphy in health and constipation using oral iodine-131-cellulose. J Nucl Med 1990;31:985–9.
41. Basile M, Neri M, Carriero A, et al. Measurement of segmental transit through the gut in man: a novel approach by the biomagnetic method. Dig Dis Sci 1992;37:1537–43.
42. Wald A. Colonic transit and anorectal manometry in chronic idiopathic constipation. Arch Intern Med 1986;146:1713–6.
43. Schang JC. Colonic motility in subgroups of patients with the irritable bowel syndrome. In: Poitras P, editor. Proceedings of the First International Symposium on Small Intestinal and Colonic Motility. Montreal; Centre de Recherches Clinique, Hôpital Saint-Luc and Jouveinal Laboratoires/Laboratories; 1985. p. 101–12.
44. Kuijpers HC. Application of the colorectal laboratory in diagnosis and treatment of functional constipation. Dis Colon Rectum 1990;33:35–9.

45. Corazziari E, Dani S, Pozzessere C, et al. Colonic segmental transit times in non-organic constipation. Rend Gastroenterol 1975;7:67–9.

46. Marzio L, Del Bianco R, Delle Donne M, et al. Mouth-to-cecum transit time in patients affected by chronic constipation: effect of glucomannan. Am J Gastroenterol 1989;84:888–91.

47. Cann PA, Read NW, Brown C, et al. Irritable bowel syndrome: relationship of disorders in the transit of a single solid meal to symptom patterns. Gut 1983;24:405–11.

48. Bassotti G, Gaburri M, Clausi GG, et al. Can idiopathic megacolon cause functional motor abnormalities in the upper gastrointestinal tract? Hepatogastroenterology 1987;34:186–9.

49. Tomlin J, Read NW. Laxative properties of indigestible plastic particles. BMJ 1988;297:1175–6.

50. Devroede G, Girard G, Bouchoucha M, et al. Idiopathic constipation by colonic dysfunction: relationship with personality and anxiety. Dig Dis Sci 1989;34:1428–33.

51. Cummings JH, Wiggins H. Transit through the gut measured by analysis of a single stool. Gut 1976;17:219–23.

52. Papoolis A. Signal analysis. New York: McGraw-Hill; 1977.

53. Verduron A, Devroede G, Bouchoucha M, et al. Megarectum. Dig Dis Sci 1988;33:1164–74.

54. Waldron D, Bowes KL, Kingma YL, Cote KR. Colonic and anorectal motility in young women with severe idiopathic constipation. Gastroenterology 1988;95:1388–9.

55. Watier A, Devroede G, Duranceau A, et al. Constipation with colonic inertia. A manifestation of systemic disease? Dig Dis Sci 1985;28:1025–33.

56. Waller SL. Differential measurement of small and large bowel transit times in constipation and diarrhoea: a new approach. Gut 1975;16:371–8.

57. Ducrotte P, Rodomanska B, Weber J, et al. Colonic transit time of radiopaque markers and rectoanal manometry in patients complaining of constipation. Dis Colon Rectum 1986;29:630–4.

58. Eastwood MA, Kirkpatrick JR, Mitchell WD, et al. Effects of dietary supplements of wheat bran and cellulose of faeces and bowel function. BMJ 1973;4:392–4.

59. Melkersson M, Andersson H, Bosaeus I, Falkheden T. Intestinal transit time in constipated and nonconstipated geriatric patients. Scand J Gastroenterol 1983;18:593–7.

60. Arhan P, Sesboue B, Devroede G, et al. Colonic transit in soccer players. J Clin Gastroenterol 1995;20:211–4.

61. Hinds JP, Stoney B, Wald A. Does gender or the menstrual cycle affect colonic transit? Am J Gastroenterol 1989;84:123–6.

62. Chaussade S, Gosselin A, Hostein J, et al. Détermination du temps de transit colique (TTC) global et segmentaire dans une population de 96 sujet solontaires sains. Gastroenterol Clin Biol 1990;14:95–7.

63. Bautista CA, Varela CA, Villanueva J, et al. Measurement of colonic transit time in children. J Pediatr Gastroenterol Nutr 1991;13:42–5.

# CHAPTER 20

# Scintigraphy

*Charlene M. Prather*

Patients frequently present with symptoms of disturbed transit of the gastrointestinal transit. The need for quantitative information about gastrointestinal transit in these situations has led to the development of a variety of gastrointestinal transit tests. Colonic transit techniques have evolved from the use of nonabsorbable markers to radiopaque markers and now scintigraphy. Scintigraphic colon transit was developed from the need for a simple, noninvasive test that provided regional and overall colonic transit information. Tests of gastrointestinal transit are employed to quantitate the severity of disturbed transit in patients with a variety of functional gastrointestinal symptoms such as constipation, diarrhea, or bloating. Colonic transit is traditionally measured using radiopaque markers (Chapter 29). Although robust and inexpensive, the information from radiopaque markers is somewhat limited by the duration of the test (5–7 days) and the requirement for the patient to abstain from laxatives or other medications that alter transit. The desire for more precise measurements of regional and overall colonic transit and the need for a test with a shorter duration led to the use of nuclear medicine technology and the development of several scintigraphic techniques.

Scintigraphic colonic transit involves administering a radioactive substance (isotope) and following the progression of the isotope with a gamma camera through the gastrointestinal tract at specific time points. Early strategies to characterize colonic transit using scintigraphy have included the antegrade instillation of the radionuclide indium 111-diethylenetriamine pentaacetic acid ([111]In-DTPA) by means of an oral-cecal tube[1]

and the retrograde instillation of isotope into the colon through a tube placed by colonoscopy.[2] Although these two techniques provided more direct measures of colon transit than prior techniques, the invasiveness of their methodologies relegated them to remain research tools. A move toward more physiologic and noninvasive techniques followed, using the oral transit of the liquid isotope [111]In-DTPA as a surrogate measure of colonic transit.[3,4] This technique includes transit through the esophagus, stomach, and small bowel before reaching the colon. To facilitate a more direct measure of regional and overall colonic transit, a coated, pH-sensitive capsule was designed to deliver the isotope in a bolus fashion to the cecum.[5] These latter two techniques have gained acceptance as useful research and clinical tools for the evaluation of patients with altered bowel habits.[4,6]

## INDICATIONS

Colonic scintigraphy is used in the evaluation of patients with symptoms of altered colonic transit including constipation, abdominal bloating, and refractory irritable bowel syndrome. Measurement of colonic transit can be expected to identify the presence and severity of transit abnormalities and to assess response to therapies. Although used predominantly to evaluate suspected slow colonic transit, scintigraphic measurement of colonic transit has also been used to document rapid colonic transit.[7] In addition, scintigraphic colonic transit is used when more specific regional colonic transit information is desired. Patients with slow colonic transit may be identified as having predominant delay of right colon transit, left colon transit, or overall transit.[8] This information may become increasingly important as pharmaceutical agents are developed that target specific transit abnormalities such as slow proximal colon emptying or slow rectosigmoid emptying. Measures of colonic transit may also be used to provide objective evidence of the efficacy of medical and surgical therapies.

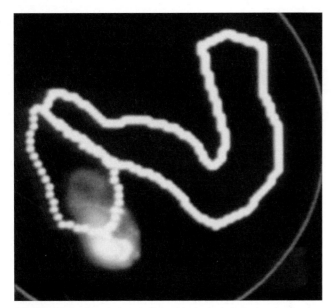

**FIGURE 20.1.** Dissolution of pH-sensitive capsule in ileum-releasing isotope. The broken line indicates the cecum and ascending colon; the solid line outlines the transverse colon. Just below the broken line, the isotope can be seen filling the terminal ileum.

## TECHNIQUES

### Coated, pH-Sensitive Capsule Technique

The pH-sensitive capsule method of measuring colonic transit is at least as sensitive as the radiopaque marker method for detecting delayed colonic transit and has been used successfully to identify accelerated transit.[9,10] This technique was originally described using a methacrylate-coated capsule containing resin pellets labeled with isotope.[11] The methacrylate coating is pH sensitive and dissolves in the relatively alkaline pH of the ileum (ileal pH = 7.4). The distal ileum empties solid residue in a bolus fashion.[12] Thus, the capsule dissolves in the ileum and the isotope is delivered in a bolus fashion to the cecum (Fig. 20.1). This provides a more direct measure of colonic transit. The radiolabeled pellets used in the initial description of the pH-sensitive capsule technique are not readily available, leading to a modification of the originally described technique. Activated charcoal is substituted for the resin pellets, providing nearly identical results to the resin pellet technique.[13] The use of charcoal makes this technique more generally available for clinical and research applications.[13] Although the more economical and readily available isotope technetium 99m ($^{99m}$Tc) can be used in place of $^{111}$In, most centers use $^{111}$In because of its longer half-life (67 hours), allowing procurement of multiple scans over several days. By contrast, the half-life of $^{99m}$Tc is only 6 hours. Use of iodine 131 has also been described, although its use is not widespread.[14,15]

### Technical Details

The following supplies are needed for capsule preparation:
- 5-mg activated charcoal
- 0.1-mCi (3.7 MBq) $^{111}$In-DTPA
- Size 1 gelatin medication capsule
- Warming plate
- Methacrylate
- Granular dextrose

The capsule must be prepared in the laboratory setting with appropriate radiation safety precautions in place. Limited air circulation is preferred as care must be taken to

**A** 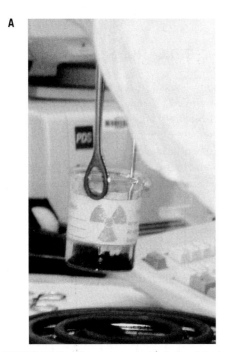  **B** 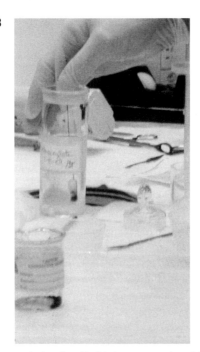  **C**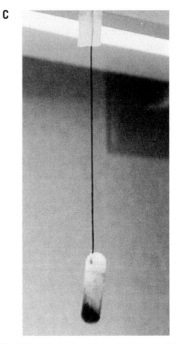

**FIGURE 20.2.** Pharmacy-grade charcoal and the isotope are mixed and gently dried over a warming plate (**A**). After the charcoal is packed in a gelatin capsule, the capsule is dipped in methacrylate (**B**). The capsule is then hung to dry (**C**).

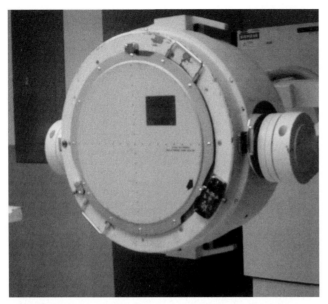

**FIGURE 20.3.** A single-headed large-field-of-view gamma camera.

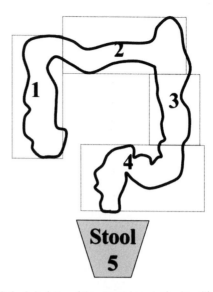

**FIGURE 20.4.** Calculation of the geometric center begins with dividing the colon into the four segments, with a fifth segment representing excreted stool.

keep the charcoal particles from becoming aerosolized. The charcoal is placed in a Pyrex glass container and the $^{111}$In is added with a small amount of 0.1-N HCl, saturating the charcoal. The amount of $^{111}$In added is calculated using standard decay tables so that 0.1 mCi is remaining at the start of the anticipated study. This allows for efficient use of the amount of isotope contained per unit vial and stream-lining of the production process. For example, all capsules could be prepared on Friday for the following week (Table 20.1). Using a warming plate and metal stirring spatula, the charcoal is gently dried over the warming plate (Fig. 20.2A). The charcoal is scraped into the gelatin capsule, and any remaining space is filled with granular dextrose. The capsule is submerged into methacrylate solution with three separate dips (Fig. 20.2B). The capsule is then hung to air dry for a period of 1 hour (Fig. 20.2C).[13]

The capsule is ingested following an overnight fast. Subjects are fed a standard breakfast, lunch 4 hours later, and dinner 4 hours after that. Images are obtained using a large-field-of-view gamma camera with a medium-energy, parallel-hole collimator (Fig. 20.3). For clinical studies, anterior and posterior images are obtained with the subjects standing for

**TABLE 20.1.** Isotope Amount for Advanced Preparation

| Number of Days Ahead | Activity ± 10% (µCi) |
| --- | --- |
| Three days (Monday) | 208 |
| Four days (Tuesday) | 266 |
| Five days (Wednesday) | 340 |
| Six days (Thursday) | 435 |
| Seven days (Friday) | 558 |

For convenience, several capsules can be prepared in advance, adjusting the amount of isotope for the day it will be administered. The table illustrates the amount of isotope required if the capsules were made on a Friday for the following week.

60 seconds in each position at time periods 4 hours and 24 hours. During research studies or when more detailed information is desired, additional time periods may be studied.

### Colonic Transit Analysis

The scans are analyzed using standard region-of-interest programs, separating the colon into anatomic sections. These sections are given numeric values: cecum and ascending = 1, transverse = 2, descending = 3, rectosigmoid = 4, and stool = 5 (Fig. 20.4). Using these sections, a weighted average of counts is determined. This weighted average is called the geometric center. To calculate the geometric center, the percentage of radioactivity in these five regions is determined and a composite score is calculated using the formula

$$(\%AC*1 + \%TC*2 + \%DC*3 + \%RS*4 + \%Stool*5)/100$$

The percentage of istope is determined in each segment and multiplied by the corresponding number assigned to the segment (eg, if 20% of the isotope resided in the transverse colon, multiply 20 by 2). These are added together and divided by 100 to determine the geometric center. A low geometric center indicates slow colonic transit (Fig. 20.5). A high geometric center indicates more rapid colonic transit (Fig. 20.6). In healthy subjects, the 4-hour geometric center is 1.14 ± 0.07 and the 24 geometric center is 2.83 ± 0.25 (mean ± SEM) (Fig. 20.7).[16] A large number of subjects across centers have not been studied to provide the most accurate assessment for normal colonic transit values. Table 20.2 reviews data gleaned from several published studies.[1,13,16–18] Direct comparisons between techniques and investigators are difficult because of different meal nutrient and fiber composition during the study and the number of colonic regions used for the assessment of the geometric center. The correlation between scintigraphic and radiopaque

**TABLE 20.2.** Normal Values for Scintigraphic Transit

| Lead Author | Technique | Subjects | No. of Colonic Regions* | 4-Hour GC | 24-Hour GC | 48-Hour GC |
|---|---|---|---|---|---|---|
| Krevsky[1] | Cecal instillation | 7 | 7 | 4.8 (5 h) | 5.3 | 6.3 |
| Burton[13] | Coated capsule—charcoal | 10 | 5 | 1.1 | 2.7 | NA |
| Camilleri[16] | Coated capsule—pellets | 22 | 5 | 1.1 | 2.8 | NA |
| Krevsky[18] | PO liquid isotope | 15 | 7 | NA | 4.2 | 6.2 |
| Notghi[19] | Coated capsule—pellets | 8 | 5 | 1.4 | 2.9 | 4.1 |

*Number of colonic regions plus stool.

GC, geometric center; NA, not available.

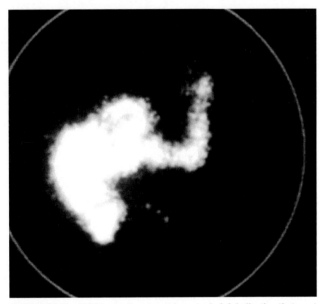

**FIGURE 20.5.** At 24 hours, the geometric center is 1.4, indicating that most of the isotope resides in the proximal colon.

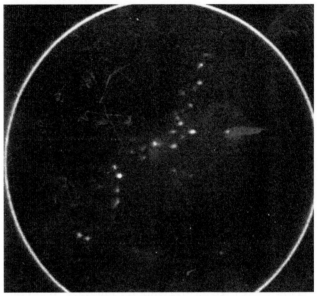

**FIGURE 20.6.** At 24 hours, the geometric center is 4.9, indicating that most of the isotope has already been excreted in the stool.

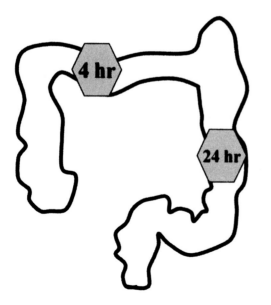

**FIGURE 20.7.** The hexagons show the expected location of the geometric center in healthy subjects at 4 and 24 hours.

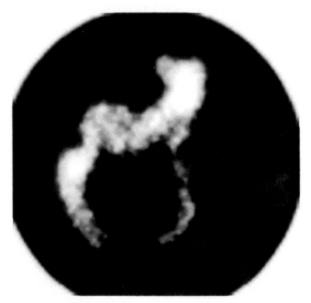

**FIGURE 20.8.** Mildly slow colonic transit at 24 hours with a geometric center past the splenic flexure.

**TABLE 20.3.** Comparison of Scintigraphic Techniques for Measuring Colonic Transit

| Method | Advantages | Disadvantages | Comments |
|---|---|---|---|
| Orocecal intubation | Direct instillation of isotope into the colon | Orocecal intubation necessary | Invasive<br>Research tool |
| Cecal instillation | Direct instillation of isotope into the colon<br>Can show retrograde movement | Colonoscopy necessary<br>Fluoroscopy<br>Prepared colon | Invasive<br>Research tool |
| Oral liquid transit | Simple<br>Minimal preparation | Liquid rather than solid label<br>Small bowel—terminal ileum<br>overlap with cecum | Noninvasive<br>Multiple scans without increased<br>radiation exposure |
| Coated capsule | Physiologic<br>Solid-phase label<br>No colon preparation required | Preparation of capsule<br>Failure of capsule dissolution (5%) | Noninvasive<br>Acceptable radiation exposure |

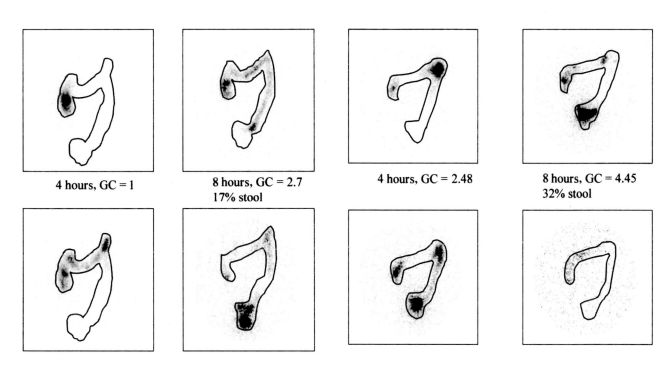

4 hours, GC = 1

8 hours, GC = 2.7
17% stool

4 hours, GC = 2.48

8 hours, GC = 4.45
32% stool

**FIGURE 20.9.** Normal colonic transit with images obtained at 4, 6, 8, and 24 hours. Note the predominance of isotope located in the rectosigmoid at 24 hours.

**FIGURE 20.10.** Rapid colonic transit with images obtained at 4, 6, 8, and 24 hours. Note the near complete emptying of the colon at 24 hours.

marker colonic transit results in normal and constipated patients is good. However, when comparing the coated capsule method containing 1-mm particles to the 6-mm radiopaque marker method, the larger markers moved significantly faster through the proximal colon.[9] In the calculation of the geometric center, isotope count corrections are also made for depth (geometric mean of the anterior and posterior scans), isotope decay, and Compton scattering.[9] In addition to the geometric center method of quantifying colonic transit, regional transit or emptying can also be measured for specific colonic sections. These methods of measuring colonic transit have provided additional insight into the normal physiology of the colon. The coated capsule technique illustrated that the ascending colon acts as a reservoir for solid materials and exhibits a two-phase emptying

profile. There is an initial lag phase when minimal emptying occurs, followed by a phase of linear emptying.[11]

The coated capsule method of measuring colonic transit provides a more direct measure of colonic transit. Additional advantages conferred with using this method include studying the colon in its natural state (ie, the unprepared colon) and the ability to procure multiple scans or images of the colon without increasing the radiation exposure to the subject. The primary disadvantage is the need for capsule preparation and access to a gamma camera. In addition, the capsule fails to dissolve in the ileum in about 5% of subjects. The advantages and disadvantages of the scintigraphic techniques are reviewed in Table 20.3. Figures 20.8 to 20.10 show slow, normal, and rapid colony transit.

## Orocecal Transit of [111]In-DTPA

The preparation of the specialized capsules has proved difficult for many centers to incorporate. An alternative method for measuring colonic transit has been described using [111]In-DTPA in 10-mL water.[19] This is administered with a solid meal that has been labeled with [99m]Tc. The Tc is used to measure gastric and small bowel transit of solids. The [111]In-DTPA provides a measure of liquid gastric emptying and small bowel transit. The average abdominal counts are measured at a specified time point, typically between 2 and 3 hours, and taken as 100% of the radioactivity. Scintigraphic scans are obtained at 24 and 48 hours, and the geometric center is determined. Investigators describing this technique have further subdivided the colon into smaller regions using seven areas for the calculation of the geometric center: 1 = cecum and ascending colon, 2 = hepatic flexure, 3 = transverse colon, 4 = splenic flexure, 5 = descending colon, 6 = rectosigmoid, and 7 = stool. The normal geometric center at 24 hours is $4.2 \pm 0.5$ and $6.2 \pm 0.2$ at 48 hours.[17] The results with this technique show that women have slower colonic transit than men do, with 68% retention at 24 hours versus 36.3% in men. Age did not influence colonic transit. Using the geometric center method of analyzing colonic transit, normal values at 24 hours were $4.6 \pm 1.5$ (splenic flexure) and $6.2 \pm 1.0$ (rectosigmoid) at 48 hours.[17]

Scintigraphic colonic transit provides physiologic, quantitative information about overall and regional colonic transit. The methodologies for these techniques have been simplified, making them generally applicable for both the clinical and research laboratories. The scintigraphic transit measures accurately separate normal from rapid and delayed transit. This allows more reliable targeting of therapy for patients with similar complaints but abnormalities of transit localized to different regions of the gastrointestinal tract.

## REFERENCES

1. Krevsky B, Malmud LS, D'Ercole F, et al. Colonic transit scintigraphy. A physiologic approach to the quantitative measurement of colonic transit in humans. Gastroenterology 1986;91:1102–12.
2. Moreno-Osset E, Bazzocchi G, Lo S, et al. Association between postprandial changes in colonic intraluminal pressure and transit. Gastroenterology 1989;96:1265–73.
3. Maurer AH, Krevsky B. Whole-gut transit scintigraphy in the evaluation of small-bowel and colon transit disorders. Semin Nucl Med 1995;25:326–38.
4. Bonapace ES, Maurer AH, Davidoff S, et al. Whole gut transit scintigraphy in the clinical evaluation of patients with upper and lower gastrointestinal symptoms. Am J Gastroenterol 2000;95:2838–47.
5. Camilleri M, Colemont LJ, Phillips SF, et al. Human gastric emptying and colonic filling of solids characterized by a new method. Am J Physiol 1989;257:G284–90.
6. Charles F, Camilleri M, Phillips SF, et al. Scintigraphy of the whole gut: clinical evaluation of transit disorders. Mayo Clin Proc 1995;70:113–8.
7. Charles F, Phillips SF, Camilleri M, Thomforde GM. Rapid gastric emptying in patients with functional diarrhea. Mayo Clinic Proc 1997;72:323–8.
8. Notghi A, Hutchinson R, Kumar D, et al. Simplified method for the measurement of segmental colonic transit time. Gut 1994;35:976–81.
9. Stivland T, Camilleri M, Vassallo M, et al. Scintigraphic measurement of regional gut transit in idiopathic constipation. Gastroenterology 1991;101:107–15.
10. Barrow L, Steed KP, Spiller RC, et al. Quantitative, noninvasive assessment of antidiarrheal actions of codeine using an experimental model of diarrhea in man. Dig Dis Sci 1993;38:996–1003.
11. Proano M, Camilleri M, Phillips SF, et al. Transit of solids through the human colon: regional quantification in the unprepared bowel. Am J Physiol 1990;258:G856–62.
12. Spiller RC, Brown ML, Phillips SF. Emptying of the terminal ileum in intact humans. Influence of meal residue and ileal motility. Gastroenterology 1987;92:724–9.
13. Burton DD, Camilleri M, Mullan BP, et al. Colonic transit scintigraphy labeled activated charcoal compared with ion exchange pellets. J Nucl Med 1997;38:1807–10.
14. McLean RG, Smart RC, Gaston-Parry D, et al. Colon transit scintigraphy in health and constipation using oral iodine-131-cellulose. J Nucl Med 1990;31:985–9.
15. Smart RC, McLean RG, Gaston-Parry D, et al. Comparison of oral iodine-131-cellulose and indium-111-DTPA as tracers for colon transit scintigraphy: analysis by colon activity profiles. J Nucl Med 1991;32:1668–74.
16. Camilleri M, Zinsmeister AR. Towards a relatively inexpensive, noninvasive, accurate test for colonic motility disorders. Gastroenterology 1992;103:36–42.
17. Krevsky B, Maurer AH, Niewiarowski T, Cohen S. Effect of verapamil on human intestinal transit. Dig Dis Sci 1992;37:919–24.
18. Notghi A, Hutchinson R, Kumar D, et al. Simplified method for the measurement of segmental colonic transit time. Gut 1994;35:976–81.
19. McLean RG, Smart RC, Lubowski DZ, et al. Oral colon transit scintigraphy using indium-111 DTPA: variability in healthy subjects. Int J Colorectal Dis 1992;7:173–6.

CHAPTER 21

# Manometry

*Arnold Wald*

## ANATOMY AND FUNCTION

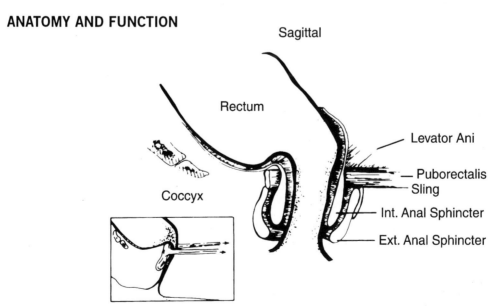

**FIGURE 21.1.** Anatomy of the anorectum. The major structures of the anorectum are the rectum, the anorectal angle formed by the puborectalis muscle, and the internal and external anal sphincters surrounding the anal canal. The rectal wall includes both inner circular and outer longitudinal smooth muscle layers; the internal anal sphincter consists of thickened circular smooth muscle that is innervated by the enteric nerves. Both the puborectalis and external anal sphincter muscles are striated muscles for which innervation is provided from the sacral nerves, the former innervated by S3 and S4, whereas the latter receives its nerve supply from the pudendal nerves (S2, 3, and 4). Sensory mechanoreceptors in the perirectal tissues allow awareness of rectal filling or distention, whereas anal nerve endings permit discrimination of gas, liquids, or solid rectal contents.

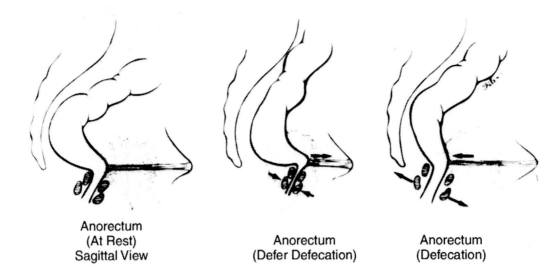

Anorectum
(At Rest)
Sagittal View

Anorectum
(Defer Defecation)

Anorectum
(Defecation)

**FIGURE 21.2.** Anatomic changes during continence and defecation. At rest (*left*), the anorectal angle approximates 85 to 105 degrees and normally is at the level of an imaginary line drawn from the symphysis pubis to the tip of the coccyx. About 80% of the resting pressure in the anal canal is derived from the internal anal sphincter, and this greatly exceeds intrarectal pressure. The movement of fecal wastes to the rectum reflexively but temporarily relaxes the internal anal sphincter. Defecation is deferred (*center*) by contraction of both the puborectalis muscle and external anal sphincter, the former narrowing the anorectal angle and the latter increasing resistance pressures in the anal canal until the rectum accommodates to its increased contents and propulsive forces are diminished. During defecation (*right*), increased intra-abdominal pressures help to propel bowel contents toward the anal canal while relaxation of striated muscles results in perineal descent, widening of the anorectal angle, and decreasing pressures in the anal canal. After defecation is completed, anorectal structures return to their normal positions at rest.

## METHODS OF OBTAINING MANOMETRIC RECORDINGS OF THE ANORECTUM

Various methods exist for recording anorectal motility, each with advantages and potential drawbacks. All of these catheters are connected to a physiograph recorder via transducers.

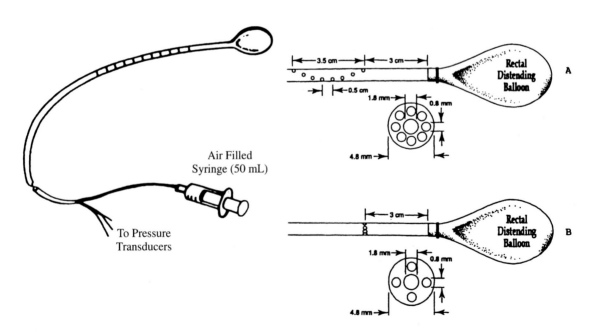

Air Filled
Syringe (50 mL)

To Pressure
Transducers

**FIGURE 21.3.** Perfusion manometry catheter. For recording resting and squeeze pressures of the anal canal, open-tipped perfusion catheters of small diameter (*arrows*) provide the most physiologic measurements. Distention of a balloon at the end of the catheter with different volumes of air allows determination of rectal sensory thresholds and is used to elicit reflexive internal anal sphincter relaxation. Solid-state transducers may also be used but are more fragile and expensive to repair. They are particularly useful for ambulatory recordings.

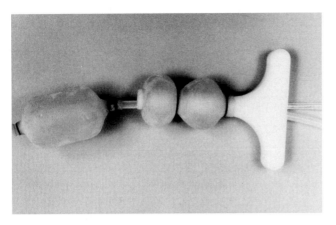

**FIGURE 21.4.** Schuster-type balloon manometer. This manometer consists of a hollow cylinder surrounded by a double balloon with the rectal distention balloon passing through the cylinder. This is most efficient for eliciting internal anal sphincter and external anal sphincter responses and for evaluating anorectal responses when the patient attempts to expel the manometer (pseudodefecation). It is also useful when performing biofeedback for both fecal incontinence and pelvic floor dyssynergia.

**FIGURE 21.5.** Rectal compliance catheter. A latex balloon 10 cm in length constructed from commercial nonlubricated condoms and tied to a polyethylene tube is used to study rectal compliance. This is useful in detecting megarectum, rectal hypotonia, and conditions in which rectal viscoelasticity is reduced, such as inflammatory and ischemic diseases.

## PREPARATION AND MANOMETRIC TECHNIQUES

One or two small enemas may be administered approximately 2 hours before anorectal manometry in constipated patients to ensure that the study can be performed satisfactorily, but this is optional. With the patient lying on his/her side, a digital examination is performed to assess anorectal structures and to relax the external anal sphincter. Catheter insertion techniques vary according to the apparatus that is used.

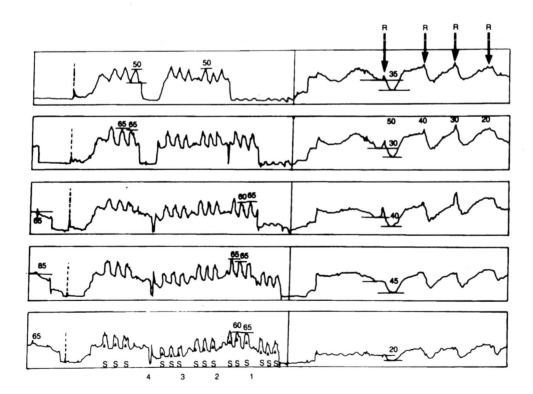

**FIGURE 21.6.** Perfusion catheter tracing. This catheter is inserted into the anus using the index finger as a guide and is slowly passed to approximately 15 cm from the anal verge. After several minutes elapse, the catheter is withdrawn at 0.5- to 1.0-cm intervals (station pull-through technique) to assess resting pressures (*R*), as shown in the tracings. The patient is asked to tighten (squeeze) the anal sphincters at each level once step-up pressures are observed to assess maximal squeeze (*S*) pressures. Then a series of rectal distentions (RD) with 50, 40, 30, and 20 mL of air in decreasing volumes is administered to measure internal anal sphincter relaxation and obtain the threshold of rectal sensation, defined as the smallest volume of transient distention sensed.

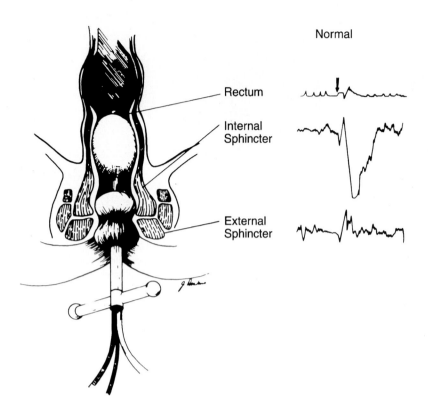

Normal

Rectum

Internal
Sphincter

External
Sphincter

**FIGURE 21.7A.** Balloon manometer tracings. First, the rectal balloon is gently inserted using the index finger, as with the perfusion catheter. Using the rectal balloon passed through the hollow cylinder to guide insertion, the manometer is then gently slid into the rectum. When the external sphincter balloon is just visible outside the anus, first the internal and then the external anal balloons are inflated with 10 mL of air. The catheter is shown in position within the anorectum in the accompanying illustrations. **A,** The rectal balloon is first rapidly inflated and deflated with 50 mL of air (*arrow*) using a syringe attached to a three-way stopcock. Reflex relaxation of the internal anal sphincter and simultaneous contraction of the external anal sphincter are recorded as well as the ability of the patient to sense rectal distention. Distentions are repeated using 5- to 10-mL decrements until the lowest volume that elicits each parameter is recorded. Voluntary squeeze pressures and responses to cough and perianal scratch are also obtained (see Table 21.1).

**TABLE 21.1** Representative Normal Values (Mean ± SEM)

|  | Women | n | Men | n |
|---|---|---|---|---|
| Length of anal canal (cm) | 4.0 ± 1.0 | 18 | 4.0 ± 1.0 | 18 |
|  | 3.7 ± 0.2 | 10 | 4.0 ± 0.6 | 12 |
| Resting anal canal pressures (mm Hg) | 58 ± 3 | 22 | 66 ± 6 | 15 |
|  | 54 ± 5 | 12 | Not studied |  |
|  | 50 ± 13 | 18 | 63 ± 12 | 18 |
|  | 49 ± 3 | 12 | 49 ± 3 | 7 |
| Maximal squeeze pressures (mm Hg) | 135 ± 15 | 22 | 218 ± 18 | 15 |
|  | 90 ± 9 | 12 | Not studied |  |
|  | 159 ± 45 | 18 | 238 ± 38 | 18 |

| Duration of EAS Maximum Squeeze (Mean ± SEM) | | |
|---|---|---|
| Duration (s) | n | Criteria |
| 49 ± 1 | 16 | Mean 3 trials 10 mm Hg in lower anal canal |

Reproduced with permission from Diamant NE, Kamm MA, Wald A, Whitehead WE. AGA technical review on anorectal testing techniques. Gastroenterology 1999;116:735–60.

**TABLE 21.2** Representative Normal Values (Mean ± SEM)

| Thresholds of IAS Relaxation | | |
|---|---|---|
| Thresholds (mL) | n | Characteristics of Distending Balloon |
| 14 ± 1 | 16 | 5 cm long, 5 cm from anal verge |
| 20 (10–30) | 11 |  |
| 22 ± 3 (10–40) | 12 |  |
| 25 ± 2 | 17 |  |

| Thresholds of Conscious Perception of Rectal Distention | | |
|---|---|---|
| Rectal Sensation (mL) | n | Technique |
| 13 ± 2 (10–30) | 11 | Balloon 5 cm from anal verge |
| 13 ± 3 (5–30) | 12 |  |
| 14 ± 3 | 17 |  |
| 17 ± 9 | 36 |  |

| Rectal Compliance | | |
|---|---|---|
| Rectal Compliance (mL/mm Hg) | n | Technique |
| 14 ± 2 | 34 | Balloon 5 cm long, 5 cm from anal verge; 50–250 mL |

Reproduced with permission from Diamant NE, Kamm MA, Wald A, Whitehead WE. AGA technical review on anorectal testing techniques. Gastroenterology 1999;116:735–60.

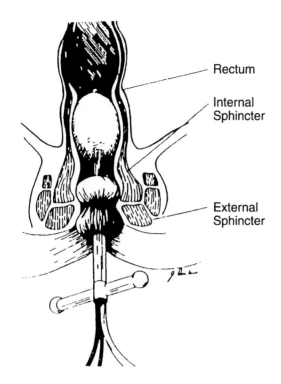

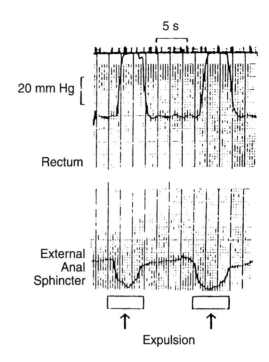

**FIGURE 21.7B.** The patient is then asked to attempt to expel the manometer (pseudodefecation); normally, increased pressures are recorded from the rectal balloon, whereas decreased pressures are observed on the external sphincter balloon. This is performed three times to ensure a reproducible pattern.

## Rectal Compliance (dV/dP)

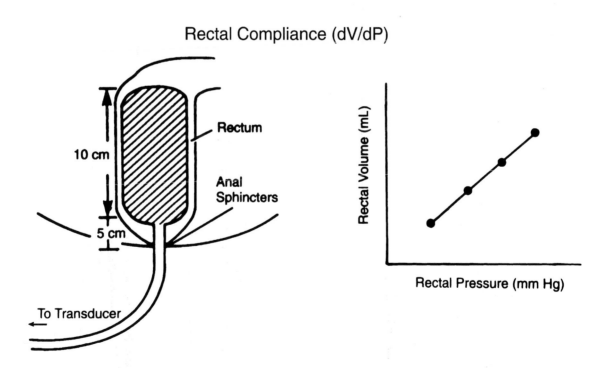

**FIGURE 21.8.** Rectal compliance (dV/dP). Rectal compliance is obtained by progressively inflating a cylindrical latex balloon (illustrated in Fig. 21.5 and positioned in the rectum 5 cm from the anal verge) with air in 50-mL increments to a maximum of 250 mL, as illustrated in the figure. Pressures within the balloon are measured by an external transducer and are corrected by subtracting pressures obtained when inflated with the same volumes in ambient air. This corrects for pressures derived from the resistance of the balloon itself. A compliance curve is then constructed, as illustrated in the figure, in which compliance equals dV/dP for 50 to 250 mL. The range in normal subjects is from 6 to 20 mL/mm Hg. Reproduced with permission from Wald A. Disorders of defecation and fecal continence. Cleve Clin J Med 1989;56:491–501(See Table 21.2).

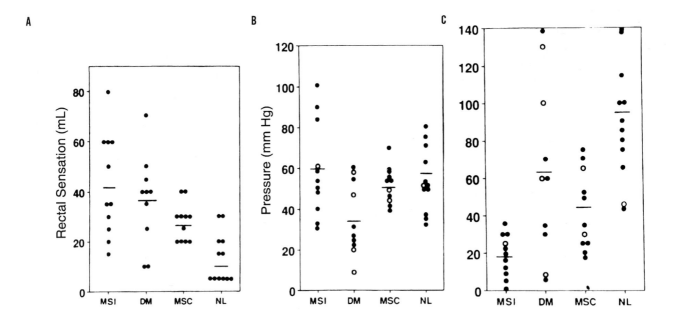

## MANOMETRIC PATTERNS IN DISORDERS ASSOCIATED WITH FECAL INCONTINENCE

**FIGURE 21.9.** Anorectal function in diabetes mellitus and multiple sclerosis. **A**, Rectal sensory thresholds in patients with diabetes mellitus with fecal incontinence (DM) and multiple sclerosis with fecal incontinence (MSI), continent MS patients (MSC), and normal controls (NL). Over 50% of patients with fecal incontinence caused by diabetes or MS have thresholds of rectal sensation exceeding 30 mL. All study groups have mean sensory thresholds that are significantly higher than that of the control subjects. **B**, Resting anal sphincter pressures in the same groups of subjects. Patients with MS have

normal pressures, whereas diabetics with fecal incontinence often have diminished pressures at rest, presumably reflecting autonomic nerve dysfunction. **C**, Anal squeeze pressures in the study groups. Incontinent patients with MS uniformly have decreased squeeze pressures compared with normal controls, whereas continent patients with MS have squeeze pressures that are modestly impaired. Diabetics with fecal incontinence vary greatly with respect to squeeze pressures, making manometric studies important when assessing continence mechanisms. Reproduced with permission from Caruana BJ, Wald A, Hinds JP, Eidelman BH. Anorectal sensory and motor function in neurogenic fecal incontinence: comparison between multiple sclerosis and diabetes mellitus. Gastroenterology 1991;100:465–70.

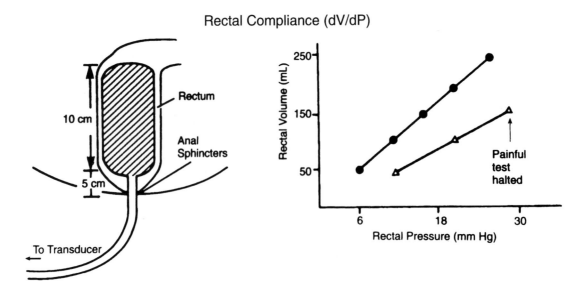

**FIGURE 21.10.** Rectal compliance in a normal subject and in a patient with ulcerative proctitis. In inflammatory or ischemic diseases of the rectum, higher pressures are generated at all volumes of rectal distention of the compliance balloon, and intolerance to progressive distention occurs at lower volumes compared with that in normal subjects. Such patients may experience fecal incontinence associated with urgency despite normal anal sphincteric function.

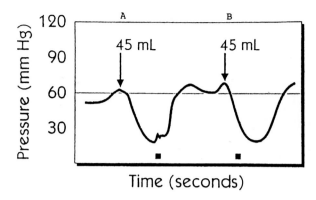

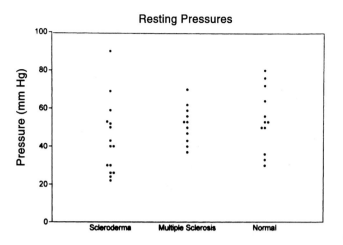

**FIGURE 21.11.** Recognition of rectal distention in a normal subject and in a patient with fecal incontinence. In a normal subject (**B**), inflation of a rectal balloon is recognized promptly (■), whereas in many patients with fecal incontinence (**A**), recognition is delayed by 2 seconds or more. Reproduced with permission from Miner PB. Management of fecal incontinence. In: Winawer SJ, editor. Management of gastrointestinal diseases. New York: Gower Medical Publishing; 1992. p. 36.1–20.

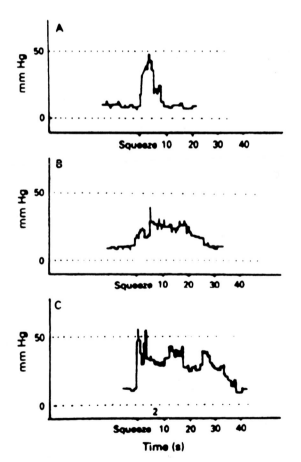

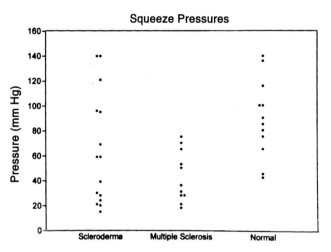

**FIGURE 21.13.** Rest and squeeze anal sphincter pressures in normal subjects, patients with scleroderma, and those with multiple sclerosis. As a group, patients with multiple sclerosis have normal resting pressures but decreased squeeze pressures (see Fig. 21.9). Some patients with scleroderma have decreased resting pressures, whereas others have weak squeeze pressures, but the range is quite broad, as is true with normal subjects.

**FIGURE 21.12.** Duration of external anal sphincter contraction in a normal subject and in a patient with fecal incontinence before and after biofeedback. In these tracings, external sphincter contractions in a patient with fecal incontinence (*top*) are not sustained compared with a normal subject (*middle*). After biofeedback, the patient is able to sustain contractions for a longer period of time (*bottom*). Reproduced with permission from Chiaroni G, Scattolini C, Bonfante F, Vantini I. Liquid stool incontinence with severe urgency: anorectal function and effective biofeedback treatment. Gut 1993;34:1576–80.

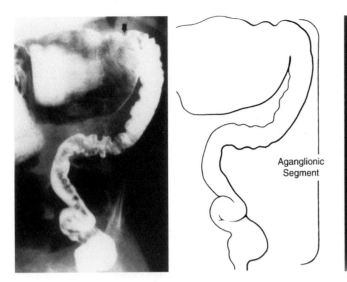

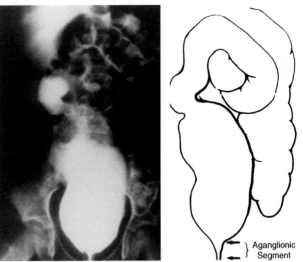

**FIGURE 21.14.** Hirschsprung's disease: barium enema. In patients with Hirschsprung's disease (congenital aganglionosis), varying lengths of distal bowel receive no enteric innervation. The aganglionic bowel is narrowed and spastic, whereas the normally innervated proximal bowel is dilated and filled with fecal material. In cases of suspected aganglionosis, it is preferable not to cleanse the colon prior to barium studies to accentuate the transition zone from aganglionic to normally innervated bowel. *Left*, Barium enema in a patient with aganglionosis to the splenic flexure. *Right*, an 11-year-old boy with involvement of only the distal 1 to 2 cm of rectum (ie, short segment disease). It is important to remove the insertion catheter used to instill barium to avoid missing short segment disease.

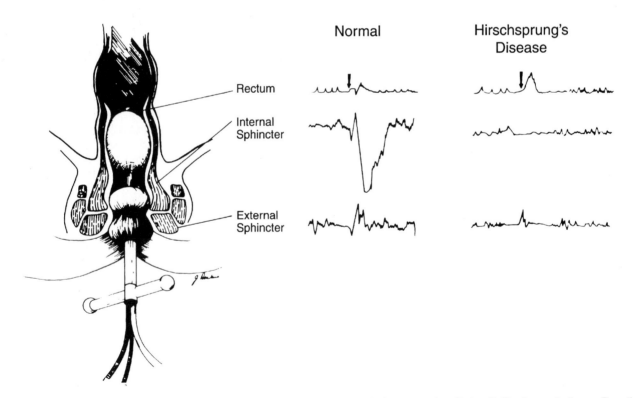

**FIGURE 21.15.** Hirschsprung's disease: balloon manometry. Internal anal sphincter responses to rectal distention in a patient with Hirschsprung's disease are compared with those in a normal subject using the Schuster-type balloon manometer. The congenital aganglionosis of Hirschsprung's disease invariably affects the internal anal sphincter. In contrast to normal reflexive relaxation of the internal anal sphincter following rectal distention (*arrows*), no such relaxation occurs in patients with Hirschsprung's disease. Thus, the presence of internal anal sphincter relaxation in a constipated patient excludes Hirschsprung's disease from consideration. However, the failure to detect internal sphincter relaxation is not specific for Hirschsprung's disease, and the diagnosis should be confirmed using histologic or neurohistochemical assessment of biopsy material.

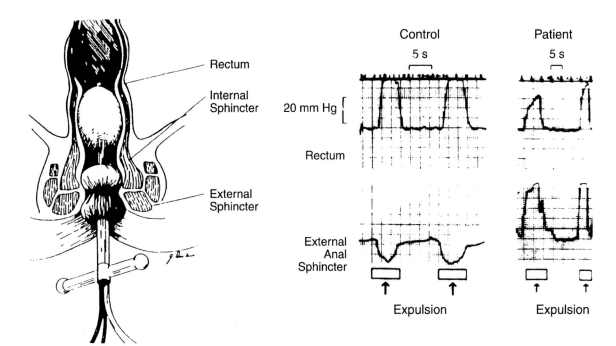

**FIGURE 21.16.** Pelvic floor dyssynergia (anismus). With the Schuster-type balloon manometer in place, the patient is asked to attempt to expel the manometer as he/she would when attempting to defecate. In contrast to the characteristic decrease in external anal sphincter pressure observed when a patient attempts to expel the balloon manometer, patients with pelvic floor dyssynergia unconsciously contract or fail to relax the external anal sphincter and puborectalis muscle, resulting in increased pressures on the external sphincter balloon. This manometric pattern can be distinguished from simple voluntary squeezing by observing the increased pressures in the rectal balloon as the patient bears down during pseudodefecation. However, this study is not ideal as the patient is lying on the side and false positives may occur if the buttocks are large. Diagnostic precision can be enhanced if simultaneous electromyographic (EMG) recordings of the external anal sphincter are made during this maneuver.

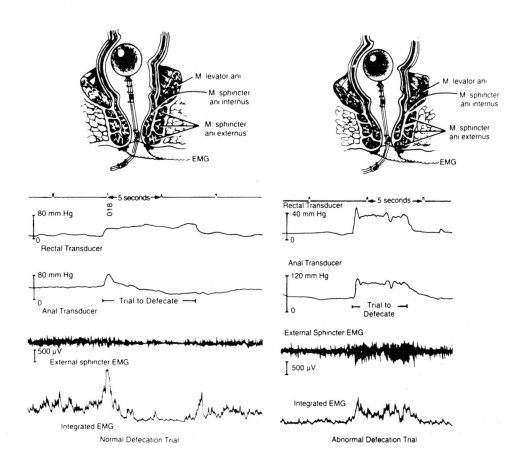

**FIGURE 21.17.** Normal defecation versus pelvic floor dyssynergia. Pressure changes in the rectum and anal canal and EMG recordings from the external anal sphincter during pseudodefecation. Normal defecation is characterized by increased rectal (intra-abdominal) pressure, decreased anal pressure, and decreased direct and integrated EMG activity as measured by surface electrodes (*left*). In a patient with pelvic floor dyssynergia (*right*), there is increased anal pressure and EMG activity of the external sphincter during attempted defecation. Courtesy of Dr. Vera Loening, University of Iowa Hospitals, Iowa City, IA.

## Rectal Compliance (dV/dP)

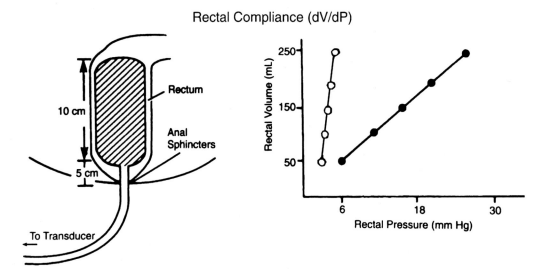

**FIGURE 21.18.** Rectal compliance in idiopathic megarectum (dV/dP). The graphs plot the rectal pressures obtained by incremental distention of the compliance balloon in the rectum in a normal subject (●—●) and in a patient with megarectum (○—○). In patients with megarectum, rectal pressures at volumes of 50 to 250 mL are lower than those of normal subjects, and compliance (ΔV/ΔP) is higher. In addition, a sense of rectal filling or urge to defecate occurs at much higher volumes of rectal distention (if it occurs at all) when compared to normal subjects. In our laboratory, a compliance of >20 mL/mm Hg suggests rectal hypotonia or megarectum and correlates well with the finding of megarectum as determined with radiologic studies. In contrast, a compliance of <6 mL/mm Hg suggests rectal hypertonia.

## OTHER DISORDERS

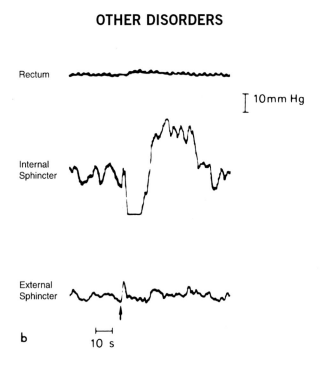

**FIGURE 21.19.** Anal fissures. High resting anal sphincter pressures occur in patients with anal fissures. In addition, rectal distention results in normal internal anal sphincter (Int. Sphinct.) relaxation and external anal sphincter (Ext. Sphinct) contractions, but relaxation is often followed by an immediate overshoot contraction of the internal anal sphincter. This overshoot contraction disappears following successful treatment of the anal fissures. Reproduced with permission from Nothmann BJ, Schuster MM. Internal anal sphincter derangement with anal fissures. Gastroenterology 1974;67:216–30.

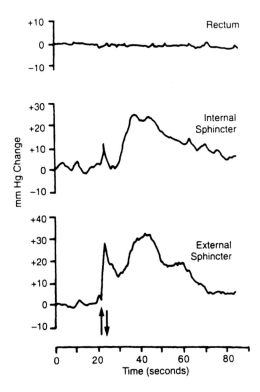

**FIGURE 21.20.** Myotonic dystrophy. This disorder often affects both the striated external anal sphincter muscle and the smooth internal anal sphincter muscle. Rectal distention (*arrows*) induces a myotonic response of both anal sphincters in this tracing. Reproduced with permission from Schuster MM, Tow DE, Sherbourne DH. Anal sphincter abnormalities characteristic of myotonic dystrophy. Gastroenterology 1965;49:641–8.

## STUDIES OF PELVIC FLOOR NEUROPHYSIOLOGY

### Electromyography of External Anal Sphincter and Puborectalis Muscle

In this technique, the patient is placed on the side and a ground electrode is strapped to the thigh. A standard concentric needle EMG electrode is inserted, without anesthesia, into the superficial portion of the external sphincter or the puborectalis muscle. Alternatively, surface electrodes are placed on the skin over the superficial part of the external anal sphincter. The myoelectric activity recorded by the concentric needle EMG electrode is displayed on an oscilloscope at rest, with voluntary squeeze, and after a supramaximal stimulus is applied by a biopolar stimulating electrode to the perianal area or transrectally to the terminal portion of the pudendal nerves, which supply the sphincters.

Concentric needle electrodes are more painful than surface EMG electrodes but provide assurance that muscle activity is obtained from the specific muscle to be studied. Moreover, surface electrodes cannot be used to obtain recordings from the puborectalis muscle. The need for meticulous technique and experience with the performance and interpretation of EMG activity make this test highly operator dependent.

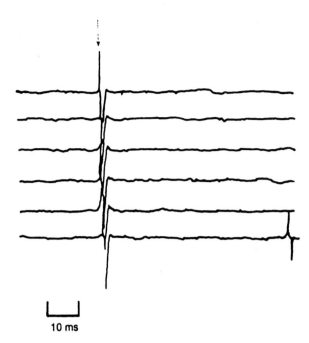

**FIGURE 21.21.** Normal external sphincter EMG pattern. An example of motor unit potentials of short duration obtained by a concentric needle electrode placed in the external anal sphincter of a normal subject. Reproduced with permission from Bartolo DCC, Jarratt JA, Read MG, et al. The role of partial denervation of the puborectalis in idiopathic faecal incontinence. Br J Surg 1983;70:664–7.

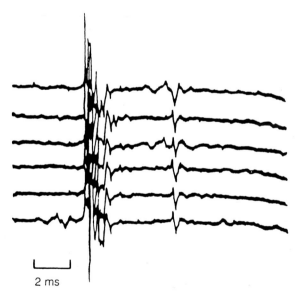

**FIGURE 21.22.** Denervation pattern. An example of a motor unit potential obtained by a concentric needle electrode inserted into the puborectalis muscle of a patient with idiopathic fecal incontinence. The first component of the motor unit potential shows prominent jitter (significant variation of the intervals between motor unit potentials) and intermittent blocking caused by failure of conduction across immature motor nerve end plates. The finding of prominent jitter and blocking using conventional EMG techniques implies recent and perhaps continuing injury of the motor nerve supplying the muscle. Reproduced with permission from Bartolo DCC, Jarratt JA, Read MG, et al. The role of partial denervation of the puborectalis in idiopathic faecal incontinence. Br J Surg 1983;70:664–7.

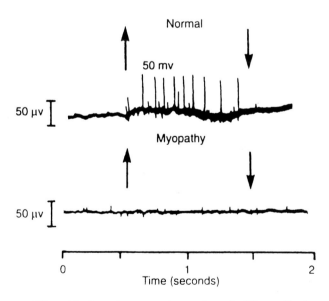

**FIGURE 21.23.** Myopathic pattern. Concentric needle EMG recording in a normal subject and a patient with ocular myopathy demonstrating normal and absent spike potentials in the external anal sphincter during rectal distention (*arrows*). Reproduced with permission from Teasdall RD, Schuster MM, Walsh FB. Sphincter involvement in ocular myopathy. Arch Neurol 1964;10:446–8.

**FIGURE 21.24.** Pudendal nerve stimulating and recording glove with electrodes. Digitally directed pudendal nerve terminal motor latency measuring device. The distance from the stimulating cathode at the top of the index finger (S) to the recording electrode (R) at the base of the finger is 3 cm. Repeated stimuli are applied to the left and right pudendal nerves by the operator while the recording electrode identifies the motor responses of the left and right external sphincter muscles. Latencies are calculated by averaging at least five separate nerve stimuli.

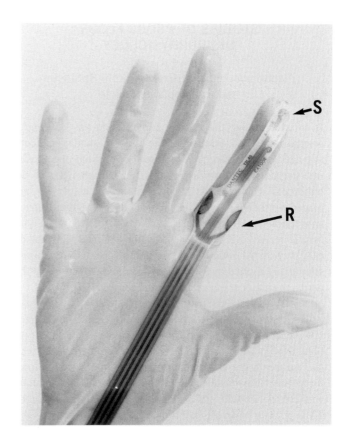

## Pudendal Nerve Terminal Motor Latency

In this technique, the operator inserts the gloved index finger containing the stimulating cathode into the rectum. A stimulus is applied to the right and left pudendal nerves at the level of the ischial tuberosities, and motor unit potentials are recorded at the right and left external sphincter muscles, respectively. Pudendal nerve conduction is measured by calculating the time between application of the stimulus and the sphincter muscle response and is called the latency period. Latency periods in normal subjects range up to 2 milliseconds.

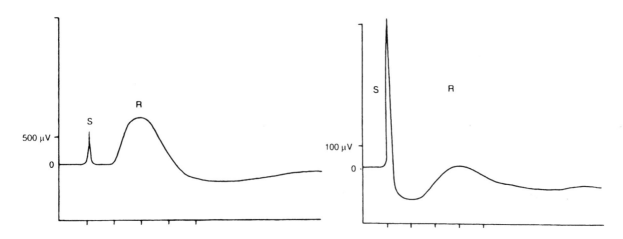

**FIGURE 21.25.** Normal versus "idiopathic" fecal incontinence. Motor unit action potential in a normal subject (*left*) and in a patient with idiopathic fecal incontinence (*right*). The latency period is measured from stimulus (S) to motor response (R). In normal subjects, latency periods range up to 2 milliseconds, whereas in patients with idiopathic fecal incontinence, latencies often exceed these values. This indicates damage to the motor portion of the pudendal nerves, which leads to impaired function of the external anal sphincter muscles. Thus, patients with idiopathic fecal incontinence appear to have a form of neurogenic external anal sphincter and/or puborectalis dysfunction caused by injury to the pudendal nerves. Reproduced with permission from Kiff ES, Swash M. Slowed conduction in the pudendal nerves in idiopathic (neurogenic) fecal incontinence. Br J Surg 1984;71:614–6.

## RADIOGRAPHIC STUDIES

Dynamic radiographic studies can be used to assess both the structure and function of the anorectum at rest, during attempts to retain rectal contents (continence), and during expulsion of radiographic contrast (defecography, defecating proctography). These techniques require meticulous attention to detail and are highly operator dependent.

Moreover, universal agreement concerning measurements (ie, the best way to determine the longitudinal axis of the rectum) has not been established, and concern has been expressed about interobserver variability. Finally, these tests are not physiologic in that barium or barium paste is not comparable to normal stool. Despite these concerns, potentially important information concerning anorectal structure and function may be obtained.

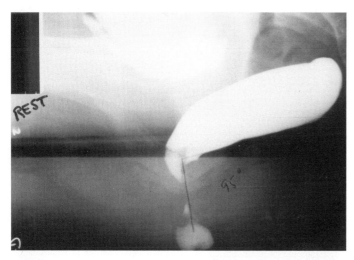

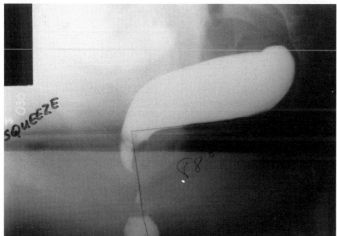

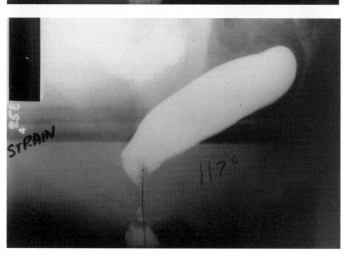

**FIGURE 21.26.** Dynamic proctography in normal subjects. With the patient in the left lateral recumbent position, 200 to 250 mL of barium contrast medium (40% w/v) is instilled to fill the rectum and distal sigmoid colon. Lateral radiographs are obtained at rest (*top*), when the patient squeezes maximally (*middle*), and when the patient strains (*bottom*) while attempting to retain the barium. The anorectal angle is calculated from the intersection of a line drawn along the posterior rectal wall or the mid-rectum with a line drawn along the axis of the anal canal. The position of the pelvic floor is determined by the junction of the anorectal angle and compared with its normal position, which approximates a line drawn from the symphysis pubis to the tip of the coccyx.

## DEFECOGRAPHY (DEFECATING PROCTOGRAPHY)

Approximately 45 minutes prior to the procedure, 240 mL of barium contrast medium (40% w/v) is administered orally to opacify the small intestine. With the patient in the lateral position, approximately 200 mL of thickened barium paste is administered into the rectum using a wide-tipped syringe. The paste consists of barium contrast (20% w/v) mixed with a thickening agent such as instant potato flakes or hydrophilic psyllium colloid (Metamucil), which is beaten with a whisk until a smooth paste is formed. Once the rectum has been filled, the syringe tip is gradually withdrawn without stopping the instillation in order to opacify the anal canal. A tampon soaked with iodinated contrast material is often inserted into the vagina of female patients to study the rectovaginal wall during evacuation.

The patient is then seated on a thick plastic ring containing a calibrated receptacle mounted on the footboard of the fluoroscopy table. Lateral films are obtained at rest and during expulsion of the barium paste, which the patient is asked to do as quickly and as completely as possible. Evacuation is recorded on spot film for subsequent evaluation.

The anorectal angle is defined as the angle between lines drawn through the central axis of the anal canal and the posterior wall of the rectum and is measured at rest, with voluntary squeeze, and during straining. Rectal emptying is defined as the percentage of barium paste expelled during a defined period of time, usually 60 to 120 seconds. Normal emptying of 200 mL of barium contrast ranges from 40 to 100% (median 50%).

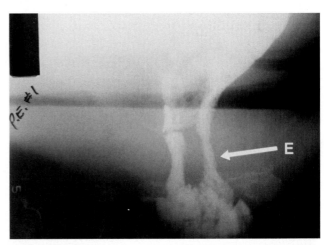

**FIGURE 21.28.** Enterocele. An enterocele (E) is seen descending between the anterior rectal and posterior vaginal walls. Courtesy of Department of Radiology, University of Pittsburgh Medical Center, Pittsburgh, PA.

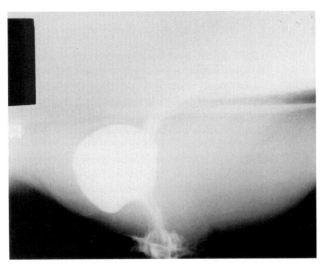

**FIGURE 21.27.** Defecography: recotocele. During expulsion, a large anterior rectocele fills with barium, but expulsion of contrast appears normal. (Courtesy of Department of Radiology, University of Pittsburgh Medical Center, Pittsburgh, PA.) Several studies have demonstrated that rectoceles are common in women without defecatory complaints so that caution is necessary before implicating a rectocele as the cause of defecatory difficulty. Reproduced with permission from Wald A, Caruana BJ, Freimanis MG, et al. Contributions of evacuation proctography and anorectal manometry to the evaluation of adults with constipation and defecatory difficulty. Dig Dis Sci 1990;35:481–7.

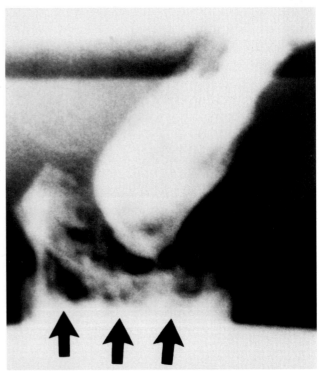

**FIGURE 21.29.** Intussusception. During attempted evacuation, inversion of the rectal mucosa and intussusception into the lower rectum occurs during maximal straining (*arrows*). No further passage of contrast into the anal canal occurs in this patient. Courtesy of Department of Radiology, University of Pittsburgh Medical Center, Pittsburgh, PA.

## RECTAL SCINTIGRAPHY

Artificial stool is prepared by adding 2 mCi of technetium 99m–labeled sulfur colloid to 400 mL of water at 37°C. Fifty grams of aluminum magnesium silicate powder are added slowly while constantly stirring to produce a smooth, thick, paste-like gel.

With the patient in a lateral recumbent position, 100 or 200 mL of artificial stool are inserted into the rectum using a rectal tube attached to a wide-tipped syringe. A right lateral scan is obtained for 2 minutes using a gamma camera with a low-energy collimator linked to a computer while the patient is seated on a specially constructed commode. The subject is then asked to evacuate the rectum while dynamic 2-second images are acquired for 2 minutes. Counts are analyzed using regions of interest drawn about areas of maximal activity, and dynamic curves of rectal emptying are obtained.

The potential advantages of this technique are the ability to more precisely quantitate rectal emptying over time and to assess the effect of different volumes of artificial stool on evacuation dynamics. However, similar to dynamic proctography, the artificial stool differs from normal stool, and care must be used when interpreting such studies in patients with defecatory complaints.

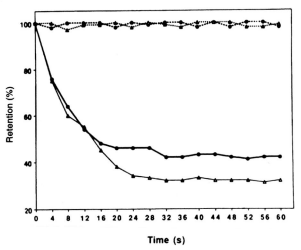
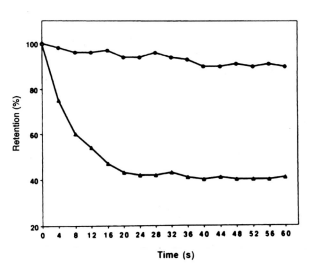

**FIGURE 21.30. A**, Normal and inhibited defecation. Normally, artificial stools of 200 mL (△—△) and 100 mL (●—●) are emptied rapidly from the rectum in an exponential fashion. An example of such a pattern of emptying in a normal subject and one with inhibited defecation is illustrated. Normal emptying is ≥30% for 200-mL volumes and ≥12% for 100-mL volumes. **B**, Volume-related inhibited defecation. A patient with this pattern empties 200 mL of contrast normally (△—△) but exhibits decreased emptying of the 100-mL volume (●—●). In contrast to patients with inhibited defecation, pelvic floor dyssynergia is not seen on anorectal manometry. Reproduced with permission from Wald A, Jafri F, Rehder J, Holeva K. Scintigraphic studies of rectal emptying in patients with constipation and defecatory difficulty. Dig Dis Sci 1993;38:353–8.

## SUMMARY

Proper evaluation of patients with fecal incontinence and disorders of defecation requires an understanding of anorectal physiology and appropriate use of currently available techniques for assessing anorectal function.

No single test can characterize all of the important mechanisms that govern continence and defecation. This chapter illustrates the various tests that are currently available and some of the clinical circumstances in which they can provide insights into the pathogenesis and treatment of patients with anorectal disorders.

### SELECTED READINGS

Caruana BJ, Wald A, Hinds JP, Eidelman BH. Anorectal sensory and motor function in neurogenic fecal incontinence: comparison between multiple sclerosis and diabetes mellitus. Gastroenterology 1991;100:456–70.

Cheong DMO, Vaccaro CA, Salanga VD, et al. Electrodiagnostic evaluation of fecal incontinence. Muscle Nerve 1995;18.612–9.

Diamant NE, Kamm MA, Wald A, Whitehead WE. AGA technical review on anorectal testing techniques. Gastroenterology 1999;116:732–60.

Hamel-Roy J, Devroede G, Arhan P, et al. Comparative esophageal and anorectal motility in scleroderma. Gastroenterology 1985;88:1–7.

Meunier PD, Gallaverdin D. Anorectal manometry: the state of the art. Dig Dis 1993;11:252–69.

Müller-Lissner SA, Bartolo DCC, Christiansen J, et al. Interobserver agreement in defecography—an international study. Z Gastroenterol 1998; 36:2734–9.

Wald A. Colonic and anorectal motility testing in clinical practice. Am J Gastroenterol 1994;89:2109–15.

Wald A. Fecal incontinence. In: Brandt LJ, editor. Clinical practice of gastroenterology. Philadelphia: Current Medicine; 1998. p. 637–45.

Wald A, Caruana BJ, Freimanis MG, et al. Contributions of evacuation proctography and anorectal manometry to the evaluation of adults with constipation and defecatory difficulty. Dig Dis Sci 1990;35:481–7.

Wald A, Jafri F, Rehder J, Holeva K. Scintigraphic studies of rectal emptying in patients with constipation and defecatory difficulty. Dig Dis Sci 1993;38:353–8.

Whitehead WE, Schuster MM. Anorectal physiology and pathophysiology. Am J Gastroenterol 1987;82:487–97.

CHAPTER 22

# Ultrasonography

*Volker F. Eckardt, Moritz A. Konerding and Paul Enck*

With the introduction of anal endosonography and endoanal magnetic resonance imaging, new dimensions have been added to the investigation of patients with functional and organic disorders of the anal canal. First attempts to evaluate anal and perianal morphology by endosonographic imaging were made in 1986 using low-frequency transducers.[1] However, only when the water-filled balloons covering the transducers were replaced by hard sonolucent plastic cones and when higher-frequency transducers (7–10 MHz) became available did endosonography allow more accurate imaging of an undistorted anal canal.[2–6] This chapter describes the normal endosonographic morphology of the anal canal and compares these findings with those obtained in anatomic preparations. Furthermore, examples of clinical applications for anal endosonography will be presented. Finally, the relationship between anal morphology and anorectal functions as measured by manometry and electromyography (EMG) will be discussed.

## TECHNICAL PERFORMANCE

Currently, the most frequently used transducers for anal endosonography are the Brüel & Kjaer endoprobe (Naerum, Denmark) and the Kretz multiplane rectal transducer (Zipf, Austria). Both are covered with a hard sonolucent endpiece that allows direct acoustic coupling without distortion of the anal canal. Acoustic coupling is intensified by covering the endpiece with a latex finger tip and ultrasound gel. The frequency of the transducers ranges from 7 (Brüel & Kjaer) to 7.5 to 10 MHz (Kretz). Both instruments differ in the diameter of the recording endpiece (Brüel & Kjaer = 1.7 cm, Kretz = 2.1 cm), maximum penetration depth (Brüel & Kjaer = 4.5 cm, Kretz = 5 cm), and size of the sector scan display (Brüel & Kjaer = 360 degrees, Kretz = 355 degrees). However, none of these differences appears to affect their clinical applicability, and both methods produce comparable images.

At the beginning of the procedure, patients are placed in a left lateral position with their hips and knees flexed at a 90-degree angle. The rigid probe is first introduced into the distal rectum and is then preferably placed on a fixed device that allows withdrawal of the instrument in regular intervals without changing its axial position (Fig. 22.1). To secure the most

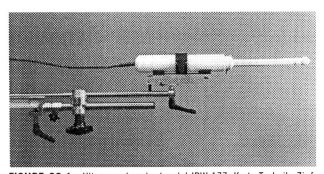

**FIGURE 22.1.** Ultrasound probe (model IRW 177; Kretz Technik, Zipf, Austria) positioned on a fixed device allowing withdrawal of the instrument at regular intervals.

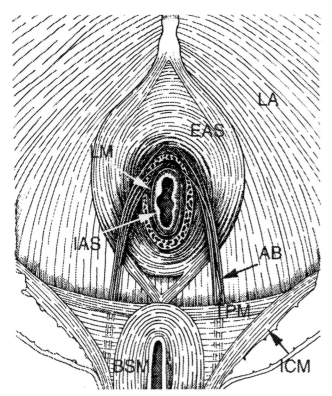

**FIGURE 22.2.** Schematic drawing of the pelvic floor musculature, demonstrating structures that may be visualized endosonographically. EAS, external anal sphincter; LM, longitudinal muscle; IAS, internal anal sphincter; AB, anterior bands; TPM, transverse perineal muscle; ICM, ischiocavernosus muscle; BSM, bulbospongiosus muscle.

accurate axial positioning, either the prostate gland or the uterine cervix can be used as orientation points when the probe is first inserted into the rectum. The transducer is then withdrawn in 0.5-cm increments. After each withdrawal, the ultrasonographic image is frozen to obtain videoprints or photographs. In addition, measurements of muscle thickness and/or the size of certain defects may be performed with a cursor on the monitor screen.

With one exception (Fig. 22.2), the images presented in this chapter were obtained with the Kretz rectal transducer. Images are oriented such that the anterior portion of the anal canal appears on the bottom, whereas the posterior portion is seen on the top of each photograph. Figure 22.2 schematically outlines the muscle structures that may be visualized by endoluminal ultrasonography. Similar to the endosonographic images, the drawing depicts the anatomic structures as being viewed from a knee-elbow position.

## ANAL ENDOSONOGRAPHY VERSUS CROSS-SECTIONAL ANATOMY

### Proximal Anal Canal

In the proximal anal canal, the puborectalis muscle is visualized as an array of clearly demarcated fiber bundles of low echogenicity that surround the dorsal anal canal in a horseshoe-like fashion and radiate into an anterolateral

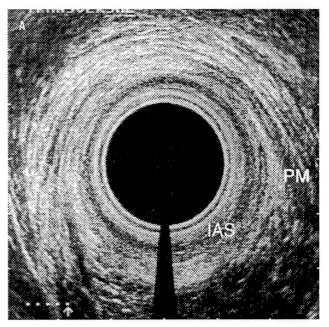

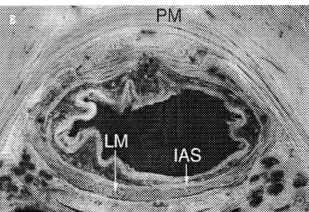

**FIGURE 22.3.** Endosonographic (**A**) and anatomic images (**B**) of the proximal anal canal showing the puborectalis muscle (PM) as an array of muscle fibers that surround the dorsal anal canal in a horseshoe-like fashion. In addition, anatomic sections demonstrate the internal anal sphincter (IAS) and the longitudinal muscle (LM), whereas endosonography only recognizes the IAS as an additional muscular structure.

direction (Fig. 22.3). Interposed between these fiber bundles are streaky areas of high echogenicity that are believed to represent fibrous tissue.

### Mid Anal Canal

On withdrawing the transducer from the upper into the mid anal canal, the organized fiber arrangement of the puborectalis muscle disappears, and three main layers of varying echogenicity become apparent (Fig. 22.4A). The first (inner) layer is hyperechoic and represents the mucosa and subepithelial tissue (the available transducers do not allow a clear differentiation between mucosal and submucosal tissue). The second layer is a well-defined hypoechoic ring that surrounds the anal canal in a circular fashion and represents the internal anal sphincter (IAS). The IAS is not always sym-

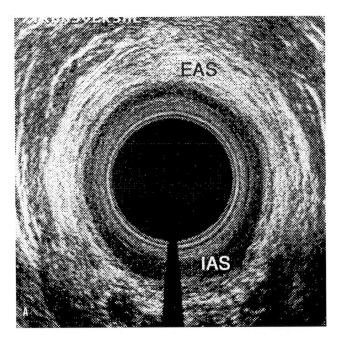

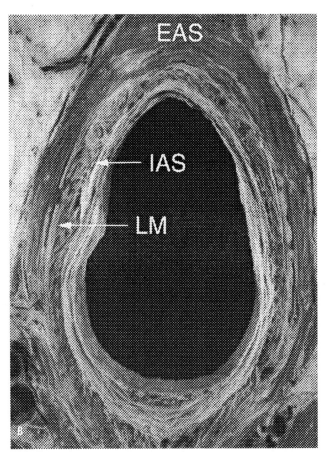

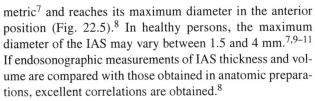

**FIGURE 22.4.** Endosonographic (**A**) and anatomic images (**B**) of the mid anal canal. Again, endosonography clearly outlines two muscular structures, namely, the internal anal sphincter (IAS), characterized by its low echogenicity, and the external anal sphincter (EAS), which has a mixed or high echogenicity. Between the two structures, an additional ring-like structure is faintly recognizable and may represent the longitudinal muscle (LM). However, because of the high echogenicity of this muscle, its clear endosonographic identification remains difficult or even impossible.

metric[7] and reaches its maximum diameter in the anterior position (Fig. 22.5).[8] In healthy persons, the maximum diameter of the IAS may vary between 1.5 and 4 mm.[7,9–11] If endosonographic measurements of IAS thickness and volume are compared with those obtained in anatomic preparations, excellent correlations are obtained.[8]

Greater difficulties are encountered in defining the boundaries of the external anal sphincter (EAS). It is commonly believed that the third endosonographic layer, which is characterized by a mixed echogenicity, represents the EAS.[3,6,7,12] However, one group of authors has described an additional zone of high echogenicity within the inner aspects of this third endosonographic layer.[13,14] It is assumed that this area of high echogenicity represents the longitudinal muscle. Although it may be difficult or even impossible to identify this structure by endosonography, anatomic studies regularly reveal the presence of a longitudinal muscle (see Fig. 22.4B).[8] In the literature, this muscular structure is frequently referred to as the conjoint longitudinal muscle, assuming that it results from a fusion of striated pubococcygeal fibers with the longitudinal smooth muscle of the rectum.[15] However, at least in the mid and lower anal canal, immunohistologic studies have failed to show any striated muscle fibers within this longitudinal muscle[8] but reveal an intermingling of longitudinal and circular smooth muscle fibers at its inner aspects. The difficulties encountered in clearly identifying the longitudinal muscle by endosonogra-

phy may be related to its rich content of fat and fibrous tissue (Fig. 22.6), which is comparable to that observed within the EAS. Such similarities may lead to almost identical echogenicities of the two muscles and thus to a similar appearance during endosonographic imaging. Finally, owing to the fact that the outer borders of the EAS exhibit a shaggy appearance and are difficult to delineate when imaged by endosonography, measurements of EAS thickness are poorly reproducible[16] and should be viewed with great caution.

### Lower Anal Canal

On withdrawal of the endosonographic probe into the distal anal canal, the IAS becomes thinner, and asymmetries of the EAS are more pronounced. In its anterior aspect, the EAS is often deficient in females and becomes tapered in men.[2] At this level, endosonographic delineation of the EAS is further impaired by the rich vascular supply (Fig. 22.7) of the perineum and by the presence of the transverse perineal muscle, which often crosses the anterior portion of the EAS and therefore interferes with its clear endosonographic imaging. All of these anatomic features may give rise to significant difficulties if one attempts to define the boundaries of the "normal" EAS and to differentiate between traumatic muscular defects and normal anatomic variations. Such difficulties are most frequently encountered in the anterior portion of the anal canal, where most sphincter defects occur.

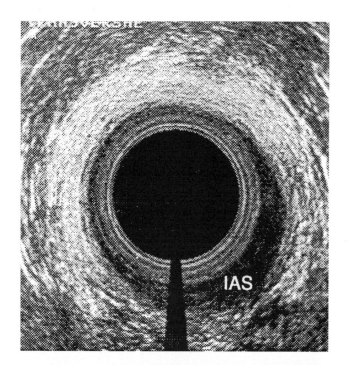

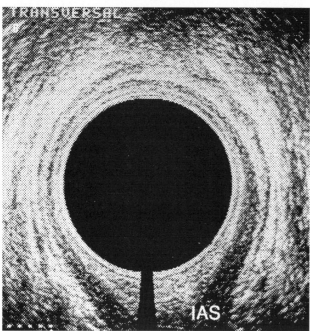

**FIGURE 22.5.** The internal anal sphincter (IAS) often reaches its greatest diameter in the anterior position (**A**), an area where submucosal tissue may also become thicker (**B**).

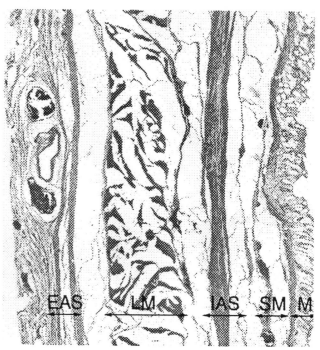

**FIGURE 22.6.** Histologic sections through the mid anal canal clearly outline three different muscle layers: the internal anal sphincter (IAS), longitudinal muscle (LM), and external anal sphincter (EAS). The LM and EAS exhibit similar contents of fat and fibrous tissue, which possibly explains their similar echogenicity and the difficulties encountered on separating these two structures by endosonography.

In the mid and lower portions of the anal canal, endosonography frequently demonstrates fiber bundles of low echogenicity that appear to originate from the IAS, traverse the longitudinal muscle and EAS, and finally radiate into an anterolateral position to the urogenital diaphragm (Fig. 22.8A). These fiber bundles, which have been named anterior bands, consist mainly of smooth muscle[8,17] and seem to represent an anchoring mechanism in the ventral portion of the anal canal, where the thickness of the EAS diminishes (Fig. 22.8B).

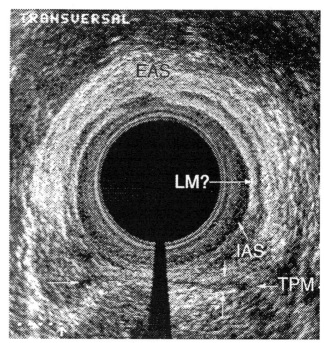

**FIGURE 22.7.** Endosonographic image of the lower anal canal. In its anterior portion, the external anal sphincter (EAS) is difficult to delineate and is often crossed by a linear structure of low echogenicity representing the transverse perineal muscle (TPM). Again, this figure shows a ring-like structure interposed between the IAS and EAS, which possibly represents the longitudinal muscle (LM).

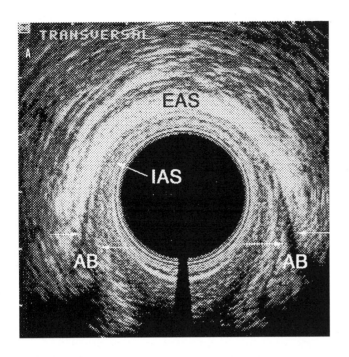

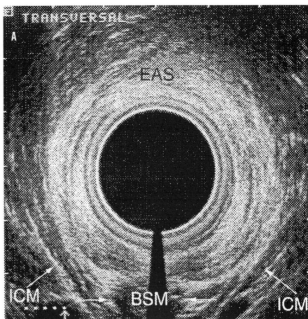

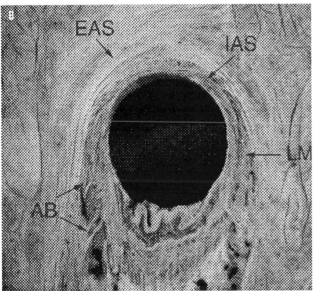

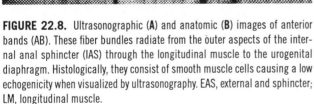

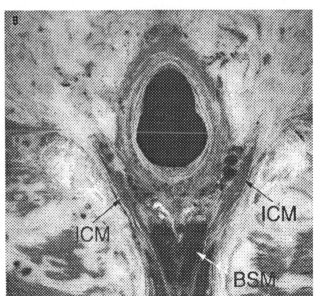

**FIGURE 22.8.** Ultrasonographic (**A**) and anatomic (**B**) images of anterior bands (AB). These fiber bundles radiate from the outer aspects of the internal anal sphincter (IAS) through the longitudinal muscle to the urogenital diaphragm. Histologically, they consist of smooth muscle cells causing a low echogenicity when visualized by ultrasonography. EAS, external and sphincter; LM, longitudinal muscle.

**FIGURE 22.9.** Ultrasonographic (**A**) and anatomic (**B**) images of the most distal end of the anal canal. At this level, the internal anal sphincter is barely recognized as a small rim of low echogenicity surrounding the anal lumen. In the anterior aspect of the anal canal, additional structures become more prominent, namely, the ischiocavernosus (ICM) and bulbospongiosus muscle (BSM). EAS, external and sphincter.

In nearly half of all endosonographic examinations, endosonography identifies oblique fiber bundles of low echogenicity that border the anterior portions of the EAS (Fig. 22.9A). A comparison of these images with those obtained in anatomic preparations (Fig. 22.9B) reveals that these oblique fibers represent the ischiocavernosus muscle. In addition, in the most anterior aspect of the anal canal, the bulbospongiosus muscle is endosonographically visualized as an ovular area of low echogenicity.

## ENDOSONOGRAPHIC VISUALIZATION OF ANAL LESIONS

### Sphincter Defects

The integrity of the anal sphincters can be assessed by either digital examination, EMG, or anal endosonography. Digital examination is the most simple procedure but only detects large defects with a sensitivity of less than 60%.[18,19]

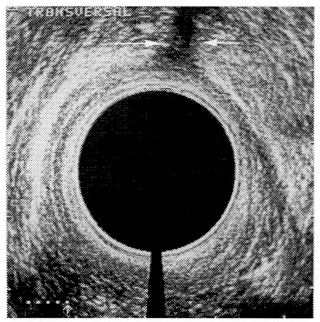

**FIGURE 22.10.** Localized defect of the external anal sphincter (EAS) in its posterior portion (*arrows*). The mixed echogenicity of the EAS is interrupted by a narrow scar of low echogenicity.

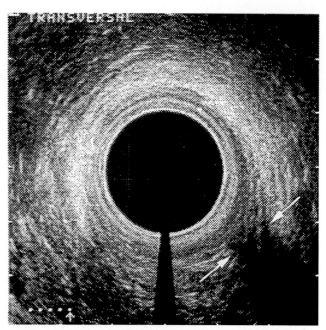

**FIGURE 22.11.** Anterior defect of the external anal sphincter (*arrows*). Because of the more complicated anatomy of the anterior anal canal, delineation of such defects may be more difficult than those occurring in the posterior portion.

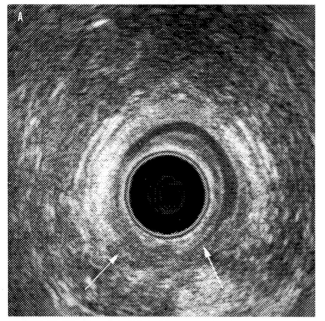

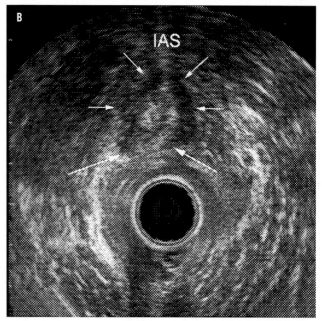

**FIGURE 22.12.** Traumatic defect of the external and internal anal sphincter (IAS) as viewed from the anus (**A**) and the vagina (**B**) with the Brüel and Kjaer Diagnostic Ultrasound System. In the anterior portion, a disruption of the normal texture of both muscles is demonstrated (*long arrows*) but perhaps more clearly seen when viewed from the vagina. Since vaginal endosonography leaves the anal canal unstretched and undistorted, the IAS appers thicker when viewed from this aspect. Courtesy of Dr. Richelle J.F. Felt-Bersma, Department of Gastroenterology, Academic Hospital Rotterdam "Dijkzigt," Rotterdam, The Netherlands.

Electromyography has a higher sensitivity, but its disadvantages are that it is a painful procedure and allows only the localization of EAS defects. In contrast, anal endosonography has an almost 100% sensitivity, is no more painful than digital examination, and may determine EAS and IAS defects. Comparisons between EMG and endosonographic studies have consistently shown that there is a high correlation between these two techniques.[18,20,21] In addition, anal endosonography may also detect deep lesions that are frequently missed by concentric needle EMG.[22] All of these features suggest that endosonography represents the most useful screening tool in selecting patients for the surgical repair of sphincteric defects.

External anal sphincter defects are endosonographically

recognized as sharp interruptions of the normal texture of this muscle. Surprisingly, most of these scars are of low echogenicity, a phenomenon that largely facilitates their endosonographic detection. This is especially true for defects that occur in the highly echogenic posterior and lateral aspects of the EAS (Fig. 22.10). However, greater difficulties are encountered in attempting to clearly delineate anterior defects. In this area, the normal EAS may be deficient or may be crossed by blood vessels and by the transverse perineal muscle. All of these features may not only interfere with the endosonographic delineation of the normal EAS but also especially with a clear delineation of sphincteric defects (Fig. 22.11). For females, it has been suggested that such difficulties may be overcome if the endosonographic probe is inserted into the vagina instead of the anus.[23,24] This procedure has the advantage that it can also be used when perianal pain prevents the insertion of an anal probe. In addition, viewing the undistorted anal canal from the vagina (Fig. 22.12) may increase the diagnostic yield of endosonography by up to 25%.[24]

Anal endosonography is the only widely available method that allows the detection of IAS defects. Such defects are easily recognized as breaks in the ring of the IAS. Trauma to the anal canal such as dilation may lead to fragmentation (see Fig. 22.13) of this muscle and occasionally to its almost total disappearance.

### Perianal Sepsis

Anal endosonography may facilitate the localization of perianal abscesses and fistulas and may therefore assist in the surgical treatment of these lesions. Inflammatory infiltrates and abscess formations are visualized as hypoechoic lesions that are located either between the IAS and EAS or within the extrasphincteric space (Figs. 22.14 to 22.17). The fistula tract is usually recognized as a sharply demarcated area of high echogenicity surrounded by a hypoechoic inflammatory infiltrate (see Fig. 22.14). Although most fistula tracts are easily recognized by conventional ultrasonography, their visualization may be enhanced by injecting hydrogen peroxide into the external opening.[25]

The accuracy of anal endosonography for the detection and localization of perianal fistulas and abscesses exceeds 90%.[26,27] However, a potential disadvantage of this method may be related to the fact that patients with inflammatory lesions poorly tolerate the insertion of the probe into the anal canal and distal rectum. In women, such problems may be overcome by imaging the perianal structures through vaginal endosonography.

### Anal Neoplasms and Perianal Cysts

The clinical value of anal ultrasonography in the staging of anal carcinoma has been studied only in small patient numbers.[28–30] However, these studies have uniformly shown that there is a clear correlation between transanal ultrasonographic

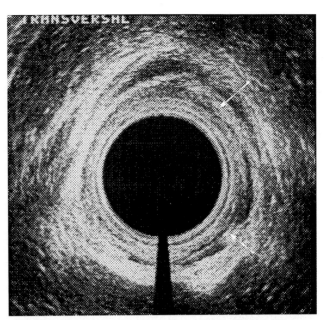

**FIGURE 22.13.** Internal anal sphincter defect with fragmentations of this muscle in its right lateral portion (*arrows*) and poor visibility in its left lateral aspects.

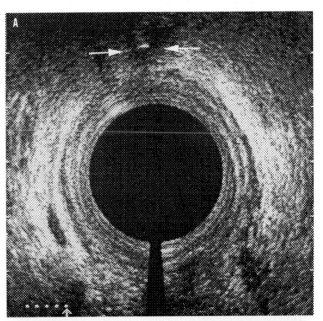

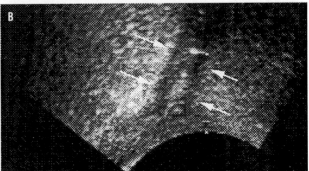

**FIGURE 22.14.** Sonogram of a transsphincteric fistula. **A**, Transverse sections show a pinpoint lesion of high echogenicity that is surrounded by a hypoechoic inflammatory infiltrate (*arrows*). **B**, A longitudinal section through the same area demonstrates that the fistula tract crosses the external anal sphincter.

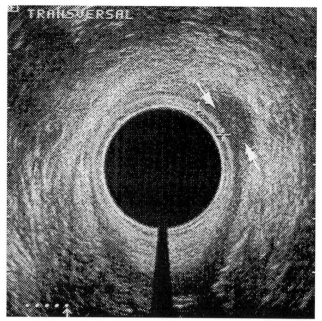

**FIGURE 22.15.** Anal endosonography of the distal anal canal showing a small intersphincteric abscess (*arrows*) in the posterior portion of the anal canal.

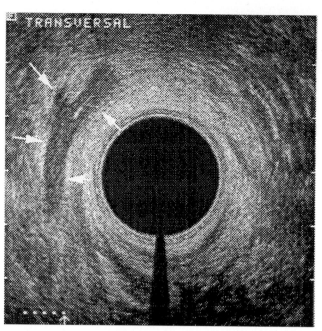

**FIGURE 22.16.** Transanal sonogram showing an extrasphincteric inflammatory lesion (*arrows*). The central fistula tract is visualized as a hyperechoic pinpoint structure.

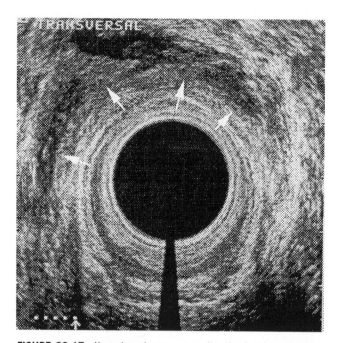

**FIGURE 22.17.** Horseshoe-abscess surrounding the dorsal portion of the anal canal. Endosonographically, the abscess is characterized as a zone of low echogenicity (*arrows*) bordering and infiltrating the external anal sphincter.

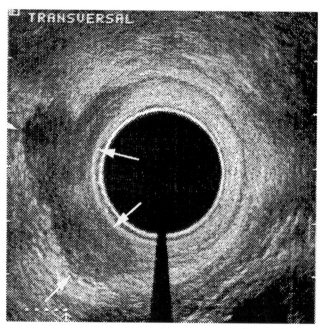

**FIGURE 22.18.** Anal epidermoid carcinoma (*arrows*) infiltrating through the internal and external anal sphincter into the perianal fat.

images and the intraoperative findings with regard to tumor size, estimated volume, and depth of infiltration. Endosonographically, these tumors are characterized by a low echogenicity and irregular contours extending through the different layers of the anal muscular coat (Fig. 22.18). Anal endosonography has also been recommended as a follow-up procedure in patients with anal neoplasms undergoing radiochemotherapy, but so far it remains to be determined whether this technique allows a reliable differentiation between tumor recurrence and scar tissue.

On rare occasions, endosonography may detect perianal cysts. They can be differentiated from neoplasms and inflammatory lesions by their regular surface and a very low echogenicity (Fig. 22.19).

## ANAL MORPHOLOGY AND FUNCTION

As soon as anal endosonography became available to the research community, it raised hopes that with this new tool, a direct link between sphincter morphology and sphincter performance would become accessible, especially in those cases in which sphincter dysfunction (incontinence) could not be explained based on functional assessment (manometry and/or EMG) alone.[2] Two aspects of such an association between anal morphology and its functions have been questioned and have found a preliminary answer: morphology and manometric measures and morphology and EMG mapping of sphincter defects. Both will be briefly presented here.

### Morphology and Manometry

The first[31] and all subsequent reports of a significant correlation between IAS and EAS morphology, especially sphincter muscle diameter on the one hand and anal sphincter restings and squeeze pressures, respectively, as assessed by anal manometry on the other hand, have raised doubts about its validity since, usually, correlations reported were weak ($r$ = .5–.7) despite their occasional significance with increasing number of patients included. This indicated that factors others than muscle thickness are contributing to muscle performance as well (eg, age and gender). Inversely, muscle diameter, especially of the EAS, decreased with increasing age and was lower in women as compared to men but never predicted the overall muscle performance.[32]

A second reason accounting for this dissociation between morphology and function has already been addressed above, namely, that identifying the outer delineation of the EAS muscle with ultrasonography appears to be especially difficult because of its shaggy appearance. Consequently, in a study

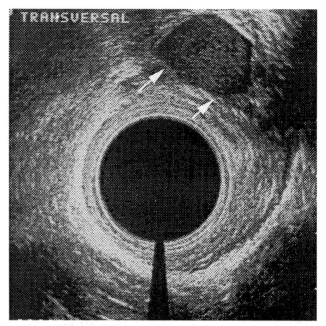

**FIGURE 22.19.** Endosonographic image of a perianal cyst (*arrows*). This rare lesion is characterized by an almost round configuration, a clearly delineated surface, and a very low echogenicity.

comparing repeated measures of the sphincter muscle diameters by different investigators and with different sonography machines,[16] the within- and between-investigator agreement was especially poor for the EAS.

Therefore, clinical routine morphometric assessment of the exact IAS and EAS diameter has almost entirely been given up, except in a few cases in which the muscle diameters appear to be exceeding the normal range (eg, in patients with muscular hypertrophy.[4,33] It specifically cannot replace anorectal manometry for the measurement of anal functions.

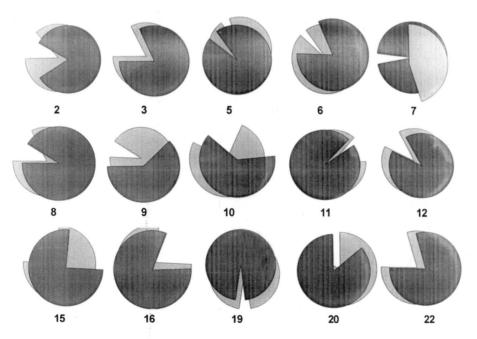

**FIGURE 22.20.** Agreement in defect localization between sphincter EMG (*lighter circles*) and anal ultrasonography (*darker circles*) in 15 of 22 patients with asssumed sphincter defects. Missing sections represent muscle gaps identified by the respective method; except for case 15, agreement was good.

## Sphincter Mapping Compared to Electromyography

The second approach comparing anal sonogram to sphincter function was related to the possibility of replacing the invasive needle EMG procedure by the non- or less invasive sonographic alternative. As has already been stated, agreement between the sonographic sphincter defect identification and the mapping of defects in the EAS muscle circumference by EMG was excellent, irrespective of whether the comparison was made independently,[13,20,21,34] simultaneously,[7,22] or intraoperatively.[14] Also, histologic[14,18] or postmortem comparison between the sonographic and the morphologic appearance of the sphincter muscles was reported to be excellent. In only a few cases, discrepancies of results were found between the two investigations (Fig. 22.20).[21,22]

However, since EMG provides insights into anal sphincter function other than the identification and localization of muscle defects, it cannot and has not entirely replaced EMG evaluation during the diagnostic work-up of patients with sphincter dysfunction.

## REFERENCES

1. Cammarota T, Discalzo L, Corno F, et al. First experiences with transrectal echotomography in perianal abscess pathology. Radiol Med (Torino) 1986;72:837–40.
2. Law PJ, Bartram CI. Anal endosonography: technique and normal anatomy. Gastrointest Radiol 1989;14:349–53.
3. Nielsen MB, Pedersen JF, Hauge C, et al. Endosonography of the anal sphincter: findings in healthy volunteers. AJR Am J Roentgenol 1991;157:1199–202.
4. Eckardt VF, Nix W. The anal sphincter in patients with myotonic muscular dystrophy. Gastroenterology 1991;100:424–30.
5. Cuesta MA, Meijer S, Derksen EJ, et al. Dis Colon Rectum 1992;35:59–63.
6. Tjandra JJ, Milsom JW, Stolfi VM, et al. Endoluminal ultrasound defines anatomy of the anal canal and pelvic floor. Dis Colon Rectum 1992;35:465–70.
7. Wong RF, Bonapace ES Jr, Chung CY, et al. Simultaneous endoluminal sonography and manometry to assess anal sphincter complex in normal subjects. Dig Dis Sci 1998;43:2363–72.
8. Konerding MA, Dzemali O, Gaumann A, et al. Correlation of endoanal sonography with cross-sectional anatomy of the anal sphincter. Gastrointest Endosc 1999;50:804–10.
9. Eckardt VF, Dodt O, Kanzler G, Bernhard G. Anorectal function and morphology in patients with sporadic proctalgia fugax. Dis Colon Rectum 1996;39:755–62.
10. Burnett SJD, Bartram CI. Endosonographic variations in the normal internal anal sphincter. Int J Colorectal Dis 1991;6:2–4.
11. Schäfer A, Enck P, Fürst G, et al. Anatomy of the anal sphincters. Comparison of anal endosonography to magnetic resonance imaging. Dis Colon Rectum 1994;37:777–81.
12. Papachrysostomou M, Pye SD, Wild SR, Smith AN. Significance of the thickness of the anal sphincters with age and its relevance in faecal incontinence. Scand J Gastroenterol 1994;29:710–14.
13. Sultan AH, Kamm MA, Hudson CN, et al. Endosonography of the anal sphincters: normal anatomy and comparison with manometry. Clin Radiol 1994;49:368–74.
14. Sultan AH, Nicholls RJ, Kamm MA, et al. Anal endosonography and correlation with in vitro and in vivo anatomy. Br J Surg 1993;80:508–11.
15. Williams P, Warwick R, Dyson M, Bannister LH, editors. Gray's anatomy. 37th ed. Edinburgh: Churchill Livingstone; 1989. p. 1369–73.
16. Enck P, Heyer Th, Gantke B, et al. How reproducible are measurements of the anal sphincter muscle diameter by endoanal ultrasound? Am J Gastroenterol 1997;92:293–6.
17. Eckardt VF, Jung B, Fischer B, Lierse W. Anal endosonography in healthy subjects and patients with idiopathic fecal incontinence. Dis Colon Rectum 1994;37:235–42.
18. Sultan AH, Kamm MA, Talbot IC, et al. Anal endosonography for identifying external sphincter defects confirmed histologically. Br J Surg 1994;81:463–5.
19. Nielsen MB, Hauge C, Rasmussen OO, et al. Anal endosonographic findings in the follow-up of primary sutured sphincteric ruptures. Br J Surg 1992;79:104–6.
20. Law PJ, Kamm MA, Bartram CI. A comparison between electromyography and anal endosonography in mapping external anal sphincter defects. Dis Colon Rectum 1990;33:370–3.
21. Enck P, von Giesen HJ, Schäfer A, et al. Comparison of anal sonography with conventional needle electromyography in the evaluation of anal sphincter defects. Am J Gastroenterol 1996;91:2539–43.
22. Burnett SJD, Speakman CTM, Kamm MA, Bartram CI. Confirmation of endosonographic detection of external anal sphincter defects by simultaneous electromyographic mapping. Br J Surg 1991;78:448–50.
23. Alexander AA, Liu JB, Merton DA, Nagle DA. Fecal incontinence: transvaginal US evaluation of anatomic causes. Radiology 1996;199:529–32.
24. Poen AC, Felt-Bersma RJ, Cuesta MA, Meuwissen GM. Vaginal endosonography of the anal sphincter complex is important in the assessment of faecal incontinence and perianal sepsis. Br J Surg 1998;85:359–63.
25. Cheong DM, Nogueras JJ, Wexner SD, Jagelman DG. Anal endosonography for recurrent anal fistulas: image enhancement with hydrogen peroxide. Dis Colon Rectum 1993;36:1158–60.
26. Law PJ, Talbot RW, Bartram CI, Northover JMA. Anal endosonography in the evaluation of perianal sepsis and fistula in ano. Br J Surg 1989;76:752–5.
27. Deen KI, Williams JG, Hutchinson R, et al. Fistulas in ano: endoanal ultrasonographic assessment assist decision making for surgery. Gut 1994;35:391–4.
28. Goldman S, Norming U, Svensson C, Glimelius B. Transanorectal ultrasonography in the staging of anal epidermoid carcinoma. Int J Colorectal Dis 1991;6:152–57.
29. Herzog U, Boss M, Spichtin HP. Endoanal ultrasonography in the follow-up of anal carcinoma. Surg Endosc 1994;8:1186–9.
30. Roreau G, Palazzo L, Colardelle P, et al. Endoscopic ultrasonography in the staging and follow-up of epidermoid carcinoma of the anal canal. Gastrointest Endosc 1994;40:447–50.
31. Pittman JS, Benson JT, Summers JE. Physiologic evaluation of the anorectum. A new ultrasound technique. Dis Colon Rectum 1990;33:476–8.
32. Schäfer R, Heyer T, Gantke B, et al. Anal endosonography and manometry: comparison in patients with defecation problems. Dis Colon Rectum 1997;40:293–7.
33. Kamm MA, Hoyle CH, Burleigh DE, et al. Hereditary internal anal sphincter myopathy causing proctalgia fugax and constipation. A newly identified condition. Gastroenterology 1991;100:805–10.
34. Tjandra JJ, Milsom JW, Schroeder T, Fazio VW. Endoluminal ultrasound is preferable to electromyography in mapping anal sphincter defects. Dis Colon Rectum 1993;36:689–92.

CHAPTER 23

# Gall Bladder and Biliary Tract: Normal Function and Clinical Disorders

*Walter J. Hogan and Reza Shaker*

## CLINICAL STUDIES OF GALLBLADDER MOTILITY

Impaired gallbladder motility has been shown to produce recurrent biliary-type pain in some patients without documented gallstones. This has been referred to as acalculous cholecystitis or acalculous biliary pain. These patients typically have no etiology for pain demonstrable by standard ultrasonography, cholecystography, cholescintigraphy, or endoscopic retrograde cholangiopancreatography (ERCP) with sphincter of Oddi (SO) manometry. Gallbladder dysmotility as a cause of pain remains somewhat controversial from the viewpoint of clinicopathologic correlation. However, as technology to assess gallbladder motor function continues to develop, the role of functional disorders of the gallbladder in the spectrum of a clinical pain syndrome may be appropriately defined.

The challenge that clinicians face currently is how to accurately diagnose gallbladder dysfunction. Although no uniformly acceptable standard has been established, several methods to assess gallbladder motility have been developed, and many of these have been reviewed recently.[1,2]

### Technique

#### Gallbladder Stimulation

It goes without saying that to measure gallbladder motility and specifically its emptying capability, the organ must first be stimulated. Endogenous cholecystokinin (CCK) appears to be the main stimulant involved in gallbladder contraction. Clinically, the gallbladder can be stimulated by ingesting a standardized fatty meal (eg, Lipomul, Mead Johnson Laboratories, Evansville, IN; 3.3 mL/kg) to increase endogenous CCK levels or by infusing low-dose CKK octapeptide (CCK-8) intravenously (eg, Kinevac). However, impaired gastric emptying or malabsorption could cause a false "abnormal" gallbladder response to a fatty meal; hence, exogenous CCK-8 is probably the more reliable and reproducible stimulant of gallbladder motility.

Studies have demonstrated that optimal gallbladder emptying occurs with a continuous infusion rate of 20 ng/kg/h.[3] (Rapid bolus CCK-8 infusion may elicit gallbladder spasm and block the ejection process early.[4–6]) In addition, bolus injection of CCK-8 may cause abdominal discomfort.[7]

### Gallbladder Imaging

Cholecystography has been used extensively in the past in conjunction with various stimulants to assess gallbladder motility. Unfortunately, because it provides only two-dimensional images, gallbladder emptying cannot be determined.

Two noninvasive relatively accurate methods of assessing gallbladder motility exist: cholescintigraphy and ultrasonography. Neither method directly measures smooth muscle contraction or volume. Their correlation with each other and with in vitro gallbladder emptying remains controversial.[8] For example, nuclear medicine demonstrated continued excretion of bile at 45 and 60 minutes, whereas ultrasonography did not show significant volume variations in these time frames.[9–11]

## Cholescintigraphy

Cholescintigraphy monitors the hepatic excretion of a radionuclide technetium 99m ($^{99m}$Tc)-labeled iminodiacetic acid analogs in the bile and specifically measures radioactivity over the gallbladder.[12] The study measures gallbladder emptying by computer-generated time-activity curves in response to a stimulus. The following methodology is generally used.

**CHOLESCINTIGRAPHY WITH CCK-8 STIMULATION.** The patient fasts overnight. Then 1.0 mCi of $^{99m}$Tc-diaminodiacetic acid is administered intravenously followed by 5 mL of saline flush. Scan 1 is obtained with the patient supine using a gamma camera with a multipurpose resolution collimator over 60 to 90 minutes until gallbladder activity is maximal and most of the radioactivity is cleared from the liver. Without changing the patient's position, CCK-8 (Kinevac) is administered as a continuous intravenous infusion (20 ng/kg/h) over 45 minutes. Data obtained from the anterior projection are adequate for cholescintigraphy studies.[13] Scan 2 is obtained starting 5 minutes before CCK-8 infusion using computer imaging and data acquisition over the gallbladder at 5-minute intervals until 20 minutes post–CCK-8 infusion (total scan time 70 minutes).

The gallbladder ejection fraction (GBEF) is calculated by the following formula:

$$GBEF \% = \frac{\text{change in gallbladder activity}}{\text{baseline gallbladder activity}} \times 100$$

## Ultrasonography

Real-time ultrasonography can be used to determine gallbladder volume serially in response to a stimulus. However, this technique is used much less frequently in clinical practice. The degree of operator variability is very important with this technique but may be useful in those patients in whom radiation exposure is a concern (eg, the pregnant woman).

Gallbladder volume can be calculated by the sum of cylinders method or the ellipsoidal method, as described by Dodds and others.[8] The former method is time consuming, cumbersome, and rarely used in clinical practice. The ellipsoidal method is easier to perform and correlates well with the sum of cylinders method and cholescintigraphy studies. Absolute gallbladder volume can be assessed during fasting as well as residual and refilling volumes after emptying.

**GALLBLADDER EMPTYING DETERMINED BY ULTRASONOGRAPHY.** The patient is fasted overnight. Gallbladder volume is calculated by the ellipsoidal method:

$$\text{Volume} = \frac{\text{maximum length (L)} \times \text{maximum width (W)}}{6}$$
$$\times \text{maximum height (H)} = 0.52 \times (L \times W \times H)$$

Gallbladder emptying is stimulated by CCK-8 infusion or a fatty meal (eg, Lipomul).

The gallbladder volume is recalculated at 5- to 10-minute intervals for a total of 45 to 60 minutes:

$$GBEF \% = \frac{\text{gallbladder volume after stimulus}}{\text{gallbladder volume before stimulus}} \times 100$$

## Interpretation

Several studies have reported good to excellent therapeutic results following cholecystectomy in patients with biliary pain and abnormal GBEF determined by CCK-stimulated cholescintigraphy. In a seminal study validating the efficacy of the CCK cholescintigraphy study, 103 patients with biliary (acalculus) pain were screened.[14] Twenty-one patients had a mean GBEF <40%, a value ± 3 SD below the mean GBEF value of 75% determined in a group of 40 volunteer subjects (Table 23.1 and Figure 23.1). These 21 patients were prospectively randomized to elective cholecystectomy versus no operation. Subsequently, 10 of the 11 patients undergoing surgery were without pain after a mean follow-up period of 34 months; the other patient had improvement of symptoms. All nonoperated patients remained symptomatic at follow-up. Gallbladder histology demonstrated chronic cholecystitis in all patients based on predetermined criteria.

In a retrospective report encompassing a 5-year period, a group of 53 patients with suspected biliary dyskinesia and

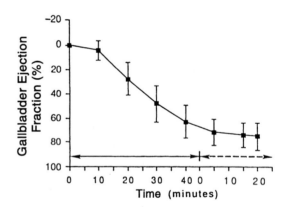

**FIGURE 23.1.** Cholecystokinin (CCK) cholescintigraphy: percentage of gallbladder ejection fraction in 40 normal volunteers. Mean gallbladder ejection fraction values ± SD are shown. *Solid arrow* indicates indicates duration of CCK infusion; *broken arrow* indicates time since CCK infusion was stopped. Reproduced with permission from Yap L, Wycherley AG, Morphett AD, Toouli J. Acalculus biliary pain: cholecystectomy alleviates symptoms in patients with abnormal cholescintigraphy. Gastroenterology 1991;101:786–93.

**TABLE 23.1.** GBEF in Normal Volunteers

|  | Males (n = 19) | Females (n = 21) | Total (n = 40) |
|---|---|---|---|
| GBEF (%) | 79.3 ± 12.6 | 70.1 ± 10.1 | 74.5 ± 12.2 |
| 95% CL (%) | > 54 | 50–90 | > 51 |
| 99% CL (%) | > 42 | > 40 | > 40 |

Gallbladder ejection fraction (GBEF %) 15 minutes after completion of a 45-minute cholecystokinin infusion (20 ng/kg/h) in normal volunteers.
All numbers expressed as mean ± SD. CL, confidence limit.

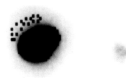

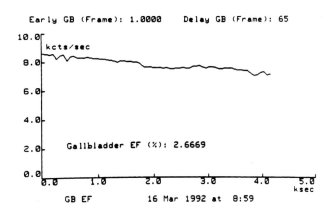

**FIGURE 23.2.** Cholecystokinin (CCK) cholescintigraphy study in a patient with acalculous cholecystitis. *Top*, early and delayed (post-CCK) frames with gallbladder (GB) and background area outlined. *Right*, plot of changing counts over the GB with time. Gallbladder ejection fraction was calculated as <3%. EF, ejection fraction.

negative conventional diagnostic studies had an abnormal GBEF <35% on CCK cholescintigraphy study.[15] Twenty-seven patients underwent cholecystectomy. Twenty-four patients (89%) improved significantly; 2 patients improved partially, whereas 1 patient improved minimally. (Interestingly, the gallbladder specimens in 9 of the 10 patients who showed significant improvement were normal histologically.) The 6 patients who did not have surgery did not improve significantly. A more recent report demonstrated the usefulness of the CCK-stimulated hepatobiliary scan in a group of 69 patients with biliary-like symptoms but no sonographic evidence of gallstones.[16] Twenty-nine of these patients had a GBEF <35%; 17 patients had cholecystectomy. Fifteen of the pathologic specimens demonstrated evidence of chronic cholecystitis. At mean follow-up of 11 months, 8 patients (47%) in the operative group had complete resolution of their symptoms, 6 patients (35%) had significant improvement, 2 patients (12%) were unchanged, and 1 patient (6%) was worse. Twelve of the 29 patients did not have gallbladder surgery. At 11 months, 4 patients (33%) had improved, whereas 8 patients (66%) reported no change or worsening of their symptoms. Of note in this study is the report of symptom reproduction following CCK gallbladder stimulation in 53% of patients in the operative group and 33% of patients in the nonoperative group; average GBEF determined in these two groups was 10% versus 23%, respectively.

Other retrospective studies have reported the usefulness of the CCK-stimulated hepatobiliary scan in screening adult patients with suspected biliary-type pain categorized as dyskinesia or acalculous disease[17,18] and in children diagnosed with gallbladder dyskinesia.[19]

Not all investigators find the CCK-stimulated cholescintigraphy study to be a clinically discriminating test, however. In a group of 57 patients referred to surgeons with demonstrated cholelithiasis, the CCK scintigraphy test was used in an attempt to identify those patients whose symptoms were "nonbiliary" from those patients with real "biliary distress."[20] Despite analysis of several parameters of gallbladder function from the CCK cholescintigraphy study, the authors were unable to accurately separate those patients who benefited from subsequent cholecystectomy from those who improved without surgery. Less convincing results were

reported in another nonrandomized study of patients with chronic right upper quadrant pain, but shorter data acquisition times may have underestimated GBEF.[21] However, clinicians and surgeons have found a low GBEF determined by CCK cholescintigraphy to be clinically useful as an objective method to confirm their diagnosis. An abnormally low GBEF is not specific for acalculous gallbladder disease, however. Numerous other diseases, concurrent therapeutic drugs, and improper CCK infusion methodology are associated with low GBEF. A caveat concerning the CCK scintigraphy test has been raised recently.[22] Patients who have been investigated in publications confirming the usefulness of CCK cholescintigraphy demonstrated a high pretest likelihood of a gallbladder disorder; they underwent extensive work-up and follow-up. Cholecystokinin cholescintigraphy is now being used by clinicians to shorten diagnostic work-up time and confirm or exclude the diagnosis of dyskinesia. The positive predictive value of the CCK scintigraphy test will likely be lower and the false-positive rate will likely be higher in this "new group" of referral patients. The proper use of this study by the clinician, the use of optimal methodology in performing CCK cholescintigraphy, and the interpretation of results in the global perspective of the patient's history and clinical setting will result in the lowest possible false-positive rates.

### Examples of Studies with Interpretation

In normal individuals, the GBEF at 15 minutes following a 45-minute period of infusion is 75% (see Fig. 23.1) This response of the gallbladder to CCK-8 slow infusion is highly reproducible and approximates the normal response of the gallbladder to the ingestion of a meal.

A marked decrease in GBEF is demonstrated in a patient with acalculous cholecystitis (Fig. 23.2) who had a 3-year history of intermittent right upper quadrant abdominal pain and negative routine diagnostic evaluation. The patient's symptoms resolved following cholecystectomy and have been absent during an 8-year follow-up period.

Figure 23.3 demonstrates results from an ultrasonographic recording of gallbladder volume during CCK-8 infusion. The gallbladder volume is reduced 70% over the course of 45 to 60 minutes.

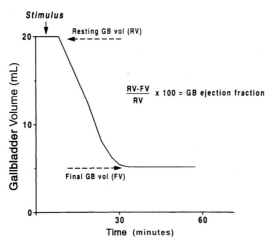

**FIGURE 23.3.** Gallbladder (GB) volume response to stimulation by chole-cystokinin-8 infusion. The formula for calculating gallbladder ejection fraction is shown in the text.

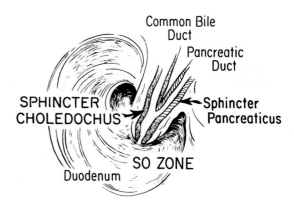

**FIGURE 23.5.** Schema of the anatomy of the sphincter of Oddi (SO) showing the confluence of "sphincteric" zones, which entwine the distal biliary and pancreatic ductal systems. Manometrically, there are no discrete segments or minisphincters appreciated within the SO zone. The pressure profile is a continuum within each ductal segment.

## CLINICAL STUDIES OF SPHINCTER OF ODDI MOTOR FUNCTION

Prior to the introduction of biliary endoscopy in the early 1970s, the human SO motor function could be measured only indirectly through a choledochal access at the time of surgery. Sphincter of Oddi manometry came of age in 1975 as an extension of diagnostic ERCP examination. Subsequently, SO manometry has developed as the primary diagnostic modality for determining pressures within the major pancreaticobiliary ductal system and motor activity within the SO zone.

Initial manometric studies, using a syringe-pump catheter perfusion technique only recorded a pressure plateau between the common bile duct (CBD) and the duodenum. However, with the introduction of the minimally compliant capillary infusion pump system and the triple-lumen manometric catheter, dynamic features of the SO pressure zone became more clearly defined.[23] There are three components associated with the SO pressure profile: the duct-to-duodenum pressure gradient, basal SO pressure, and phasic SO contractions (Fig. 23.4).

The SO zone extends, manometrically, over an 8- to 10-mm distance in a "Y" configuration encompassing the confluence of the distal pancreaticobiliary tract (Fig. 23.5). The SO zone forms a pressure gradient between the duodenum and the respective ductal systems. The resting pressure within the CBD and pancreatic duct (PD) averages 15 mm Hg. Sphincterotomy of the appropriate SO segment completely abolishes this pressure gradient. In normal subjects, the SO pressure profile is similar whether the manometry catheter is directed into the CBD SO segment or the PD SO segment.[24] It is important to remember that the ductal orientation of the manometry catheter should be determined at the time of SO pressure recording because SO motor dysfunction may be confined to a single segment or "limb" of the Y-shaped SO zone.

During slow catheter pull-through from the duct into the duodenum, the basal SO high-pressure zone is established. The length of the SO zone and reproduction of the pressure profile in two and preferably all three recording tips are accomplished during consecutive catheter pull-throughs. The normal basal SO pressure averages 20 mm Hg above resting duodenal pressure. Superimposed on the basal SO pressure plateau are phasic SO contractions, which occur at a rate of approximately 4/min and have a mean amplitude of 150 mm Hg. This contractile activity of the SO has been demonstrated during radiologic studies for decades. Phasic SO contractions propagate predominantly in an antegrade direction toward the duodenum.[25] Standard values for SO motor activity have been established by several investigators throughout the world using ERCP manometry (Table 23.2).[26,27] Abnormal basal SO pressure appears to be the most important diagnostic feature detected by SO manom-

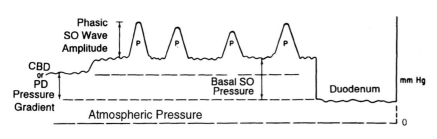

**FIGURE 23.4.** Sphincter of Oddi pressure profile demonstrating the features that are relevant to manometric recording (ie, duct to duodenum pressure gradient, basal SO pressure, and phasic SO contractions). P indicates phasic SO waves superimposed on basal SO pressure. Note that baseline is atmospheric pressure, which allows monitoring of duodenal pressure variations. CBD, common bile duct; PD, pancreatic duct.

**TABLE 23.2.** Standard Values for SO Motor Activity

| | | | Phasic Contraction | | |
| Author | Patients No. | Basal Pressure (mm Hg) | Amplitude (mm Hg) | Frequency (p/min) | Antegrade Sequence (%) |
|---|---|---|---|---|---|
| Toouli[26] (1985) | 10 postcholecystectomy | 41 | 389 | 7 | ≥50 |
| Geenen[45] (1987) | 27 abdominal pain | 40 | 350 | 8 | ≥50 |
| Gelrud[27] (1988) | 50 healthy | 35 | 220 | 10 | <50 |

*Values: mean ± 3 SD.

**TABLE 23.3.** SO Dysfunction: Operational Distinction Between SO Stenosis versus SO Dysfunction

| | SO Dysfunction | |
| Manometry Criteria | Stenosis | Dyskinesia |
|---|---|---|
| Tachyoddia | − | + |
| Paradoxical CCK-OP response | − | + |
| High basal SO pressure | + | + |
| Smooth muscle effect (relaxation) | | |
|    CCK-OP | − | + |
|    Amyl nitrite | − | + |
|    Glucagon | − | + |

SO, sphincter of Oddi; CCK, cholecystokinin; OP, octapeptide.
(−) absent; (+) present.

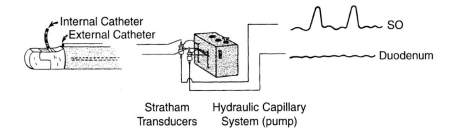

**FIGURE 23.6.** Endoscopic retrograde cholangiopancreatography manometric recording system. The manometry catheter is shown exiting the biopsy channel of the duodenoscope; the duodenal pressure recording catheter is attached to the shaft of the endoscope by parafilm wrap. The pneumohydraulic capillary pump system and trace recording complete the system.

etry. Other alterations of SO motor function that have been considered to be diagnostic of SO dysfunction[28] have not been validated to date.[29]

### Indications

Sphincter of Oddi manometry is performed as a diagnostic procedure in patients with pancreaticobiliary disorders and suspected SO dysfunction. At the outset, terminology requires definition. A structural alteration of the SO mechanism has been termed SO stenosis. A functional alteration of the SO mechanism has been labeled SO dyskinesia. Because it is often difficult or impossible to distinguish a structural from a functional SO disorder, the all-encompassing term SO dysfunction has been used. However, an operational distinction between stenosis versus dyskinesia can sometimes be determined by SO manometry (Table 23.3).

### Technique

#### Sphincter of Oddi Manometry Catheters

PERFUSED CATHETER SYSTEM. Pressure recording from the CBD and SO segment is accomplished using a triple-lumen polyethylene catheter with an outer diameter of 1.7 mm, a luminal diameter of 0.5 mm, and a length of 200 cm. The recording catheter is extruded as a single tube. A lateral orifice (0.5 mm) is cut for each lumen. The most distal orifice is 5 mm from the end of the catheter, and the three orifices are spaced 2 mm apart so that the distance between the distal and proximal orifices spans 4 mm. The catheter lumen beyond each

side hole is sealed with a plug. The end of the catheter, starting from the most distal orifice, is tattooed with circumferential black marks, spaced 2 mm apart to permit endoscopic observation of the depth of catheter penetration in the SO zone. A small sleeve ensemble is attached to the distal shaft of the catheter to allow insertion over a guidewire. The catheter is passed through the biopsy channel of the duodenoscope over the guidewire and inserted through the papilla and into the duct. Perfused SO manometry catheters are manufactured by Arndorfer Industries (Greendale, WI) and Wilson-Cook Co. (Durham, NC). Continuous recording of intraluminal duodenal pressure is obtained by a single-lumen Teflon catheter attached to the endoscope with parafilm so that its recording orifice is 4 mm proximal to the biopsy channel opening. Duodenal pressure transients can be recognized during recording periods, which can cause trace artifacts. This Teflon catheter has an outer diameter of 1.7 mm and an inner diameter of 0.8 mm (Fig. 23.6)

During recordings, each catheter lumen is infused with bubble-free saline at a rate of 0.25 mL/min by a minimally compliant hydraulic capillary infusion system using a reservoir pressure of 350 mm Hg. The performance of the recording system at the selected reservoir pressure and infusion rate are tested as follows: The inherent postocclusion rise rate of the infused catheter system is determined by abruptly obstructing the recording orifice of each recording lumen (Fig. 23.7). The pressure rise rate (mm Hg/sec) is measured to caps of 100, 200, and 300 mm Hg pressure. The postocclusion rise rates are as follows: 0 to 100 mm Hg (100–1,200 mm Hg/s), 0 to 200 mm Hg (550–1,000 mm Hg/s), and 0 to 300 mm Hg (350–500 mm Hg/s). The frequency response

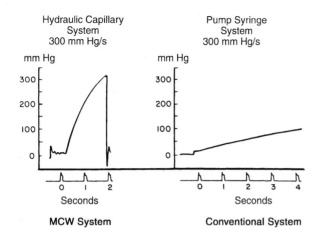

**FIGURE 23.7.** Comparison of postocclusion rise rate response between the hydraulic system and the pump syringe system. Note the rapid rise rate of the former (*left*) and the "dampened" response of the latter (*right*). The pressure rise rate (mm Hg/s) is measured to a plateau of 300 mm Hg in this illustration.

for each recording lumen of the triple-lumen catheter is flat to 4 or 5 Hz, with a measurement accuracy of 5%.

The effect of bubbles in the fluid column of the catheter has been evaluated by injecting 2- to 5-μL volumes of air into the transducer port and allowing the bubble to flow into the catheter. A small 5-μL air bubble in the catheter or transducer deteriorates the pressure rise rate and linear frequency response by more than 50%. Therefore, caution must be exercised to avoid air leaks (bubbles) during SO manometric recording.

### Aspirating Manometry Catheter
The conventional triple-lumen SO manometry catheter has been adapted so that one lumen is used for aspirating pancreaticobiliary juice during the SO recording period to avoid ductal overdistention.[30] The incidence of post-ERCP pancreatitis is significantly decreased using this catheter, but SO pressure is recorded from only two ports, not three, with this method.

**INTRALUMINAL MICROTRANSDUCER CATHETER.** Manometry catheters with a miniature solid-state intraluminal transducer(s) located at the distal tip have been used to measure pancreaticobiliary duct pressure.[31] This system avoids the infusion of fluid and enables recording of intraductal pressure for prolonged periods of time. However, these catheters are often unsuitable for measuring SO pressure dynamics per se because of the difficulty maintaining the sensor tip within the sphincteric zone. Additionally, solid-state transducers are notorious for baseline "drift," which can occur over prolonged recording periods.

### The SO Manometrist
An understanding of basic manometric recording principles, equipment, operation, and recording technique is essential to perform SO manometry. In addition to this fundamental knowledge, on-the-job experience and knowledgeable technical assistance are prime prerequisites for the task. Finally, familiarity with diagnostic ERCP and the vicissitudes of cannulation affords a valuable background experience for the manometrist.

The most critical skill for the manometrist is developing an effective interaction with the endoscopist. During the actual recording period, the manometrist controls the action. The manometrist frequently must "slow the action" to obtain an SO trace that is accurate and interpretable. The manometrist must be able to tell the endoscopist when to "freeze" catheter movement advance or withdraw it to obtain the best trace and to describe the quality of trace that is evolving during the procedure. The dialogue between these two principles should be constant, informative, and relevant. Vigorous respirations of the patient can cause "to/fro" catheter movement and "sliding" through the SO zone; this can result in considerable trace artifact. Appropriate annotation should be made on the trace and/or corrective action should be taken by the endoscopist relative to catheter stabilization or repositioning. Active duodenal contractions may result in significant catheter displacement or transmission of the duodenal contractions into the recording segment of the SO. Difficulties with catheter insertion, angulation, or resistance need to be conveyed and dutifully recorded in an appropriate temporal framework onto the trace itself. With the advent of videoendoscopy, the manometry catheter position, visible markings, and alignment can now be seen by both principles. This enables the manometrist to interact more intelligently with the endoscopist and also to note events of significance onto the trace recording.

Concerns have been raised about the use of paramedical technicians or "across the table" interpretation by the endoscopist who is already occupied performing the ERCP procedure. Recording technique and artifact recognition may be compromised in these situations. Because abnormal SO pressures inevitably result in an endoscopic sphincterotomy, it is imperative that appropriately trained and experienced personnel are dedicated to obtaining as accurate an SO manometric recording as possible.

### The Endoscopist
Without the patience and skill of the endoscopist, manometric pressure recording from the SO zone is impossible. The endoscopist must be experienced. He or she must be able to selectively and freely cannulate the duct of choice with a frequency approximating 95%. The endoscopist needs to have perceptive abilities, which translate to awareness of traction, tension, or angulation on the manometry catheter. The endoscopist must be able to continually reposition and align the catheter parallel to the long axis of the duct into which the catheter is inserted. Finally, the endoscopist must have the patience and interest to obtain an SO manometric pressure recording. The quality of the SO manometric tracing is directly proportional to the latter attributes.

### Techniques of SO Pressure Recording
Immediately prior to endoscopy, all patients are sedated with incremental (intravenous) doses of midazolam or

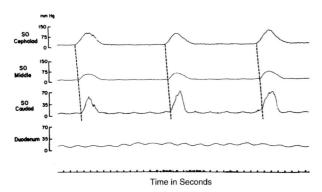

**FIGURE 23.8.** Sphincter of Oddi (SO) manometry tracing of phasic SO contractions recorded from the three catheter tips (proximal, middle, and distal), which span a 4-mm distance. With the polygraph paper speed increased to 5 cm/s, separation of the wave onset is better appreciated. Antegrade sequence of wave contractions (toward the duodenum) is demonstrated in these three series of SO contractions.

diazepam. Recently, meperidine has been shown by several investigators to influence phasic SO wave frequency but not the basal SO pressure.[32] For that reason, intravenous meperidine is frequently used in association with sedatives prior to ERCP manometry.

Following completion of the diagnostic ERCP examination, the intraductal contrast medium is allowed to escape into the duodenum. Performing diagnostic ERCP prior to SO manometry does not alter the validity of the recording and is cost effective.[33] The diagnostic cannula is removed over a guidewire and subsequently replaced by the manometry catheter. The guidewire is removed during the SO recording period because it often causes trace artifact. At the completion of the manometric recording, a small amount of contrast medium can be introduced through the manometric catheter to verify its position in the CBD or PD if this is necessary. Frequently, the ductal orientation of the manometry catheter is judged on the basis of the color of fluid aspirated. However, the accuracy of this technique has never been validated.

During the manometric study, the recording orifices of the triple-lumen catheter are initially stationed for 2 to 3 minutes in the duct to record pressure and to allow a "stabilization" period for the SO sphincteric mechanism. The catheter is then withdrawn across the SO in 2-mm increments using the circumferential rings on the catheter as reference points for depth insertion. At each "station," pressure recording is obtained for at least 60 to 90 seconds. When the catheter is stationed so that all three orifices record basal SO pressure and/or phasic SO contractions, a 3- to 5-minute recording is obtained with the polygraph paper speed increased to 5 cm/sec. The temporal relationship of the phasic pressure waves recorded by the three recording orifices can be determined much more accurately at the higher paper speed (Fig. 23.8).[34]

### Interpretation: SO Manometric Trace

The manometric trace is scored as follows (Table 23.4).[35] Common bile duct (or PD) and basal SO pressures are refer-

**TABLE 23.4.** Interpretation of SO Tracings

| Overview: Reference Points | |
|---|---|
| Duodenal pressure | Three tips average (pre-post study) or duodenal (4th) tip recording concurrently |
| Ductal pressure | Three tips averaged for 30–60 s |
| Duct/duodenal | Subtract mean duodenal pressure from mean ductal pressure |
| Basal SO pressure | Recorded and averaged from all three tips; measured from plateau between phasic waves to duodenal pressure |
| Phasic SO waves | Amplitude: (mm Hg) height from basal plateau to peak of SO contraction<br>Frequency (per minute) and duration (in seconds)<br>Propagation sequence:<br>Contraction onset proximal tip to distal tip; mean value three tips for 2 min |
| Provocative tests | CCK-OP: 20 ng/kg/IV; basal and phasic SO activity observed 3–5 min before and after administration<br>Amyl nitrite ampule: 4 sniffs after breakage; observe pulse change; monitor basal and phasic SO activity for 2–3 min |
| Variables | Allow baseline trace to stabilize for 2–3 min after entering duct<br>Identify duct, ie, CBD or PD at completion<br>Caveats: respiration; patient positioning, morbid obesity, movement, and retching; duodenal contractions; catheter "wedge"; catheter "tightness"; catheter torque/attitude change |

SO, sphincter of Oddi; CCK, cholecystokinin; OP, octapeptide; CBD, common bile duct; PD, pancreatic duct.

enced to duodenal pressure. Since atmosphere is zero point, we are able to record "true" duodenal pressure from the catheter affixed to the endoscope. The ductal pressure is obtained by subtracting the resting duodenal pressure from the resting ductal pressure from each of the three SO recording ports. Basal SO pressure is also calculated by subtracting the duodenal pressure from the baseline SO pressure obtained between phasic SO waves for each recording orifice. A basal SO pressure is obtained from at least 2 minutes of recording from each tip. The mean of these three values determines the final basal SO pressure. The frequency, amplitude, and duration of phasic waves are calculated over the same recording period, and a mean value is determined for each minute. Amplitude of the phasic contractions is calculated by subtracting the basal SO pressure from peak wave pressure. The direction of propagation of SO wave sequences is determined by drawing a line between the onset of the major upstroke of the phasic wave in the proximal recording orifice to the onset of each corresponding phasic wave in the distal recording orifice. In this manner, phasic wave sequences over a 4-mm span are classified as antegrade (ie, toward the duodenum), retrograde (ie, away from the duodenum), or simultaneous (Fig. 23.9). The number of phasic waves occurring over a 3-minute period is calculated. For each type of wave (simultaneous,

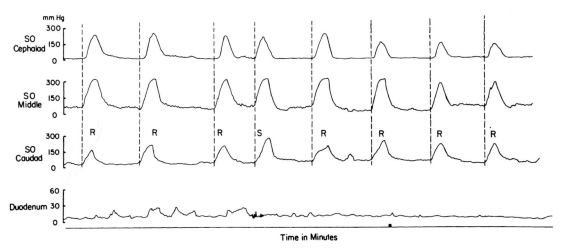

**FIGURE 23.9.** Triple-lumen catheter recording from the sphincter of Oddi (SO) zone showing in this series phasic SO contraction propagation occurring in retrograde (R) or simultaneous (S) sequence. In this instance, the patient had demonstrated common duct calculi at the time of SO manometry study.

antegrade, or retrograde), we calculate the percentage of total phasic waves recorded within the 3-minute period. Analysis of SO pressure shows no difference in values recorded from control patients or volunteers with or without a gallbladder.[36] A sample SO manometry report form used in our hospital is shown in Figure 23.10.

Some investigators have developed a different system of SO manometric pressure recording using the aspirating catheter. Sphincter of Oddi pressure was obtained for a minimum of 30 seconds and generally more than 1 minute; pressures were recorded in at least two leads. The "four-point method" is used to determine the most representative segment for measurement of the basal pressures. The four lowest points in the highest sustained sphincter pressure zone are read and averaged by this method. The mean of all basal sphincter recordings combining all leads and all pull-throughs is taken as the basal SO pressure for data analysis.[37]

### Reproducibility of SO Manometry

Several investigators around the world have demonstrated the reproducibility of SO manometric pressure recording in the same patient or groups of patients.[38,39] Figure 23.11 compares basal SO pressures in a group of 47 patients studied on two occasions over a 12-month period. There is a significant correlation in the reproducibility of basal SO pressure in patients with normal and patients with high basal SO pressures

### Examples of Recordings with Interpretation

#### Normal

An example of a normal SO pressure obtained by the triple-lumen manometric catheter pull-through from the steady, CBD pressure through the SO zone (elevated plateau pressure with superimposed phasic contractions) into the low-pressure duodenum is shown in Figure 23.12. Figure 23.13 demonstrates phasic SO contractions recorded in all three catheter tips. The normal frequency of phasic SO contractions is

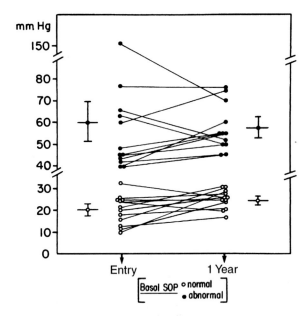

**FIGURE 23.11.** Reproducibility of sphincter of Oddi (SO) motor function. Comparison of basal SO pressures recorded in 47 patients after a 1-year interval. The patient groups were subdivided into those with high basal SO pressure (SOP) versus those with normal basal SOP. There was a significant correlation in basal SOP obtained on two occasions over the year period in both groups.

approximately 4 to 6/min; the wave duration is 4 to 5 seconds. The wave sequencing can be variable, but the majority of sequences are antegrade or simultaneous.

Normal subjects and patients who approximate normals have pressure profiles that are similar in the pancreatic segment of the SO and the CBD segment of the SO.[27] Figure 23.14 shows a catheter pull-through from the PD into the duodenum (left) and a catheter pull-through from the CBD into the duodenum (right) in the same patient.

## ERCP MANOMETRY REPORT

**Patient Name:** Mary Jones                **Procedure Date:**                **Med. Rec. #:** 00-97-60
**Endoscopist:** Bill Smith, M.D.          **Referring M.D.:** Edgar Poe, M.D.

I. **CLINICAL NOTATION:** Recurrent abdominal pain-history suggestive of biliary dyskinesia. No documented epidosdes of fever, but LFT's and amylase have been elevted trasiently on three occasions.

II. **PROCEDURE:**
ERCP Manometry is performed with a triple-lumen catheter with recording tips spaced 2 mm apart. The catheter is passed through the biopsy channel of the duodenscope and inserted through the papilla. The Common Bile Duct (CBD) or Pancreatic Duct (PD) is cannulated freely and pressures are obtained during slow pull-through of the sphincter of Oddi (SO) zone. Each tip is perfused with water by a non-compliant pump (0.25 ml/min). A separate catheter, attached to the endoscope, measure duodenal pressure concurrently. Certain drugs/hormones may be administered I.V. during SO pressure recording.

III. **SPHINCTER OF ODDI PRESSURES—NORMAL VALUES**

Gradient: CBD/Duodenum: 15 mm Hg          Basal SO: $15 \pm 10$ mm Hg
PD/Duodenum: 17 mm Hg          Phasic SO: Amplitude $130 \pm 16$ mm Hg
                                                                     Frequency $4 \pm 0.5$ p/min
**NOTE:** Ductal structures and contrast drainage time normal          Duration $4.3 \pm 1.5$ sec

IV. **STUDY RESULTS**

Manometry Catheter Orientation: CBD    X          PD    X

| Catheter | PRESSURES | | | Gradients | | SO PHASIC | | | | | | | |
|---|---|---|---|---|---|---|---|---|---|---|---|---|---|
| | | | | | | SO Basal | | Amplitude | | Frequency | | Duration | |
| | Duo | CBD | PD | CBD | PD | CBD | PD | CBD | PD | CBD | PD | CBD | PD |
| Tip 1 (prox) | 10 | 25 | 30 | 15 | 20 | 100 | 160 | 170 | 250 | 6 | 8 | 3 | 3 |
| Tip 2 (mid) | 20 | 25 | 30 | 5 | 10 | 150 | 100 | 180 | 135 | 6 | 8 | 3 | 3 |
| Tip 3 (dist) | 22 | 25 | 30 | 3 | 8 | 55 | 165 | 180 | 150 | 6 | 8 | 3 | 3 |
| Mean | 17 | 25 | 30 | 8 | 13 | 105 | 142 | 177 | 178 | 6 | 8 | 3 | 3 |

(PD basal SO: 142 – 17 = 125mm Hg)          CBD basal SO: 105 – 17 = 88 mm Hg)

**DRUG RESPONSE:** A decreases in pressure with Amyl Nitrite inhalation; CCK ablated SO phasic/basal SO pressure temporarily.

V. **INTREPRETATION:** Abnormal basal SO pressure elevation recorded from both PD/CBD segments of the SO. There is relaxation of SO basal pressure with Amyl Nitrite and the CCK. This response suggests a muscular rather than structural cause for abnormal pressure.

Staff Signature

**FIGURE 23.10.** Endoscopic retrograde cholangiopancreatography (ERCP) manometry report: patient with recurrent abdominal pain and history of dyskinesia. Both common bile duct (CBD) and pancreatic duct (PD) portions of the sphincter of Oddi (SO) were evaluated by manometric pressure recording, and elevated basal SO pressure was demonstrated in both segments. LFT, liver function test; CCK, cholecystokinin.

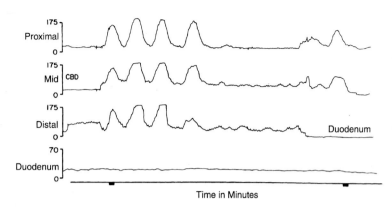

**FIGURE 23.12.** Normal sphincter of Oddi (SO) pressure profile obtained by the triple-lumen manometric catheter pull-through from a steady common bile duct (CBD) pressure through the SO zone (elevated pressure plateau with superimposed phasic contractions) into the low-pressure duodenum. Pressure (mm Hg) is shown on the vertical axis for each of the three recording tips (proximal, middle, and distal). The duodenal pressure recording is shown in the bottom trace. Time interval (minutes) is designated by the *square black marks* on the horizontal axis. The transient pressure "peaks" in the proximal and middle tip recordings immediately preceding catheter exit into the duodenum are attributable to angulation of the catheter at the papillary "hood" as it leaves the SO zone and is artifactual.

**FIGURE 23.13.** An example of triple-lumen manometric pressure recording within the zone of the sphincter of Oddi (SO) demonstrating phasic SO contractions. Peak amplitude of the contractions ranges from 100 mm Hg (proximal recording tip) to 60 mm Hg (distal recording tip). The frequency of phasic SO contractions is 3/min; the wave duration is 4 seconds. The phasic SO wave sequences are simultaneous in this tracing. The duodenal pressure is recorded concurrently and shown in the bottom trace. This is an example of a normal SO manometric tracing.

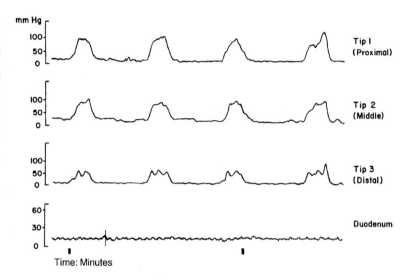

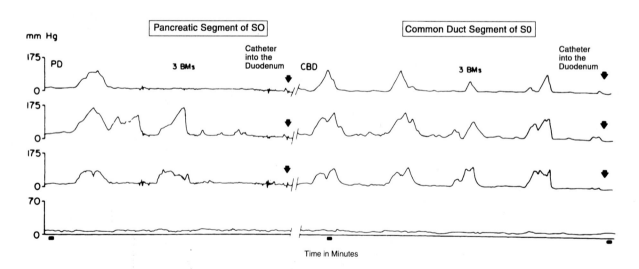

**FIGURE 23.14.** A comparison of manometric pressures from both segments of the sphincter of Oddi (SO) in the same patient is shown in these two adjacent tracings. Pressures (mm Hg) are shown on the vertical axis. Time (minutes) is noted on the horizontal axis. On the left trace, the catheter records pressure from the pancreatic duct (PD) at an insertion depth of three black marks (BM). The *black arrows* indicate the pressure "step-down" into the duodenum. A similar recording sequence is shown on the right from the common bile duct (CBD). Basal SO pressures are identical in both SO segments. Although the wave contraction contour and sequencing in the pancreatic duct segments appear less uniform than in the CBD segment in this tracing, average phasic SO amplitudes and durations were very similar.[27]

*Pathologic States*

Examples of SO stenosis are shown in Figures 23.15 and 23.16. Dyskinesia in the PD segment of the SO is shown in Figure 23.17. Elevated basal SO pressure is recorded in all tips: phasic SO contractions are superimposed. The elevated basal SO pressure relaxed temporarily following amyl nitrite inhalation, suggesting a muscular "spasm" rather than a structural cause for the elevated pressure. We define this as "dyskinesia."

Cholecystokinin-octapeptide (CCK-OP) may infrequently cause a "paradoxical" increase in basal SO pressure (Fig. 23.18).[40–42]

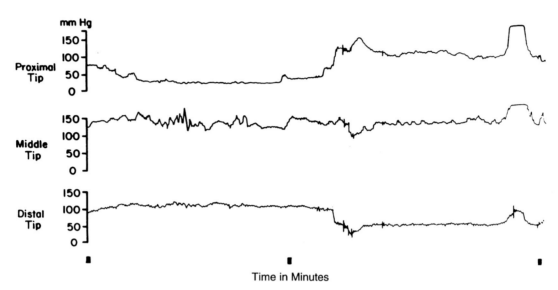

**FIGURE 23.15.** Triple-lumen pressure recording with the catheter "stationed" within the sphincter of Oddi (SO) segment of the common bile duct (CBD) demonstrating elevated basal SO pressure in a patient with suspected papillary stenosis (there is no phasic SO activity present in this portion of the tracing). Basal SO pressure is markedly elevated and sustained in the middle recording tip (>130 mm Hg) during this 2-minute recording period. This elevated basal SO pressure appears to "rise and fall" within tips 1 and 3, but there is a 4-mm distance "spanned" by these three recording tips. Respiration and subtle catheter movement cause transient catheter tip displacement from a relatively short high-pressure zone accounting for the unique appearance of this trace. The high basal SO pressure was not affected by intravenous administration of cholecystokinin-octapeptide.

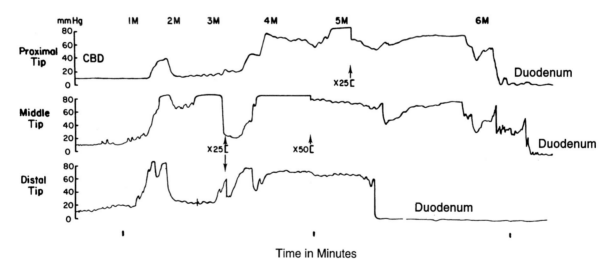

**FIGURE 23.16.** Another example of elevated basal sphincter of Oddi (SO) pressure caused apparently by stenosis and demonstrated during manometric pull-through of the SO zone from the common bile duct (CBD) into the duodenum. (There is no continuous duodenal pressure recording in this portion of the trace.) Pressures (mm Hg) are noted on the vertical axis at the initiation of the pull-through from the CBD. Peak pressure scale is 80 mm Hg. Circumferential marks (M) visible to the endoscopist are annotated at the top of the tracing and indicate catheter depth insertion. At 5 marks in the proximal tip, basal SO pressure becomes markedly elevated and requires attenuation of pressure sensitivity (×25) to a peak scale of 200 mm Hg. In the middle tip, recording pressure sensitivity requires downscaling at 3 (200 mm Hg peak scale) and 4 marks (400 mm Hg peak scale). Basal SO pressure is also elevated in the distal recording tip, but attenuation of pressure sensitivity was not required. The average of all three recording tips for basal SO pressure sustained for 2 minutes during this pull-through was 108 mm Hg.

Normally, a CCK-OP bolus completely ablates phasic SO activity and decreases basal SO pressure. Figure 23.19 shows an example of the effect of CCK-OP (20 ng/kg/IV) on SO pressures.

An example of SO tachyoddia is shown in Figure 23.20. Tachyoddia or rapid phasic SO contractions have been demonstrated at the time of duodenal phase III motor activity in humans and animals.[43] Infrequently, rapid phasic SO contractions (>8/min) are recorded without concurrent duodenal contractions signifying phase III MMC activity. Figures 23.21 and 23.22 demonstrate this phenomenon.

The effects of endoscopic sphincterotomy on SO motor function in a patient with biliary dyskinesia are shown in Figure 23.23. Following completion of the sphincterotomy

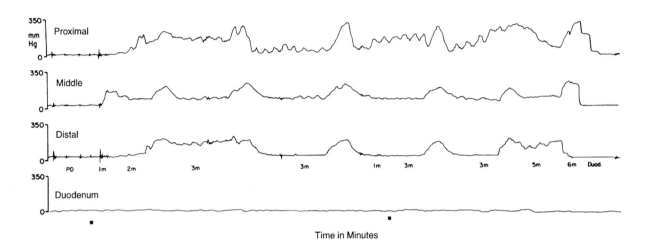

**FIGURE 23.17.** Triple-lumen catheter pull-through of the sphincter of Oddi (SO) zone from the pancreatic duct (PD) into the duodenum. Note that the pressure sensitivity scale (vertical axis) is 350 mm Hg. The position of the manometry catheter within the SO is noted by the marks (m) designation. There is a sustained basal SO pressure elevation in the proximal and middle recording tips with superimposed phasic SO contractions. Basal SO pressure is less consistently elevated in the distal recording tip, but this probably reflects relative asymmetry of the SO zone. Basal SO pressure is quite stable (*bottom tract*). The PD/duodenum pressure gradient is very well shown in this example. The basal SO pressure partially relaxed following amyl nitrite inhalation, suggesting a muscular "spasm" rather than a structural cause for the elevated pressure.

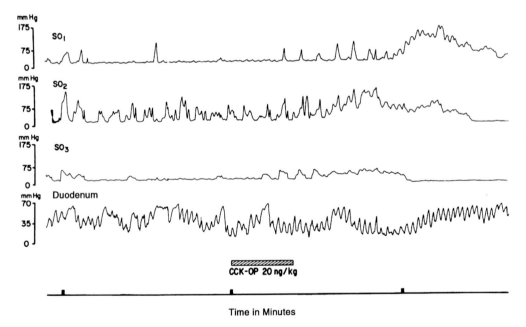

**FIGURE 23.18.** Cholecystokinin-octapeptide (CCK-OP) administration (horizontal bar) causes a "paradoxical" increase in basal sphincter of Oddi (SO) pressure especially in the proximal (SO$_1$) and middle (SO$_2$) recording tips during manometric pressure recording while stationed within the SO zone. Following CCK-OP (20 mg/kg/IV) within 30 seconds, basal SO pressure increased from 40 to 175 mm Hg (SO$_1$) and 40 to 160 mm Hg (SO$_2$). Increase in basal SO pressure in SO$_3$ is less dramatic. The sustained basal SO contraction appears to move in an orad direction following CCK, and this is attributable to catheter movement caused by sphincteric spasm. The duodenal pressure is moderately elevated throughout the recording period (which is not unusual) but appears to decrease transiently for 20 seconds after CCK-OP injection.

incision, manometric catheter pull-through of the SO zone (from the CBD into the duodenum) shows complete obliteration of the basal SO pressure, phasic SO contractions, and duct-to-duodenal pressure gradient in this sequence.

### Clinical Results

Sphincter of Oddi manometry is a diagnostic modality used to evaluate SO motor function in patients with suspected SO dysfunction. The test should be used only when there is a high degree of suspicion of this disorder.

Patients with suspected SO dysfunction frequently present with abdominal pain characteristic of biliary or pancreatic origin. Additionally, there may be transient elevation of liver function tests, dilation, and/or delayed contrast emptying of the CBD or PD at ERCP study, or recurrent episodes of pancreatitis. Because of the variable clinical presentation, patients with suspected SO dysfunction have been arbitrarily divided into three clinically descriptive groups (types I–III) for both the biliary and pancreatic systems according to the abdominal pain pattern and a graded scale of associated clin-

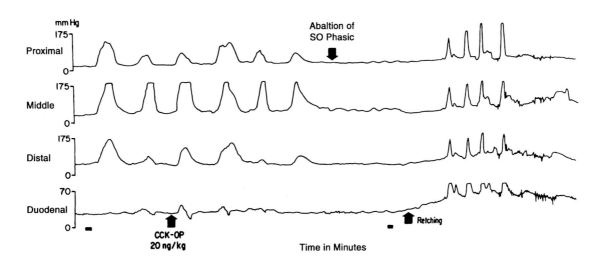

**FIGURE 23.19.** A bolus of cholecystokinin-octapeptide (CCK-OP) (*bottom arrow*) completely ablates phasic sphincter of Oddi (SO) activity in all three recording tips 30 seconds after administration (*top arrow*). Subsequently, there is a rapid, simultaneous pressure rise in all SO recording tips (including the duodenum) associated with patient retching (*second bottom arrow*). This is not a paradoxical response to CCK and reflects transmission of intra-abdominal pressure increase to all recording tips.

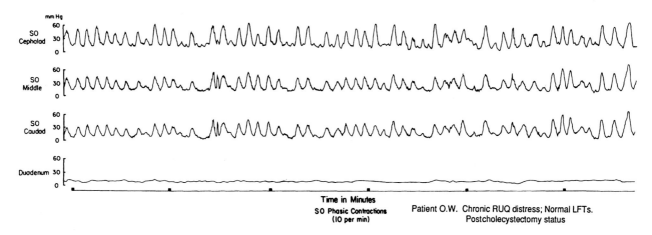

**FIGURE 23.20.** This is a 5-minute sphincter of Oddi (SO) tracing in a patient with a 4-year history of chronic right upper quadrant (RUQ) pain that persisted despite a cholecystectomy and was not associated with elevated serum, liver, or pancreatic enzymes. At the time of SO manometric recording, rapid phasic SO contractions (~10 per minute) were recorded over a sustained period. Although rapid phasic SO contractions have been recorded in human and animal models during passage of the migrating myoelectric activ-ity (phase 3) through the duodenum, no equivalent contractile activity is recorded within the duodenum. This trace represents an example of SO tachy-oddia, which is the occurrence of rapid (≥8/min) phasic contractions for a sustained period of time. It is postulated that this rapid SO contractile activity may cause functional obstruction to flow and result in clinical symptoms. Following endoscopic sphincterotomy, this patient has been asymptomatic for 6 years. LFT, liver function test.

ical features (Table 23.5).[44] This clinical classification has been quite useful in determining therapeutic outcomes of diagnostic studies and treatments in at least two of the three groups (biliary type I and II).

### Biliary SO Segment Dysfunction

Group I patients have been shown to have dysfunction of the SO mechanism in 65 to 80% of cases. A minority of these group I patients, however, have normal ERCP manometry of the SO.[45] The explanation for this finding is not fully under-

stood but may relate to structural alterations occurring above the zone of the sphincter. Group I patients have routinely responded to sphincterotomy, albeit endoscopic or operative. The underlying etiology in this patient group is generally accepted to be structural alteration of the distal choledochus.

Group II patients with biliary disorders have been more critically and extensively evaluated in a prospective, randomized outcome study.[46] Forty-seven patients (45 females, 2 males) who met the criteria for group II were extensively evaluated by conventional diagnostic and laboratory test prior to

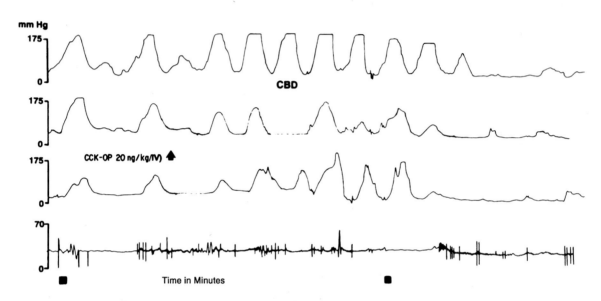

**FIGURE 23.21.** Rapid (9/min) phasic sphincter of Oddi (SO) contractions (tachyoddia) are recorded from the common bile duct (CBD) segment of the SO by the triple-lumen catheter. Intravenous cholecystokinin-octapeptide (CCK-OP) (*arrow*) rapidly ablates phasic SO contractions and decreased basal SO pressure within 45 seconds after administration. The bottom trace records duodenal pressure, which is quiescent.

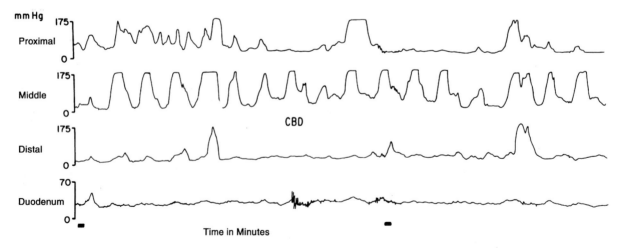

**FIGURE 23.22.** Discordant motor activity within the sphincter of Oddi (SO) is shown in this triple-lumen manometric recording from the common bile duct (CBD) segment of the SO. The middle recording tip demonstrates rapid SO contractions (10/min) while less frequent and unrelated contractile activity is noted in the adjacent proximal and distal recording tips. The duodenal pressure recording is the bottom trace and demonstrates no con-

tractile activity of significance. This patient had intermittent epigastric and right upper quadrant postcholecystectomy pain but demonstrated no abnormality in basal SO pressure. This unusual sequence of phasic SO activity was not sustained and may reflect alteration of the SO contractile frequency gradient demonstrated in the animal model. The clinical significance of this motor activity is not known.

**A**

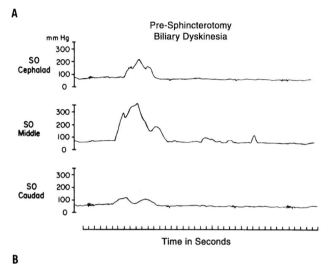

**B**

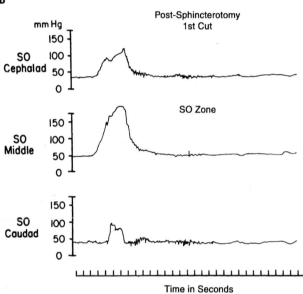

**TABLE 23.5.** SO Dysfunction: Patient Classification

Patients with suspected SO dysfunction related to biliary tract disorders are classified as follows:

- Biliary Type I SO Dysfunction
  Patients have "typical" biliary-type pain, dilated (≥ 12 mm) or delayed (>45 min) CBD drainage, and documented liver function test abnormalities (alkaline phosphatase and transaminase values (>2  normal ≥ 2 separate occasions).
- Biliary Type II SO Dysfunction
  Patients have typical biliary-type pain and one or two of criteria for I.
- Biliary Type III SO Dysfunction
  Patients have only typical biliary-type pain and no objective abnormalities.

Patients with suspected SO dysfunction related to pancreatic tract disorders are classified as follows:

- Pancreatic Type I SO Dysfunction
  Patients have idiopathic recurrent pancreatitis and/or "typical" pancreatic-type pain, amylase/lipase values (>2  normal ≥ 2 occasions), dilated (>6 mm) pancreatic duct, and prolonged (>10 min) pancreatic duct drainage time.
- Pancreatic Type II SO Dysfunction
  Patients have pancreatic-type pain and one or two of the criteria for I.
- Pancreatic Type III SO Dysfunction
  Patients have pancreatic-type pain and no objective abnormalities.

SO, sphincter of Oddi; CBD, common bile duct.

**FIGURE 23.23.** The effects of endoscopic sphincterotomy on sphincter of Oddi (SO) motor function in a patient with SO dyskinesia is shown in above three trace sequences. **A**, High-amplitude phasic SO contractions are shown in the middle recording tip exclusively, although basal SO pressure of 50 mm Hg is recorded from all three tips. **B**, Following initial sphincterotomy incision, phasic SO contraction amplitudes and basal SO pressure are only modestly affected. Vertical scale to 180 mm Hg. **C**, Following extension of the sphincterotomy incision, manometric catheter pull-through of the SO zone from the common bile duct (CBD) into the duodenum shows complete obliteration of the basal SO pressure, phasic SO contractions, and duct-to-duodenal pressure gradient.

**C**

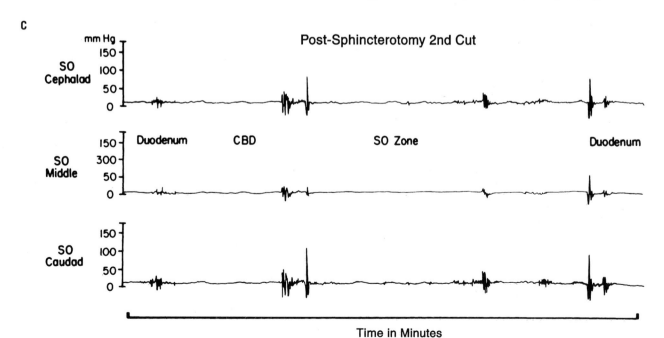

randomization to endoscopic sphincterotomy or sham endoscopic sphincterotomy. A number of potential outcome predictors were evaluated (eg, liver function tests, CBD diameter and drainage, response to the morphine prostigmine challenge, and SO manometry). At the 1-year follow-up period, only the group of patients who had abnormal SO pressures and endoscopic sphincterotomy were doing well. Ten of 12 patients were completely well, and 1 patient was much improved. These results were based on both subjective and objective criteria. The outcomes of patients in both sham and SO sphincterotomy groups who had normal basal SO pressure were not significantly different from each other at 1-year follow-up. Only the SO manometric study results (ie, an abnormal basal SO pressure) appeared to be predictive of positive clinical outcome. After 1 year, several of the patients from the sham group with elevated basal SO pressure were offered endoscopic sphincterotomy. In those patients with elevated SO pressures, the sensitivity and specificity of the SO manometric study was 71% and 89%, respectively, at the 1-year period. At 4-year follow-up, patient well-being based on symptomatic evaluation was very good; the correlation between elevated basal SO pressure and therapeutic outcome was even stronger (17 of 19 patients were markedly improved). This study has been continued for 12 years now, and these results have persisted. The patients who had abnormal basal SO pressure and endoscopic sphincterotomy have continued to do well.[47]

Group III patients, those defined as SO dyskinesia, are the most difficult clinical group because the presumption of SO dysfunction is based only on quality and location of pain. The results of treatment in group III patients are much less impressive. An appropriately controlled study has not been performed on patients with suspected SO dysfunction. Endoscopic sphincterotomy performed on the basis of elevated basal SO pressure in this group has not shown results that were significant.

Recently, the Australian Group has performed a randomized prospective study of patients defined by ERCP manometry as "SO stenosis" versus "SO dyskinesia."[29]

The effects of sphincterotomy were evaluated in patients randomized on the basis of endoscopic SO biliary manometric pressure measurements. Endoscopic retrograde cholangiopancreatography was performed in 1981 on postcholecystectomy patients with entry criteria including recurrent biliary-type pain for at least 6 months and one or more of the following: transient increases in serum transaminase with episodes of pain, dilation of the bile duct >12 mm at ERCP examination, and a positive response to the morphine neostigmine test. The manometric record was categorized as (1) normal, (2) "stenosis" (a category defined by a basal SO pressure >40 mm Hg), and (3) SO dyskinesia based on an increased incidence of phasic SO contractions (>7/min), an increased incidence of retrograde propagated SO phasic contractions (>50%), and a paradoxical contraction response of the SO to CCK-OP bolus injection. Sphincter of Oddi manometry was repeated at 3 and 24 months.

Patients were stratified within the three categories based on the results of the SO manometry and subsequently randomized to sham or endoscopic sphincterotomy. Stenosis was diagnosed when basal SO pressure averaged >40 mm Hg in all three recording channels. The criteria for dyskinesia have been detailed above. Other features evaluated during the long-term study included the presence or absence of a dilated CBD, elevated liver function tests, and a positive response to the morphine provocation test. The latter was considered positive when it reproduced biliary-type pain and was associated with elevation of either aminotransferase, amylase, or both in blood samples.

The effects of sham or endoscopic sphincterotomy on the individual patient's pain required the use of a linear analog pain chart, which was administered before and during each follow-up visit. A clinician followed the patients for a 3-month interval for a period of 2 years. This clinician was not involved with the endoscopy and was unaware of the results of manometry or randomization. The patient's symptoms and pain diaries were evaluated at each visit, and symptoms were categorized as "no change/worse," "improved," or "asymptomatic."

Twenty-six of a total of 81 patients (32%) had SO stenosis based on manometric results. In the SO stenosis group (predominantly type II), 11 of 13 patients (85%) showed long-term improvement after the sphincterotomy. In the sham group with "stenosis," only 5 of 13 patients (30%) improved —an insignificant number. The other manometric categories defined as SO dyskinesia and SO normal showed no significant symptomatic improvement. Interestingly, symptomatic outcome was independent of bile duct dilation, alteration of liver enzymes, or the results of the morphine neostigmine provocation test. This is the same disassociation seen in the earlier American study of 47 type II patients. None of the diagnostic test results have been found to be predictors of an outcome to sphincterotomy other than the SOM measurement. This second randomized study reiterates the finding that patients with presumed SO dysfunction categorically classified as type II or higher who have manometric features characteristic of SO stenosis have a significant chance of a positive clinical outcome after sphincterotomy. Clinical outcome appears to be unrelated to the number of associated positive entry criteria, however.

## Pancreatic SO Segment Dysfunction

Although dysfunction of the SO is most commonly associated with disorders of the biliary tract, renewed interest has been focused on the SO and its association with patients who have idiopathic recurrent acute pancreatitis or "pancreaticobiliary pain."

Recurrent acute pancreatitis is an inflammatory condition often manifested by unpredictable, intermittent episodes of disabling abdominal pain that may occur over a protracted period of time. The attacks of pancreatitis frequently require hospitalization and may have significant complications. Often the etiology for the pancreatitis escapes routine diagnostic studies. Recently, SO dysfunction has been promoted as a possible cause of idiopathic recurrent pancreatitis[48] and post-ERCP pancreatitis.[49] Investigators have also shown that pancreatic disorders may be related to SO dysfunction, which involves either the pancreatic sphincter, the biliary sphincter, or both.

Chen et al have recently demonstrated an association between SO dysfunction and idiopathic recurrent pancreatitis in a prospective, randomized study.[48] Sphincter of Oddi manometric disorders were detected in 25 of 28 patients with this problem. The most common manometric finding was an abnormally elevated basal SO pressure suggesting a structural abnormality, although features of SO dyskinesia were also present in some of these patients. Subsequent operative sphincterotomy resulted in long-term cure or a noticeable reduction in the symptoms of these patients.

Tarnasky et al reported an increased risk of post-ERCP pancreatitis when hypertension was demonstrated in the pancreatic segment of the SO in 10 of 32 patients with suggested SO dyskinesia.[49] Patients with increased basal SO pressure in the pancreatic duct were 10 times more likely to develop pancreatitis than those patients with normal PD manometric pressures following biliary sphincterotomy. Subsequently, Tarnasky et al have most recently reported their results following stenting of the hypertensive SO pancreatic segment after biliary sphincterotomy.[50] Pancreatic stenting significantly reduced the risk of pancreatitis from 26 to 7% (10 of 39 in the patient group with stenting versus 3 of 41 in the stent group). It was strongly suggested that stenting of the hypertensive pancreatic duct segment should be considered after biliary sphincterotomy.

A group of 360 patients was evaluated with SO manometry to determine the frequency of motor abnormality in both the pancreatic and biliary SO sphincter and to correlate the results with a "clinical suspicion" of SO dysfunction. This study took place between 1993 and 1996.[51] Manometric recordings in this group were obtained from both a pancreatic and a biliary portion of the SO at the same session using the aspirating-type catheter.

Overall, the frequency of SO dysfunction was observed to differ according to whether patients were typed by biliary or pancreatic criteria. Approximately 65% of biliary type II patients and 59% of biliary type III patients had SO disorders. Fifty-five percent of patients without pancreatitis had an abnormal basal SO pressure. Sphincter of Oddi dysfunction was present in 72.3% of patient with idiopathic pancreatitis and 53.9% of patients with chronic pancreatitis.

At the Rome II Consensus meeting, it was estimated from the accumulated experience of the members that predictability of SO dysfunction was highest in biliary type I (65–95%) and II (50–63%) patients.[52] Sphincter of Oddi dysfunction was less common in type III, ranging from 12 to 28%. This new study from the United States cites figures that far exceed these estimates in the type III patient category. The authors have suggested a number of reasons for the marked differences in frequencies of abnormal basal SO pressure from previously published series. First, they suggest that the selection of patients with a pain pattern that is typical of the biliary tract versus a nonspecific pain pattern similar to that of

patients with irritable bowel will probably increase the percentage of patients with SO dysfunction. It is noteworthy, however, that the patients in this study with pancreaticobiliary pain have never been adequately defined and add a new dimension to any upper gastrointestinal pain syndrome. Second, the authors recognize that if abnormal sphincter pressure is required in two or three recording channels to make the diagnosis of SO dysfunction, the frequency of SO dysfunction will be lower. Third, differences in design of the manometric pressure recording catheter and the recording technique will also be factors that significantly influence the results of the SO manometry study.

### Complications of SO Manometry

Similar to other diagnostic and therapeutic ERCP procedures, potentially serious complications may be associated with SO manometry study. The major complication is pancreatitis. This is more often associated with cannulation and pressure recording from the PD portion of the SO. The overall incidence of pancreatitis following SO manometry has been reported to range from 5 to 19% (mean 7.3%).[34,35,53] Procedure-induced pancreatitis may be severe, and reported complications include pancreatic phlegmon, pseudocyst formation, or protracted hospitalization with associated complications. Sphincter of Oddi manometry is not indicated in patients with a recent episode of acute pancreatitis (2–3 weeks) or pseudocyst formation. Although the incidence of postmanometry pancreatitis has been reported to be increased in patients with "chronic pancreatitis," this has not been our experience when performing SO manometry.

Preventive measures to avoid post-SO manometry pancreatitis include limiting the time of pancreatic manometry (<3 minutes) or avoiding pancreatic manometry altogether when the clinical problem points to the biliary tract and decreasing the perfusion rate to 0.05 to 0.1 mL/lumen/min while recording within the pancreatic segment of the SO or possibly using the microtransducer recording technique. However, no specific studies have been done to compare the post-SO manometric pancreatitis rate between the microtransducer and the perfused manometric system to ascertain the safety of one technique over the other.[54] Finally, an aspiration manometry catheter has been developed by modifying the triple-lumen SO catheter (such catheters are commercially available from the previously mentioned vendors).[55] The catheter permits standard perfusion through two lumens but aspiration from the third lumen from both end and side ports. In a comparison of the aspirating manometry catheter system versus the conventional triple-lumen catheter recorder, 76 patients were prospectively randomized and evaluated for postmanometry pancreatitis.[56] Patients studied by the aspiration technique had a 3% incidence of pancreatitis; patients evaluated by the standard triple-lumen perfusion technique had a 23% incidence of pancreatitis following the study. Perfusion manometry of the PD exclusively was associated with a pancreatitis rate of 31% in this study. (The frequency of mild pancreatitis following SO manometry at our institution has been less than 10% overall.) Because of the potential serious complications of SO manometry, it is highly recommended that patients routinely be informed of these risks and their potential significance prior to this diagnostic study.

### Correlation with Other Techniques

Fatty meal sonography (FMS) has been advocated as a noninvasive diagnostic method of evaluating SO dysfunction. Fatty meal sonography, in theory, is a biliary "stress test" that is proposed to distinguish the nonobstructed from the obstructed CBD. Fatty meal ingestion (Lipomul, 3.3 mL/kg) stimulates the duodenal release of CCK. Subsequently, CCK causes increased hepatic bile flow, contraction of the gallbladder (when present), and relaxation of the SO mechanism. Sonographic measurement of the CBD diameter is made before ingestion of the fatty meal and again at 45 minutes following the meal. A normal FMS response is generally accepted as no change or a decrease in the diameter of the CBD. A positive test response has been defined as a ≥2-mm increase in CBD diameter at 45 minutes following the fatty meal. Using these criteria, a test sensitivity of 74% and specificity of 100% have been reported for detecting partial CBD obstruction arising from a number of causes (eg, stones, strictures, or dyskinesia).[57] When the results of FMS were compared to the results of SO manometry study in a group of biliary type III patients, however, correlation was poor.[58] Five of 32 patients demonstrated abnormal SO motor function; FMS test results were abnormal in only 1 patient in this group.

Quantitative hepatobiliary scintigraphy (QHBS) has also been used to evaluate SO dysfunction.[59] The test consists of the intravenous administration of 5 mCi of diisopropyl-phenyl-carbamoyl-aminoacetic acid and determination of radioactive counts of isotope distribution over the liver and biliary tract. A variety of quantitative criteria (computer-generated time-activity curves for the hepatobiliary system and duodenum) have been used in hepatobiliary scintigraphy to diagnose partial CBD obstruction. Hepatic clearance (the percentage of radiolabeled isotopic activity excreted at 45–60 minutes) was the more reliable indicator in one study. A sensitivity of 67% and a specificity of 85% for the QHBS were reported in patients with partial CBD obstruction. A reduced hepatic isotope clearance (<63%) at 45 minutes was the most sensitive indicator of a positive examination in another report.[60] Quantification of bile transit time from hepatic hilum to the duodenum demonstrated a satisfactory reproducibility and diagnostic sensitivity in detecting delayed bile flow from the CBD to the duodenum in another report.[61] Prolongation of hepatic hilum-duodenal isotopic transit time is strongly suggestive of SO dysfunction in patients with nondilated CBD. Unfortunately, the test does not discriminate possible SO obstruction/dysfunction in patients with a dilated CBD or a functioning gallbladder. The latter acts as a bile reservoir, thus affecting transit of bile from liver to duodenum. The effect of hepatic parenchymal disease on the hepatic hilum to duodenal transit time (because of interference with hepatic uptake) has not been evaluated.

The diagnostic efficacy of QHBS was recently compared with SO manometry in patients with suspected biliary types II and III SO dysfunction.[62] Twenty postcholecystectomy patients with suspected types II and III SO dysfunction and 20 asymptomatic postcholecystectomy control patients were evaluated by both diagnostic modalities. Cholecystokinin was administered during scintigraphy. Sphincter of Oddi manometry was performed in 15 symptomatic patients (5 type II, 10 type III). Nine of the 15 patients had elevated basal SO pressure. The QHBS parameters were significantly increased in the 9 patients compared to asymptomatic patients. In the 6 patients with normal SO pressure, QHBS results were also within normal limits. The hilum duodenal transit time was the most sensitive scintigraphic parameter (89%) to identify SO dysfunction, whereas the combined sensitivity of peak tracer activity and half-time of tracer excretion in the CBD reached 100%.

Further application of the QHBS test in similar clinical studies with appropriate patient stratification is necessary before this test is recommended as the screening procedure of choice to diagnose SO dysfunction.

### REFERENCES

1. Brugge WR. Motor function of the gallbladder: measurement and clinical significance. Semin Roentgenol 1991;26:226–31.
2. Toouli J. Biliary motility. Curr Opin Gastroenterol 1991;7:758–64.
3. Spellman SJ, Shaffer EA, Rosenthal L. Gallbladder emptying in response to cholecystokinin: a cholescintigraphy study. Gastroenterology 1979;77:115–20.
4. Hopman WPM, Jansen JBMJ, Rosenbusch G. Gallbladder contraction induced by cholecystokinin: bolus injection or infusion? BMJ 1986;292:375–6.
5. Masclee AA, Hopman W, Corstens F, et al. Simultaneous measurement of gallbladder emptying with cholescintigraphy and US during infusion of physiologic doses of cholecystokinin: a comparison. Radiology 1989;173:407–10.
6. Pauletzki J, Cicala M, Spengler U, et al. Gallbladder emptying during high dose cholecystokinin infusions. Effects in patients with gallstone disease and healthy controls. Scand J Gastroenterol 1995;30:128–32.
7. Toftdahl DB, Hojgaard L, Winkler K. Dynamic cholescintigraphy inductions and description of gallbladder emptying. J Nucl Med 1996;37:261–6.
8. Dodds WJ, Groh WJ, Danweesh RM, et al. Sonographic measurement of gallbladder volume. Am J Radiol 1985;145:1009–11.
9. Buchpiquel CA, Sapienza MT, Vezzozzo DP, et al. Gallbladder emptying in normal volunteers. Comparative study between cholescintigraphy and ultrasonography. Clin Nucl Med 1996;21:208–12.
10. Siegel A, Kuhn JC, Crow H, Holtzman. Gallbladder ejection fraction; correlation of 3 scintigraphic and ultrasonographic techniques. Clin Nucl Med 2000;25:1–6.
11. Wedmann B, Schmidt G, Wegener M, et al. Sonographic evaluation of gallbladder kinetics: in vitro and in vivo comparison of different methods to assess gallbladder emptying. J Clin Ultrasound 1991;19:341–9.
12. Krishnamurthy GT, Bobba VR, Kingston E. Radionuclide ejection fraction: a technique for quantitative analysis of motor function of the human gallbladder. Gastroenterology 1981;80:482–90.
13. Patankar R, Ozmen MM, Aldous A, et al. Standardization of a technique for BRIDA cholescintigraphy. Nucl Med Commun 1996;17:724–8.
14. Yap L, Wycherley AG, Morphett AD, Toouli J. Acalculus biliary pain: cholecystectomy alleviates symptoms in patients with abnormal cholescintigraphy. Gastroenterology 1991;101:786–93.
15. Yost F, Margenthaler J, Presti M, et al. Cholecystectomy is an effective treatment for biliary dyskinesia. Am J Surg 1999;178:462–5.

16. Skipper K, Slyh S, Dunn E, Schwartz A. Laparoscopic cholecystectomy for an abnormal hepato-iminodiacetic acid scan; a worthwhile procedure. Am Surg 2000;66:30–2.

17. Canfield AJ, Hetz SP, Schriver JP, et al. Biliary dyskinesia: a study of more than 200 patients and review of the literature. J Gastrointest Surg 1998;5:443–8.

18. Adams DB, Tarnasky PR, Hawes RH, et al. Outcome after laparoscopic cholecystectomy for chronic acalculous cholecystitis. Am Surg 1998; 64(1):1–5.

19. Lugo-Vicente HL. Gallbladder dyskinesia in children. J Soc Laparoendosc Surg 1997;1(1):61–4.

20. Gani JS. Can sincolide cholescintigraphy fulfil the role of gallbladder stress test for patients with gallbladder stones? Aust N Z J Surg 1998; 68:514–9.

21. Westlake PJ, Hershfield NB, Kelly JK, et al. Chronic right upper quadrant pain without gallstones: does HIDA scan predict outcome after cholecystectomy? Am J Gastroenterol 1990;85:986–9.

22. Ziessman HA. Cholecystokinin cholescintigraphy: victim of its own success? J Nucl Med 1999;40:2038–42.

23. Geenen JE, Hogan WJ, Dodds WJ, et al. Intraluminal pressure recording from the human sphincter of Oddi. Gastroenterology 1980;78:317–24.

24. Raddawi H, Geenen JE, Hogan WJ, et al. Pressure measurements from biliary and pancreatic segments of sphincter of Oddi: comparison between patients with functional abdominal pain, biliary or pancreatic disease. Dig Dis Sci 1991;36:71–4.

25. Toouli J, Geenen JE, Hogan WJ, et al. Sphincter-of-Oddi motor activity: a comparison between patients with common bile duct stones and controls. Gastroenterology 1982;82:111–7.

26. Toouli J, Roberts-Thomson IC, Dent J, Lee J. Manometric disorders in patients with suspected sphincter-of-Oddi dysfunction. Gastroenterology 1985;88:1243–50.

27. Guelrud M, Mendoza S, Rossiter G, et al. Sphincter of Oddi manometry in healthy volunteers. Dig Dis Sci 1992;35:38–42.

28. Hogan WJ. Sphincter-of-Oddi: physiology and pathophysiology. Regul Pept Lett 1991;III(2):23–8.

29. Toouli J, Roberts-Thomson IC, Kellow J, et al. Manometry based randomized trial of endoscopic sphincterotomy for sphincter of Oddi dysfunction. Gut 2000;46:98–102.

30. Sherman S, Troiano FP, Hawes RH, Lehman GA. Sphincter of Oddi manometry: decreased risk of clinical pancreatitis with the use of a modified aspirating catheter. Gastrointest Endosc 1990;36:462–6.

31. Tanaka M, Ikeda S, Nakayama F. Non-operative measurement of pancreatic and common bile duct pressure with a microtransducer catheter and effects of duodenoscopic sphincterotomy. Dig Dis Sci 1981;26: 545–52.

32. Sherman S, Gottlieb K, Uzer MF, et al. Effect of meperidine on the pancreatic and biliary sphincter. Gastrointest Endosc 1996;44:239–42.

33. Blaut U, Sherman S, Fogel E, Lehman GA. Influence of cholangiography on biliary sphincter of Oddi manometric parameters. Gastrointest Endosc 2000;52:624–9.

34. Corazziari E, Biliotti D, International Congress for Sphincter of Oddi Study. Sphincter of Oddi manometry. Gastroenterol Int 1989;2:180–4.

35. Corazziari E, Torsoli A. Manometry of the sphincter of Oddi: methodology and standardization. Z Gastroenterol Vehr Bd 1988;23: 214–67.

36. Funch-Jensen P. Pre-operative sphincter of Oddi manometry. Ital J Gastroenterol 1985;17:347–9.

37. Damian E, Fogel EL, Rusche M, et al. Frequency of abnormal pancreatic and biliary sphincter manometry compared with clinical suspicion of sphincter of Oddi dysfunction. Gastrointest Endosc 1999;50:637–41.

38. Funch-Jensen P, Kruse A, Raunsback J. Reproducibility and estimation of minimal recording duration in endoscopic sphincter of Oddi manometry. Ital J Gastroenterol 1986;18:37–8.

39. Corazziari E, Habib FI, Biliotti D, et al. Reading error and time variability of sphincter of Oddi recordings. Gastroentrology 1988;17:343–7.

40. Toouli J, Hogan WJ, Geenen JE, et al. Action of cholecystokinin-octapeptide on sphincter-of-Oddi basal pressure and phasic wave activity in humans. Surgery 1980;92:497–503.

41. Hogan WJ, Geenen JE, Dodds WJ, et al. Paradoxical motor response to cholecystokinin-octapeptide (CCK-OP) in patients with suspected sphincter-of-Oddi dysfunction. Gastroenterology 1982;82:1085.

42. Rolny P, Arleback A, Funch-Jensen P, et al. Paradoxal response of sphincter-of-Oddi to intravenous injection of cholecystokinin or ceruletide. Manometric findings and results of treatment in biliary dyskinesia. Gut 1986;27:1507–11.

43. Torsoli A, Corazziari E, Habib FI, et al. Frequencies and cyclic pattern of the human sphincter-of-Oddi phasic activity. Gut 1986;27:363–9.

44. Hogan WJ, Geenen JE. Biliary dyskinesia. Endoscopy 1988;20: 179–83.

45. Rolny P, Geenen JE, Hogan WJ, et al. Clinical features, manometric findings and endoscopic therapy results in group I patients with sphincter of Oddi dysfunction. Gastrointest Endosc 1991;37:252–3.

46. Geenen JE, Hogan WJ, Dodds WJ, et al. The efficacy of endoscopic sphincterotomy after cholecystectomy in patients with sphincter of Oddi dysfunction. N Engl J Med 1989;320:82–7.

47. Kaikaus RM, Jacob L, Geenen JE, et al. Long-term outcome of endoscopic sphincterotomy in patients with group II sphincter of Oddi dysfunction. Gastroenterology 1995;108:A419.

48. Chen J, Saccone G, Toouli J. Sphincter of Oddi dysfunction and acute pancreatitis. Gut 1998;43:305.

49. Tarnasky P, Cunningham J, Cotton P, et al. Pancreatic sphincter hypertension increases the risk of post-ERCP pancreatitis. Endoscopy 1997;29:252.

50. Tarnasky P, Palesch Y, Cunningham J, et al. Pancreatic stenting prevents pancreatitis after biliary sphincterotomy in patients with sphincter of Oddi dysfunction. Gastroenterology 1998;115:1518.

51. Eversman D, Fagel EL, Rusche M, et al. Frequency of abnormal pancreatic and biliary sphincter of Oddi dysfunction. Gastrointest Endosc 1999;50:637–641.

52. Rome II: a multinational consensus document on functional gastrointestinal disorders. Gut 1999;45(1).

53. Rolny P, Anderberg B, Kluse I et al. Pancreatitis after sphincter of Oddi manometry. Gut 1990;31:821–4.

54. Sherman S, Ruffolo TA, Hawes RH, Lehman GA. Complications of endoscopic sphincterotomy: a prospective series with emphasis on the increased risk associated with sphincter of Oddi dysfunction and non dilated bile duct. Gastroenterology 1991;101:1068–75.

55. Sherman S, Troiano FP, Hawes PH, et al. Does continuous aspiration from an end and side port in a sphincter of Oddi manometry catheter alter recorded pressures? Gastrointest Endosc 1990;36:500–3.

56. Sherman S, Troiano FP, Hawes PH, et al. Sphincter of Oddi manometry: decreased risk of clinical pancreatitis with use of a modified aspirating catheter. Gastrointest Endosc 1990;36:462–466.

57. Darweesh RMA, Dodds WJ, Hogan WJ, et al. Fatty-meal sonography for evaluating patients with suspected partial common duct obstruction. AJR Am J Roentgenol 1988;151:63.

58. Dean RS, Geenen JE, Stewart ET, et al. Sphincter of Oddi (SO) manometry and ultrasound (US) fatty meal test in patients with suspected SO dyskinesia: a comparison of test results. Gastro-enterology 1990;100:A314.

59. Darweesh RMA, Dodds WJ, Hogan WJ, et al. Efficacy of quantitative hepatobiliary scintigraphy and fatty-meal sonography for evaluating patients with suspected partial common duct obstruction. Gastroenterology 1988;94:779–86.

60. Shaffer ED, Hershfield NB, Logan K, et al. Cholescintigraphic detection of functional obstruction of the sphincter of Oddi. Gastroenterology 1986;90:728–33.

61. Cicala M, Scopinaro F, Corraziari E, et al. Quantitative cholescintigraphy in the assessment of choledochoduodenal bile flow. Gastroenterology 1991;100:1106–13.

62. Madacsy L, Middelfort H, Matzien P, et al. Quantitative hepatobiliary scintigraphy and endoscopic sphincter of Oddi manometry in patients with suspected sphincter of Oddi dysfunction: assessment of flow-pressure relationship in the biliary tract. Eur J Gastroenterol Hepatol 2000;12:777–86.

# Dysautonomia

*Ramesh K. Khurana*

The motor, transport, secretory, storage, and excretory functions of the gastrointestinal tract depend on the intrinsic and extrinsic autonomic innervation. The enteric nervous system (ENS), an integrated neural network within the walls of the digestive tract, comprises intrinsic innervation. The ENS is semiautonomous; it can carry out its motor function after complete extrinsic denervation. Extrinsic innervation consists of the parasympathetic vagal and sacral nerves (S2–S4) and thoracolumbar sympathetic nerves (T5–L3). The parasympathetic and sympathetic divisions of the autonomic nervous system supply sensory and motor innervation to regulate the function of the digestive tract. In addition, the central nervous system modulates the gastrointestinal function. The interactions among the brain, parasympathetic and sympathetic nerves, and ENS integrate activity in different regions of the gut and coordinate activity between the digestive tract and other organs.[1]

Gastrointestinal motility disorders may be caused by a myopathic (smooth muscle) or a neuropathic (intrinsic or extrinsic innervation) process. Disorders of the smooth muscle include infiltrative amyloidosis, hollow visceral myopathy, and muscular dystrophy. A neuropathic dysmotility may result from the involvement of intrinsic and/or extrinsic autonomic innervation. Achalasia of the cardia, Hirschsprung's disease, Chagas' disease and paraneoplastic enteric neuronopathy result from the involvement of the ENS.[1,2] Autonomic neuropathies constitute disorders of extrinsic innervation. These may affect both the parasympathetic and the sympathetic systems (pandysautonomia) or may selectively involve cholinergic (parasympathetic and sympathetic sudomotor fibers) or adrenergic functions.[3,4] The central nervous system disorders associated with gastrointestinal dysmotility include parkinsonism, Shy-Drager syndrome, brainstem tumors, and spinal cord transection.[1]

Patients with a history of gastrointestinal motility disorders without autonomic symptoms may be clinically observed, whereas those with autonomic symptoms should undergo autonomic assessment. An algorithm outlining a stepwise approach to such patients is presented in Figure 24.1. History taking and physical examination are the twin elements of clinical autonomic evaluation that guide appropriate laboratory tests. The patient should be asked in some detail about the cardinal symptom(s). This should be followed by questions pertaining to the various categories of autonomic symptoms since autonomic dysfunction may present with protean and at times banal manifestations. Dizziness caused by low blood pressure (BP) is the most common complaint, with severity ranging from lightheadedness to syncope. It can be judged from the duration of standing time to the onset of orthostatic symptoms.[5] Vasomotor symptoms provide clues to the under-

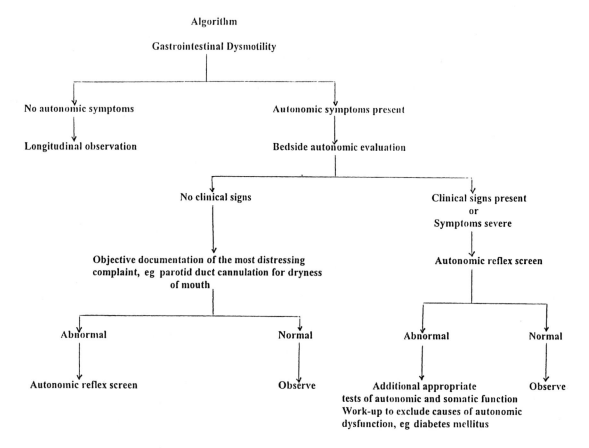

**FIGURE 24.1.** A stepwise approach to autonomic evaluation in patients with gastrointestinal dysmotility.

lying condition. Examples are generalized flushing on exposure to a hot environment in patients with anhidrosis and a purplish lace-like pattern affecting the lower limbs in patients with orthostatic tachycardia.[6] A generalized loss of sweating may present with heat intolerance, but patients with a patchy loss of sweating may instead complain of increased focal sweating caused by compensatory hyperhidrosis. Occurrence of facial sweating during eating but with decreased perspiration elsewhere is not uncommon in patients with diabetic autonomic dysfunction.[7] Salivation, an important secretomotor function, affects taste perception, oral lubrication, and antimicrobial activities. If a patient has to sip liquids to aid in the swallowing of food or to aid in articulation, it indicates a more than 50% decrease in salivary function.[8] Dryness of the mouth can be seen in patients with Shy-Drager syndrome, postganglionic cholinergic dysautonomia, and pandysautonomia.[3,9] The patient should be asked in detail about gastrointestinal symptoms pertaining to the different regions of the gut. Symptoms of urinary bladder involvement may range from a lack of sensation of bladder fullness, hesitancy, and infrequent micturition to urinary retention.[10] Sexual dysfunction is a frequent and early symptom in men with autonomic disorders. Patients may report retrograde ejaculation as voiding of milky urine after intercourse. Male patients may initially experience a partial failure with infrequent and ill-sustained erections and impaired morning erections, eventually evolving into full-

blown impotence. Sleep disturbances are more common than realized. Excessive snoring at night in patients with Shy-Drager syndrome may indicate vocal cord paralysis. Hypersomnolence may be a feature of hypothalamic involvement. Additionally, history taking is incomplete without the review of medication use, especially psychotropic drugs, antihypertensives, and calcium channel blockers.[10,11]

A full somatic neurologic examination is essential since autonomic dysfunction is usually associated with involvement of the central or peripheral nervous systems.[10] Patients with autonomic symptoms should undergo bedside autonomic evaluation. Some autonomic signs such as facial flushing, regional hyperhidrosis, and Horner's syndrome can be observed even during the interview with the patient. Other signs such as sexual immaturity and type of obesity require careful observations.[12] Blood pressure (BP) and heart rate (HR) should be checked with the patient recumbent; patients with orthostatic hypotension may demonstrate supine hypertension, and those with vagal neuropathy may present with resting tachycardia.[13] Loss of sweating may cause dry skin. Involvement of the mucosal membranes should be assessed by examining the conjunctiva for redness, the cornea for ulceration, and the oral cavity for dryness. Vasomotor changes affecting the face and limbs should be noted. Gastrointestinal function assessment should include examination for stomach fullness, succussion splash, bowel sounds, and rectal tone. A distended urinary bladder is readily palpable as a suprapubic swelling and is dull to percussion. Of the various autonomic reflexes, the light reflex is easily evaluated. For proper evaluation, use a bright penlight and ask the patient to look afar to avoid the influence of the near reflex. Miosis may indicate Horner's syndrome. If a large pupil does not react to direct light, the response of the pupil to a sustained stimulus for at least 1 minute should be employed to demonstrate a tonic pupil.[14] To assess the baroreceptor reflex, the BP and HR should be checked in the supine position and then periodically for 3 to 10 minutes in the standing position. A normal subject should demonstrate the following changes: systolic blood pressure (SBP), $-6.5 \pm 0.5$ mm Hg; diastolic blood pressure (DBP), $+5.6 \pm 0.4$ mm Hg; and HR, $+12.3 \pm 0.5$ beats per minute (bpm). A fall in BP of 20/10 mm Hg with symptoms indicates orthostatic hypotension, and tachycardia > 28 bpm above baseline value along with orthostatic intolerance indicates orthostatic tachycardia.[15]

Evaluation of the patient may reveal a history of autonomic symptoms without any obvious clinical signs suggestive of either psychosomatic complaints or subclinical dysfunction. The laboratory approach to such patients should seek objective evidence of the single, most distressing complaint before using a standard battery of simple and noninvasive tests (see Fig. 24.1). Patients with advanced symptoms and prominent clinical signs (eg, orthostatic hypotension) require a detailed evaluation. Autonomic assessment is aimed at the following aspects: (a) to detect and verify suspected autonomic impairment; (b) to determine the involvement of various organs; (c) to assess the severity of autonomic dysfunction; (d) to apportion sympathetic and parasympathetic or adrenergic and cholinergic involvement of a particular organ or several organs; (e) to localize the site of a lesion in the peripheral autonomic nervous system (ie, preganglionic versus postganglionic); (f) to evaluate response to therapy; and (g) to monitor the longitudinal course of the illness.[16]

Anatomic inaccessibility precludes direct physiologic testing of the autonomic nervous system. The investigations of the autonomic nervous system are therefore based on the following principles: (a) abnormalities of reflex responses to physiologic and pharmacologic stimuli; (b) altered pharmacologic responses of the denervated target tissues; (c) immunohistochemical changes in the tissues following denervation; (d) measurement of levels of the neurotransmitters in the plasma, cerebrospinal fluid, and urine; and (e) quantification of autonomic receptor affinity and density. Tissue immunohistochemistry and receptor studies require specialized research laboratories, but most of the other investigations can be carried out in clinical autonomic laboratories. A large number of tests are available for the evaluation of various organs, and several tests are sometimes available to assess a single organ system. The selection of the tests for a particular patient should be based on a differential diagnosis list, the repertoire of tests available, and the therapeutic questions raised. How many tests are essential for a particular patient remains debatable. Because of the confounding variables

(training laboratory personnel, variations in protocol, laboratory conditions, etc) and because of the possibility of patchy involvement of the autonomic nervous system, a single function should not be ascribed to a single test. Furthermore, most of the autonomic tests are continuous (ie, a range with a predetermined cutoff for abnormality) and not dichotomous (ie, positive or negative). Therefore, the clinical importance of one abnormal test remains uncertain. Hence, a battery of tests is recommended.[17,18] In 1996, a consensus report by the Therapeutics and Technology Subcommittee of the American Academy of Neurology recommended the following tests[19]:

*Tests of Cardiovagal Function*
1. Heart rate response to deep breathing ($HR_{DB}$)
2. Valsalva's ratio (VR)
3. Heart rate response to standing

*Tests of Adrenergic Function*
1. Beat-to-beat BP recording of the Valsalva's maneuver (VM)
2. Blood pressure and heart rate response to standing/tilt table test (TTT)

*Tests of Sudomotor Function*
1. Thermoregulatory sweat test (TST)
2. Quantitative sudomotor axon reflex test
3. Sympathetic skin response
4. Sweat imprint method

In this chapter, four commonly performed tests used to document autonomic function (autonomic reflex screen) will be discussed in detail. These are $HR_{DB}$, VM, TTT, and TST. These tests have been accepted by the medical community at large and assigned current procedural terminology codes. Moreover, the equipment for these tests can be either easily assembled or is easily available at affordable prices.

Patient preparation is essential to produce consistent results. A thorough review of medications taken by the patient should be conducted several days in advance of the laboratory studies, and the patient should be instructed to avoid anticholinergics, diuretics, sympathomimetics, $\alpha$-adrenergic antagonists, $\beta$-adrenergic antagonists, alcohol, and fludrocortisone for 48 to 72 hours. Some patients may require tapering of drugs before discontinuation. The patient should not consume nicotine or caffeine for 3 to 4 hours. If the patient is in moderate to severe pain or a diabetic individual has had symptoms of hypoglycemia within the previous 12 hours, testing should be withheld. These tests are usually performed 3 to 4 hours after a light breakfast, after emptying the urinary bladder, in a quiet room with subdued lighting, and at an ambient temperature of 22 to 24°C.[20] The subject is familiarized with the equipment and reminded to report any symptoms during the test. The tests for cardiovascular autonomic function should be performed in the following sequence with a minimum 2-minute rest between them: $HR_{DB}$, VM, and TTT. The TTT is performed at the end to avoid the influence of redistribution of blood volume. We prefer to perform the TST on a separate day.

## HEART RATE RESPONSE TO DEEP BREATHING

Heart rate response to deep breathing is a cyclical shortening and lengthening of heart periods corresponding to the inspiratory and expiratory phases of the respiratory cycle. Introduced by Wheeler and Watkins in 1973, this is an established, simple, sensitive, noninvasive, and reproducible test of cardiovagal function.[21]

### Scientific Basis

The afferent impulses carried by the vagus nerve originate chiefly from the pulmonary stretch receptors.[22] A central gating mechanism located in the medulla oblongata in association with both the nucleus tractus solitarius and the nucleus ambiguus interacts with afferent impulses to generate this response.[23] The efferent pathway is vagal in origin since administration of an atropine bolus at a dose of 0.02 mg/kg body weight abolishes this response.[24]

### Technique

The HR is monitored with a standard electrocardiograph or a cardiac monitor. The subject practices respiratory maneuvers for 30 seconds and then rests supine for a period of 5 minutes. For the test, the subject breathes evenly at a rate of six breaths per minute, 5 seconds in and 5 seconds out, with the help of a metronome or verbal instructions for eight respiratory cycles.[25] The rate and depth of breathing are carefully monitored since the maximum change of heart rate has been demonstrated at breathing frequencies between 5.5 and 7.0 per minute and at a maximum voluntary depth.[26]

### Analysis

Aberrant beats or other artifacts are excluded, and six consecutive respiratory cycles are selected. Of the several time domain measures available, the following two are easily measurable indices of HR variability (Fig. 24.2):

1. Maximum – minimum heart rate: The maximum minus minimum HR during each 10-second breathing cycle is determined. The difference constitutes the HR response variability (see Fig. 24.2). The mean of the differences during six consecutive breathing cycles provides the HRDB in bpm, which in our laboratory is 25.63 ± 2.3 SE (age 23–49 years).[24] The HR response to deep breathing declines with age; therefore, using a simple cutoff point without considering the age effect might produce false-negative results. Masaoka and colleagues studied 143 subjects (age range 20 to 80 years) and published the following normative data: 20 to 29 years, 29.7 ± 5.8 SD; 30 to 39 years, 25.5 ± 8.8 SD; 40 to 49 years, 18.5 ± 7.0 SD; 50 to 59 years, 16.1 ± 5.8 SD; and 60+ years, 11.8 ± 5.4 SD.[27]

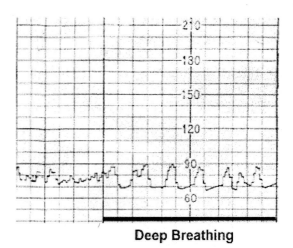

**Deep Breathing**

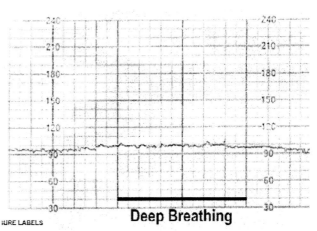

**Deep Breathing**

**FIGURE 24.2.** Heart rate variation on deep breathing at five to seven breaths per minute in a normal subject (*top panel*) and in a patient with Shy-Drager syndrome (*lower panel*). Analysis by maximum – minimum heart rate method.

2. Expiration-to-inspiration ratio (E:I ratio)

E:I ratio =

$$\frac{\text{mean value for longest R-R interval(s) during each expiration}}{\text{mean value for shortest R-R interval(s) during each inspiration}}$$

Normal subjects show an E:I ratio of 1.33 ± 0.04, with a proposed lower limit of 1.1.[28]

## VALSALVA'S MANEUVER

This maneuver, presumably introduced by Antonio Maria Valsalva to inflate the middle ear almost 300 years ago, has only recently become popular for evaluating human autonomic function.[29] It is a safe, reproducible, and quantitative test.

### Scientific Basis

Valsalva's maneuver evaluates the change in cardiovascular response to an acute and transient rise in intrathoracic pres-

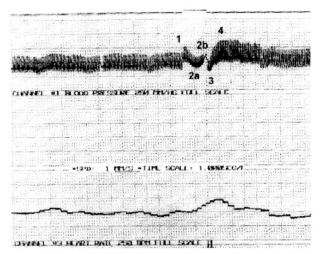

**FIGURE 24.3.** Beat-to-beat blood pressure and heart rate changes during the Valsalva's maneuver in a normal subject showing four phases of the response.

sure. Hamilton and colleagues divided the normal cardiovascular response to VM (50 mm Hg expiratory strain for 10 seconds) into four sequential phases (Fig. 24.3)[30]:

- *Phase 1.* At the onset of forced expiration, there is a sudden initial rise in SBP and DBP, with a variable 1 to 2 beats decrease in heart rate.
- *Phase 2.* This phase follows phase 1 during continued expiratory strain and is subdivided into early and late components. During the early component, there is a decrease in SBP, DBP, mean blood pressure (MBP), and the pulse pressure (PP). It is accompanied by acceleration of the HR. During the later component, there is a quick leveling of BP to a steady state followed by a partial recovery. It is associated with tachycardia.
- *Phase 3.* A brief, abrupt decline in BP to resting or below resting levels occurs immediately after termination of expiratory strain, followed by an additional small increase in heart rate.
- *Phase 4.* A marked increase in SBP, DBP, and PP occurs that exceeds the resting levels. It is associated with bradycardia.

The cardiovascular responses during phases 1 and 3 are primarily determined by the mechanical effects of forced expiration, whereas responses to phases 2 and 4 are associated with a baroreflex control. An acute rise in intrathoracic pressure during phase 1 blocks the venous inflow and compresses the aorta, thereby forcing the blood into the periphery. Conversely, during phase 3, an acute decline in the level of intrathoracic pressure suddenly relieves compression from the aorta, allowing reperfusion of the pulmonary vascular circuit.[31] Phases 2 and 4 are dependent on a complex interaction between arterial baroreceptors, chemoreceptors, cardiopulmonary receptors, and both end-organs—heart and vasculature. Hypotension as a result of impaired venous return during phase 2 stimulates the sympathetic nervous system via the barosensory input.[32] Tachycardia during this phase is

mediated by cardiovagal inhibition with a late contribution from sympathetic cardioacceleratory output.

Phase 4 is characterized by resumption of normal cardiac output into an intensely constricted peripheral arteriolar bed giving rise to systolic overshoot within 4 seconds of release of strain.[30] As aortic pressure rises, baroreceptors are stimulated, producing a reflex bradycardia.

### Technique

The equipment for VM is a disposable mouthpiece attached by a connecting tubing to a mercury or aneroid manometer. A needle placed in the tubing permits a small fixed leak during the expiratory strain, thus forcing the subject to maintain an open glottis, and ensures persistent elevation of intrathoracic pressure. A heart rate monitor or an electrocardiograph is used to record the beat-to-beat change in HR. The BP was previously recorded either intermittently by a sphygmomanometer or continuously with an indwelling arterial catheter. Recently, equipment capable of recording BP noninvasively and continuously has become available. Examples are Finapres (Ohmeda 2300, Denver, CO) and Pilot (Colin Medical Instruments Corp., San Antonio, TX).

The semirecumbent subject is instructed to expire forcefully at the end of a normal inspiration against the column of a manometer to 40 mm Hg for 10 or 15 seconds. He/she is then asked to begin the expiratory strain abruptly, maintain expiratory strain as steadily as possible, terminate it quickly, and breathe quietly after release of the strain. The subject practices the maneuver as explained until a reproducible hemodynamic response is obtained. After a rest period of 5 minutes, the subject performs the VM three times at 2-minute intervals. The HR and BP are recorded before, during, and at least 2 minutes after the VM.[33,34]

### Analysis

Valsalva's maneuver provides a measure of three autonomic functions: cardiovagal, cardiovascular sympathetic, and baroreceptor sensitivity.

The VR has been employed as an index of vagal activity. It is calculated by the longest beat-to-beat R-R interval immediately after the strain divided by the shortest R-R interval during the strain or maximal tachycardia during the strain divided by maximal bradycardia after the strain (see Fig. 24.3).[35] The VR is recorded three times to document consistency. Some investigators use a mean of three responses, whereas others recommend using the highest of three responses to reduce the effect of performance error.[36,37] The mean VR in our laboratory (40 mm Hg expiratory strain for 10 seconds) is $1.8 \pm 0.3$ SD.[34] The VR is reduced in patients with afferent (tabes dorsalis), medullary, or efferent lesions. The VR is a simple and quantifiable test that correlates well with HR responses to other vagotonic (simulated diving response) and vagolytic stimuli (atropine blockade). Recent data suggest that the VR is not as selective a test of cardiovagal function as previously believed. In addition, there is an age-related linear decrease in VR. Low and colleagues reported a decline in VR of .01 per year and suggested the following formula:

$$y = 2.27 - 0.01x$$

where y = VR and x = age in years.[38]

The normal pattern consists of a rise in BP (phase 1), a fall in BP (phases 2 and 3), and another rise in BP (phase 4). There are two broad groups of abnormal responses recognized: the blocked response and the partially blocked response. The blocked response is characterized by a continuous fall of BP throughout phase 2 without any evidence of leveling off and a gradual recovery of BP to baseline level over a period of about 30 seconds (Fig. 24.4). In brief, both late phase 2 and phase 4 are absent. This response is seen in cases of severe autonomic failure resulting from afferent (tabes dorsalis), central (cervical spinal cord transection), or efferent (diabetic polyneuritis or pure dopamine β-hydroxylase deficiency) lesions.[39–41]

The term "partially blocked" response is applied to the BP changes seen in patients with mild to moderate adrenergic impairment. This response is infrequently noted. It is characterized by reduced or absent late phase 2 and reduced phase 4.[36]

Baroreflex sensitivity is determined by correlating a rise or fall in BP with the consequent beat-to-beat R-R interval change. It can be studied during phase 4, starting with the lowest SBP just after the release of strain to the highest SBP attained several beats later. The change in SBP is plotted against the corresponding R-R interval and a regression analysis is performed. The slope of the regression line allows quantification of the baroreflex sensitivity; a high slope indicates good sensitivity and a relatively flat slope indicates a weak reflex.[42]

## TILT TABLE TEST

Head-up tilt (HUT) has been used for over 50 years to diagnose orthostatic insufficiency, and the list of its indications has expanded vastly over the past 15 years. It is now an established test to detect propensity toward vasovagal syncope. Other indications include orthostatic intolerance, chronic fatigue, recurrent unexplained falls, recurrent dizziness, and recurrent transient ischemic attacks.[43]

### Scientific Basis

A change from a recumbent to an upright position results in a gravitational shift of 500 to 1,000 mL of venous blood from the central circulation to the dependent capacitance vessels of the abdomen, pelvis, and lower limbs. Despite this redistribution of blood volume, the BP is maintained acutely by the neurohumoral systems and on a relatively long-term basis by the capillary-fluid-shift and the renin-angiotensin systems.[44]

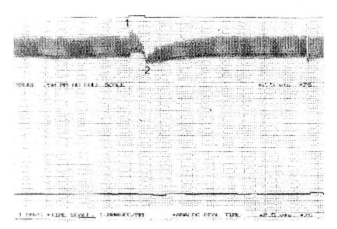

**FIGURE 24.4.** Beat-to-beat blood pressure changes in a patient with pure autonomic failure showing a blocked response (continuing fall of blood pressure during phase 2 followed by a slow recovery). VM, Valsalva's maneuver.

Of the neurohumoral responses, the arterial baroreflex is the key regulatory mechanism for a beat-to-beat control of BP. The baroreceptor reflex arc consists of the arterial (aortic arch and carotid sinus) baroreceptors and cardiopulmonary baroreceptors. In humans, the baroreceptor pathway from the carotid sinus is more important for neural cardiovascular control. The carotid sinus afferents travel via the glossopharyngeal nerve, and the aortic arch afferents travel via the vagus nerve to terminate in the nucleus of the tractus solitarius in the medulla. There is a complex wiring in the brain stem that integrates signals from the hypothalamus and higher cortical centers and from the nucleus of the tractus solitarius and ends in the nucleus ambiguus (vagal, parasympathetic) and rostral ventrolateral medulla (sympathetic), which, in turn, innervate the heart and blood vessels, respectively.[45]

A decrease in BP owing to a centrifugal shift in blood volume diminishes transmural pressure and unloads inhibitory baroreceptor influence, thereby activating the sympathetic outflow and reducing the vagal activity. The increased sympathetic activity leads to vasoconstriction of the resistance and capacitance vessels in the splanchnic, musculocutaneous, and renal vascular beds. The withdrawal of vagal influence and increased sympathetic activity produce reflex acceleration of heart rate. Additional vasoconstriction is achieved through a local sympathetic C-fiber–mediated axon reflex called the venoarteriolar reflex.[46] Hormones that help maintain BP include norepinephrine, vasopressin, endothelin, and angiotensin.[47]

### Technique

The HUT without intravascular instrumentation is preferred. An electrically operated table with a foot support is used. The table can be raised or lowered to a final angle within 10 to 20 seconds. Blood pressure is measured continuously by means of an automated device or intermittently by the cuff auscultation method using a stethoscope and a calibrated sphygmomanometer. Heart rate and rhythm are recorded continuously using a beat-to-beat monitor or a standard electrocardiographic machine.

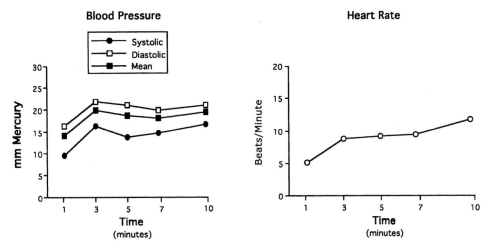

**FIGURE 24.5.** Blood pressure and heart rate responses to the 90-degree head-up tilt in the normal subjects (change from baseline). Reproduced with permission from Khurana RK, Nicholas EM. Head-up tilt table test: how far and how long? Clin Auton Res 1996;6:335–41. ©1996 Lippincott Williams & Wilkins.

The subject is strapped loosely to the tilt table across the knees, thighs, and the chest with noninvasive instrumentation in place. Baseline BP and heart rate measurements are obtained during resting conditions for a period of 5 to 10 minutes. A supine BP measurement just before the tilt is used as a baseline. The subject is tilted up to a specified angle for a predetermined period. The angle and duration of tilt vary considerably between laboratories. We use a 90-degree tilt for a duration of 10 minutes except for patients with suspected neurally mediated syncope, who require a tilt duration of 30 to 45 minutes.[43] Blood pressure and heart rate are measured during the tilt and for 2 minutes after the tilt-back maneuver. The subject reports symptoms as they occur, and the physician observes the clinical signs such as tachypnea, facial pallor, and acral discoloration. The test is terminated early if presyncopal symptoms and appropriate cardiovascular changes appear.[48]

## Analysis

Hemodynamic responses to passive HUT in normal subjects (Fig. 24.5) consist of a slight decrease or a slight rise in SBP, a gradual rise in DBP by about 10%, little change in MBP, and a gradual rise in HR by approximately 10 bpm.[44] For proper analysis, the timing of the BP reading after postural change and orthostatic symptoms should be taken into account. In our laboratory, passive HUT to 90 degrees (n = 19, age range 22–55 years) produced the hemodynamic responses in Table 24.1 at various times after the stimulus onset.

**TABLE 24.1** Hemodynamic Responses Produced by Head-up Tilt

| Time (min) | SBP (mm Hg) | DBP (mm Hg) | MBP (mm Hg) | HR Beats |
|---|---|---|---|---|
| 1 | −2.89 ± 4.63 | 4.44 ± 2.75 | 2.0 ± 3.27 | 12.0 ± 2.39 |
| 5 | 5.68 ± 6.30 | 7.89 ± 4.02 | 7.16 ± 4.66 | 19.53 ± 2.63 |
| 10 | 5.74 ± 7.09 | 10.95 ± 3.33 | 9.21 ± 4.11 | 18.79 ± 2.27 |

SBP, systolic blood pressure; DBP, diastolic blood pressure; MBP, mean blood pressure; HR, heart rate.

At 10 minutes, the SBP change varied from −8 to 20 mm Hg, the DBP increase ranged from 4 to 18 mm Hg, the MBP increase ranged from 1 to 17 mm Hg, and the heart rate accelerated from 14 to 23 bpm.[48]

Based on the orthostatic cardiovascular changes and symptoms, a spectrum of abnormal responses has been recognized (Fig. 24.6).

### Orthostatic Hypotension

According to a consensus statement, orthostatic hypotension is defined as a reduction of SBP > 20 mm Hg and DBP > 10 mm Hg within 3 minutes of 60-degree HUT.[49] A borderline reduction in SBP and DBP with orthostatic symptoms, however, may be significant. Heart rate changes that accompany orthostatic hypotension provide useful information. Occurrence of normal tachycardia suggests intact cardiac innervation, an attenuated heart rate increase favors intact cardiovagal control with sympathetic insufficiency, and a fixed heart rate indicates advanced autonomic failure affecting both sympathetic and cardiovagal fibers. Occurrence of excess tachycardia may also indicate autonomic dysfunction.

Orthostatic hypotension is a sign, with fainting as its most recognized symptom. In our experience, lightheadedness and weakness of the legs are frequent symptoms.[5] Orthostatic hypotension can produce a large variety of symptoms including impaired cognition, blurred vision, fatigue, headache, and neck discomfort (labeled as coat hanger–type pain).[50,51] Common causes of orthostatic hypotension include volume depletion, drugs (α-adrenergic blockers, postganglionic blockers, neuroleptics, antidepressants, vasodilators), endocrine dysfunction, and autonomic insufficiency affecting central or peripheral sympathetic pathways.

### Vasovagal Syncope

The alternative terms used to describe this condition include neurocardiogenic syncope and neurally mediated hypotension. In 1986, Kenny and colleagues discovered that they could reproduce clinical symptoms and hypotension with or

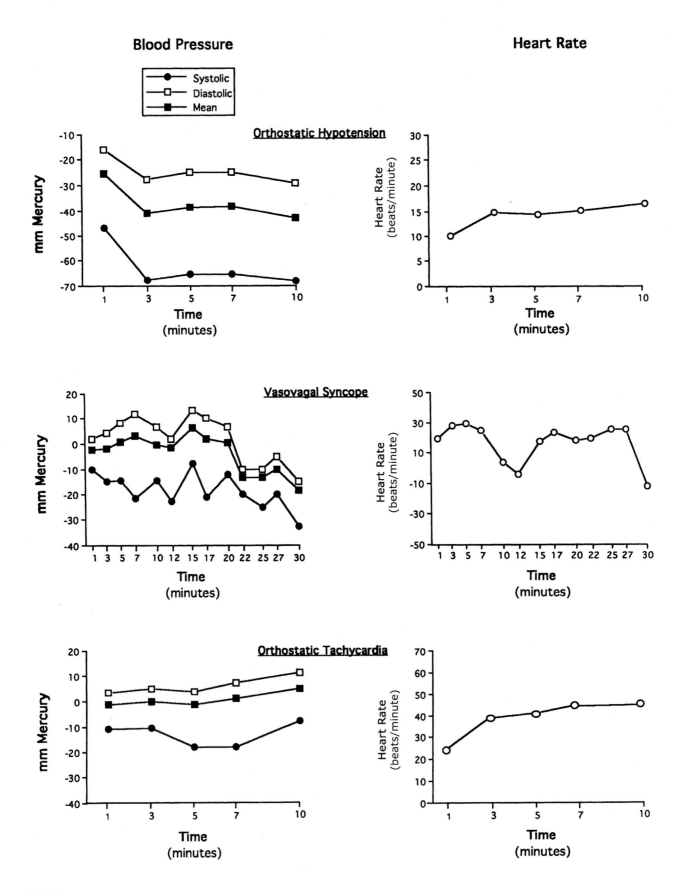

**FIGURE 24.6.** Changes in the blood pressure and heart rate to the 90-degree head-up tilt in the patient groups. Reproduced with permission from Khurana RK, Nicholas EM. Head-up tilt table test: how far and how long? Clin Auton Res 1996;6:335–41.

without bradycardia in 67% of patients with unexplained syncope after a HUT of 29 ± 19 minutes.[52] There may be an initial phase of elevated heart rate and BP or a gradual decline in SBP before the withdrawal of sympathetic influence at the time of syncope and development of bradycardia.[48] The bradycardia and hypotension exhibit different time courses, with hypotension developing earlier and coinciding more closely with symptoms of presyncope or syncope.[53]

### Orthostatic Tachycardia

POTS (postural tachycardia syndrome) is a popular acronym. The syndrome is characterized by the occurrence of orthostatic tachycardia and orthostatic intolerance.[6] The heart rate increase during 10-minute HUT should exceed 2 SD above normal for that laboratory. Novak and colleagues proposed a heart rate increase >30 bpm during HUT or a heart rate value >120 bpm.[54] Orthostatic tachycardia is usually accompanied by a mild decrease in SBP, a rise in DBP, and narrowed PP. In some patients, supine normotension (DBP <90 mm Hg) is converted into orthostatic and sustained hypertension (DBP >90 mm Hg), producing a pattern of orthostatic tachycardia and orthostatic hypertension.[55]

Symptoms of orthostatic intolerance include dizziness, palpitations, nausea, fatigue, clammy skin, anxiety, difficulty breathing, and paresthesiae. The patients may manifest panic-like symptoms and emotional incontinence. Orthostatic discoloration of the limbs is common.[6,54,55]

## THERMOREGULATORY SWEAT TEST

The TST is a qualitative test of high sensitivity and low specificity. It is useful in assessing the integrity of central and peripheral sympathetic sudomotor pathways. It provides an important ability to examine the whole anterior body surface for the pattern and degree of sweat loss.

### Scientific Basis

Sweating, a reflex activity, is mediated by the afferent, central, and efferent pathways. An increase in skin temperature from the periphery and an increase in the core temperature are the two main afferent stimuli for thermal sweating. These impulses travel via A-δ and C fibers from the body surface and via the trigeminal nerve from the face to the contralateral spinothalamic tract, hypothalamus, and cerebral cortex. The central sudomotor control consists of excitatory and inhibitory components. Of the various sweat centers, the anterior hypothalamus is the most powerful excitatory center and the bulbar ventromedial reticular formation is the most powerful inhibitory center. These efferent pathways descend as crossed and uncrossed fibers from the hypothalamus and travel via the tegmentum of the pons and the lateral reticular substance of the medulla to end on the cells of the intermediolateral column. The axons of these cells pass as preganglionic fibers to the neurons in the paravertebral ganglia at the corresponding and several adjacent levels. The postganglionic fibers for the general body surface travel via the gray rami communicantes and the peripheral nerves to the sweat glands.[56] The postganglionic fibers for the face originate from the superior cervical ganglion and travel around the external and internal carotid arteries to join the divisions of trigeminal nerve distal to the gasserian ganglion.[7] The approximate sudomotor "dermatomes" supplying the various regions are T1 to T2, ipsilateral head and neck; T2 to T6, upper limbs; T5 to T12, trunk; and T10 to L3, lower limbs.[56–59]

### Technique

Patients should not wear tight stockings and ace bandages or undergo tests requiring the placement of electrodes on the skin for 24 hours before the TST. Additionally, they should not shave the skin, use deodorant, or apply skin lotion or cosmetics for 1 day before the test.

The subject lies unclothed on a table, and the baseline oral temperature and skin temperature are recorded. To detect subtle sweating, several chemicals that change color when moist can be used. We use an iodine and starch combination. A commercially available iodine is painted over the body and allowed to dry. The cornstarch is sprinkled in a powdering manner over the dried iodine areas. Other investigators spray soluble starch treated with iodine or alizarin red. The patient is exposed to a heated environment in a sweat chamber or heat cradle. In addition, overhead infrared lamps are used to heat the skin. The skin temperature is maintained between 39 and 40°C, air temperature between 45 and 50°C, and relative humidity between 35 and 40%. The test is continued until profuse generalized sweating occurs or a rise in oral temperature by 1°C above baseline or to at least 38°C is observed. The duration of heating required to produce sweating varies from 15 to 45 minutes. The pattern of sweating is recorded manually or photographically, and then the patient is helped to wash off the indicator.[59–61]

### Analysis

Contrary to the traditional presumption of a uniform and generalized response, the topographic distribution of sweating differs in normal subjects. Hertzman observed profuse sweating in the paramedian regions of the trunk and reduced sweating along the medial aspect of thighs in five normal subjects.[62] Fealey tested thermal sweating in 50 control subjects in the supine position (age range 20–75 years). He noted areas of "normal" anhidrosis over bony prominences such as the patellae, clavicles, lateral calves, and inner thighs and relative hypohidrosis over proximal extremities when compared with distal regions. He found left-to-right symmetry and described three patterns of normal sweating[59]:

- *Type 1*—generalized and profuse sweating. This is more common in men.
- *Type 2*—generalized and profuse sweating except for hypohidrosis over proximal limbs. This is more common in women.

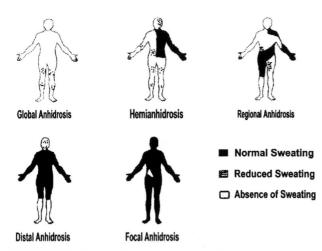

**Global Anhidrosis**     **Hemianhidrosis**     **Regional Anhidrosis**

■ **Normal Sweating**

▨ **Reduced Sweating**

▢ **Absence of Sweating**

**Distal Anhidrosis**     **Focal Anhidrosis**

**FIGURE 24.7.** Diagram of thermoregulatory sweating showing various patterns of anhidrosis in various autonomic disorders. Global anhidrosis, pure autonomic failure; hemianhidrosis, glioma, postsurgery, at the cervicomedullary junction; regional anhidrosis, diabetic dysautonomia and right thoracic sympathectomy; distal anhidrosis, diabetic dysautonomia; focal anhidrosis, postsurgical.

- *Type 3*—generalized and profuse sweating except for hypohidrosis over proximal upper limbs and the lower body.

Sweating may be diminished (hypohidrosis) or absent (anhidrosis) in response to an adequate thermal stimulus. The pattern of anhidrosis may not only suggest the diagnosis of autonomic disorder but may also point toward the level of involvement along the sympathetic sudomotor pathway. Furthermore, the degree of anhidrosis and an excess rise in core body temperature may provide evidence of the severity of the thermoregulatory impairment. There are several recognized patterns of anhidrosis (Fig. 24.7)[59]:

1. *Global anhidrosis.* An area of anhidrosis exceeding 80% of the body surface seen in patients with hypothalamic lesions, multiple system atrophy,[63] or a spinal cord transection above the first thoracic level. Global anhidrosis may also occur in patients with primary autonomic failure or chronic idiopathic anhidrosis.
2. *Hemianhidrosis.* Incomplete hemianhidrosis usually follows unilateral lesions of the brain stem or spinal cord. It is mostly ipsilateral.[64]
3. *Regional anhidrosis.* There are large areas of anhidrosis that are not contiguous. For example, patients with dysautonomia may show anhidrosis of the trunk or anhidrosis of proximal parts of all extremities.
4. *Segmental anhidrosis.* This pattern displays involvement of large areas of anhidrosis that are usually contiguous and asymmetric and have sharply demarcated borders. This is seen in patients with Ross's syndrome or truncal neuropathy.
5. *Distal anhidrosis.* Initially, sweat loss is evident in the distal lower limbs. With progression of neuropathy, the anterior abdominal wall and fingers are affected. This pattern is seen in length-dependent neuropathies. The TST is espe-

cially useful in the diagnosis of small fiber neuropathies for which routine electrophysiologic studies are normal.
6. *Focal anhidrosis.* Loss of sweating is confined to isolated dermatomes, peripheral nerves, or small localized skin areas. Involvement in the distribution of a peripheral nerve is characterized by a central zone of anhidrosis, an intermediate zone of hypohidrosis, and a peripheral zone of perilesional hyperhidrosis.[65] The injury from radiation or surgical incision can produce sharply localized areas of anhidrosis.
7. *Multifocal anhidrosis.* This pattern may be seen in patients with mononeuritis multiplex or leprosy.

The pattern of sweat loss depends on the site of lesion along the sudomotor pathway. A few patterns (eg, global anhidrosis) may occur with involvement of central or peripheral components. On the other hand, some patterns are quite specific for the location of lesion (eg, medial supraorbital anhidrosis in patients with unilateral or bilateral involvement of the cephalic sympathetic pathway).[66] Therefore, recognition of lesion-related patterns may be useful from a clinical perspective.

## OTHER TESTS TO DOCUMENT AND QUANTIFY AUTONOMIC FUNCTION

The $HR_{DB}$, VR, TTT, and TST are simple, noninvasive, and reproducible tests. They constitute a limited representative battery of autonomic functions providing information about quantitative baroreceptor and qualitative sudomotor responses. The tests comprising this battery are deceptively simple but have complex underlying mechanisms. Moreover, the performance and analyses of these tests are easily influenced by the confounding variables. Since the autonomic nervous system innervates every organ, autonomic impairment in patients with generalized disorders may affect several additional organs, whereas focal or multifocal involvement may spare sudomotor or baroreceptor functions. Therefore, autonomic evaluation should be individualized by using several diverse tests, physiologic and pharmacologic, to complement the battery and to quantify the autonomic deficit in terms of severity and organ involvement.[67]

These cardiovagal reflexes ($HR_{DB}$ and VM) have been considered a general representative of the vagal function because of the close concordance between abdominal vagal dysfunction and cardiovagal neuropathy in patients with diabetes mellitus.[68] We found discordance between cardiovagal function tests and gastrointestinal motility in 3 of 10 patients with chronic intestinal pseudo-obstruction unrelated to the duration of illness.[4] The vagus nerve supplies several control systems including aortic arch baroreceptors, respiration, and the gastrointestinal tract. It is likely that the vagal fibers of one system may be affected earlier than others because of selective vulnerability, length-dependent involvement, or scattered pathology. Therefore, tests of vagal function concerned specifically with regional or individual organ function such as pancreatic polypeptide levels may be more appropriate in an individual patient.

In brief, the tests of sympathetic and parasympathetic function that do not involve baroreceptors (eg, isometric hand-grip test, and cold face test), the tests that provide specific information about the affected organs (eg, Schirmer's test for lacrimation, urodynamic studies for bladder dysfunction), and the tests that provide answers to specific questions (eg, isoproterenol test for ß-receptor supersensitivity) should supplement the autonomic reflex screen to make an appropriate diagnosis and develop a reasonable plan of treatment. These tests should be performed in the regional autonomic laboratories where such expertise is available. Presumed pathways and normal responses of various tests of autonomic function are described in Tables 24.2, 24.3, and 24.4.[69–112]

## LOCALIZATION OF THE LESION

Autonomic dysfunction may affect afferent, central, efferent sympathetic, and efferent parasympathetic pathways. The majority of tests of autonomic function neither differentiate the site(s) of dysfunction nor exclude changes in the effector organs. To dissect the pathways involved in autonomic failure, tests of autonomic function based on either changes in BP or HR are employed. Some of these tests are invasive and complex. Usually, several tests with different afferent and efferent pathways are performed, and the integrity of the nontested limb of the reflex is deduced by process of exclusion.

There are no clinically applicable autonomic tests that isolate the function of afferent pathway. Valsalva's maneuver, HUT, and heart rate response to an increase or decrease in BP may reveal abnormality of the baroreceptor reflex arc. A normal response to tests that bypass baroreceptors such as the cold pressor test indicates a preserved sympathetic efferent pathway. Similarly, a normal response to a test without a known afferent pathway (pressor response to the mental arithmetic test or sweating in response to thermal stimulation) provides evidence of an intact efferent pathway. These tests allow the investigator to infer abnormality of the afferent pathway.[113] For the parasympathetic involvement in patients with abnormal baroreflex responses, a normal heart rate rise in response to atropine or bradycardia in response to the cold face test suggests the possibility of an afferent lesion.

Until recently, there were no reliable tests to distinguish between central and peripheral autonomic dysfunction. Measurement of vasopressin levels and response of growth hormone to administration of clonidine may be helpful (Table 24.5). A lack of rise in vasopressin levels in response to baroreflex stimuli (eg, TTT) suggests disconnection between the brain stem and neurohypophysis.[98] Intravenous administration of insulin or the $\alpha 2$ adrenoreceptor agonist clonidine causes an increase in growth hormone levels, and an absence of this response suggests central involvement.[103,104]

Evaluation of sympathetic efferent vasomotor and cardiovascular, sudomotor, and pupillomotor fibers helps in localizing the lesion to the efferent pathway (see Table 24.5).

Orthostatic hypotension results from an alteration in the baroreflex at any level as shown by abnormal responses to the VM or TTT. An absence of BP elevation in response to mental arithmetic stimulus favors efferent involvement. No sweating with body heating but with normal sweating in response to intradermal pilocarpine administration indicates a preganglionic involvement. A subnormal level of supine plasma norepinephrine suggests a postganglionic abnormality. Tyramine, an indirectly acting sympathomimetic amine, requires adequate norepinephrine stores in the nerve endings for its action. A lack of rise in plasma norepinephrine indicates the inability of postganglionic neurons to elaborate norepinephrine—a postganglionic defect. Pupils following denervation fail to respond to cocaine or hydroxyamphetamine but dilate markedly in response to 1% phenylephrine.

Parasympathetic pupillomotor fibers are assessed by constriction in response to dilute pilocarpine, indicating denervation supersensitivity. A subnormal rise in HR in response to a pharmacologic dose of atropine indicates efferent cardiovagal involvement.[114]

It is important to localize the lesion along autonomic pathways for prognostic, diagnostic, and therapeutic purposes. In patients with generalized autonomic dysfunction, involvement of postganglionic sympathetic and parasympathetic neurons, especially in the initial stage of the disorder, favors the diagnosis of pure autonomic failure, which progresses slowly and does not significantly affect the life span of the patient. Patients with preganglionic involvement, however, suffer from multiple system atrophy, a condition that causes rapid deterioration and limited life expectancy.[113] Localization of the lesion allows identification of a disease often associated with a specific type of abnormality. For example, afferent involvement of the baroreceptor reflex pathways narrows the list of differential diagnoses to conditions such as tabes dorsalis and Holmes-Adie syndrome.[114,115] Similarly, documentation of a preganglionic type of Horner's syndrome indicates the need for work-up of neoplasm as a likely cause of the disorder.[91] At the least, in patients with gastrointestinal dysfunction, involvement of sympathetic and parasympathetic functions separates neuropathic dysfunction restricted to bowels from a more widespread and generalized involvement, thus improving the sensitivity and specificity of the diagnosis.

The localization of the lesion and study of the pharmacologic characteristics of the disorder permit the selection of an appropriate therapeutic plan. In patients with orthostatic hypotension, the choice of pressor drugs is affected by the presence of pre- or postganglionic involvement. For a patient with a "flat" or minimal norepinephrine response to edrophonium, it would be inappropriate to recommend a drug that stimulates norepinephrine release. Conversely, in a patient with a normal norepinephrine response to edrophonium, drugs increasing the release of norepinephrine may be combined with those that reduce uptake such as tyramine and monoamine oxidase inhibitors.[116] In patients with a postganglionic lesion, there may be supersensitivity to drugs mimicking neurotransmitters. This may indicate the need for a graduated prescription of a sympathomimetic drug. In patients with cholinergic dysfunction, hypersensitivity to cholinomimetic drugs may be generalized rather than organ specific. Subcutaneous administration of bethanechol in a patient with Shy-Drager syndrome has been shown to produce tearing, copious salivation, and sweating besides improving esophageal, bowel, and bladder function.[63]

In brief, involvement of the smooth muscle, ENS, sympathetic nervous system, or parasympathetic nervous system may cause gastrointestinal dysmotility. Motility studies eval-

uate functions of the smooth muscle and the ENS. Tests of sympathetic and parasympathetic functions, discussed in this chapter, are necessary to study the integrity of extrinsic innervation. Analysis of these tests may allow distinction between myopathic and neuropathic processes that may be generalized or restricted to the gut. Generalized neuropathic disorders can be further dissected into cholinergic versus adrenergic and preganglionic versus postganglionic, thus permitting selection of appropriate management.

**TABLE 24.2** Tests Based on Autonomic Reflexes

| Test | Pathways | Normal Responses and Remarks |
| --- | --- | --- |
| Isometric hand-grip[69,70] | Afferents from activated muscles and central command from motor cortex → rostral ventrolateral medulla → sympathetic efferents | Change in DBP is the most sensitive and specific measurement, 5 min is the most important time measurement<br>DBP for men: ↑ 27.55 ± 1.82 mm Hg (mean ± SE)<br>DBP for women: ↑ 22.39 ± 1.78 mm Hg SE<br>Individuals with a 30% MVC of 7 kg or less had a lower increase in DBP. It is a sensitive, specific, and reproducible test of adrenergic function. |
| Cold pressor[71–73] | Sensory afferents → spinothalamic tracts → suprapontine and infrathalamic relays → sympathetic efferents | Mean SBP ↑ = 16.2 mm Hg<br>Mean DBP ↑ = 13.2 mm Hg<br>DBP more reliable in diagnosing sympathetic dysfunction; not well validated in autonomic disorders |
| Heart rate response to standing (30:15 ratio)[74] | IX and X afferents → brain stem → vagal and sympathetic efferent responses | HR ↑ initially around 15th beat, then relative ↓ HR around 30th beat; normal ratio < 1.04 below age of 59 yr, declines with age; a test of cardiovagal function |
| Cold face[75,76] | Trigeminal afferents → brain stem → vagal efferents | HR ↓ 21.4 ± 16.6 SD, measures vagal activity independent of baroreceptor functions; response is reproducible. |
| Mental arithmetic[77,78] | Cerebrum → sympathetic efferents → end organ | Increase in systolic BP ~ 15 mm Hg |
| Sympathetic skin response[79–81] | Somatic afferents → suprabulbar somatosympathetic interactions → sympathetic efferents → sweat glands | Latencies: palms 1.57 ± 0.05 s<br>soles 2.09 ± 0.04 s<br>Enormously variable; habituates; absent in axonal neuropathies but present in demyelinating disorders; of limited specificity |
| Schirmer's[82–84] | Trigeminal afferents → lacrimal nucleus in the pons → greater superficial petrosal nerve → vidian nerve → sphenopalatine ganglion → lacrimal gland | Normal wetting: > 15 mm in 5 min<br>Bilateral difference significant if lesser value is at least 27% smaller than the larger one |
| Salivation[8,85] | Inferior salivatory nucleus → cranial nerve IX → lesser petrosal nerve → otic ganglion → parotid gland | Unstimulated secretion, 9–12 drops/2 min<br>Stimulated (lemon juice) secretion, 43–49 drops/2 min |
| Gastrointestinal dysmotility | Parasympathetic vagal and sacral neurons stimulate motility and relax the internal rectal sphincter<br>Sympathetic innervation slows motility, contracts esophageal and internal rectal sphincters | See this atlas for normal and abnormal patterns |
| Urinary bladder cystometry[86,87] | Frontal cortex → pontine detrusor nucleus → sacral parasympathetic neurons → detrusor muscle; bladder afferents → pudendal nuclei → detrusor muscle | Initial sensation of filling, low intravesicle pressure during collection of urine, urgency to void when bladder reaches capacity and ability to suppress the detrusor contraction with a decline in intravesicle pressure |

DBP, diastolic blood pressure; MVC, maximum voluntary contraction; SBP, systolic blood pressure; HR, heart rate; BP, blood pressure; →, leads to; ↑, increase; ↓, decrease.

**TABLE 24.3.** Altered Pharmacologic Responses of Denervated Tissues

| Test | Pathways | Normal Responses and Remarks |
|---|---|---|
| **Cardiovascular** | | |
| Norepinephrine infusion[88,89] | Direct action of $\alpha$-adrenoreceptor agonist on end-organ | Normal: BP proportional to the log of plasma norepinephrine level, exaggerated BP response and gain of the dose-response curve measure baroreceptor modulation; a shift to the left of the dose-response curve (decreased threshold) implies denervation supersensitivity |
| Isoproterenol infusion[90] | Direct action of $\beta$2-adrenoreceptor agonist on end-organ | Normal: HR $\uparrow$ at 0.03 ug/kg/min is 10 ± 2 SD<br>Exaggerated increase suggests $\beta$-receptor hyperresponsiveness |
| Atropine bolus[24] | Muscarinic cardiac blockade | HR $\uparrow$ from 72.15 ± 4.7 SE to 112.92 ± 5.39 SE to 0.02 mg/kg/dose —the minimum vagolytic dose; diminished to absent increase in vagal hypoactivity |
| **Pupils** | | |
| Phenylephrine solution[91–93] | Sympathetic end-organ response to $\alpha$1 receptor agonist | Normal: minimal dilation<br>Denervation supersensitivity: marked dilation<br>Mydriasis increases with age in normal subjects<br>Age-related normal range should be used |
| Dilute pilocarpine[94,95] | An end-organ muscarinic agonist | Normal: 0.5- to 1.0-mm constriction<br>Denervation supersensitivity: marked pupillary constriction of dilated or normal-sized pupil<br>Does not differentiate preganglionic from postganglionic lesion |

BP, blood pressure; HR, heart rate; $\uparrow$, increase.

**TABLE 24.4.** Measurement of Neurotransmitters and Neuropeptides in Various Biologic Fluids

| Test | Pathways | Normal Responses and Remarks |
|---|---|---|
| Plasma NE levels[96,97] | Baroreflex mediated increase in sympathetic neuronal activity releases NE from the nerve terminals | Normal: recumbent plasma NE 250–350 pg/mL and a 2- to 3-fold increase on standing; low levels when recumbent and no rise when standing suggests postganglionic autonomic failure, considerable overlap between central and peripheral autonomic failure group |
| Plasma AVP levels[98,99] | $\downarrow$ Blood volume $\rightarrow$ stimulation of atrial stretch receptors $\rightarrow$ vagus nerve nucleus tractus solitarius $\rightarrow$ paraventricular nucleus of hypothalamus $\rightarrow$ posterior hypophysis $\rightarrow$ systemic circulation | Normal: small but significant rise (1.3 ± 0.2 to 3.2 ± 0.3 pmol/L)<br>Postganglionic autonomic failure: marked rise in AVP levels (1.1 ± 0.3 to 38.0 ± 8.0 pmol/L)<br>Central autonomic failure (multiple system atrophy): a small rise in AVP (0.5 ± 0.1 to 1.5 ± 0.3 pmol/L)<br>Failure to increase AVP during hypotension but with normal response to infusion of hypertonic saline suggests involvement of baroreceptor afferents in the vagus nerve or their central connections |
| Urinary NE metabolites[100] | Intraneuronal NE is deaminated<br>Extraneuronal or released NE is predominantly O-methylated to NMN | Provides a measure of secretion over a longer period, NMN reflects the amount of NE released into active form; patients with peripheral autonomic failure show a decrease in all metabolites; patients with multiple system atrophy show a disproportionate reduction in urinary NMN excretion, indicating inability to release NE |
| Pancreatic polypeptide[101,102] | An index of cholinergic efferent vagal activity | Significant increase in levels in normals<br>Minimal or no increase in patients with PAF |

NE, norepinephrine; AVP, arginine vasopressin; NMN, normetanephrine; PAF, pure autonomic failure; $\downarrow$, decrease; $\rightarrow$, leads to.

**TABLE 24.5** Tests Useful in Localizing Autonomic Dysfunction

| Test | Pathway | Normal Responses and Remarks |
|---|---|---|
| **Neuroendocrine**<br>Clonidine infusion[103,104] | An α2-adrenoreceptor agonist stimulates GH-RH neurons in the hypothalamus → anterior pituitary → GH | ↑ GH peaked at 60 min in normals and in patients with peripheral autonomic dysfunction; no increase in patients with MSA, a central disorder; GH ↑ in MSA patients following L-dopa administration indicates intact GH-RH neurons and the anterior pituitary |
| Edrophonium bolus[105,106] | Edrophonium, a short-acting cholinesterase inhibitor, does not cross blood-brain barrier and amplifies endogenous cholinergic activity → stimulates nicotinic receptors within paravertebral ganglia | Normal: NE increase from 153 ± 15 to 234 ± 29 pg/mL at 4 min after injection; MSA patients show a 35–60% increase in NE; PAF patients show none to minimal increase in NE (−6 ± +11%); differentiates central from peripheral autonomic dysfunction |
| **Cardiovascular**<br>Tyramine bolus [88,107] | Tyramine releases NE from both the vesicles and the cytosol within the sympathetic nerve terminal; also inhibits reuptake | Normals: minimal change in MBP until 30 ug/kg/dose; MBP increases proportional to the log of the tyramine dose; SBP increases lower in patients with PAF when compared with MSA; tyramine-induced NE rises above baseline almost same in normal and MSA patients but reduced in patients with PAF; difficult to interpret in patients with early or incomplete lesions |
| **Pupils**<br>Cocaine[108] | Cocaine blocks reuptake of NE in the axonal terminal of the postganglionic neuron; NE acts on the end-organ | Normals: pupil dilation of 1.84 ± 0.8 mm SD<br>Impaired or absent dilation indicates sympathetic denervation; Post cocaine aniscoria of 1.0 mm when compared with normal pupil predicts Horner's syndrome |
| Hydroxyamphetamine[92,109] | Hydroxyamphetamine releases NE from the cytoplasmic pool of the postganglionic nerve terminals; NE acts on the end-organ | Normals: pupillary dilation<br>Normal responses of no value in localization<br>No dilation indicates postganglionic lesion |
| **Sudomotor**<br>Quantitative sudomotor axon reflex[110,111] | Measures axon reflex stimulated postganglionic sweat output | A prolonged latency or diminished sweat output indicates postganglionic sudomotor dysfunction; an increase in the ratio of sweating in the forearm/sweating below the waist can detect early involvement; a sensitive, dynamic, and reproducible test; requires a special apparatus |
| Sweat imprint method[112] | Direct action of pilocarpine, a muscarinic agonist, on fully or partially innervated sweat glands | A decrease in sweat output indicates early or partial involvement; no sweating is elicited from chronically denervated sweat glands; absence of sweating indicates postganglionic lesion |

GH, growth hormone; GH-RH, growth hormone–releasing hormone; MSA, multiple system atrophy; NE, norephinephrine; PAF, pure autonomic failure; MBP, mean blood pressure; →, leads to; ↑, increase.

# REFERENCES

1. Wingate DL. Autonomic function and dysfunction in the gastrointestinal tract. In: Mathias CJ, Bannister R, editors. Autonomic failure. 4th ed. New York: Oxford University Press; 1999. p. 271–82.
2. Khurana RK. Paraneoplastic autonomic dysfunction. In: Low PA, editor. Clinical autonomic disorders. 2nd ed. Philadelphia: Lippincott-Raven; 1997. p. 545–54.
3. Khurana RK. Acute and subacute autonomic neuropathies. In: Bannister R, editor. Autonomic failure. 2nd ed. New York: Oxford University Press; 1988. p. 624–31.
4. Khurana RK, Schuster MM. Autonomic dysfunction in chronic intestinal pseudo-obstruction. Clin Auton Res 1998;8:335–40.
5. Khurana RK. Orthostatic hypotension. NY State J Med 1988;88:570–2.
6. Khurana RK. Orthostatic intolerance and orthostatic tachycardia: A heterogeneous disorder. Clin Auton Res 1995;5:12–18.
7. Watkins PJ. Facial sweating after food: a new sign of diabetic neuropathy. BMJ 1973;1:583–7.
8. Wolff A. Salivary gland disorders associated with autonomic dysfunction. In: Korczyn AD, editor. Handbook of autonomic nervous system dysfunction. New York: Marcel Dekker; 1995. p. 293–309.
9. Khurana RK, Nelson E, Azzarelli B, et al. Shy-Drager syndrome: diagnosis and treatment of cholinergic dysfunction. Neurology 1980;30:805–9.
10. Low PA, Suarez GA, Benarroch EE. Clinical autonomic disorders: classification and clinical evaluation. In: Low PA, editor. Clinical autonomic disorders. 2nd ed. Philadelphia: Lippincott-Raven; 1997. p. 3–15.
11. Chokroverty S. Sleep apnea and autonomic failure. In: Low PA, editor. Clinical autonomic disorders. 2nd ed. Philadelphia: Lippincott-Raven; 1997. p. 633–47.
12. Plum F, Uitert RV. Neuroendocrine diseases and disorders of the hypothalamus. In: Reichlin S, Baldessarini RJ, Martin JB, editors. The hypothalamus. New York: Raven Press; 1978. p. 415–73.
13. Ridley A, Hierons R, Cavanagh JB. Tachycardia and the neuropathy of porphyria. Lancet 1968;2:708–10.
14. Smith SA. Pupil function: tests and disorders. In: Bannister R, Mathias CJ, editors. Autonomic failure. 3rd ed. Oxford: Oxford Medical Publishers; 1992. p. 421–41.
15. Streeten DHP. Orthostatic disorders of the circulation. Mechanisms, manifestations, and treatment. New York: Plenum Medical Book Company; 1987. p. 111–26.
16. Low PA, Polinsky RJ, Kaufmann HC, et al. Autonomic function and dysfunction. Continuum 1998;4:7–40.
17. Weissler AM. A perspective on standardizing the predictive power of noninvasive cardiovascular tests by likelihood ratio computation: mathematical principles. Mayo Clin Proc 1999;74:1061–71.
18. Wieling W. Impaired vagal heart rate control in diabetics: relationship to long-term complications. Neth J Med 1988;30:260–9.
19. Clinical autonomic testing report of the Therapeutics and Technology Assessment Subcommittee of the American Academy of Neurology. Neurology 1996;46:873–80.
20. Low PA, Pfeiffer MA. Standardization of autonomic function. In: Low PA, editor. Clinical autonomic disorders. 2nd ed. Philadelphia: Lippincott-Raven; 1997. p. 287–95.
21. Wheeler T, Watkins PJ. Cardiac denervation in diabetes. BMJ 1973;4:584–6.
22. Anrep GV, Pascual W, Rossler R. Respiratory variations of the heart rate. 1. The reflex mechanisms of the respiratory arrhythmia. Proc Royal Soc 1936;119:191–217.
23. Lopes OU, Palmer JF. Proposed respiratory gating mechanisms for cardiac slowing. Nature 1976;264:454–6.
24. Khurana RK, Jones AD. Assessment of minimum vagolytic dose of atropine. Neurology 1999;52:A343.
25. Harry JD, Freeman R. Determining heart-rate variability comparing methodologies using computer simulation. Muscle Nerve 1993;16:267–77.
26. Hirsch JA, Bishop B. Respiratory sinus arrhythmia in humans: how breathing pattern modulates heart rate. Am J Physiol 1981;241:H260–9.
27. Masaoka S, Lev-Ran A, Hill LR, et al. Heart rate variability in diabetes: relationship to age and duration of the disease. Diabetes Care 1985;8:64–8.
28. Sundkvist G, Almér L-O, Lilja B. Respiratory influence on heart rate in diabetes mellitus. BMJ 1979;1:924–5.
29. Corbett JL. Some aspects of the autonomic nervous system in normal and abnormal man [dissertation]. Oxford (UK): Univ. of Oxford; 1969.
30. Hamilton WF, Woodbury RA, Harper HT Jr. Physiologic relations between intrathoracic, intraspinal, and arterial pressure. JAMA 1936;107:853–6.
31. Eckberg DL. Parasympathetic cardiovascular control in human disease: a critical review of methods and results. Am J Physiol 1980;239:H581–93.
32. Porth CJM, Bamrah VS, Tristani FE, et al. The Valsalva maneuver: mechanisns and clinical implications. Heart Lung 1984;13:507–18.
33. Benarroch EE, Sandroni P, Low PA. The Valsalva maneuver. In: Low PA, editor. Clinical autonomic disorders. Boston: Little Brown & Co.; 1993. p. 209–15.
34. Khurana RK. Valsalva ratio: a noninvasive and quantifiable test of vagal function. Trans Am Neurol Assoc 1981;106:107–9.
35. Levin AB. A simple test of cardiac function based upon heart rate changes induced by the Valsalva maneuver. Am J Cardiol 1966;18:90–9.
36. Sandroni P, Benarroch EE, Low PA. Pharmacological dissection of components of the Valsalva maneuver in adernergic failure. J Appl Physiol 1991;71:1563–7.
37. Baldwa VS, Ewing DJ. Heart rate response to the Valsalva manoeuvre: reproducibility in normals, and relation to variation in resting heart rate in diabetics. Br Heart J 1977;39:641–4.
38. Low PA, Opfer-Gehrking TL, Proper CJ, et al. The effect of aging on cardiac autonomic and postganglionic sudomotor function. Muscle Nerve 1990;13:152–7.
39. Sharpey-Schafer EP, Taylor PJ. Absent circulatory reflexes in diabetic neuritis. Lancet 1960;1:1559–62.
40. Watson WE. Some circulatory responses to Valsalva's manoeuvre in patients with polyneuritis and spinal cord disease. J Neurol Neurosurg Psychiatry 1962;25:19–23.
41. Biaggioni I, Goldstein DS, Atkinson T, et al. Dopamine-ß hydroxylase deficiency in humans. Neurology 1990;40:370–3.
42. Palmero HR, Caeiro TF, Iosa DJ, et al. Baroreceptor reflex sensitivity index derived from phase 4 of the Valsalva manoeuvre. Hypertension 1981;3:134–7.
43. Benditt DG, Ferguson DW, Grubb BP, et al. Tilt table testing for assessing syncope. Am Coll Cardiol 1996;28:263–75.
44. Smit AAJ, Halliwill JR, Low PA, et al. Pathophysiological basis of orthostatic hypotension in autonomic failure. J Physiol 1999;519:1–10.
45. Wieling W, Karemaker JM. Measurement of heart rate and blood pressure to evaluate disturbances in neurocardiovascular control. In: Mathias CJ, Bannister R, editors. Autonomic failure. 4th ed. Oxford (UK): Oxford University Press; 1999. p. 196–210.
46. Henriksen O, Skagen K, Haxholdt O, et al. Contribution of local blood flow regulation mechanisms to the maintenance of arterial pressure in upright position during epidural blockade. Acta Physiol Scand 1983;118:271–80.
47. Ziegler MG, Lake CR, Kopin IJ. The sympathetic nervous system defect in primary orthostatic hypotension. N Engl J Med 1977;296:293–7.
48. Khurana RK, Nicholas EM. Head-up tilt table test: how far and how long? Clin Auton Res 1996;6:335–41.
49. Consensus Committee on the American Consensus statement on the definition of orthostatic hypotension, pure autonomic failure, and multiple system atrophy. Neurology 1996;46:1470.

50. Low PA, Opfer-Gehrking TL, McPhee BR, et al. Prospective evaluation of clinical characteristics of orthostatic hypotension. Mayo Clin Proc 1995;70:617–22.

51. Robertson D, Kincaid DW, Haile V, et al. The head and neck discomfort of autonomic failure: an unrecognized aetiology of headache. Clin Auton Res 1994;4:99–103.

52. Kenny RA, Ingram A, Bayliss J, et al. Head-up tilt: a useful test for investigating unexplained syncope. Lancet 1986;2:1352–4.

53. Khurana RK. Vasovagal syncope. In: Sinha KK, Chandra P, editors. Advances in clinical neurosciences. Ranchi (India): The Catholic Press; 1999. p. 441–69.

54. Novak V, Novak P, Opfer–Gehrking TL, et al. Clinical and laboratory indices that enhance the diagnosis of postural tachycardia syndrome. Mayo Clin Proc 1998;73:1141–50.

55. Khurana RK, Yao MD. Orthostatic intolerance with orthostatic hypertension: clinical and autonomic profile. Neurology 2000;54:A161.

56. Ogawa T, Low PA. Autonomic regulation of temperature and sweating. In: Low PA, editor. Clinical autonomic disorders. 2nd ed. Philadelphia: Lippincott-Raven; 1997. p. 83–96.

57. Wang GH. The neural control of sweating. Madison (WI): University of Wisconsin Press; 1964.

58. List CF, Peet MM. Sweat secretion in man. IV sweat secretion of the face and its disturbances. Arch Neurol Psychiatry 1938;40:443–70.

59. Fealey RD. Thermoregulatory sweat test. In: Low PA, editor. Clinical autonomic disorders. 2nd ed. Philadelphia: Lippincott-Raven; 1997. p. 245–57.

60. Guttman L. The management of the Quinizarin test. Postgrad Med J 1947;23:353–66.

61. Sato KT, Richardson A, Timm DE, et al. One-step iodine starch method for direct visualization of sweating. Am J Med Sci 1988;295:528–31.

62. Hertzman AB. Individual differences in regional sweating. J Appl Physiol 1957;10:242–8.

63. Khurana RK. Cholinergic dysfunction in Shy-Drager syndrome: effect of the parasympathomimetic agent, bethanechol. Clin Auton Res 1994;4:5–13.

64. List CF, Peet MM. Sweat secretion in man. V. Disturbances of sweat secretion with lesions of the pons, medulla and cervical portion of the cord. Arch Neurol Psychiatry 1939;42:1098–127.

65. Guttman L. Topographic studies of disturbances of sweat secretion after complete lesions of peripheral nerves. J Neurol Psychiatry 1940;3:197–210.

66. Khurana RK. Oculocephalic sympathetic dysfunction in post-traumatic headaches. Headache 1995;35:614–20.

67. Low PA. Pitfalls in autonomic testing. In: Low PA, editor. Clinical autonomic disorders. 2nd ed. Philadelphia: Lippincott-Raven; 1997. p. 391–401.

68. Buysschaert M, Donckier J, Dive A, et al. Gastric acid and pancreatic polypeptide responses to sham feeding are impaired in diabetic subjects with autonomic neuropathy. Diabetes 1985;34:1181–5.

69. Khurana RK, Setty A. The value of the isometric hand-grip test—studies in various autonomic disorders. Clin Auton Res 1996;6:211–8.

70. Ewing DJ, Irving JB, Kerr F, et al. Cardiovascular responses to sustained handgrip in normal subjects and in patients with diabetes mellitus: a test of autonomic function. Clin Sci Mol Med 1974;46:295–306.

71. Lovallo W. The cold pressor test and autonomic function: a review and integration. Psychophysiology 1975;12:268–82.

72. Hines EA Jr. Significance of vascular hyperreaction as measured by cold pressor test. Am Heart J 1940;19:408–16.

73. Saymalp S, Sözen T, Özdougan M. Cold pressor test in diabetic autonomic neuropathy. Diabetes Res Clin Pract 1994;26:21–8.

74. Wieling W, Karemaker JM. Measurement of heart rate and blood pressure to evaluate disturbances in neurocardiovascular control. In: Mathias CJ, Bannister R, editors. Autonomic failure. 4th ed. New York: Oxford University Press; 1999. p. 196–210.

75. Khurana RK, Watabiki S, Hebel JR, et al. Cold face test in the assessment of trigeminal-brainstem-vagal function in humans. Ann Neurol 1980;7:144–9.

76. Heath ME, Downey JA. The cold face test (diving reflex) in clinical autonomic assessment: methodological considerations and repeatability of responses. Clin Sci 1990;78:139–47.

77. LeBlanc J, Cote J, Jobin M, et al. Plasma catecholamines and cardiovascular responses to cold and mental activity. J Appl Physiol 1979;47:1207–11.

78. Ludbrook J, Vincent A, Walsh JA. Effects of mental arithmetic on arterial pressure and hand blood flow. Clin Exp Pharmacol Physiol 1975;2 Suppl 2:67–70.

79. Shahani BT, Halperin JJ, Boulu P, et al. Sympathetic skin response—a method of assessing unmyelinated axon function in peripheral neuropathies. J Neurol Neurosurg Psychiatry 1984;47:536–42.

80. Hoeldtke RD, Davis KM, Hshieh PB, et al. Autonomic surface potential analysis: assessment of reproducibiilty and sensitivity. Muscle Nerve 1992;15:926–31.

81. Knezevic W, Bajada S. Peripheral autonomic surface potential. A quantitative technique for recording sympathetic conduction in man. J Neurol Sci 1985;67:239–51.

82. Hanson J, Fikentscher R, Roseburg B. Schirmer test of lacrimation, its clinical importance. Arch Otolaryngol 1975;101:293–5.

83. Miller NR. Anatomy, physiology, and testing of normal lacrimal secretion. In: Miller NR, editor. Walsh and Hoyt's clinical neuro-ophthalmology. 4th ed. Baltimore: Williams & Wilkins; 1985. p. 458–68.

84. Feldman F, Wood MM. Evaluation of the Schirmer tear test. Can J Ophthalmol 1979;14:257–9.

85. White KD. Salivation: a review and experimental investigation of major techniques. Psychophysiology 1977;14:203–12.

86. Bradley WE, Yang CC. Autonomic regulation of urinary bladder. In: Low PA, editor. Clinical autonomic disorders. 2nd ed. Philadelphia: Lippincott-Raven; 1997. p. 117–27.

87. Yang CC, Bradley WE. The diagnosis and treatment of urinary bladder dysfunction. In: Low PA, editor. Clinical autonomic disorders. 2nd ed. Philadelphia: Lippincott-Raven; 1997. p. 613–31.

88. Polinsky RJ, Kopin IJ, Ebert MH, et al. Pharmacologic distinction of different orthostatic hypotension syndromes. Neurology 1981;31:1–7.

89. Bannister R, Davies B, Holly E, et al. Defective cardiovascular reflexes and supersensitivity to sympathomimetic drugs in autonomic failure. Brain 1979;102:163–76.

90. Fouad FM, Tadena-Thome L, Bravo EL, et al. Idiopathic hypovolemia. Ann Intern Med 1986;104:298–303.

91. Miller NR. Disorders of pupillary dysfunction, accommodation, and lacrimation. In: Miller NR, editor. Walsh and Hoyt's clinical neuro-ophthalmology. 4th ed. Baltimore: Williams and Wilkins; 1985:469–556.

92. Thompson HS, Mensher JH. Adrenergic mydriasis in Horner's syndrome. Am J Ophthalmol 1971;72:472–80.

93. Smith SA, Smith SE. Pupil function: tests and disorders. In: Mathias CJ, Bannister R, editors. Autonomic failure. 4th ed. New York: Oxford University Press; 1999. p. 245–53.

94. Cohen DN, Zakov ZN. The diagnosis of Adie's pupil using 0.0625% pilocarpine solution. Am J Ophthalmol 1975;79:883–5.

95. Ponsford JR, Bannister R, Paul EA. Methacholine pupillary responses in third nerve palsy and Adie's syndrome. Brain 1982;105:583–97.

96. Ziegler MG, Lake CR, Kopin IJ. The sympathetic-nervous-system defect in primary orthostatic hypotension. N Engl J Med 1977;296:293–7.

97. Goldstein DS, Polinsky RJ, Garty M, et al. Patterns of plasma levels of catechols in neurogenic orthostatic hypotension. Ann Neurol 1989;26:558–63.

98. Kaufmann H, Oribe E, Miller M, et al. Hypotension-induced vasopressin release distinguishes between pure autonomic failure and multiple system atrophy with autonomic failure. Neurology 1992;42:590–3.

99. Williams TDM, Lightman SL, Bannister R. Vasopressin secertion in

progressive autonomic failure: evidence for defective afferent cardio-vascular pathways. J Neurol Neurosurg Psychiatry 1985;48:225–8.

100. Kopin IJ, Polinsky RJ, Oliver JA, et al. Urinary catecholamine metabolites distinguish different types of sympathetic neuronal dysfunction in patients with orthostatic hypotension. J Clin Endocrinol Metab 1983;57:632–7.

101. Schwartz TW. Pancreatic polypeptide: a hormone under vagal control. Gastroenterology 1983;85:1411–25.

102. Polinsky RJ, Taylor IL, Chew P, et al. Pancreatic polypeptide responses to hypoglycemia in chronic autonomic failure. J Clin Endocrinol Metab 1982;54:48–52.

103. Thomaides TN, Chaudhari KR, Maule S, et al. Growth hormone response to clonidine in central and peripheral primary autonomic failure. Lancet 1992;340:263–6.

104. Kimber JR, Watson L, Mathias CJ. Distinction of idiopathic Parkinson's disease from multiple-system atrophy by stimulation of growth-hormone release with clonidine. Lancet 1997;349:1877–81.

105. Leveston SA, Shah SD, Cryer PE. Evidence of sympathetic postganglionic axonal lesion in diabetic adrenergic neuropathy. J Clin Invest 1979;64:374–80.

106. Gemmill JD, Venables GS, Ewing DJ. Noradrenaline response to edrophonium in primary autonomic failure: distinction between central and peripheral damage. Lancet 1988;1:1018–21.

107. Demanet JC. Usefulness of noradrenaline and tyramine infusion tests in the diagnosis of orthostatic hypotension. Cardiology 1976;61:213–24.

108. Kardon RH, Denison CE, Brown CK, et al. Critical evaluation of the cocaine test in the diagnosis of Horner's syndrome. Arch Ophthalmol 1990;108:384–7.

109. Van der Weil HL, Van Gijn J. Localization of Horner's syndrome: use and limitations of hydroxyamphetamine test. J Neurol Sci 1983;59:229–35.

110. Low PA, Caskey PE, Tuck RR, et al. Quantitative sudomotor axon reflex test in normal and neuropathic subjects. Ann Neurol 1983;14:573–80.

111. Hoeldtke RD, Bryner KD, Horvath GG, et al. The redistribution of sudomotor responses is an early sign of sympathetic dysfunction in type I diabetes. Clin Autonom Res 2000;10:229.

112. Kennedy WR, Sakuta M, Sutherland D, et al. Quantitation of the sweating deficiency in diabetes mellitus. Ann Neurol 1984;15:482–8.

113. Low PA, Polinsky RJ, Kaufmann HC, et al. Multiple system atrophy (MSA), pure autonomic failure (PAF), and related extrapyramidal disorders. Continuum 1998;4:41–58.

114. Johnson RH, McLellan DL, Love DR. Orthostatic hypotension and the Holmes-Adie syndrome. J Neurol Neurosurg Psychiatry 1971;34:562–70.

115. Sharpey-Schafer EP. Circulatory reflexes in chronic disease of the afferent nervous system. J Physiol 1956;134:1–10.

116. Bannister R. Treatment of progressive autonomic failure. In: Bannister R, editor. Autonomic failure. 1st ed. New York: Oxford University Press; 1983. p. 316–34.

# CHAPTER 25

# Postoperative Motility Disorders

*Nancy N. Baxter and John H. Pemberton*

Gastrointestinal motility is sometimes disturbed by operative procedures, either in a temporary or permanent fashion. Despite this, unaltered postoperative function is the norm after most surgical procedures because of the tremendous reserve and potential for adaptation of the digestive tract. Perhaps because of this, our knowledge regarding the impact of various surgical procedures on motility is less than complete. This chapter discusses what is known about temporary disorders of gastrointestinal motility, which may follow any operative procedure, and common disorders resulting from specific procedures, which may produce long-term dysfunction.

## TEMPORARY DISORDERS OF GASTROINTESTINAL MOTILITY

### Ileus

Ileus is the most common postoperative motility disorder, occurring in virtually all patients undergoing major abdominal surgery.[1,2] In addition, ileus may be associated with nonabdominal surgery and other nonoperative causes. Ileus generally refers to nonmechanical bowel obstruction that results from aperistalsis or failure of coordinated peristalsis of the gastrointestinal tract.[3] The patient with ileus presents with abdominal distention, failure to pass flatus or feces, and nausea/vomiting with oral intake. After abdominal surgery, a period of ileus is expected. Typically, peristaltic activity returns rapidly in the small bowel, with activity returning within 12 hours. Gastric peristalsis and function return within 24 hours. Colonic activity, however, requires 48 to 72 hours to return to normal and does so in a proximal to distal fashion (Fig. 25.1).[1,4,5] Thus, the typical postoperative ileus is largely the function of colonic aperistalsis (Fig. 25.2).[1,6] Return of function with the passage of flatus is generally observed after approximately 4 days; therefore, ileus lasting up to 5 days after abdominal surgery may be considered normal.[2] The cause of typical postoperative ileus has not been well delineated; however, the evidence suggests that it is a dysfunction of the autonomic nervous system. Colonic motility via the enteric nervous system is largely mediated by the autonomic nervous system. Sympathetic stimulation leads to inhibition of colonic motility, whereas parasympathetic stimulation has the reverse effect. Ileus is thought to occur when the balance between sympathetic and parasympathetic output is lost, with the overall result being inhibition of colonic motility. Prolonged postoperative ileus occurs when disruption of normal patterns of contraction lasts beyond 5 days. The causes are very poorly understood; however, numerous factors are known to be associated with prolonged ileus (Table 25.1). Prolonged postoperative ileus occurs in up to 15% of patients after major abdominal surgery, and the costs of treating this condition are substantial. As postoperative ileus is a major determinant of length of hospital stay, numerous studies have evaluated methods of shortening this period.

### Nasogastric Decompression
Gastric decompression with a nasogastric tube was widely believed to shorten periods of ileus, and this led to the routine

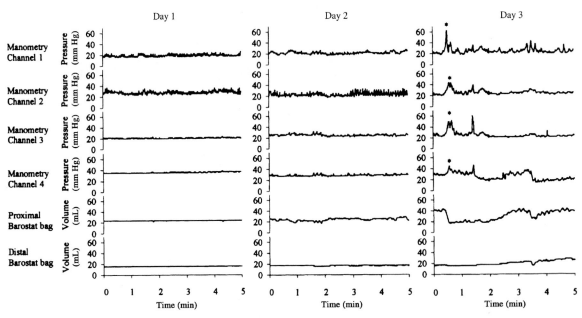

**FIGURE 25.1.** Representative recordings during postoperative days 1, 2, and 3. *Upper traces:* manometry pressure curves. Channel 1 is positioned most proximally in the colon and the subsequent channels further distally. The asterisk indicates a propagated contraction. *Lower traces:* barostat bag volume curves. Reproduced with permission from Huge A, Kreis M, Zittel T, et al. Postoperative colonic motility and tone in patients after colorectal surgery. Dis Colon Rectum 2000;43:932–9.

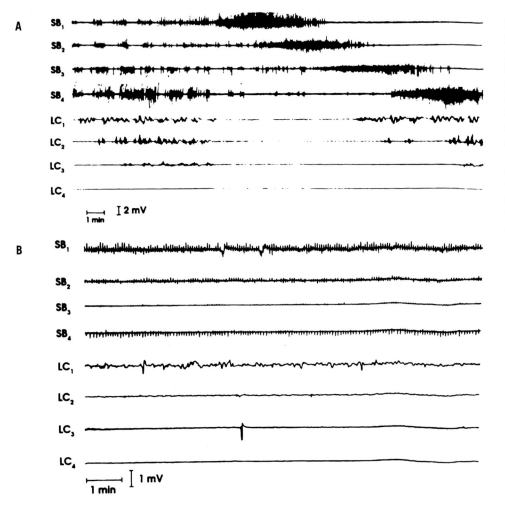

**FIGURE 25.2. A,** Typical recording made at baseline, demonstrating a migrating myoelectric complex ($SB_1$–$SB_4$) with phase 1, 2, and 3 and a migrating colonic complex ($LC_1$–$LC_3$). **B,** Typical recording made during the early postoperative period, demonstrating normal slow waves in the small intestine ($SB_1$–$SB_4$) and large bowel ($LC_1$–$LC_4$) with no spiking activity. Reproduced with permission from Ludwig K, Frantzides C, Carlson M. et al. Myoelectric motility patterns following open versus laparoscopic cholecystectomy. J Laparoendosc Surg 1993;3:461–6.

**TABLE 25.1.** Factors That May Increase the Incidence and Duration of Postoperative Ileus

Sepsis
Wide exposure of the abdominal cavity (laparotomy versus laparoscopy)
Multisystem trauma
Prolonged operative time
Inhalation anesthesia, especially nitrous oxide
Electrolyte imbalance (especially hypokalemia)
Prolonged intraoperative hypoxemia or hypotension
Opioid analgesia
Orthopedic surgery (eg, spinal)

Reproduced with permission from Woods M. Perspect Colon Rect Surg 2000;12:57–76.

use of nasogastric drainage after laparotomy.[7] Numerous randomized controlled trials[8–12] and a meta-analysis[13] have demonstrated no increase in the length of ileus or complications when nasogastric suction was omitted. Thus, these studies do not support the routine use of nasogastric tubes after laparotomy. Given that the major determinant of postoperative ileus is colonic motility, the lack of efficacy of nasogastric decompression is not surprising.

### Delay in Oral Intake

Surgeons have traditionally delayed oral intake after laparotomy until the resolution of ileus is evidenced by the passage of flatus. Return to a solid diet then occurs, usually over a 3-day period of time. As the typical postoperative ileus lasts 4 to 5 days, this has necessitated a 7- to 8-day hospital stay even in an uneventful recovery after major abdominal surgery. With the advent of laparoscopic techniques and early feeding in these patients, obligatory starvation after laparotomy has been questioned. Five randomized controlled trials have been performed after colorectal surgery to evaluate the effect of early feeding.[14–18] Although these studies have demonstrated that early feeding is safe, with no difference in complication rates, interestingly, only one study demonstrated a significant difference in the length of ileus or hospital stay.

### Effect of Narcotic Analgesic

Parenteral narcotics are commonly used in the postoperative period, particularly after laparotomy. Narcotics are known to have an adverse effect on gut motility.[19–22] A single dose of intravenous narcotic is known to delay gastric emptying.[23,24] Morphine is known to decrease propulsive contractions in the colon (Fig. 25.3).[25,26] The use of non-narcotic analgesia postoperatively has been demonstrated to decrease the length of ileus when compared to narcotic analgesics.[27,28] Although the use of narcotics increases the duration of postoperative ileus, adequate analgesia is necessary after major surgery and justifies the use of these medications.[19,28]

The method of parenteral delivery of narcotic analgesics may also affect gastrointestinal motility. Three retrospective studies have matched groups of postoperative patients receiving patient-controlled analgesia (PCA) to groups receiving intermittent dosing of narcotics. Patients with PCA resolved

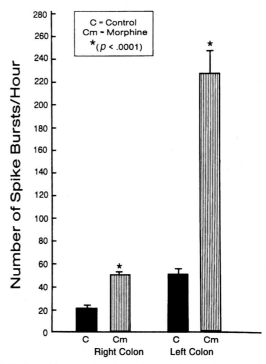

**FIGURE 25.3.** Mean number of spike bursts per hour at two colon recording sites before and after intravenous administration of morphine. Differences are significant at both sites. Reproduced with permission from Frantzides C, Cowles V, Salaymeh B, et al. Morphine effects on human colonic myoelectric activity in the postoperative period. Am J Surg 1992;163:144–9.

**TABLE 25.2.** Mechanisms by Which Thoracic Epidural Anesthesia May Promote Gastrointestinal Motility

Blockade of nociceptive afferent nerves
Blockade of thoracolumbar sympathetic efferent nerves
Unopposed parasympathetic efferent nerves
Reduced need for postoperative opiates
Increased gastrointestinal blood flow
Systemic absorption of local anesthetic

Reproduced with permission from Steinbrook R. Epidural anesthesia and gastrointestinal motility. Anesth Analg 1998;86:837–44.

their postoperative ileus on average 1 day later than the group receiving intermittent doses of analgesia.[29–31] The higher steady-state levels of narcotics in individuals receiving PCA may explain the prolongation of ileus; however, not all studies have replicated this finding.

### Effect of Epidural Analgesia

Epidural analgesia has been evaluated as a narcotic-sparing method of postoperative pain control. Numerous mechanisms have been proposed by which epidural anesthesia may promote early return of gastrointestinal motility (Table 25.2).[32] Thoracic epidurals have been shown to reduce postoperative pain and the length of ileus after abdominal surgery (Fig. 25.4).[32–37] This has not, however, always translated into a reduced length of stay. When the epidural catheter is placed below T12, improvements in gastrointestinal motility are less

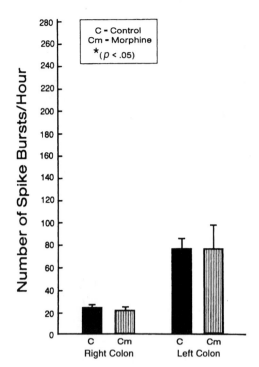

**FIGURE 25.4.** Mean number of spike bursts per hour at two colon recording sites before and after epidural administration of morphine. Epidural morphine has no significant effect on colon myoelectric activity. Reproduced from Am J Surg, Vol. 163, Frantzides C, Cowles V, Salaymeh B, et al. Morphine effects on human colonic myoelectric activity in the postoperative period, 144–9, Copyright 1992, with permission from Excerpta Medica Inc.

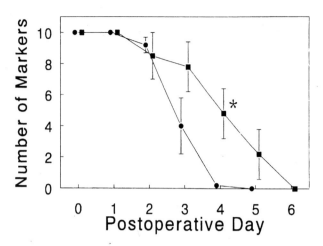

**FIGURE 25.5.** Results of transit time studies after colon surgery in dogs. Significantly larger numbers of markers remained after open surgery (■) as compared to laparoscopic (●) colon resection on postoperative day 4. *$p < .05$ by Mann-Whitney U test. Reproduced with permission from Hotokezaka M, Combs M, Schirmer B. Recovery of gastrointestinal motility following open versus laparoscopic colon resection in dogs. Dig Dis Sci 1996;41:705–10.

consistent. Although fewer studies have been conducted, those that compare epidural narcotics to epidural local anesthetics demonstrate that patients receiving epidural local anesthetics had greater gastrointestinal motility, with improved gastric emptying, acetaminophen absorption, and more rapid resolution of ileus.[32]

### Ambulation

Although widely assumed to have beneficial effects, no studies have demonstrated that early ambulation is associated with a shortened duration of ileus. Patients mobilized on day 1 after major abdominal surgery did not have an improved return of function as compared with those mobilized on day 4.[38]

### Effect of Surgery

The influence of surgical factors on ileus has been evaluated. Laparotomy with manipulation of the small bowel has been shown to result in ileus. Although the degree of dissection and the length of the incision have not been shown to be a determinant,[39] ileus may be worsened by the presence of blood, peritonitis, or retroperitoneal irritation.[40] Recently, with the advent of laparoscopic techniques, the impact of minimally invasive surgery on the degree of ileus has been evaluated. Decreased incision size and lesser bowel manipulation have been proposed as mechanisms for a reduction in ileus after minimally invasive surgery. The

reduced need for narcotics after laparoscopic surgery has also been cited as a possible factor. In most studies comparing laparoscopic to open colectomy using canine models, the length of postoperative ileus was reduced in the laparoscopic group (Fig. 25.5).[41–43] In humans, some authors have shown a more rapid return of gut function after laparoscopic colectomy,[44–46] whereas others have not found substantial benefits of laparoscopic surgery with respect to the reduction of ileus.[47,48] Multicentered trials comparing open to laparoscopic colectomy are currently ongoing and should help answer this question.

### Preoperative Suggestion

Interestingly, there may be some impact of suggestion on the length of postoperative ileus. In a randomized study, patients who had heard a short presentation discussing the importance of a rapid resolution of ileus had a faster return of bowel function as measured by passage of flatus and a decreased length of stay compared with those hearing an unrelated presentation.[49] These findings may, in part, explain the shortened length of ileus found in some studies of laparoscopic surgery, where preoperative education is generally given regarding shortened hospital stay and rapid refeeding.

### Treatment

Prolonged postoperative ileus is generally treated supportively, with nasogastric suction, intravenous fluid, and nutritional support. The administration of promotility agents such as erythromycin, cisapride, and metoclopramide has also been investigated. In a thorough review of the literature, no evidence was found for the benefit of metoclopramide or erythromycin in the treatment of postoperative ileus. Some benefit has been found after administration of cisapride; however, this drug is no longer available for use.[50]

**TABLE 25.3.** Factors Contributing to the Development of Ogilvie's Syndrome

Obstetric/vaginal delivery
Pelvic/retroperitoneal operations
Cardiopulmonary failure
Sepsis
Multiple trauma
Central nervous system/orthopedic operations
Neurologic problems
Hepatic failure
Carcinomatosis
Renal failure
Cardiothoracic operations
Burns
Drugs
    Opiates
    Antidepressants (tricyclics)
    Chlorpromazine
    Nimodipine
    Steroids (renal transplant patients)
Lead poisoning
Tick bite
Herpes zoster
Scleroderma
Mesenteric ganglionitis/hypogenesis
Renal cell carcinoma
Mesenteric vein thrombosis
Tuberculous peritonitis
Visceral myopathy

Reproduced with permission from Sgambati S, Armstrong D, Ballantyne G. Management of acute colonic psuedo-obstruction (Ogilvie's syndrome). Perspect Colon Rect Surg 1994;7:77–96.

### Colonic Pseudo-obstruction

One extreme example of ileus is colonic pseudo-obstruction, or Ogilvie's syndrome, in the postoperative state. In Oglivie's syndrome, there is colonic obstruction in the absence of any mechanical blockage. Patients present with abdominal distention (which may be massive), inactive bowel sounds, nausea/vomiting, and obstipation. Patients are often elderly and debilitated. Plain films of the abdomen show massive colonic distention that may be difficult to differentiate from mechanical colonic obstruction (Fig. 25.6). Colonic pseudo-obstruction occurs commonly after pelvic surgery and nonabdominal surgery, particularly cardiovascular and orthopedic surgery, and numerous conditions predispose its development (Table 25.3).

Colonic pseudo-obstruction is thought to be attributable to aperistalsis of the colon caused by disturbance in neurologic regulation[1,51]; again, excess sympathetic stimulation results in functional obstruction of the colon.[1] If untreated, the distention may become massive, resulting in cecal ischemia and perforation. When treating pseudo-obstruction, mechanical obstruction by tumor or stricture must first be ruled out. Because this is often impossible on plain film radiography, water-soluble contrast is often used to rule out a distal colonic obstruction (Fig. 25.7). Conservative measures, including nasogastric suction, enemas, correction of electrolyte abnor-

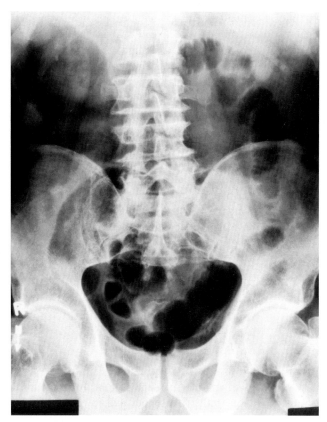

**FIGURE 25.6.** Abdominal radiograph in a patient with colonic pseudo-obstruction.

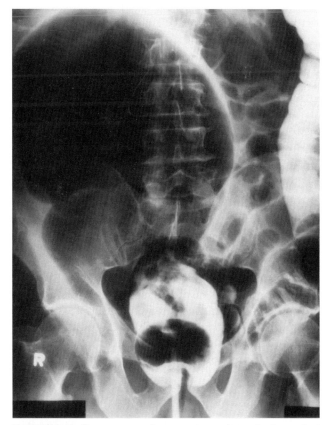

**FIGURE 25.7.** Hypaque enema demonstrating no obstruction in a patient with colonic pseudo-obstruction.

malities, limiting narcotic use, and treating underlying medical disorders, may be effective if colonic distention is not marked. Often, however, intervention is required to prevent progression and potential perforation. Neostigmine, a parasympathomimetic agent, has been used in the treatment of colonic pseudo-obstruction and has been shown to be dramatically effective.[52–54] In a clinical trial of 21 patients with pseudo-obstruction, administration of 2 mg of neostigmine over 3 to 5 minutes was associated with immediate clinical response, with a significant decrease in girth and a 5-cm average decrease in cecal diameter.[52] Administration of neostigmine mandates cardiac monitoring and may be contraindicated for patients with underlying bradyarrhythmia. In those who have failed neostigmine, colonoscopic decompression may be required.

## POSTOPERATIVE MOTILITY DISORDERS AFTER SPECIFIC PROCEDURES

### Esophageal Procedures

#### Normal Motility

The esophagus facilitates passage of food from mouth to stomach without reflux. An upper and lower esophageal sphincter bound the esophagus. Swallowing results in relaxation of the upper esophageal sphincter, allowing passage of the food bolus into the esophagus. A peristaltic contraction is then initiated, propelling the food bolus rapidly distally. This is termed primary peristalsis. The lower esophageal sphincter relaxes in response to primary peristalsis, allowing the food bolus to enter the stomach. The basal pressure of the upper and lower esophageal sphincter prevents reflux. Secondary peristalsis of the esophagus is initiated by esophageal distention and continues in an orderly fashion until the esophagus is cleared. Tertiary peristaltic waves occur in disease states. They are high amplitude and irregular.

#### Myotomy

Heller's myotomy for achalasia requires some mobilization of the esophagus at the hiatus. Any procedure requiring esophageal mobilization may inadvertently enlarge the esophageal hiatus, dividing the hiatal attachments to the gastroesophageal junction. This may reduce the length of esophagus exposed to abdominal pressures, disturbing native antireflux mechanisms. In a review of 5,002 patients undergoing Heller's myotomy reported in 75 articles, an average of 8.6% of patients (range 0–29%) had significant gastroesophageal reflux. The risk was found to be higher with an abdominal versus a thoracic approach, and the addition of a fundoplication to abdominal myotomy has been recommended.[55]

#### Esophagectomy

Esophagectomy for malignancy is a major procedure with significant morbidity and mortality. The stomach is the most commonly used conduit to replace the esophagus and re-establish intestinal continuity. Delayed gastric emptying of the intrathoracic neo-esophagus may occur in a large percentage of patients after esophagectomy with gastric pull-through.[56] Patients have symptoms of fullness and may experience reflux. As the vagus is usually divided during esophagectomy, delayed emptying likely relates to functional obstruction of the stomach at the pylorus.[56] In a randomized trial of 200 patients, pyloroplasty has been shown to reduce the incidence of delayed gastric emptying.[56] Patients with a pyloroplasty had improved tolerance for solids both in the early postoperative period and at 6 months compared to patients who did not have a pyloroplasty. Another study compared pyloroplasty, pyloromyotomy, and pyloric stretching and found all three to be equally effective in preventing gastric outlet obstruction.[57]

The technique of esophagectomy may also influence the degree of reflux. A retrospective study of 295 patients after esophagectomy for cancer demonstrated a higher incidence of delayed gastric emptying and pneumonia after esophagectomy through a right thoracotomy as opposed to a transhiatal or left thoracotomy approach.[58]

#### Fundoplication

Fundoplication is a commonly performed procedure for the treatment of gastroesophageal reflux disease, and its use may be increasing now as laparoscopic Nissens are quite popular. In the most commonly performed Nissen fundoplication, the fundus is wrapped 360 degrees around the esophagus. The esophageal hiatus is also plicated. Although fundoplication is a well-tolerated procedure, problems may arise. The wrapped fundus creates a one-way valve-like mechanism, allowing food to enter into the stomach, but does not allow gastric contents to reflux into the esophagus. This valve-like mechanism may function too well, preventing passage of air. When eructation is impossible, air accumulates in the stomach, resulting in symptoms of distention and bloating. This has been referred to as the "gas bloat" syndrome and may occur in up to 50% of patients in the early postoperative period.[59–61] Patients with gastroesophageal reflux disease tend to swallow air to relieve reflux symptoms. After fundoplication, this tendency exacerbates gas accumulation.[62] Injuries to the vagus during esophageal mobilization lead to gastric outlet obstruction and gastric atony, which also exacerbates gas bloat symptoms. Gas bloat generally improves with time but occasionally may be prolonged and severe, necessitating further therapy. Before intervention, it is essential to rule out small bowel obstruction as a cause of symptoms. Also, patients should undergo testing for vagal function, ruling out inadvertent vagotomy as a cause. Motility agents may be of use in these patients, and a period of months of watchful waiting is recommended given the natural history of the problem. A small number of people will require further surgical intervention for intractable gas bloat. Generally, surgical therapy involves taking down the Nissen fundoplication and substituting a more limited fundoplication, enabling vomiting and eructation. The condition of gas bloat

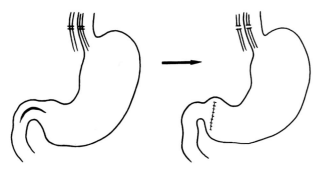

**FIGURE 25.8.** Truncal vagotomy and Heineke-Mikulicz pyloroplasty. Reproduced with permission from Sachdeva A, Zaren H, Sigel B. Surgical treatment of peptic ulcer disease. Med Clin North Am 1991;75:999–1012.

**A**

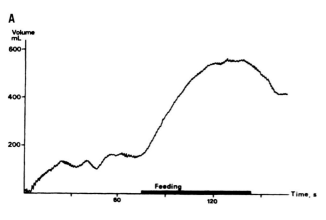

**B**

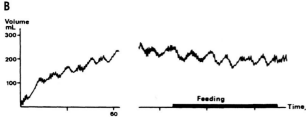

**FIGURE 25.9.** Continuous gastric volume recording at a pressure load of 10 cm of water. Effect of feeding before (**A**) and after (**B**) vagotomy. The marked relaxatory response to feeding is abolished by vagotomy. Reproduced with permission from Jahnberg T, Abrahamsson H, Jansson G, Martinson J. Gastric relaxatory response to feeding before and after vagotomy. Scand J Gastroenterol 1977;12:225–8.

may, in part, reflect preexisting abnormalities in gastric emptying as well: in a study of 81 patients undergoing antireflux surgery, preoperative delayed gastric emptying was associated with symptoms of bloating, inability to belch, and relief of bloating with belching.[63]

## Gastric Procedures

Motility disorders after gastric procedures are intriguing and have been widely studied. Fortunately, with the advent of effective medical therapy for peptic ulcer disease, the need for surgery has declined dramatically; therefore, these complications have become much less frequent.

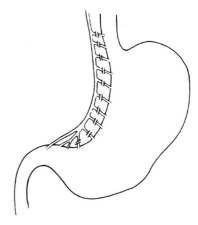

**FIGURE 25.10.** Highly selective vagotomy. Reproduced with permission from Sachdeva A, Zaren H, Sigel B. Surgical treatment of peptic ulcer disease. Med Clin North Am 1991;75:999–1012.

### Gastric Motility

Distal esophageal distention results in reflex relaxation of the gastric fundus. Relaxation allows gastric volume to increase without large increases in gastric pressure, enabling the stomach to fulfill a reservoir role after ingestion of a meal. Gastric distention stimulates gastric motility. Gastric contents are propelled distally from the fundus to the antrum and then to the pylorus. The pylorus closes prior to the arrival of the food bolus, opening just enough to pass small amounts of liquid and food particles less than 1 mm in diameter. The remainder of the food bolus returns to the proximal antrum, and this pattern continues, churning the contents, mixing them with digestive juices, and morselizing them.

Three aspects of gastric surgery impact on the development of motility disorders: vagotomy; destruction of a functional pylorus, and gastric resection. The vagus has many functions in the regulation of gastric motility in addition to innervating the acid-secreting parietal cells of the stomach. The vagus mediates receptive relaxation of the stomach. Antral activity in response to gastric distention is a vagally mediated response. The vagus is also important in mediating gastric emptying through coordinating relaxation of the pylorus. This coordinated relaxation allows controlled release of gastric contents into the duodenum and is destroyed functionally by vagotomy and structurally by pyloroplasty, pyloromyotomy, and distal gastrectomy.

Truncal vagotomy (Fig. 25–8), performed at the esophageal hiatus, leads to vagal denervation of the abdominal viscera. The effects on the stomach include loss of reflexive relaxation of the fundus (Fig. 25.9), a decrease in antral motility, and a lack of coordinated pyloric emptying. Because of the undesired effects of truncal vagotomy, more selective procedures have been developed. In the highly selective vagotomy (Fig. 25.10), only vagal fibers to the acid-producing portion of the stomach are divided, from the esophagus proximally to the junction of the body and antrum distally. This preserves hepatic, pancreatic, antral, pyloric, and small bowel vagal innervation and obviates the need for gastric drainage procedure.

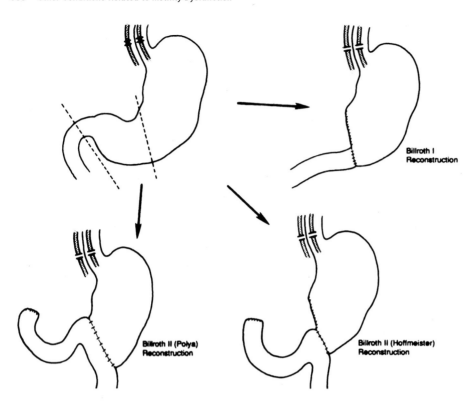

**FIGURE 25.11.** Gastric procedures with Billroth I and Billroth II reconstructions. Reproduced with permission from Sachdeva A, Zaren H, Sigel B. Surgical treatment of peptic ulcer disease. Med Clin North Am 1991;75:999–1012.

**TABLE 25.4.** Motility Disorders Related to Gastric Procedures

| Disorder | Cause | Treatment | Course |
|---|---|---|---|
| Gastric atony | Vagotomy with loss of tonic contractions of proximal stomach | Supportive therapy<br>Motility agents<br>If intractable, subtotal gastrectomy | Majority improve over time with symptomatic treatment |
| Dumping<br>Early | Rapid emptying of hyperosmolar contents due to loss of reservoir and pylorus lead to massive fluid shifts | Small, frequent meals<br>Avoid carbohydrate loads<br>May try octreotide | Improvement over time; most better by 6 mo |
| Late | Rapid emptying leads to insulin hypersecretion and ultimate hypoglycemia | Same; if intractable, consider reversed jejunal segment | Majority improve with time |
| Diarrhea | Vagotomy<br>? Alterations in secretion of bile acids | Cholestyramine; consider reversed jejunal segment if intractable | Majority improve with time |
| Alkaline reflux | Destruction of pylorus<br>Failure of gastric clearance | Often requires surgical intervention with Roux-en-Y | Most improve with surgical intervention |
| Roux stasis | Ectopic pacemakers in Roux limb | Prevent with "uncut" Roux; try motility agents, consider completion gastrectomy and Roux-en-Y esophagojejunostomy if intractable | Very difficult to treat; most have some relief with surgery |

Motility disorders after gastric surgery (Fig. 25.11) may be divided into (1) those in which transit is too rapid (dumping), (2) those in which transit is too slow (gastric atony), (3) those with reflux of bowel content (alkaline reflux gastritis), and (4) those of unknown etiology (postvagotomy diarrhea). In addition, when large amounts of the stomach are resected, the lack of an adequate gastric reservoir leads to symptoms of early satiety, reflux, and bloating (Table 25–4).

RAPID TRANSIT. Rapid gastric emptying, especially of carbohydrate-rich food through an incompetent pylorus, leads to the syndrome of dumping in up to 15% of individuals undergoing vagotomy and pyloroplasty (Fig. 25–12). The rates of dumping are even higher after vagotomy and distal antrectomy. Dumping may be divided into an early and late form. In early dumping, symptoms of diaphoresis, weakness, palpitations, and flushing develop 10 to 30 minutes after the

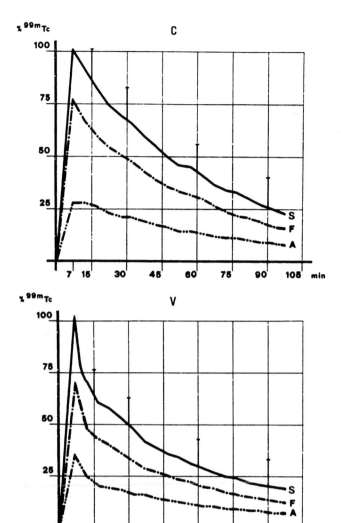

**FIGURE 25.12.** Gastric emptying of radioactivity-labeled liquids in controls (**C**) and patients after truncal vagotomy and pyloroplasty (**V**). Note the extremely rapid emptying of liquids after vagotomy, especially in the initial phase. S, total stomach; F, proximal area representing fundal activity; A, distal area representing antral activity; $^{99m}$Tc, technetium 99m. Reproduced with permission from Calabuig R, Carrio I, Mones J, et al. Gastric emptying after truncal vagotomy and pyloroplasty. Scand J Gastroenterol 1988;23:659–64.

ingestion of a meal. These may be accompanied by gastrointestinal symptoms including nausea, vomiting, and explosive diarrhea. The cardiovascular effects are secondary to rapid fluid shifts into the small bowel lumen in response to a high osmotic load. The gastrointestinal effects may be secondary to gastrointestinal hormone release in response to the rapid efflux of carbohydrates.

In late dumping, vasomotor symptoms present 2 to 4 hours after eating. The high carbohydrate load leads to an overstimulation of enteroglucagon release that, in turn, stimulates release of insulin. The resulting hyperinsulinemia and hypoglycemia lead to the palpitations, diaphoresis, weakness, and flushing experienced by these patients.

The diagnosis of the dumping syndrome is usually made on history. In the case of late dumping, it is important to exclude insulinoma as a potential cause of the hyperinsulinemia in the presence of hypoglycemia. Conservative therapy is generally successful and consists of dietary modification including separating liquids and solids, avoiding carbohydrate-rich foods, and taking frequent small-volume meals. Most patients improve over the first 6 months. Octreotide, a long-acting somatostatin analogue, has been used with some success in the treatment of dumping.[64,65] Rarely, patients have intractable symptoms, necessitating further intervention.

### SLOW TRANSIT.

*Gastric Atony.* This complication develops in up to 10% of patients after truncal vagotomy.[66] The loss of gastric vagal innervation leads to a loss of coordination of peristalsis. This leads to a disruption of antral mixing and subsequent gastric distention and inadequate propulsion. Patients have symptoms of bloating, distention, epigastric fullness, and nausea. Tolerance for liquids is generally much better than for solids. Patients with severe gastric atony will vomit undigested food that may have been eaten days previously, and persistent gastric atony may lead to the development of bezoars. Obstruction should be ruled out as a cause of symptoms with barium studies and/or endoscopy. Patients generally improve over time, and the use of prokinetic agents may have some benefit. After 6 to 12 months, a small number of patients will continue to have severe symptoms. Near-total gastrectomy with Roux-en-Y gastrojejunostomy is the recommended treatment, with a 40% or greater response rate.[67–71]

*Roux Stasis Syndrome.* Thirty percent of patients will develop delay in gastric emptying after Roux-en-Y gastrojejunostomy reconstruction.[66] The transection of the jejunum required for Roux construction disturbs the usual pattern of arborally propagated potentials originating in the duodenum.[72] Ectopic pacemakers develop in the Roux limb, which can induce pacesetter potentials that migrate orally.[73] This leads to delayed transit through the Roux limb, resulting in symptoms similar to those of gastric atony.[74] The Roux loop itself may cause functional resistance to gastric emptying that compounds the problem.[75] Roux stasis syndrome is a difficult disorder to treat. There may be some benefit to the administration of prokinetic agents.[76,77] Surgical approaches include completion gastrectomy with Roux-en-Y esophagojejunostomy or intestinal pacing, but both have less than perfect success in ameliorating symptoms.[78] The best treatment may be prevention. The development of the "uncut Roux" limb, for which there is maintenance of continuity between the duodenum, allowing propagation of duodenal pacemaker activity to the Roux limb, has had success in preventing this complication (Fig. 25.13).[79–81]

### REFLUX.

*Alkaline Reflux Gastritis.* This is a frequent long-term complication of gastrectomy, particularly common after Billroth II reconstruction. Patients present with symptoms of vague

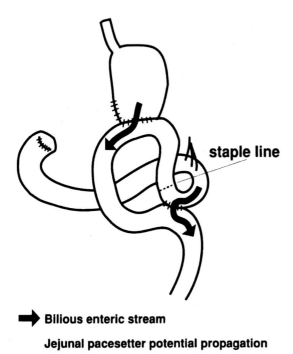

**staple line**

➡ **Bilious enteric stream**

**Jejunal pacesetter potential propagation**

➡ **Gastric enteric stream**

**FIGURE 25.13.** The "uncut" Roux gastrojejunostomy. Mucosal continuity is maintained allowing aboral transmission of pacemaker potentials. Staple line prevents reflux of enteric contents. Reproduced with permission from Eagon J, Miedema B, Kelly K. Postgastrectomy syndromes. Surg Clin North Am 1992;72:445–65.

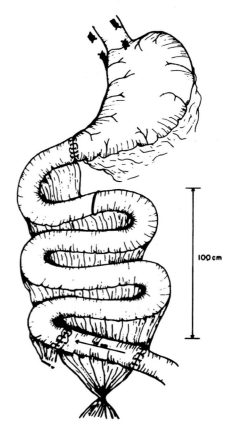

100 cm

**FIGURE 25.14.** Reversed jejunal limb for the treatment of refractory postvagotomy diarrhea. Reproduced from Am J Surg Vol. 159, Sawyers J, Management of postgastrectomy syndromes, 8–14, Copyright 1990, with permission from Excerpta Medica Inc.

abdominal pain, dyspepsia, nausea, and vomiting of bilious gastric contents that does not relieve the pain. Patients may also lose weight and have anemia. Of all postgastrectomy syndromes, severe alkaline reflux gastritis is most likely to require operative intervention.[82] This syndrome is caused by reflux of alkaline gastrointestinal content into the remaining stomach through a defunctioned or absent pylorus.[83] The gastric mucosa is injured by the presence of bile acids in the stomach, and a histologic gastritis results.[84] Treatment with conversion to a Roux-en-Y anastomosis is usually successful, although gastric stasis may result.

### UNCLEAR ETIOLOGY.

*Postvagotomy Diarrhea.* Diarrhea is a well-known complication of vagotomy, occurring in up to 25% of patients undergoing truncal vagotomy, 3% of patients undergoing selective vagotomy, and less than 1% of patients undergoing highly selective vagotomy.[85] Patients present with frequent watery stools that may be explosive. The diarrhea tends to be episodic in nature, nocturnal, and not associated with food intake. There may be a female preponderance. The diarrhea becomes incapacitating in 1 to 2% of patients.[86] When severe, this problem may result in profound weight loss and malabsorption. The etiology of postvagotomy diarrhea is not clear, although because the incidence of diarrhea is much lower after highly selective vagotomy, the loss of hepatic, pyloric,

and/or small bowel vagal innervation in truncal vagotomy may be causative. The loss of pyloric competence and receptive relaxation may lead to rapid transit of liquid gastric contents into the small bowel, leading to diarrhea.[87,88] However, the correction of rapid emptying has not been found to improve postvagotomy diarrhea. Small bowel dysmotility caused by vagotomy with subsequent bacterial colonization may contribute to the diarrhea. Abnormalities of gallbladder emptying into the duodenum may be important in the etiology of postvagotomy diarrhea. This is supported by the finding that diarrhea improves with the administration of cholestyramine, a bile-acid binding resin.[89,90] Also, patients with postvagotomy diarrhea have higher levels of fecal bile acids than controls.[91] The difference in the incidence of this complication after highly selective vagotomy versus truncal vagotomy may result from preservation of hepatic vagal fibers supplying the gallbladder in highly selective vagotomy, allowing preservation of gallbladder function.

The diagnosis of postvagotomy diarrhea is usually made clinically. Other causes of diarrheal illness should be ruled out. Patients generally improve over a 6- to 12-month period. Cholestyramine may be of benefit. In severe cases failing medical management, a reversed jejunal loop may be beneficial (Fig. 25.14).

### Operations for Gastric Cancer

Resections of gastric malignancies often require removal of 85% or more of the gastric reservoir. Despite this, metabolic and motor dysfunction are less common in this group of patients than in patients operated on for peptic ulcer disease. This is likely attributable in part to the limited life expectancy of many individuals with gastric cancer. The removal of greater than 85% of the stomach may lead to sensations of early satiety, nausea, and vomiting secondary to a lack of capacity.

## Duodenal Operations

### Pancreaticoduodenectomy

Because of the close proximity of the duodenum to the head of the pancreas and the common bile duct, isolated duodenal resections are uncommon. Resection of the duodenum is usually performed in concert with resection of the head of the pancreas and the common bile duct. Reconstruction is generally accomplished by choledochojejunostomy, pancreaticojejunostomy, and duodenojejunostomy. This is the so-called pylorus-sparing Whipple procedure. The classic Whipple procedure also includes a partial gastrectomy and necessitates a gastrojejunostomy for reconstruction. Between 9 and 46% of patients will develop delayed gastric emptying, which has been found to be the most common complication of this procedure.[92,93] There are numerous potential causes of delayed gastric emptying after pancreaticoduodenectomy. These include mechanical or functional damage to the pylorus, resection of the duodenal pacemaker, and disruption of the gastrointestinal nervous plexus.[94] Initially, pylorus-sparing pancreaticoduodenectomy was felt to increase the rate of delayed gastric emptying. Although there may be a transient delay in gastric emptying in pyorus-sparing procedures, this has not been found to be clinically significant.[95–97] In fact, the presence of postoperative complications, not pyloric sparing, was most predictive of the development of delayed gastric emptying.[96,98,99] Because of a lower incidence in marginal ulceration and dumping with preservation of the pylorus, along with the overall greater ease of the procedure, pylorus-sparing pancreaticoduodenectomy has been widely adopted. In general, patients with delayed gastric emptying after this procedure respond to prolonged nasogastric suction with nutritional support.

## Small Bowel Procedures

### Small Bowel Motility

Normal small bowel motility is characterized by two distinct patterns, corresponding to the fasting and fed states. In the fasting state, there is a cyclic migrating myoelectric complex (MMC) initiated in the stomach and duodenum that regularly propagates through the small intestine, clearing the intestine of contents. Cycles last approximately 90 to 120 minutes. In the fed state, MMC patterns are interrupted and replaced by intermittent contractions or segmentation, allowing mixing and slow distal propulsion of contents.[100] The frequency of these segmental contractions decreases distally, with the high-

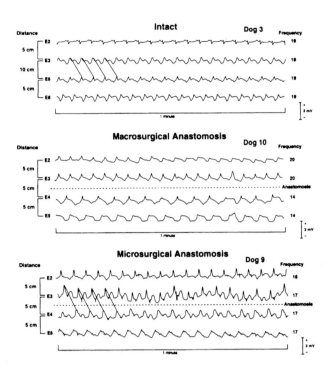

**FIGURE 25.15.** Jejunal electrical recordings in dogs. Pacesetter potentials are propagated distally (*slanted lines*) along intact jejunum and across a jejunal microanastomosis but not across a jejunal macroanastomosis. Distance = distance between electrodes (*E*); Frequency = pacesetter potential frequency (CPM). Reproduced with permission from Hart S, Nguyen-Tu B, Hould F, et al. Restoration of myoelectrical propagation across a jejunal transection using microsurgical anastomosis. J Gastrointest Surg 1999;3:524–32.

est frequency found in the duodenum. This functions to facilitate movement of material from the proximal (more rapidly contracting) to the distal (less rapidly contracting) bowel.[101]

### Bowel Resection

Bowel resection with reanastomosis leads to a disruption of the normal propagation of electrical control activity from the proximal to the distal bowel. With disruption of mucosal continuity, electrical activity from the duodenal pacemaker is no longer transmitted to bowel distal to the site of anastomosis. Pacemakers in the remaining bowel become dominant and initiate electrical control activity in the remaining intestine at a slower rate, decreasing the frequency of contractions distal to the anastomosis. In dogs, transection and reanastomosis of small intestine have been found to result in fewer distally propagating contractions, with a net result of slower intestinal transit.[102] Also, with jejunal transection, up to 25% of pacesetter potentials have been found to propagate orally in the area of the anastomosis, with slowed transit as the result.[103] Despite these findings, resection of the intestine in humans is well tolerated. With end-to-end anastomosis, propagation of the MMC returns to normal after 30 to 40 days.[104] Microsurgical anastomosis has been shown to maintain episodic propagation of pacesetter potentials across the anastomosis, preserving motility and transit distal to the transection (Fig. 25.15).[105]

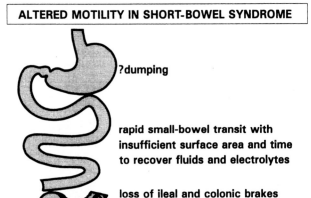

**ALTERED MOTILITY IN SHORT-BOWEL SYNDROME**

?dumping

rapid small-bowel transit with
insufficient surface area and time
to recover fluids and electrolytes

loss of ileal and colonic brakes

### Short Gut Syndrome

Owing to tremendous potential for adaptation, resections of significant amounts of small bowel may be performed with little effect. However, short gut syndrome, characterized by weight loss, diarrhea, fat malabsorption, and water and electrolyte depletion, occurs when less than 100 cm of functioning small bowel remains.[106] Changes in motility may exacerbate the syndrome (Fig. 25.16). The motor response to extensive resections has been studied in animals. Researchers have found that initially after a 75% small bowel resection in dogs, although the frequency of MMC cycling did not change, motor activity in the remaining segment became completely dominated by repetitive clusters of high-amplitude waves with elevations in basal tone. These clusters were similar to those found in the distal ileum of control animals but without the migration of clusters generally seen in the distal ileum. The cluster activity may be a response to exposure to volatile fatty acids or bile acids in the remaining bowel. These cluster patterns were abnormal and postulated to contribute to the diarrhea and malabsorption after bowel resection.[107,108] Along with mucosal and hormonal adaptations occurring after bowel resection, adaptations in small bowel motility are thought to contribute to improvements in the short gut syndrome seen over time. A decrease in the frequency of cluster activity has been found with time after massive small bowel resection.[109] The duration of the MMC cycle has been found to be shortened in humans after massive small bowel resection. This is particularly in the phase of the MMC (phase 2), during which intestinal secretions are maximal. This may be an adaptive response, resulting in a lesser amount of secretions and therefore smaller stool volumes.[110–112]

Gastric emptying may contribute to the diarrhea and malabsorption of short gut syndrome. Gastric emptying and proximal small bowel motility are slowed by the presence of fat and complex carbohydrates in the distal ileum. This reflex is termed the "ileal brake" and is likely hormonally mediated.

Patients with end jejunostomies who have lost this feedback inhibition experience increased rates of gastric emptying, exacerbating the short gut syndrome.[110]

In addition, patients with short gut syndrome may develop gastric hypersecretion caused by hypergastrinemia and parietal cell hyperplasia.[113] The cause of this is unknown but is likely hormonally mediated. Gastric hypersecretion may worsen the diarrhea in short bowel syndrome, and the excess acid delivered to the duodenum may lead to inactivation of pancreatic enzymes, worsening malabsorption.

Some of the therapeutic strategies for management of short gut syndrome target motility in an attempt to maximize fluid and nutrient absorption. Antidiarrheals and opioids are used to slow intestinal transit. Octreotide may be useful in particularly severe cases. Surgical strategies may be necessary and must be individualized and include recruitment of defunctioned bowel, intestinal lengthening procedures, reversed segments, and, finally, intestinal transplantation.

## Colonic Surgery

### Colonic Motility

In the colon, there are two main patterns of motility. Segmental contractions dominate and facilitate mixing and absorption. Material is moved forward and backward and is eventually propelled slowly in an antegrade fashion. Mass movements, the second major pattern, result from distention in the transverse and descending colon and propel contents forward more effectively and for longer distances. These mass movements occur only one to two times daily in healthy states. This allows stool to be advanced to the rectum, initiating defecation in an infrequent and socially acceptable manner.

### Segmental Colonic Resections

Different regions of the colon and rectum have different functions, and this may affect the impact of segmental resection. The ileocecal junction helps regulate the flow of intestinal contents from small to large bowel. The proximal colon functions as a reservoir and is the major site of water and electrolyte absorption in the colon. The more distal colon has a lesser absorptive role and functions mainly as a reservoir.

Generally, segmental resections of the colon are well tolerated and result in only minor changes in bowel function. However, resolution of ileus appears to be delayed by colonic anastomosis. Patients undergoing left colon resection with anastomosis were compared to individuals undergoing laparotomy for other reasons. Colonic activity was recorded using microtransducer probes. Motility in the anastomotic group was found to be significantly depressed in the first 72 hours as compared to controls (Fig. 25.17).[114] Long-term function, however, seems to be less affected. In a study of patients after right hemicolectomy with resection of the ileocecal valve, isotope movement into the colon was similar to that of controls. Intermittent ileocolic transfer of chyme was maintained after resection of the ileocecal valve, indicating that propulsive forces of the ileum are able to compensate for the loss of the

## Control

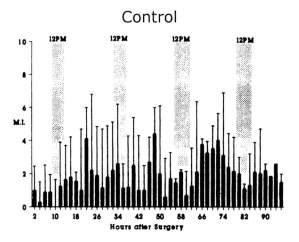

## Anastomotic

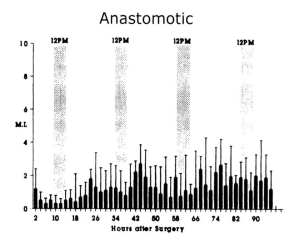

**FIGURE 25.17.** Median and upper quartile range motility. MI sum = amplitude x duration of waveforms)/time x 10) of all manometric colonic transducers in control and colonic anastomosis patient groups. Reproduced from Roberts J, Benson M, Rogers J, et al. Characterization of distal colonic motility in early postoperative period and effect of colonic anastomosis. Dig Dis Sci 1994;39:1961–67, with permission from Kluwer Academic/Plenum Publishers.

valve. Adaptation of the more distal colon to assume the reservoir function of the right colon was found. Patients experienced only minor changes in bowel habits, with slightly more frequent, softer stools.[115] In patients with short gut, the loss of the ileocecal valve and right colon may be more important and overall outcome worsened. The impact of left-sided colonic resections has not been well studied.

### Subtotal Colectomy

Subtotal colectomy with ileostomy or ileorectostomy is remarkably well tolerated. Following ileostomy, effluent is maximal on the fourth postoperative day[116] and gradually decreases as bowel adaptation occurs. This adaptation involves both mucosal and motility change. An increase in intestinal transit time is seen in these patients.[117] Gastric emptying of solids is found to be slower in ileostomy patients as compared to controls.[118] Individuals who have an ileorectal anastomosis after subtotal colectomy do remarkably well in terms of bowel function. These patients have three to five stools on average during the day and one bowel movement at night.[119,120]

**RESTORATIVE PROCTOCOLECTOMY.** In patients with ulcerative colitis and familial adenomatous polyposis, complete resection of the colon and rectum is necessary to cure or prevent disease. Restorative proctocolectomy with formation of a neorectum using an ileal pouch has enabled definitive treatment in these patients without the need for permanent ileostomy. A folded loop of terminal ileum is fashioned into a pouch, in the most commonly performed J pouch, and anastomosed to the anus (Fig. 25.18). Most patients experience excellent results after this procedure.

Numerous studies have evaluated motility after restorative proctocolectomy. Intestinal transit has been demonstrated to be prolonged in patients after pouch surgery as compared to controls or patients with ileostomies.[121] However, small bowel

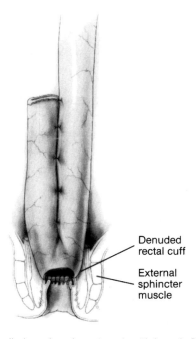

**FIGURE 25.18.** Ileal-pouch anal anastomosis with J pouch. Reproduced with permission from Gordon P, Nivatvongs S. Principles and practice of surgery for the colon, rectum, and anus. St. Louis (MO): Quality Medical Publishing; 1999.

transit time does not appear to be different in those with good versus poor pouch function,[122] indicating that more rapid small bowel transit may not be etiologic in poor pouch function. Normal contractile wave patterns do not appear to progress from the distal small bowel to the pouch.[123,124] Instead, there are two main motor responses of the pouch. As the pouch fills, long-duration waves of contraction occur, and the frequency and intensity often increase with further filling and decrease with evacuation (Fig. 25.19).[125–127] The second wave pattern consists of lower-amplitude rhythmic contraction waves.[125,128] These waves are found more commonly in

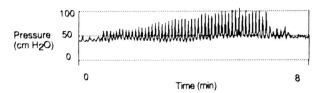

**FIGURE 25.19.** Ambulatory pouch and anal pressure recordings demonstrating a brief period of high-amplitude pouch contractions accompanied by a fall in anal pressure indicative of reflex inhibition of the internal anal sphincter. Reproduced with permission from Levitt M, Kamm K, van der Sijp J, Nicholls R. Ambulatory pouch and anal motility inpatients with ileo-anal reservoirs. Int J Colorectal Dis 1994;9:40–4.

individuals with poor pouch function. The normal contractile waves of the distal ileum are suppressed in the pouch as it fills, allowing the pouch to distend and function as a reservoir. As volume and pressure in the pouch increase and long-duration waves increase in frequency, the patient experiences the urge to evacuate. The external anal sphincter relaxes and the pouch empties, largely by Valsalva's maneuver.[129] Incomplete emptying may be associated with incontinence. Patients with poor pouch function may have a reduction in pouch compliance. Patients with poor function have been shown to have lower maximum tolerated volumes, lower volumes causing urgency, and baseline pressures above normal as compared to individuals with good pouch function.[125] The threshold volume of the pouch, the volume at which the large-amplitude propulsive waves appear, has been found to be correlated with stool frequency.[129] Diminished compliance may occur after pelvic sepsis or with pouchitis.

## Anorectal Procedures

### Anorectal Motility

The rectum is a highly compliant structure, and its distensibility functions critically in maintaining continence. The rectum is usually empty. With filling and distention, the rectoanal inhibitory reflex is initiated and the internal anal sphincter relaxes, allowing a tiny amount of rectal content to reach the transitional zone in the proximal anal canal. Sensory receptors in this area facilitate the differentiation of rectal content (ie, gas versus stool), and a conscious decision is then made regarding evacuation.[130] If the decision to evacuate is made, relaxation of the internal and external sphincters and the puborectalis occurs in conjunction with rectal contraction, and defecation occurs. This is aided by squatting and straining.

### Rectal Resections

Low anterior resection (LAR) of the rectum and anastomosis of the proximal colon to the distal rectum is a frequently performed procedure for rectal carcinoma and is commonly associated with alterations in continence, ranging from occasional inadvertent passage of flatus to frank incontinence of stool. Patients may also experience urgency and frequency. The etiology of the altered continence is multifactorial.[131] In LAR, the anastomosis is made between relatively noncompliant sigmoid colon and the more compliant rectal stump. The length of the rectum remaining is thought by most authors to be important in maintenance of normal continence.[132–134] The longer the length of normally com-

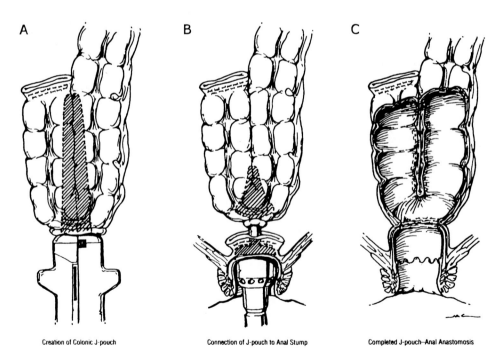

Creation of Colonic J-pouch     Connection of J-pouch to Anal Stump     Completed J-pouch–Anal Anastomosis

**FIGURE 25.20.** Coloanal J-pouch construction and pouch-anal anastomosis. **A**, The colon is folded in a J configuration and the stapler is passed through the apex of the pouch. **B**, The anvil of the stapler is secured at the apex of the pouch with a purse-string suture and the stapler is passed through the anus. **C**, Completed anastomosis. Reproduced with permission from Read T, Kodner I. Proctectomy and coloanal anastomosis for rectal cancer. Arch Surg 1999;134:670–7. Copyrighted 1999, American Medical Association.

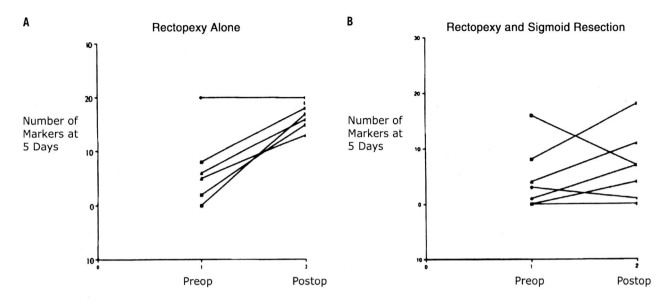

**FIGURE 25.21.** The number of colonic markers at 5 days in patients before and after surgical treatment. **A**, Rectopexy alone. **B**, Rectopexy plus sigmoid resection. Reproduced with permission from McKee R, Lauder J, Poon F, et al. A prospective randomized study of abdominal rectopexy with and without sigmoidectomy in rectal prolapse. Surg Gynecol Obstet 1992;174:145–8.

pliant rectal stump remaining, the more normal the function. Anal sphincter function may be abnormal after LAR. The volume required in the neorectum to elicit maximum inhibition of the anal sphincter has been found to be reduced after LAR at 3 months and 1 year postoperatively.[135] Anal resting pressures have been found by some authors to be decreased after LAR.[135,136] This may be attributable to direct injury to the sphincter from the insertion of the circular stapler during the anastomosis.

The creation of a colonic J pouch after ultra-low anterior resections or coloanal anastomosis has been advocated (Fig. 25.20). Creation of a 5- to 7-cm J pouch of sigmoid or descending colon has been found to improve function after rectal resection, with a decrease in stool frequency and improvements in continence as compared to those with a straight coloanal anastomosis. These differences, however, disappear over 6 to 12 months. The colonic pouch is thought to assume the reservoir function of the rectum, allowing distention without increases in intraluminal pressure, improving frequency and continence.[131,137–140]

### Rectal Prolapse

Severe constipation is a frequently reported complication of abdominal procedures for rectal prolapse. An increase in difficulty with defecation is generally reported after abdominal rectopexy without resection (Fig. 25.21)[141–146] In the Ripstein rectopexy, the rectum is mobilized and then suspended with mesh and fixed to the sacrum. The reason for the increased rate of constipation with this procedure is unclear. The correction of prolapse without resection may lead to redundancy of the sigmoid colon and kinking of the rectosigmoid junction, mechanically impairing defecation. The division of the lateral ligaments of the rectum during rec-

topexy may worsen constipation because of denervation of the rectum. In a study comparing a small group of patients after rectopexy with or without division of the lateral ligaments, those with ligament division experienced significantly more constipation and demonstrated a significantly increased rectal electrical sensory threshold.[147] Because of this, in general, when patients describe constipation preoperatively, treatment for prolapse should include a bowel resection.[148]

## SUMMARY

Postoperative motility disorders are extremely common, with transient disorders affecting nearly all patients undergoing laparotomy. Long-term alterations in gastrointestinal motility may be associated with a number of surgical procedures and reflect altered structure and function related to the specific operation performed. The variable impact of surgical procedures on motility in part reflects the tremendous adaptability of the gastrointestinal tract. This adaptation may be affected by preoperative dysfunction. More research is needed to develop a full understanding of the effect of surgery on motility and to improve both the treatment and prevention of postoperative motility disorders.

### REFERENCES

1. Livingston EH, Passaro EP Jr. Postoperative ileus. Dig Dis Sci 1990;35:121–32.
2. Resnick J, Greenwald DA, Brandt LJ. Delayed gastric emptying and postoperative ileus after nongastric abdominal surgery: part I. Am J Gastroenterol 1997;92:751–62.
3. Resnick J, Greenwald DA, Brandt LJ. Delayed gastric emptying and postoperative ileus after nongastric abdominal surgery: part II. Am J Gastroenterol 1997;92:934–40.

4. Tollesson PO, Cassuto J, Rimback G. Patterns of propulsive motility in the human colon after abdominal operations. Eur J Surg 1992;158:233–6.

5. Woods JH, Erickson LW, Condon RE, et al. Postoperative ileus: a colonic problem? Surgery 1978;84:527–33.

6. Schippers E, Holscher AH, Bollschweiler E, Siewert JR. Return of interdigestive motor complex after abdominal surgery. End of postoperative ileus? Dig Dis Sci 1991;36:621–6.

7. Sagar PM, Kruegener G, MacFie J. Nasogastric intubation and elective abdominal surgery. Br J Surg 1992;79:1127–31.

8. Nathan BN, Pain JA. Nasogastric suction after elective abdominal surgery: a randomised study. Ann R Coll Surg Engl 1991;73:291–4.

9. Bauer JJ, Gelernt IM, Salky BA, Kreel I. Is routine postoperative nasogastric decompression really necessary? Ann Surg 1985;201:233–6.

10. Olesen KL, Birch M, Bardram L, Burcharth F. Value of nasogastric tube after colorectal surgery. Acta Chir Scand 1984;150:251–3.

11. Reasbeck PG, Rice ML, Herbison GP. Nasogastric intubation after intestinal resection. Surg Gynecol Obstet 1984;158:354–8.

12. Wolff BG, Pembeton JH, van Heerden JA, et al. Elective colon and rectal surgery without nasogastric decompression. A prospective, randomized trial. Ann Surg 1989;209:670–3.

13. Cheatham ML, Chapman WC, Key SP, Sawyers JL. A meta-analysis of selective versus routine nasogastric decompression after elective laparotomy. Ann Surg 1995;221:469–76.

14. Binderow SR, Cohen SM, Wexner SD, Nogueras JJ. Must early postoperative oral intake be limited to laparoscopy? Dis Colon Rectum 1994;37:584–9.

15. Ortiz H, Armendariz P, Yarnoz C. Is early postoperative feeding feasible in elective colon and rectal surgery? Int J Colorectal Dis 1996;11:119–21.

16. Reissman P, Teoh TA, Cohen SM, et al. Is early oral feeding safe after elective colorectal surgery? A prospective randomized trial. Ann Surg 1995;222:73–7.

17. Stewart BT, Woods RJ, Collopy BT, et al. Early feeding after elective open colorectal resections: a prospective randomized trial. Aust N Z J Surg 1998;68:125–8.

18. Hartsell PA, Frazee RC, Harrison JB, Smith RW. Early postoperative feeding after elective colorectal surgery. Arch Surg 1997;132:518–20.

19. Ferraz AA, Cowles VE, Condon RE, et al. Nonopioid analgesics shorten the duration of postoperative ileus. Am Surg 1995;61:1079–83.

20. Ingram DM, Catchpole BN. Effect of opiates on gastroduodenal motility following surgical operation. Dig Dis Sci 1981;26:989–92.

21. Cali RL, Meade PG, Swanson MS, Freeman C. Effect of morphine and incision length on bowel function after colectomy. Dis Colon Rectum 2000;43:163–8.

22. Wattwil M. Postoperative pain relief and gastrointestinal motility. Acta Chir Scand Suppl 1989;550:140–5.

23. Ingram DM, Sheiner HJ. Postoperative gastric emptying. Br J Surg 1981;68:572–6.

24. Nimmo WS, Heading RC, Wilson J, et al. Inhibition of gastric emptying and drug absorption by narcotic analgesics. Br J Clin Pharmacol 1975;2:509–13.

25. Aitkenhead AR. Anaesthesia and bowel surgery. Br J Anaesth 1984;56:95–101.

26. Schang JC, Hemond M, Hebert M, Pilote M. How does morphine work on colonic motility? An electromyographic study in the human left and sigmoid colon. Life Sci 1986;38:671–6.

27. Nitschke LF, Schlosser CT, Berg RL, et al. Does patient-controlled analgesia achieve better control of pain and fewer adverse effects than intramuscular analgesia? A prospective randomized trial. Arch Surg 1996;131:417–23.

28. Cheng G, Cassissi C, Drexler PG, et al. Salsalate, morphine, and postoperative ileus. Am J Surg 1996;171:85–8.

29. LaRosa JA, Saywell RM Jr, Zollinger TW, et al. The incidence of adynamic ileus in postcesarean patients. Patient-controlled analgesia versus intramuscular analgesia. J Reprod Med 1993;38:293–300.

30. Petros JG, Realica R, Ahmad S, et al. Patient-controlled analgesia and prolonged ileus after uncomplicated colectomy. Am J Surg 1995;170:371–4.

31. Stanley BK, Noble MJ, Gilliland C, et al. Comparison of patient-controlled analgesia versus intramuscular narcotics in resolution of postoperative ileus after radical retropubic prostatectomy. J Urol 1993;150:1434–6.

32. Steinbrook RA. Epidural anesthesia and gastrointestinal motility. Anesth Analg 1998;86:837–44.

33. Rawal N, Sjostrand U, Christoffersson E, et al. Comparison of intramuscular and epidural morphine for postoperative analgesia in the grossly obese: influence on postoperative ambulation and pulmonary function. Anesth Analg 1984;63:583–92.

34. Bredtmann RD, Herden HN, Teichmann W, et al. Epidural analgesia in colonic surgery: results of a randomized prospective study. Br J Surg 1990;77:638–42.

35. Liu SS, Carpenter RL, Mackey DC, et al. Effects of perioperative analgesic technique on rate of recovery after colon surgery. Anesthesiology 1995;83:757–65.

36. Wattwil M, Thoren T, Hennerdal S, Garvill JE. Epidural analgesia with bupivacaine reduces postoperative paralytic ileus after hysterectomy. Anesth Analg 1989;68:353–8.

37. Scheinin B, Asantila R, Orko R. The effect of bupivacaine and morphine on pain and bowel function after colonic surgery. Acta Anaesthesiol Scand 1987;31:161–4.

38. Waldhausen JH, Schirmer BD. The effect of ambulation on recovery from postoperative ileus. Ann Surg 1990;212:671–7.

39. Graber JN, Schulte WJ, Condon RE, Cowles VE. Relationship of duration of postoperative ileus to extent and site of operative dissection. Surgery 1982;92:87–92.

40. Lindquist B. Propulsive gastrointestinal motility related to retroperitoneal irritation. An experimental study in the rat. Acta Chir Scand Suppl 1968;384:5–53.

41. Davies W, Kollmorgen CF, Tu QM, et al. Laparoscopic colectomy shortens postoperative ileus in a canine model. Surgery 1997;121:550–5.

42. Hotokezaka M, Combs MJ, Schirmer BD. Recovery of gastrointestinal motility following open versus laparoscopic colon resection in dogs. Dig Dis Sci 1996;41:705–10.

43. Bohm B, Milsom JW, Fazio VW. Postoperative intestinal motility following conventional and laparoscopic intestinal surgery. Arch Surg 1995;130:415–9.

44. Chen HH, Wexner SD, Iroatulam AJ, et al. Laparoscopic colectomy compares favorably with colectomy by laparotomy for reduction of postoperative ileus. Dis Colon Rectum 2000;43:61–5.

45. Milsom JW, Bohm B, Hammerhofer KA, et al. A prospective, randomized trial comparing laparoscopic versus conventional techniques in colorectal cancer surgery: a preliminary report. J Am Coll Surg 1998;187:46–54.

46. Chen HH, Iroatulam AJ, Alabaz O, et al. Laparoscopic colectomy is superior to laparotomy for reduction of disability in patients with colorectal adenoma. Chang Keng I Hsueh 1999;22:586–92.

47. Schmitt SL, Cohen SM, Wexner SD, et al. Does laparoscopic-assisted ileal pouch anal anastomosis reduce the length of hospitalization? Int J Colorectal Dis 1994;9:134–7.

48. Wexner SD, Johansen OB, Nogueras JJ, Jagelman DG. Laparoscopic total abdominal colectomy. A prospective trial. Dis Colon Rectum 1992;35:651–5.

49. Disbrow EA, Bennett HL, Owings JT. Effect of preoperative suggestion on postoperative gastrointestinal motility. West J Med 1993;158:488–92.

50. Bungard TJ, Kale-Pradhan PB. Prokinetic agents for the treatment of postoperative ileus in adults: a review of the literature. Pharmacotherapy 1999;19:416–23.

51. Longo WE, Vernava AM, III. Prokinetic agents for lower gastrointestinal motility disorders. Dis Colon Rectum 1993;36:696–708.

52. Ponec RJ, Saunders MD, Kimmey MB. Neostigmine for the treatment of acute colonic pseudo-obstruction. N Engl J Med 1999;341:137–41.

53. Stephenson BM, Morgan AR, Drake N, et al. Parasympathomimetic decompression of acute colonic pseudo-obstruction [letter]. Lancet 1993;342:1181–2.

54. Turegano-Fuentes F, Munoz-Jimenez F, Valle-Hernandez E, et al. Early resolution of Ogilvie's syndrome with intravenous neostigmine: a simple, effective treatment. Dis Colon Rectum 1997;40:1353–7.

55. Andreollo NA, Earlam RJ. Heller's myotomy for achalasia: is an added anti-reflux procedure necessary? Br J Surg 1987;74:765–9.

56. Fok M, Cheng SW, Wong J. Pyloroplasty versus no drainage in gastric replacement of the esophagus. Am J Surg 1991;162:447–52.

57. Manjari R, Padhy AK, Chattopadhyay TK. Emptying of the intrathoracic stomach using three different pylorus drainage procedures—results of a comparative study. Surg Today 1996;26:581–5.

58. Finley FJ, Lamy A, Clifton J, et al. Gastrointestinal function following esophagectomy for malignancy. Am J Surg 1995;169:471–5.

59. Hocking MP, Maher JW, Woodward ER. Definitive surgical therapy for incapacitating "gas-bloat" syndrome. Am Surg 1982;48:131–3.

60. Bushkin FL, Neustein CL, Parker TH, Woodward ER. Nissen fundoplication for reflux peptic esophagitis. Ann Surg 1977;185:672–7.

61. Woodward ER, Thomas HF, McAlhany JC. Comparison of crural repair and Nissen fundoplication in the treatment of esophageal hiatus hernia with peptic esophagitis. Ann Surg 1971;173:782–92.

62. Low DE. Management of the problem patient after antireflux surgery. Gastroenterol Clin North Am 1994;23:371–89.

63. Lundell LR, Myers JC, Jamieson GG. Delayed gastric emptying and its relationship to symptoms of "gas bloat" after antireflux surgery. Eur J Surg 1994;160:161–6.

64. Primrose JN, Johnston D. Somatostatin analogue SMS 201-995 (octreotide) as a possible solution to the dumping syndrome after gastrectomy or vagotomy. Br J Surg 1989;76:140–4.

65. Mackie CR, Jenkins SA, Hartley MN. Treatment of severe postvagotomy/postgastrectomy symptoms with the somatostatin analogue octreotide. Br J Surg 1991;78:1338–43.

66. Soybel DI, Zinner MJ. Complications following gastric operation. Maingot's abdominal operations. 10th ed. Stamford (CT): Appelton & Lange, 1997. p. 1029–56.

67. McCallum RW, Polepalle SC, Schirmer B. Completion gastrectomy for refractory gastroparesis following surgery for peptic ulcer disease. Long-term follow-up with subjective and objective parameters. Dig Dis Sci 1991;36:1556–61.

68. Forstner-Barthell AW, Murr MM, Nitecki S, et al. Near-total completion gastrectomy for severe postvagotomy gastric stasis: analysis of early and long-term results in 62 patients. J Gastrointest Surg 1999;3:15–21.

69. Eckhauser FE, Knol JA, Raper SA, Guice KS. Completion gastrectomy for postsurgical gastroparesis syndrome. Preliminary results with 15 patients. Ann Surg 1988;208:345–53.

70. Eckhauser FE, Conrad M, Knol JA, et al. Safety and long-term durability of completion gastrectomy in 81 patients with postsurgical gastroparesis syndrome. Am Surg 1998;64:711–6.

71. Karlstrom L, Kelly KA. Roux-Y gastrectomy for chronic gastric atony. Am J Surg 1989;157:44–9.

72. Richter HM III, Kelly KA. Effect of transection and pacing on human jejunal pacesetter potentials. Gastroenterology 1986;91:1380–5.

73. Karlstrom LH, Soper NJ, Kelly KA, Phillips SF. Ectopic jejunal pacemakers and enterogastric reflux after Roux gastrectomy: effect of intestinal pacing. Surgery 1989;106:486–95.

74. Herrington JL Jr, Scott HW Jr, Sawyers JL. Experience with vagotomy—antrectomy and Roux-en-Y gastrojejunostomy in surgical treatment of duodenal, gastric, and stomal ulcers. Ann Surg 1984;199:590–7.

75. Britton JP, Johnston D, Ward DC, et al. Gastric emptying and clinical outcome after Roux-en-Y diversion. Br J Surg 1987;74:900–4.

76. Petrakis J, Vassilakis JS, Karkavitsas N, et al. Enhancement of gastric emptying of solids by erythromycin in patients with Roux-en-Y gastrojejunostomy. Arch Surg 1998;133:709–14.

77. Hocking MP, Brunson ME, Vogel SB. Effect of various prokinetic agents on post Roux-en-Y gastric emptying. Experimental and clinical observations. Dig Dis Sci 1988;33:1282–7.

78. Tu BN, Kelly KA. Motility disorders after Roux-en-Y gastrojejunostomy. Obes Surg 1994;4:219–26.

79. Noh S. Improvement of the roux limb function using a new type of "uncut Roux" limb. Am J Surg 2000;180:37–40.

80. Mon RA, Cullen JJ. Standard Roux-en-Y gastrojejunostomy vs. "uncut" Roux-en-Y gastrojejunostomy: a matched cohort study. J Gastrointest Surg 2000;4:298–303.

81. Miedema BW, Kelly KA. The Roux stasis syndrome. Treatment by pacing and prevention by use of an 'uncut' Roux limb. Arch Surg 1992;127:295–300.

82. Ritchie WP Jr. Alkaline reflux gastritis. An objective assessment of its diagnosis and treatment. Ann Surg 1980;192:288–98.

83. Ritchie WP Jr. Alkaline reflux gastritis. Gastroenterol Clin North Am 1994;23:281–94.

84. Ritchie WP Jr. Postoperative alkaline reflux gastritis: a prospective clinical study of etiology and treatment. Scand J Gastroenterol Suppl 1981;67:233–5.

85. Sawyers JL. Management of postgastrectomy syndromes. Am J Surg 1990;159:8–14.

86. Carvajal SH, Mulvihill SJ. Postgastrectomy syndromes: dumping and diarrhea. Gastroenterol Clin North Am 1994;23:261–79.

87. Hartley MN, Mackie CR. Gastric adaptive relaxation and symptoms after vagotomy. Br J Surg 1991;78:24–7.

88. Parr NJ, Grime S, Brownless S, et al. Relationship between gastric emptying of liquid and postvagotomy diarrhoea [published erratum appears in Br J Surg 1988;75:500]. Br J Surg 1988;75:279–82.

89. Allan JG, Russell RI. Cholestyramine in treatment of postvagotomy diarrhoea—double-blind controlled trial. BMJ 1977;1:674–6.

90. Allan JG, Russell RI. Proceedings: double-blind controlled trial of cholestyramine in the treatment of post-vagotomy diarrhoea. Gut 1975;16:830.

91. Allan JG, Gerskowitch VP, Russell RI. The role of bile acids in the pathogenesis of postvagotomy diarrhoea. Br J Surg 1974;61:516–8.

92. Yeo CJ, Cameron JL, Sohn TA, et al. Six hundred fifty consecutive pancreaticoduodenectomies in the 1990s: pathology, complications, and outcomes. Ann Surg 1997;226:248–57.

93. Yamaguchi K, Tanaka M, Chijiiwa K, et al. Early and late complications of pylorus-preserving pancreatoduodenectomy in Japan 1998. J Hepatobil Pancreat Surg 1999;6:303–11.

94. Berge Henegouwen MI, Van Gulik TM, Moojen TM, et al. Gastrointestinal motility after pancreatoduodenectomy. Scand J Gastroenterol Suppl 1998;225:47–55.

95. Grace PA, Pitt HA, Longmire WP. Pylorus preserving pancreatoduodenectomy: an overview. Br J Surg 1990;77:968–74.

96. Berge Henegouwen MI, Van Gulik TM, DeWit LT, et al. Delayed gastric emptying after standard pancreaticoduodenectomy versus pylorus-preserving pancreaticoduodenectomy: an analysis of 200 consecutive patients. J Am Coll Surg 1997;185:373–9.

97. Kingsnorth AN, Berg JD, Gray MR. A novel reconstructive technique for pylorus-preserving pancreaticoduodenectomy: avoidance of early postoperative gastric stasis. Ann R Coll Surg Engl 1993;75:38–42.

98. Horstmann O, Becker H, Post S, Nustede R. Is delayed gastric emptying following pancreaticoduodenectomy related to pylorus preservation? Langenbecks Arch Surg 1999;384:354–9.

99. Fabre JM, Burgel JS, Navarro F, et al. Delayed gastric emptying after pancreaticoduodenectomy and pancreaticogastrostomy. Eur J Surg 1999;165:560–5.

100. Otterson MF, Sarr MG. Normal physiology of small intestinal motility. Surg Clin North Am 1993;73:1173–92.

101. Sarna SK. Cyclic motor activity; migrating motor complex: 1985. Gastroenterology 1985;89:894–913.

102. Johnson CP, Sarna SK, Zhu YR, et al. Delayed gastroduodenal emptying is an important mechanism for control of intestinal transit in short-gut syndrome. Am J Surg 1996;171:90–5.

103. Cullen JJ, Eagon JC, Hould FS, et al. Ectopic jejunal pacemakers after jejunal transection and their relationship to transit. Am J Physiol 1995;268:G959–67.

104. Telford GL, Walgenbach-Telford S, Sarna SK. Pathophysiology of small intestinal motility. Surg Clin North Am 1993;73:1193–9.

105. Hart SC, Nguyen-Tu BL, Hould FS, et al. Restoration of myoelectrical propagation across a jejunal transection using microsurgical anastomosis. J Gastrointest Surg 1999;3:524–32.

106. Thompson JS, Edgar J. Poth Memorial Lecture. Surgical aspects of the short-bowel syndrome. Am J Surg 1995;170:532–6.

107. Quigley EM, Thompson JS. The motor response to intestinal resection: motor activity in the canine small intestine following distal resection. Gastroenterology 1993;105:791–8.

108. Thompson JS, Quigley EM, Adrian TE. Factors affecting outcome following proximal and distal intestinal resection in the dog: an examination of the relative roles of mucosal adaptation, motility, luminal factors, and enteric peptides. Dig Dis Sci 1999;44:63–74.

109. Pigot F, Messing B, Chaussade S, et al. Severe short bowel syndrome with a surgically reversed small bowel segment. Dig Dis Sci 1990;35:137–44.

110. Scolapio JS, Camilleri M, Fleming CR. Gastrointestinal motility considerations in patients with short-bowel syndrome. Dig Dis 1997;15:253–62.

111. Schmidt T, Pfeiffer A, Hackelsberger N, et al. Effect of intestinal resection on human small bowel motility. Gut 1996;38:859–63.

112. Remington M, Malagelada JR, Zinsmeister A, Fleming CR. Abnormalities in gastrointestinal motor activity in patients with short bowels: effect of a synthetic opiate. Gastroenterology 1983;85:629–36.

113. Tilson MD. Pathophysiology and treatment of short bowel syndrome. Surg Clin North Am 1980;60:1273–84.

114. Roberts JP, Benson MJ, Rogers J, et al. Characterization of distal colonic motility in early postoperative period and effect of colonic anastomosis. Dig Dis Sci 1994;39:1961–7.

115. Fich A, Steadman CJ, Phillips SF, et al. Ileocolonic transit does not change after right hemicolectomy. Gastroenterology 1992;103:794–9.

116. Tang CL, Yunos A, Leong AP, et al. Ileostomy output in the early postoperative period. Br J Surg 1995;82:607.

117. Fallingborg J, Christensen LA, Ingeman-Nielsen M, et al. Gastrointestinal pH and transit times in healthy subjects with ileostomy. Aliment Pharmacol Ther 1990;4:247–53.

118. Robertson MD, Mathers JC. Gastric emptying rate of solids is reduced in a group of ileostomy patients. Dig Dis Sci 2000;45:1285–92.

119. Madden MV, Neale KF, Nicholls RJ, et al. Comparison of morbidity and function after colectomy with ileorectal anastomosis or restorative proctocolectomy for familial adenomatous polyposis. Br J Surg 1991;78:789–92.

120. van Duijvendijk P, Slors JF, Taat CW, et al. Functional outcome after colectomy and ileorectal anastomosis compared with proctocolectomy and ileal pouch-anal anastomosis in familial adenomatous polyposis. Ann Surg 1999;230:648–54.

121. Soper NJ, Orkin BA, Kelly KA, et al. Gastrointestinal transit after proctocolectomy with ileal pouch-anal anastomosis or ileostomy. J Surg Res 1989;46:300–5.

122. Goldberg PA, Kamm MA, Nicholls RJ, et al. Contribution of gastrointestinal transit and pouch characteristics in determining pouch function. Gut 1997;40:790–3.

123. Groom JS, Kamm MA, Nicholls RJ. Relationship of small bowel motility to ileoanal reservoir function. Gut 1994;35:523–9.

124. Stryker SJ, Borody TJ, Phillips SF, et al. Motility of the small intestine after proctocolectomy and ileal pouch- anal anastomosis. Ann Surg 1985;201:351–6.

125. Levitt MD, Kamm MA, Groom J, et al. Ileoanal pouch compliance and motor function. Br J Surg 1992;79:126–8.

126. Taylor BM, Cranley B, Kelly KA, et al. A clinico-physiological comparison of ileal pouch-anal and straight ileoanal anastomoses. Ann Surg 1983;198:462–8.

127. Levitt MD, Kuan M. The physiology of ileo-anal pouch function. Am J Surg 1998;176:384–9.

128. Levitt MD, Kamm MA, van DS Jr, Nicholls RJ. Ambulatory pouch and anal motility in patients with ileo-anal reservoirs. Int J Colorectal Dis 1994;9:40–44.

129. O'Connell PR, Pemberton JH, Kelly KA. Motor function of the ileal J pouch and its relation to clinical outcome after ileal pouch-anal anastomosis. World J Surg 1987;11:735–41.

130. Uher EM, Swash M. Sacral reflexes: physiology and clinical application. Dis Colon Rectum 1998;41:1165–77.

131. Williams N, Seow-Choen F. Physiological and functional outcome following ultra-low anterior resection with colon pouch-anal anastomosis. Br J Surg 1998;85:1029–35.

132. Lewis WG, Martin IG, Williamson ME, et al. Why do some patients experience poor functional results after anterior resection of the rectum for carcinoma? Dis Colon Rectum 1995;38:259–63.

133. Lewis WG, Holdsworth PJ, Stephenson BM, et al. Role of the rectum in the physiological and clinical results of coloanal and colorectal anastomosis after anterior resection for rectal carcinoma. Br J Surg 1992;79:1082–6.

134. Karanjia ND, Schache DJ, Heald RJ. Function of the distal rectum after low anterior resection for carcinoma. Br J Surg 1992;79:114–6.

135. Williamson ME, Lewis WG, Finan PJ, et al. Recovery of physiologic and clinical function after low anterior resection of the rectum for carcinoma: myth or reality? Dis Colon Rectum 1995;38:411–8.

136. Horgan PG, O'Connell PR, Shinkwin CA, Kirwan WO. Effect of anterior resection on anal sphincter function. Br J Surg 1989;76:783–6.

137. Lazorthes F, Fages P, Chiotasso P, et al. Resection of the rectum with construction of a colonic reservoir and colo-anal anastomosis for carcinoma of the rectum. Br J Surg 1986;73:136–8.

138. Parc R, Tiret E, Frileux P, et al. Resection and colo-anal anastomosis with colonic reservoir for rectal carcinoma. Br J Surg 1986;73:139–41.

139. Nicholls RJ, Lubowski DZ, Donaldson DR. Comparison of colonic reservoir and straight colo-anal reconstruction after rectal excision. Br J Surg 1988;75:318–20.

140. Berger A, Tiret E, Parc R, et al. Excision of the rectum with colonic J pouch-anal anastomosis for adenocarcinoma of the low and mid rectum. World J Surg 1992;16:470–7.

141. Scaglia M, Fasth S, Hallgren T, et al. Abdominal rectopexy for rectal prolapse. Influence of surgical technique on functional outcome. Dis Colon Rectum 1994;37:805–13.

142. Holmstrom B, Broden G, Dolk A. Results of the Ripstein operation in the treatment of rectal prolapse and internal rectal procidentia. Dis Colon Rectum 1986;29:845–8.

143. Launer DP, Fazio VW, Weakley FL, et al. The Ripstein procedure: a 16-year experience. Dis Colon Rectum 1982;25:41–5.

144. Madden MV, Kamm MA, Nicholls RJ, et al. Abdominal rectopexy for complete prolapse: prospective study evaluating changes in symptoms and anorectal function. Dis Colon Rectum 1992;35:48–55.

145. Tjandra JJ, Fazio VW, Church JM, et al. Ripstein procedure is an effective treatment for rectal prolapse without constipation. Dis Colon Rectum 1993;36:501–7.

146. Luukkonen P, Mikkonen U, Jarvinen H. Abdominal rectopexy with sigmoidectomy vs. rectopexy alone for rectal prolapse: a prospective, randomized study. Int J Colorectal Dis 1992;7:219–22.

147. Speakman CT, Madden MV, Nicholls RJ, Kamm MA. Lateral ligament division during rectopexy causes constipation but prevents recurrence: results of a prospective randomized study. Br J Surg 1991;78:1431–3.

148. Eu KW, Seow-Choen F. Functional problems in adult rectal prolapse and controversies in surgical treatment. Br J Surg 1997;84:904–11.

# CHAPTER 26

# Effect of Sleep and Circadian Rhythms

*William C. Orr*

It is obvious that cyclic behavioral patterns such as food ingestion have a significant impact on gastrointestinal (GI) functioning. Most notable is eating, which markedly affects intestinal motor functioning. Eating tends to occur at periodic intervals during the daytime (diurnal) hours, and virtually none occurs during sleep. There is then an obvious 24-hour, or circadian, pattern to human eating behavior and the demands that behavior places on the functioning of the GI system. Although circadian rhythms have been well studied in a variety of physiologic systems, sparse data are available in the GI system and, in particular, intestinal motor functioning.

Although, until recently, circadian physiology has not been widely applied to problems of clinical medicine, some circadian patterns have been well known to clinicians for years. A good example would be the circadian pattern of cortisol secretion and the 24-hour pattern of body temperature with the peak temperature occurring in the late afternoon and the troth of the temperature cycle in the early morning hours. This cycle exhibits a profound effect on the physiology and behavior of every warm-blooded (homeothermic) mammal. For example, it is well established that mental alertness and performance effectiveness are in phase with the circadian temperature cycle. The temperature rhythm has also been shown to be critically involved in regulating sleep and waking. Even within sleep, the temperature cycle has been shown to be involved in the regulation of a specific stage of sleep, namely, rapid eye movement (REM) sleep.[1]

Profound physiologic changes occur during sleep to include marked alterations in cortical and autonomic functioning.[2] Electrocortical changes identify different stages of sleep to include four stages of non-REM (NREM) and REM sleep. Although NREM sleep is generally associated with a "slowing" of autonomic functioning such as respiration and heart rate, as well as a decrease in blood pressure, the regulation of several basic life functions is profoundly altered by REM sleep.[2] For example, the regulation of core body temperature during REM sleep is such that warm-blooded animals become poikilothermic. In addition, the control of a variety of respiratory functions is markedly altered during this unique stage of sleep. For example, REM sleep is associated with a marked depression in respiratory responsiveness to increases in arterial concentrations of carbon dioxide.

Given the complex interaction among cortical, autonomic, and myenteric neuronal functioning, it is not surprising that sleep would have substantial effects on various GI motor functions. Clinically, numerous GI symptoms are well known to be altered by or to occur exclusively during sleep. Perhaps the most commonly encountered nocturnal symptom is the epigastric pain of a patient with duodenal ulcer disease. Other peptic symptoms that manifest during sleep would include those related to nocturnal gastroesophageal reflux (GER) such as heartburn and angina-like chest pain. Nocturnal diarrhea is another symptom related to GI motor functioning, the occurrence of which during sleep would suggest the presence of organic, as opposed to functional, disease.

## SLEEP PHYSIOLOGY

### Determination of Sleep Stages

To determine the presence or absence of sleep and the various sleep stages and to correlate them with intestinal events, it is necessary to simultaneously record the intestinal parameter of interest with the electroencephalogram (EEG), electro-oculogram (EOG), and the submental electromyogram (EMG). This allows the assessment of intestinal physiologic events during sleep and the determination of any alterations in functioning that may be associated with the specific physiology of either NREM or REM sleep. The specific activity noted in the EEG, EOG, and EMG allows the determination of waking and the various stages of sleep.[2,3] Waking in the different stages of sleep is illustrated in Figures 26.1 to 26.5.

### Autonomic Changes During Sleep

These figures show that the primary change noted during different states of consciousness is in the EEG. Progressing from waking to stage III to IV sleep, progressive slowing of the EEG frequency and augmentation of the amplitude can be readily identified. Physiologically, this progression into sleep is associated with a generalized decrease in autonomic functioning; most notable are a slowing of the heart rate and respiration rate and a decrease in blood pressure.[2]

Rapid eye movement is associated with a unique pattern of physiologic activity (see Fig. 26.5). First, the EEG is a low-voltage, mixed-frequency EEG, which is more characteristic of waking than sleep. Second, there is the obvious presence of conjugate eye movements, which are indistinguishable

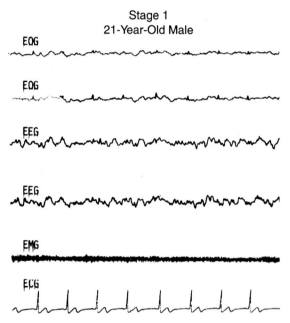

**FIGURE 26.2.** Stage 1 sleep. Note the absence of alpha activity and the predominance of theta (4–7 Hz) activity in the EEG and a reduction in the tonic activity of the chin EMG (time 20 seconds).

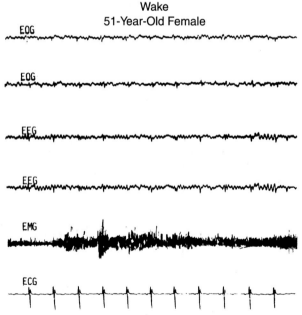

**FIGURE 26.1.** Polysomnographic (EOG, EEG, EMG, ECG) pattern of waking. Note the presence of alpha activity (8–10 Hz), the absence of eye movements, and tonic activity in the chin EMG (time 20 seconds). EOG, electro-oculogram; EEG, electroencephalogram; EMG, chin electromyogram; ECG, electrocardiogram.

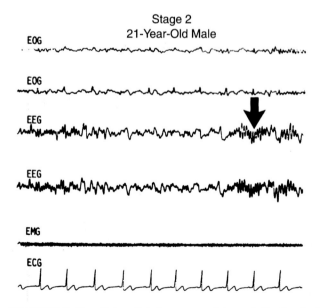

**FIGURE 26.3.** Stage 2 sleep. Note the presence of sleep spindles (bursts of 12–14 Hz activity) (time 20 seconds) in the EEG (*arrow*).

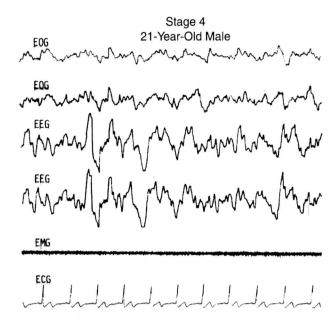

**FIGURE 26.4.** Stage 3 and 4 sleep. Note the predominance of high-voltage slowl-frequency (0.5–2 Hz) activity in the EEG. Stage 3 contains 20 to 50% of these EEG delta waves, and stage 4 contains 50% or greater in a 30-second or 1-minute epic of sleep (time 20 seconds).

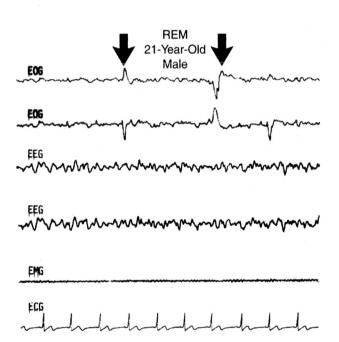

**FIGURE 26.5.** REM sleep. Note the presence of a low-voltage mixed-frequency EEG, conjugate eye movements (*arrows*), and diminished tonic activity in the EMG (time 20 seconds).

from waking ocular activity. Last, there is a profound inhibition of skeletal muscle activity, which prohibits movements during this stage of sleep. Research over the years has identified REM sleep as a unique physiologic state. For example, normal respiratory control mechanisms and temperature regulation are suspended during REM sleep.[2]

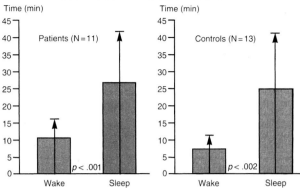

**FIGURE 26.6.** Acid clearance responses to 15 mL of acid infused into the distal esophagus during waking and sleep.

Any standard pressure, pH, or myoelectric recording can be accomplished readily in conjunction with polysomnographic monitoring. Discussion in this chapter relates to specific alterations in GI phenomena during sleep or as a function of a circadian rhythm.

## UPPER GASTROINTESTINAL FUNCTIONING DURING SLEEP

### Swallowing and Acid Clearance During Sleep

Swallowing is perhaps the single most obvious human function that is clearly related to intestinal motility. The swallow initiates the digestive process. It is obviously important in maintaining adequate nutrition, but swallowing also serves an important protective function since it is critical in facilitating the clearance of refluxed gastric contents.[4,5] Swallowing and the initiation of the peristaltic wave are necessary to producing both volume clearance and acid neutralization subsequent to GER.[5,6]

### Esophageal Motor Function During Sleep

The clearance of refluxed gastric contents is clearly dependent on adequate motor functioning of the pharynx and the esophagus. Although esophageal function does not appear to be altered during sleep, the swallowing frequency is markedly decreased.[7–9] Salivary flow is virtually nonexistent.[10] Studies by Orr and colleagues have shown that the clearance time of infused acid during sleep is significantly prolonged when compared with infusions in the waking state (Fig. 26.6).[9,11]

Esophageal motor function has not been shown to exhibit a circadian rhythmicity.[12] Lower esophageal sphincter (LES) pressure and peristaltic amplitudes were not shown to have any alteration when individuals were studied at 10 am or 10 pm (Fig. 26.7). Propagation data for the morning and the evening were similarly unaffected.

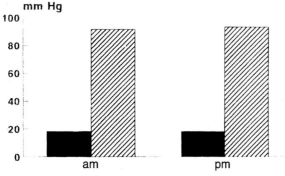

**FIGURE 26.7.** Circadian variation in esophageal function. Mean lower esophageal sphincter (LES) pressures and peristaltic amplitudes in normal volunteers studied at 10 am or 10 p.m. Adapted from Avots-Avotins AE, Ashworth WD, Stafford BD, Moore JG. Day and night esophageal motor function. Am J Gastroenterol 1990;85:683–5.

Recent studies have shown that the most common mechanism of GER is a transient relaxation of the LES.[13,14] These events occur relatively infrequently during sleep, but they have been shown to be most commonly associated with a transient arousal from sleep.[13,15] In normal volunteers and in patients with gastroesophageal reflux disease (GERD), most reflux events during sleep have been identified to occur in association with a brief arousal response.[13,15] The actual stimulus that initiates the transient relaxation response is as yet unknown. Although the majority of episodes of reflux are associated with transient arousal responses, reflux events can occur in the absence of an arousal response. This is shown in Figures 26.8 and 26.9. In Figure 26.8, the drop in esophageal pH can be seen to coincide with the transient arousal response, as documented by the movement artifact in the tracing, whereas the drop in pH in Figure 26.9 is noted to be without any alteration in the sleep tracing.

## Upper Esophageal Sphincter Functioning During Sleep

Very few studies have been done to describe the functioning of the upper esophageal sphincter (UES) during sleep since the discomfort associated with measuring this sphincter makes it very difficult to sleep. One recent study, however, has described minimal alteration in UES functioning during sleep, including REM sleep.[16] Only a modest decline in the resting pressure was noted. This observation is somewhat surprising in that the cricopharyngeus is a skeletal muscle, and if this finding can be verified, it would be one of the very few skeletal muscles in the body that does not show a substantial inhibition during REM sleep. From a purely behavioral standpoint, it makes sense that the UES does not decrease substantially during REM sleep since it provides protection of the upper airway and lungs from the aspiration of refluxed gastric contents.

## Gastric Motility and Gastric Emptying

Another measure of gastric motility, and gastric emptying, has been shown to have a marked circadian rhythm.[17] Gastric emptying studies done at 8 am and 8 pm show an appreciable slowing of gastric emptying in the evening hours (Fig. 26.10). By implication, these studies suggest a marked alteration in the drug absorption as a result of the rate of gastric emptying. Since relatively few drugs are absorbed in the stomach, the rate of gastric emptying into the small bowel would be ultimately controlled by the delivery of the drug to the absorptive areas of the small bowel. Thus, if rapid absorption of the drug is desired, it would be appropriate to administer the medication at a time when gastric emptying is most rapid (eg, in the morning). If, on the other hand, it is desired to have the peak effect of the drug delayed until the early morning hours, the late evening or bedtime drug administration would be most effective. For example, it is known that asthmatics frequently have nocturnal attacks, usually in the

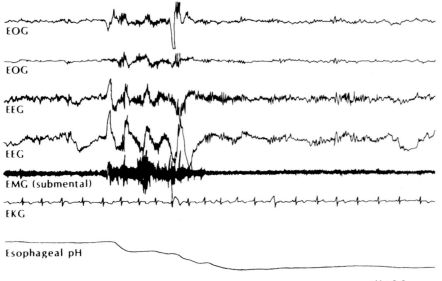

**FIGURE 26.8.** An episode of gastroesophageal reflux noted by the drop from esophageal pH to below 4 and associated with a brief arousal response. This is identified by the marked increase in the submental electromyogram (EMG) and the noted artifact in the other polygraphic recording channels. EOG, electro-oculogram; EEG, electroencephalogram; EKG, electrocardiogram.

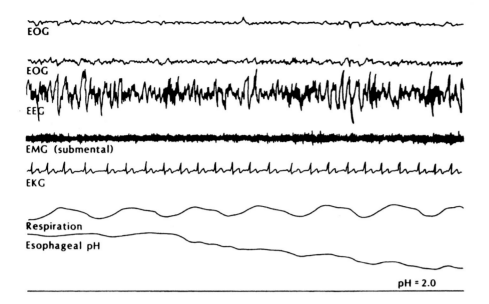

**FIGURE 26.9.** An episode of gastroesophageal reflux noted by the drop in pH below 4, which is not associated with any obvious arousal response in the polygraphic recording. EOG, electro-oculogram; EEG, electroencephalogram; EMG, electromyogram; EKG, electrocardiogram.

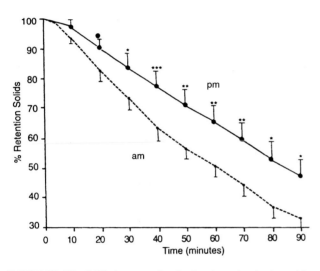

**FIGURE 26.10.** Solid-phase morning (am) and evening (pm) emptying curves. Significant differences in mean percentage retention values were noted at all timing intervals after 10 minutes (two-tailed paired $t$ test $p$ values: *.02 $< p > $.01; **.01 $< p > $.001; ***$< $.001). From Goo RH, Moore JG, Greenburg E, Alazraki NP. Circadian variation in gastric emptying of meals in humans. Gastroenterology 1987;93:515–8.

early morning hours, around 4 am. To time theophylline administration to reach a peak blood level at about that time, it would be best to delay the absorption as long as possible during the sleeping interval. This can be done by taking the medication just before bedtime.

Alterations in the electrogastrogram have been shown to be markedly altered during sleep.[18] This study demonstrated a marked decrease in the percentage of two to four cycle per minute (cpm) activity during NREM sleep. Of interest is the fact that the percentage of 2 to 4 cpm activity returned to nearly normal levels during REM sleep. These data suggest that central nervous system (CNS) arousal does seem to

"entrain" the normal pacemaker activity of the stomach. Another study has shown that patients with irritable bowel syndrome (IBS) fail to show a modulation in the amplitude or power of the gastric pacemaker during sleep.[19] Collectively, these data suggest that there are significant and important alterations in the gastric pacemaker modulated by sleep, and understanding these changes can give further understanding of normal and abnormal gastric physiology.

Also related to motility of the stomach, albeit somewhat remotely, is the mucosal susceptibility to injury. Moore and Goo have found some very interesting results in humans who were given four aspirins at 8 am and 8 pm.[20] The study found that damage to the gastric mucosa was actually 37% less in the evening, during the time gastric emptying was slowest. These are especially interesting data, but additional studies are necessary to explain the relationship between gastric emptying, motility, and mucosal susceptibility to injury. Similar studies need to be done at intervals that would allow a description of a complete circadian cycle of gastric emptying.

### Duodenal Motor Activity and Migrating Motor Complex

Finch and colleagues have described a relationship between sleep stage and duodenal motility, which probably reflect a periodicity in Phase 3 of the migrating motor complex (MMC).[21] This was not apparent with gastric motility, but they attribute this to the fact that the initiation of MMCs in the stomach appears to be somewhat less consistent when compared with those originating in the duodenum. In addition, the authors described a periodicity in the range of approximately 90 minutes shared by body movement and duodenal motor activity. They interpret this to reflect the control of these activities by a CNS mechanism that regulates other body functions in a 90-minute cycle.[22,23] In a study by David and colleagues, motor activity in the duodenum was monitored over a 24-hour period under freely ambulatory conditions and 10 healthy controls and in 10 patients with nonulcer dyspepsia.[24] Dyspeptic patients were separated into two groups: those with dyspeptic symptoms alone and those with both dyspeptic symptoms and lower bowel symptoms presumably related to IBS. The results showed a substantial decrease in the frequency of Phase 3 of the MMC during sleep in nonulcer dyspepsia patients. The patients with nonulcer dyspepsia spent the same proportion (approximately 94%) in Phase 2 regardless of whether they were asleep or awake, whereas the normal subjects showed a decrease of 84% in Phase 2 activity during sleep. Patients with dyspeptic plus IBS symptoms were not different from controls. It was also noted that Phase 2 activity in both normal subjects and patients decreases soon after going to sleep and shows a marked resumption on awakening from sleep. These data substantiate the notion that CNS arousal does affect GI motility and further reflects significant brain–gut interactions with the state of consciousness.

## LOWER GASTROINTESTINAL FUNCTIONING DURING SLEEP

### Small Bowel and MMC Activity

Alterations in lower bowel (small intestines, colon, and anorectum) motility are associated with symptoms that relate to fast or slow transit, elimination, and/or abdominal pain. Symptoms such as diarrhea, fecal incontinence, and abdominal pain are known to be altered by sleep. For example, it is well known clinically that diabetics may experience fecal incontinence during sleep, and patients with GERD often complain that heartburn awakens them from sleep.

Prolonged monitoring of the large and small bowels using a variety of sophisticated techniques, including telemetry, implanted microelectrodes, and suction electrodes, has allowed a more comprehensive description of intestinal motor activity during waking and sleep. On the basis of these studies, tonic activity in the stomach and small bowel has been described in terms of a basic electrical rhythm and more phasic phenomena, such as the MMC.[25] These studies have highlighted the extreme complexity and variability of the motor activity of the small and large bowels, and these features characterize the reviewed literature. A study of the small intestine by Thompson and colleagues found that sleep prolonged the interval between motor complexes in the small intestine.[25] A subsequent study by the same group revealed the diminution in the number of contractions of a specific type in the jejunum associated with sleep.[26] Duodenal ulcer disease and vagotomy failed to alter these findings, which suggests that this phenomenon is independent of vagal control and unaffected by duodenal disease. Kumar and his associates have described an obvious circadian rhythm in the propagation of the MMC, with the slowest velocities occurring during sleep (Fig. 26.11).[27] This finding appears to be the result of the circadian rhythm rather than a true modulation by sleep. Confirmation of these results has come from a study by Kellow and his associates, who have noted that the esophageal involvement in the MMC was decreased during sleep, with a corresponding tendency for MMCs to originate in the jejunum.[28]

### Small Bowel MMC Activity During REM and NREM Sleep

Another study by Kumar and colleagues examined the relationship between MMC cycle and REM sleep.[29] They found that, during sleep, there was a significant reduction in the MMC length and the duration of phase 2 of the MMC (Fig. 26.12). The MMCs were distributed equally among REM and NREM sleep, with no obvious alteration in the parameters of

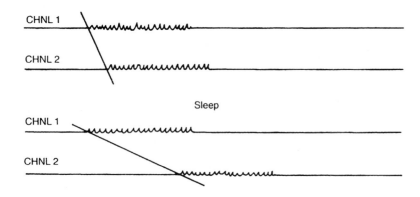

**FIGURE 26.12.** Schematic representations showing changes in the migrating motor complex cycle length depicted by the onset of Phase 3 activity during awake and sleep. Adapted from Kumar D, Idzikowski C, Wingate DL, et al. Relationship between enteric migrating motor complex and the sleep cycle. Am J Physiol 1990;259 (Gastrointest Liver Physiol, 22):G983–90.

**FIGURE 26.11.** Schematic representations showing changes in the migrating motor complex propagating velocity as noted by the onset of Phase 3 activity in two recording sites 15 mm apart. Note that sleep is associated with a marked increase in the propagating velocity of phase III activity. Adapted from Kumar D, Wingate D, Ruckebusch Y. Circadian variation in the propagation velocity of the migrating motor complex. Gastroenterology 1986;91:926–30 and Kellow JE, Borody TJ, Phillips SF, et al. Human interdigestive motility: variations in patterns from esophagus to colon. Gastroenterology 1986;91:386–95.

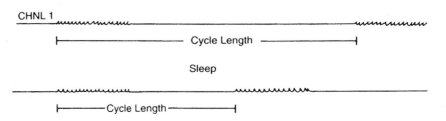

the MMC by sleep stage. These data provide evidence of periodic activity in the gut during sleep, but they are also consistent with the notion that the two cycles (eg, MMCs and REM sleep) are independent.[26] This study also documented that alterations in the MMC during sleep were similar with daytime sleep compared with nocturnal sleep, which suggests that these changes are specifically related to alterations in sleep as opposed to a circadian phenomenon.

These data would appear to be in conflict with those described above, which suggested that there was a relationship between sleep stage and duodenal Phase 3 MMC activity.[21] The same group of investigators has examined how the presence of food in the GI tract alters small bowel motility during sleep.[30] A late evening meal restored Phase 2 activity of the MMC, which is normally absent during sleep. In another study in which polysomnographic recording was used with simultaneous recording of small bowel motility, Gorard and colleagues identified an inverse relationship between the depth of sleep and small bowel motility activity.[31] Duodenal motor activity clearly diminished with decreasing levels of consciousness from waking to stage 3 and 4 sleep. Rapid eye movement sleep, which is associated with higher levels of cortical arousal, again showed an increase in duodenal motor activity toward waking levels.

## Small Bowel Activity During Sleep in Irritable Bowel Syndrome

Kellow and Phillips examined diarrhea-predominant and constipation-predominant patients with IBS and determined that patients with diarrhea-predominant IBS had a shorter period of MMCs in the daytime when compared to constipation-predominant patients.[32] All patients did show a circadian pattern in the periodicity of the MMC, with the nocturnal periodicity being somewhat shorter than in the daytime. In a subsequent study, Kellow and colleagues described a greater sensitivity in the daytime to the occurrence of Phase 3 motor activity associated with the MMC.[33] These contractions did produce awakenings from sleep, but the episodes associated with awakening from sleep were not significantly different between the patients with IBS and controls. A study of prolonged continuous recordings from the small bowel (72 hours) by the same group documented a circadian variation in the MMC propagation velocity, with the velocity being somewhat decreased during sleep.[34] These investigators documented that the MMC pattern was not different between the patients with IBS and control groups during sleep, but that during the day there were marked differences, including a shorter duration of postprandial motor activity in the patients with IBS and shorter diurnal MMC intervals in diarrhea-predominant patients when compared to constipation-predominant patients. Similarly, the previously cited study by Gorard and colleagues did not note any difference in small bowel motility in the normal subjects and patients with IBS in that both groups clearly showed an inverse relationship between the state of consciousness and the small bowel motility index.[31]

In a particularly interesting and significant study, Kumar and colleagues have described data that suggested that there were abnormalities of REM sleep in patients with IBS.[35] They documented a prolongation of REM sleep in patients with IBS. In addition, they confirmed that small bowel motility appears to be normal during sleep in patients with IBS. The results of this study were sufficiently extraordinary that it demanded attempts at replication. However, several studies have now been published that have failed to confirm these findings.[36]

## Colonic Activity

The two main functions of the colon are critically determined by motor activity, which determines the rate of transit and therefore, indirectly, the rate of absorption from the colonic lumen. Thus, alterations in colonic motility will have significant consequences in terms of transit through the colon and clinical sequelae such as constipation and diarrhea. Adler and his colleagues described a decrease in colonic motor function during sleep.[37] These results have been confirmed by two other studies, which have included measurements of transverse, descending, and sigmoid colon.[38,39] In the study by Bassotti and colleagues, inhibition on the colonic motility index is apparent in the transverse, descending, and sigmoid colon segments with a marked increase in activity on awakening (Fig. 26.13).[38] This could explain the common urge to defecate on awakening in the morning.[33] In the study by Crowell and colleagues, high-amplitude peristaltic colonic contractions were shown to be virtually absent during sleep.[39] The incidence of these contractions was markedly increased postprandially and just prior to a bowel movement, suggesting that these contractions are specifically related to colonic transit and defecation (Fig. 26.14). Neither of these studies attempted to document sleep with standard polysomnography. Colonic activity from cecum to rectum was monitored continuously for 32 hours in a study by Furukawa and colleagues.[40] These investigators also monitored sleep polygraphically according to standard electrophysiologic criteria. Further documentation of the decrease in colonic motor activity during sleep is presented in these data, but the study also describes an interesting abolition in propagating waves during slow-wave sleep (Fig. 26.15). During REM sleep, the frequency of these events rose substantially. A recent study of colonic myoelectrical activity in the human suggests a decrease in long-spike, burst activity during sleep.[41] Again, this study does not reveal whether the results are accounted for on the basis of true physiologic sleep or simply reflect a variation of colonic activity independent of sleep. Similar results have been described by Roarty and colleagues in a study that did employ polysomnographic monitoring in normal women during the follicular phase of the menstrual cycle.[42]

## Anorectal Activity

Anal canal pressures were measured continuously during sleep in a study by Orkin and colleagues.[43] They did not,

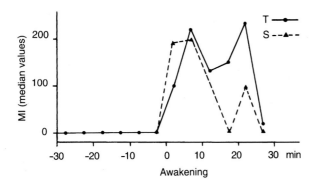

**FIGURE 26.13.** Colonic motility index per 5 minutes (expressed as medians) for transverse (T) and sigmoid (S) colon before and after sudden awakening. Adapted from Bassotti G, Bucaneve G, Betti C, Morelli A. Sudden awakening from sleep: effects on proximal and distal colonic contractile activity in humans. Eur J Gastroenterol Hepatol 1990;2:475–8.

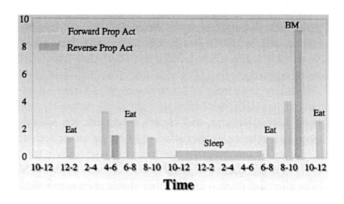

**FIGURE 26.14.** The rate of high-amplitude peristaltic contractions documented postprandially, during sleep and prior to a bowel movement. Adapted from Crowell MD, Bassotti G, Cheskin LJ, et al. Method for prolonged ambulatory monitoring of high-amplitude propagated contractions from colon. Am J Physiol 1991;261(Gastrointest Liver Physiol, 24):G263–8.

however, monitor sleep via polysomnography. The results indicated a decrease in the minute to minute variation in amplitude of spontaneous decreases in anal canal pressure during sleep. The rectum and anal canal are vital in maintaining normal bowel continence and ensuring normal defecation. In general, normal defecation is associated with sensory responses to rectal distention and appropriate motor responses of the muscles of the anal canal. These responses include a contraction of the external anal sphincter and a transient decrease in the internal anal sphincter pressure associated with rectal distention. Rao and colleagues have conducted studies that confirm the presence of an endogenous oscillation of rectal motor activity and have specifically noted that these bursts of cyclic rectal motor activity occurred in approximately 44% of the overall recording time at night.[44] They described the incidence of this motor activity to be nearly twofold greater during sleep than during the daytime. Of particular importance is the finding that the majority of contractions were propagated in a retrograde direction. This is a particularly interesting and important finding in that it offers a mechanism that may explain how the passive escape of rectal contents is prevented during sleep.

To assess the effect of sleep on these anal rectal sensory motor responses, 10 normal volunteers were studied during sleep with an anorectal probe in place.[45] This probe permits the transient distention of the rectum via a rectal balloon while the response to the internal and external anal sphincters can be simultaneously monitored. The study documented a marked decrease in the external anal sphincter response to rectal distention. The internal anal sphincter response remained unaltered (Figs. 26.16 and 26.17). In addition, there was no evidence of a conscious sensation of rectal distention up to 50 mL during sleep. Normally, a sensory response can be easily elicited with 10 to 15 mL of rectal distention. These results confirm that the external anal sphincter response to rectal distention is most likely a learned response, whereas the internal anal sphincter

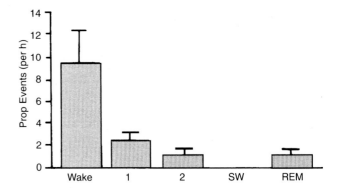

**FIGURE 26.15.** The rates of propagating colonic contractions are shown as a function of stage of sleep. Note the absence of propagating contractions during slow-wave sleep (SW). REM, rapid eye movement. Adapted from Furukawa Y, Cook, IJ, Panagopoulos V, et al. Relationship between sleep patterns and human colonic motor patterns. Gastroenterology 1994;107:1372–81.

response would appear to be a reflex response to rectal distention since it is maintained during sleep.

In an ambulatory study that monitored anorectal function, it was demonstrated by Kumar and his colleagues that external sphincter contractions occurred periodically during sleep, and these periodic bursts of activity were followed by motor quiescence.[46] These spontaneous contractions were associated with a rise in the anal canal pressure, but internal anal sphincter contractions were shown to occur independently of external anal sphincter activity. The "sampling reflex," which is a spontaneous relaxation of the internal anal sphincter, occurred frequently in the waking state but was markedly reduced during sleep. In the previously cited study by Rao and colleagues, they noted that by monitoring anal rectal functioning during sleep, a substantial proportion of rectal contractions were propagated in a retrograde fashion.[44] This would seem to make good sense in that a substantial propor-

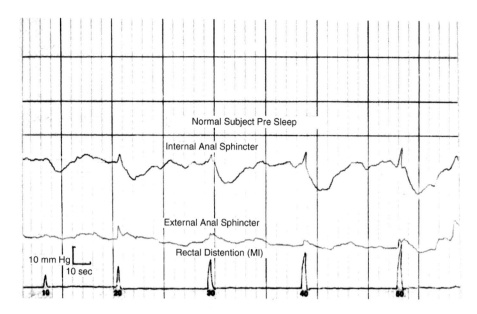

**FIGURE 26.16.** Rectal distention from 10 to 50 mL shows a clear decrease in internal anal sphincter pressure associated with each transient distention of the rectum.

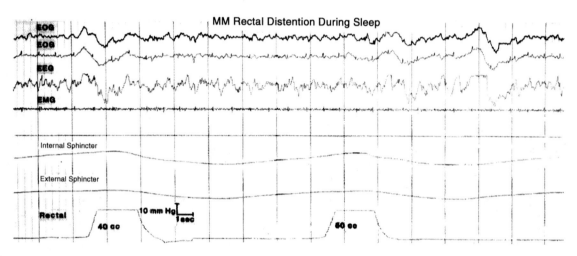

**FIGURE 26.17.** Polygraphic tracing during sleep showing the absence of an external anal sphincter response to rectal distention during sleep. (Note increase in time scale compared with Figure 26.16.) EOG, electro-oculogram; EEG, electroencephalography; EMG, electromyography.

tion of retrograde contractions during sleep would help to prevent the involuntary loss of rectal contents during sleep.

## CONCLUSIONS

This chapter presents data that describe a variety of GI motor functions that are either altered by a circadian rhythm or by sleep. It seems clear from these data that a simple understanding of intestinal function during the waking state is not sufficient to understand symptom production or pathogenesis. There are marked alterations in a number of vital biologic processes associated with different times of day and the various stages of sleep. Understanding the complexities of intestinal function and their relationship to symptoms clearly mandates an understanding of the interaction of these phenomena throughout the light/dark cycle and the profound alterations in physiologic function that occur during the one-third of our lives that is spent asleep.

### REFERENCES

1. Dinges DF. The influence of the human circadian timekeeping system on sleep. In: Kryger MH, Roth T, Dement WC, editors. Principles and practice of sleep medicine. Philadelphia: WB Saunders; 1989. p. 153–62.
2. Anch AM, Browman CP, Mitler MM, Walsh JK. Sleep: a scientific perspective. Englewood Cliffs (NJ): Prentice Hall; 1988.
3. Orr WC. Utilization of polysomnography in the assessment of sleep disorders. Med Clin North Am 1985;69:1153–67.
4. Katzka DA, DiMarino AJ. Pathophysiology of gastroesophageal reflux disease: LES incompetence and esophageal clearance. In: Castell DO, editor. The esophagus. Boston: Little, Brown & Co; 1992. p. 449–61.
5. Helm JF, Dodds WJ, Reidel DR, et al. Determinants of esophageal acid clearance in normal subjects. Gastroenterology 1983;85:607–12.
6. Helm JF, Dodds WJ, Hogan WJ, et al. Acid neutralizing capacity of human saliva. Gastroenterology 1982;83:69–74.

7. Lear CSC, Flanagan JB Jr, Moorees CFA. The frequency of deglutition in man. Arch Oral Biol 1965;10:83–96.

8. Lichter J, Muir RC. The pattern of swallowing during sleep. Electroencephalogr Clin Neurophysiol 1975;38:427–32.

9. Orr WC, Johnson LF, Robinson MG. The effect of sleep on swallowing, esophageal peristalsis, and acid clearance. Gastroenterology 1984;86:814–9.

10. Schneyer LH, Pigman W, Hanahan L, et al. Rate of flow of human parotid, sublingual, and submaxillary secretions during sleep. J Dent Res 1956;35:109–14.

11. Orr WC, Robinson MG, Johnson LF. Acid clearing during sleep in patients with esophagitis and controls. Dig Dis Sci 1981;26:423–7.

12. Avots-Avotins AE, Ashworth WD, Stafford BD, Moore JG. Day and night esophageal motor function. Am J Gastroenterol 1990;85:683–5.

13. Dent J, Doods WJ, Friedman RH, et al. Mechanism of gastroesophageal reflux in recumbent asymptomatic human subjects. J Clin Invest 1980;65:256–7.

14. Dent J, Holloway RH, Toouli J, Dodds WJ. Mechanisms of lower oesophageal sphincter incompetence in patients with symptomatic gastrooesophageal reflux. Gut 1988;29:1020–8.

15. Freiden N, Fisher MJ, Taylor W, et al. Sleep and nocturnal acid reflux in normal subjects and patients with reflux oesophagitis. Gut 1991;32:1275–9.

16. Kahrilas PJ, Dodds WJ, Dent J, et al. The effect of sleep, spontaneous gastroesophageal reflux, and a meal on upper esophageal sphincter pressure in normal human volunteers. Gastroenterology 1987;92:466–71.

17. Goo RH, Moore JG, Greenburg E, Alazraki NP. Circadian variation in gastric emptying of meals in humans. Gastroenterology 1987;93:515–8.

18. Elsenbruch S, Orr WC, Harnish MJ, Chen JDZ. Disruption of normal gastric myoelectric functioning by sleep. Sleep 1999;22:453–8.

19. Orr WC, Crowell MD, Lin B, et al. Sleep and gastric function in irritable bowel syndrome: derailing the brain-gut axis. Gut 1997;41:390–3.

20. Moore JG, Goo RH. Day and night aspirin-induced gastric mucosal damage and protection by ranitidine in man. Chronobiol Int 1987;4:111–6.

21. Finch PM, Ingram DM, Henstridge JD, Catchpole BN. Relationship of fasting gastroduodenal motility to the sleep cycle. Gastroenterology 1982;83:605–12.

22. Orr WC, Hoffman JH, Hegge FW. Ultradian rhythms in extended performance. Aerosp Med 1974;45:995–1000.

23. Lavie P. Ultradian rhythms in alertness—a pupillometric study. Biol Psychol 1979;9:49–62.

24. David D, Mertz H, Fefer L, et al. Sleep and duodenal motor activity in patients with severe non-ulcer dyspepsia. Gut 1994;35:916–25.

25. Thompson DG, Wingate DL, Archer L, et al. Normal patterns of human upper small bowel motor activity recorded by prolonged telemetry. Gut 1980;21:500–6.

26. Ritchie HD, Thompson DG, Wingate DL. Diurnal variation in human jejunal fasting motor activity. In: Proceedings of the American Physiological Society; 1980. p. 54–5.

27. Kumar D, Wingate D, Ruckebusch Y. Circadian variation in the propagation velocity of the migrating motor complex. Gastroenterology 1986;91:926–30.

28. Kellow JE, Borody TJ, Phillips SF, et al. Human interdigestive motility: variations in patterns from esophagus to colon. Gastroenterology 1986;91:386–95.

29. Kumar D, Idzikowski C, Wingate DL, et al. Relationship between enteric migrating motor complex and the sleep cycle. Am J Physiol 1990;259:G983–90.

30. Kumar D, Soffer EE, Wingate DL, et al. Modulation of the duration of human postprandial motor activity by sleep. Am J Physiol 1989;256:G851–5.

31. Gorard DA, Vesselinova-Jenkins CK, Libby GW, Farthing MJG. Migrating motor complex and sleep in health and irritable bowel syndrome. Dig Dis Sci 1995;40:2383–9.

32. Kellow JE, Phillips SF. Altered small bowel motility in irritable bowel syndrome is correlated with symptoms. Gastroenterology 1987;98:1885–93.

33. Kellow JE, Eckersley GM, Jones MP. Enhanced perception of physiological intestinal motility in the irritable bowel syndrome. Gastroenterology 1991;101:1621–7.

34. Kellow JE, Gill RC, Wingate DL. Prolonged ambulant recordings of small bowel motility demonstrate abnormalities in the irritable bowel syndrome. Gastroenterology 1990;98:1208–18.

35. Kumar D, Thompson PD, Wingate DL, et al. Abnormal REM sleep in the irritable bowel syndrome. Gastroenterology 1992;103:12–7.

36. Elsenbruch S, Harnish MJ, Orr WC. Subjective and objective sleep quality in irritable bowel syndrome. Am J Gastroenterol 1999;94:2447–52.

37. Adler HF, Atkinson AJ, Ivy AC. A study of the motility of the human colon: an explanation of dyssynergia of the colon, or of the unstable colon. Am J Dig Dis 1941;8:197–202.

38. Bassotti G, Bucaneve G, Betti C, Morelli A. Sudden awakening from sleep: effects on proximal and distal colonic contractile activity in humans. Eur J Gastroenterol Hepatol 1990;2:475–8.

39. Crowell MD, Bassotti G, Cheskin LJ, et al. Method for prolonged ambulatory monitoring of high-amplitude propagated contractions from colon. Am J Physiol 1991;261:G263–8.

40. Furukawa Y, Cook IJ, Panagopoulos V, et al. Relationship between sleep patterns and human colonic motor patterns. Gastroenterology 1994;107:1372–81.

41. Frexinos J, Bueno L, Fioramonti J. Diurnal changes in myoelectric spiking activity of the human colon. Gastroenterology 1985;88:1104–10.

42. Roarty TP, Suratt PM, Hellmann P, McCallum RW. Colonic motor activity in women during sleep. Sleep 1998;21:285–8.

43. Orkin BA, Hanson RB, Kelly KA, et al. Human anal motility while fasting, after feeding, and during sleep. Gastroenterology 1991;100:1016–23.

44. Rao SS, Welcher K. Periodic rectal motor activity: the intrinsic colonic gatekeeper? Am J Gastroenterol 1996;91:890–7.

45. Whitehead WE, Orr WC, Engel BT, Schuster MM. External anal sphincter response to rectal distention: learned response or reflex. Psychophysiology 1981;19(1):57–62.

46. Kumar D, Waldron D, Williams NS, et al. Prolonged anorectal manometry and external anal sphincter electromyography in ambulant human subjects. Dig Dis Sci 1990;35:641–8.

CHAPTER 27

# Motility as a Therapeutic Modality: Biofeedback Treatment of Gastrointestinal Disorders

*William E. Whitehead, Steven Heymen, and Marvin M. Schuster*

## THEORY OF BIOFEEDBACK LEARNING

Biofeedback training employs two types of learning: motor skills training and sensory discrimination training. In motor skills learning, the patient attempts to perform some action and uses feedback from the success or failure of each attempt to learn how to refine performance. A good example is learning to shoot a basketball: you shoot repeatedly and learn from your successful shots how to throw the ball more accurately. In the case of physiologic responses such as sphincter contractions, however, feedback on the success or failure of attempts to control the pelvic floor muscles may be difficult to perceive, especially if the muscle is initially quite weak. Consequently, biofeedback training involves detecting and transforming small changes in the muscle response to visual or auditory signals, which the patient can use to refine his/her motor skills. This is illustrated schematically in Figure 27.1. Motor skills–type biofeedback training sessions are usually supplemented by home practice (Kegel exercises), the purpose of which is to increase muscle strength by increasing the number of muscle fibers innervated by existing nerves. Biofeedback is not thought to repair or generate new neural pathways.

In other applications, biofeedback is used to teach patients to relax chronically tense muscles by providing feedback on small decreases in electromyographic (EMG) activity. This is also a type of motor skills learning, and training sessions in the laboratory or clinic are supplemented with home practice of relaxation skills on a daily basis.

A second mechanism by which biofeedback reduces symptoms, in addition to improving motor skills, is to increase the patient's awareness of somatic sensations, which are critical to biologic self-regulation. For example, one of the causes of fecal incontinence is loss of the ability to perceive rectal fullness, which is a critical cue to contract the pelvic floor muscles to avoid incontinence.[1,2] In patients with loss of rectal sensation, the goal of biofeedback training is to improve the ability to discriminate rectal filling through sensory retraining.[3,4] In other biofeedback applications, patients are taught to become more aware of muscle tension[5] so that they know when to invoke relaxation exercises or other counter-control mechanisms. Learning to discriminate somatic sensations that are cues to initiate biologic coping mechanisms is a distinctly different goal of biofeedback than motor skills training; it is relevant to some medical disorders but not others.

A wide variety of smooth muscle and secretory responses can be brought under voluntary control through the use of biofeedback training (see below). However, laboratory demonstrations of smooth muscle and secretory control have not been translated into successful clinical applications as yet; they are useful primarily for the insights they provide into brain-gut regulation of gastrointestinal physiology. On the other hand, the skeletal muscles at the two ends of the gastrointestinal tract—the pelvic floor and the proximal esophagus—have been more amenable to biofeedback training and are the basis of successful clinical applications. The bulk of the chapter will therefore be devoted to a discussion of biofeedback for fecal incontinence and outlet dysfunction–type constipation and to other potential applications that exist in the proximal (striated muscle) portion of the esophagus. Biofeedback applications to smooth muscle and secretory responses will be discussed at the end of the chapter.

## BIOFEEDBACK

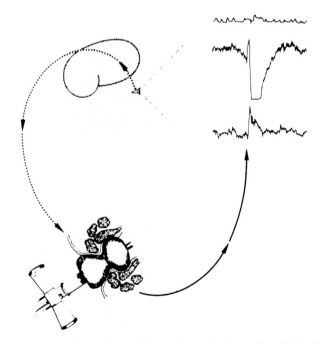

**FIGURE 27.1.** Biofeedback training requires a visual or auditory display of a physiologic event. The patient uses the augmented sensory feedback to learn, by trial and error, to improve voluntary control over the physiologic response.

## GENERAL REQUIREMENTS FOR BIOFEEDBACK

### Immediacy

Animal learning experiments show that when feedback (or punishment or reward) is delayed by more than 1 or 2 seconds, learning occurs much more slowly. In animal studies, feedback that is delayed by more than 10 seconds is completely ineffective, but in humans, learning will occur with longer delays because people are able to cognitively relate consequences to their previous actions. However, even in humans, the effectiveness of feedback decays in approximately an exponential fashion with the length of time between the physiologic event and the feedback signal. This principle of immediacy of feedback has consequences for some forms of biofeedback training. For example, it is difficult to detect a change in gastric acid secretion and convert it into a visual display rapidly, and the myoelectric slow waves and contractions of the smooth muscle of the gastrointestinal tract typically occur once every 8 to 20 seconds. This may contribute to the difficulty subjects have in learning to voluntarily control these smooth muscle and secretory responses.

### Accuracy

Physiologic recordings always include some artifact or "noise," both being terms referring to changes in the recording caused by movement, respiration, or other irrelevant sources. In addition, some methods of detecting muscle responses (especially balloon probes) make it difficult to distinguish the response of a weak muscle from the response of an adjacent strong muscle. The more artifact present in the feedback signal, the more difficult it is for the subject to make use of the feedback to learn how to control the muscle or secretory gland. Careful consideration should always be given to selecting the best physiologic transducer and then filtering the transducer's output to minimize respiration and other sources of artifact.

### Motivation

Biofeedback displays serve the function of rewards and punishments to guide learning, but only if patients are aware that control of the physiologic response will help them achieve some goal of theirs, such as recovery of continence. Biofeedback training will not occur in a poorly motivated patient. Biofeedback is therefore not a useful technique in demented or confused patients or in children younger than about 5 years of age.[6,7] Moreover, it may be helpful to explicitly motivate patients by showing them that such learning is possible and by pointing out the relationship between learning of physiologic responses and other goals they have such as continence or pain relief. In children, it is sometimes helpful to augment information feedback with material rewards or tokens (eg, stars) exchangeable for toys or privileges.

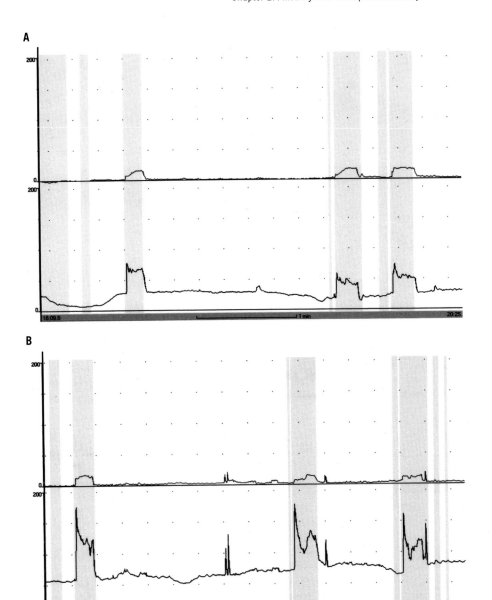

**FIGURE 27.2.** A patient with fecal incontinence shown at the beginning and end of biofeedback training. *Top channel* shows intra-abdominal pressures recorded from a balloon in the rectum, and *bottom channel* shows anal canal pressures recorded from a solid-state pressure transducer. **A,** Instructions to squeeze as if preventing a bowel movement produce weak increases in anal canal pressure averaging 50 mm Hg, and these squeezes are accompanied by increases in abdominal pressure of approximately 25 mm Hg. These increases in abdominal pressure are inappropriate responses caused by abdominus rectus contraction, and they increase the likelihood of incontinence. **B,** The same patient after a series of biofeedback training sessions. Instructions to squeeze now produce increases in anal canal pressure of approximately 120 mm Hg. Note, however, that the patient continues to show increases in abdominal pressure indicative of inappropriate abdominus rectus contractions. Further training is needed to reduce or eliminate this inappropriate response.

## FECAL INCONTINENCE

### Types of Biofeedback Training for Fecal Incontinence

Engel and colleagues first described biofeedback treatment for fecal incontinence more than 25 years ago.[8] The goal of training was to improve the patient's ability to voluntarily contract the external anal sphincter in response to rectal filling either by improving the strength of the sphincter (motor skills training) or by increasing the patient's ability to perceive weak distentions of the rectum (discrimination training) or by a combination of these two mechanisms (training in the coordination of sphincter contractions with rectal sensation). This can be accomplished through training that makes use of feedback on either anal canal pressures or pelvic floor EMG activity. These different approaches to training are described below.

### *Motor Skills Training by Pressure Biofeedback*

Biofeedback training directed at improving the strength of the external anal sphincter has most frequently been done by recording anal canal pressures and providing a visual or auditory signal that is proportional to anal canal pressure (Fig. 27.2). Anal canal pressures can be recorded by miniature balloons, solid-state pressure transducers, or perfusion ports that are connected by a continuous column of water to an external pressure transducer. The patient is asked to squeeze as if preventing defecation and is given visual feedback and verbal guidance on how to accomplish this. He/she may also be taught to inhibit inappropriate responses such as contraction of the abdominus rectus or gluteal muscles (see Fig. 27.2), which may accompany the contraction of the external anal sphincter. In most laboratories, patients have been asked to squeeze in response to distention of the rectum (accomplished by inflat-

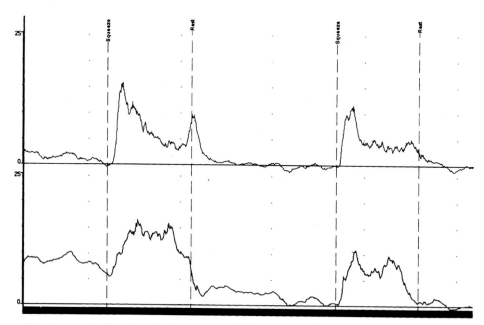

**FIGURE 27.3.** Biofeedback for fecal incontinence based on electromyography (EMG) of the pelvic floor. *Top tracing* shows averaged EMG of the external anal sphincter recorded from an intra-anal plug electrode. *Bottom tracing* shows averaged EMG activity from the abdominus rectus muscles recorded from skin surface electrodes spaced 5 cm apart over the belly of the muscle. The correct response to instructions to squeeze to prevent defecation is an increase in external anal sphincter EMG by >25 µV with little or no increase in abdominus rectus EMG. This incontinent patient shows an external anal sphincter response of approximately half normal amplitude and inappropriately contracts the abdominus rectus muscle. Visual feedback and verbal coaching are used to shape the patient's response toward a more appropriate one.

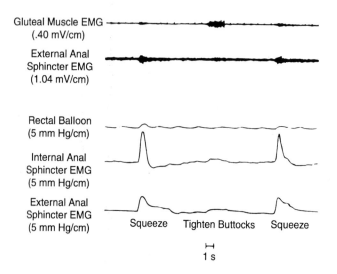

**FIGURE 27.4.** These recordings demonstrate the feasibility of recording electromyographic (EMG) activity from the pelvic floor by applying skin surface electrodes on either side of the anus (*second trace*). The *top trace* is gluteal muscle EMG recorded from similar skin surface electrodes approximately 4 cm apart over the gluteal muscles on one side. A three-balloon probe was used to record rectal pressure (*third trace*), internal anal sphincter (*fourth trace*), and external anal sphincter (*fifth trace*). When the patient is instructed to squeeze to prevent loss of stool, there is an increase in the anal sphincter EMG activity coincident with an increase in anal canal pressure (seen in both the internal and external sphincter balloons), but there is no significant increase in EMG activity recorded from the electrodes over the gluteus. Conversely, when the patient is instructed to tighten the buttocks, there is an increase in gluteal EMG activity with little change in anal sphincter EMG activity and no increase in anal canal pressure. Adapted from Whitehead WE, Schuster MM. Manometric and electromyographic techniques for assessment of the anorectal mechanism for continence and defecation. In: Hoelzl R, Whitehead WE, editors. Psychophysiology of the gastrointestinal tract: experimental and clinical applications. New York: Plenum; 1983. p. 301–29.

ing a balloon in the rectum),[9,10] but in other laboratories, the patient is asked to squeeze without rectal distention.[11]

### Motor Skills Training by EMG Biofeedback

Biofeedback training to strengthen pelvic floor muscles may also be done by showing the patient a recording of the average EMG activity recorded from the striated muscles surrounding the anal canal.[11,12] This is illustrated in Figure 27.3. In EMG biofeedback training, the patient is usually asked to squeeze and relax repeatedly without distending the rectum. Information on inappropriate abdominal wall contraction is usually not

available with this type of biofeedback training. Home exercises in which the patient is asked to repeatedly squeeze the pelvic floor muscles (Kegel exercises) to further strengthen these muscles is usually requested whether the biofeedback training employs anal canal pressure or pelvic floor EMG.

The EMG activity of the pelvic floor can be recorded using an anal plug with metal plates (electrodes) on its surface,[13] or adhesive electrodes can be applied to the skin adjacent to the anus (one electrode on either side).[11,12] Figure 27.4 shows that perianal skin electrodes give a valid recording of pelvic floor EMG activity that is not contaminated by significant amounts

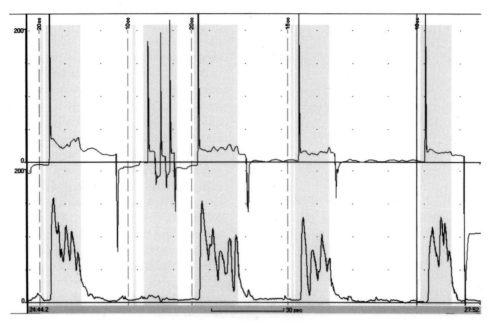

**FIGURE 27.5.** Sensory discrimination training in a patient with fecal incontinence associated with impaired ability to perceive rectal distention. The patient was instructed to squeeze the external anal sphincter whenever he perceived rectal distention. In response to a 20-mL distention, he squeezed appropriately but then failed to respond to three 10-mL distentions. The trainer presented another 20-mL distention (which the patient had previously detected) and then a 15-mL distention, and the patient responded appropriately to both of these. Finally, the 10-mL distention was introduced again, and this time the patient felt it and responded appropriately.

of gluteal EMG activity. Anal plug electrodes have the advantage that they are very easy to use and there is almost no preparation. However, some patients, especially children, are frightened by having a probe introduced into the anal canal. The advantage of the perianal skin electrodes is that they are perceived as less invasive by patients, but the disadvantage is that adhesive electrodes adhere poorly to an area that is often damp and has hair. As a result, the preparation time is longer, the electrodes are more likely to become detached, and if one has to shave the hair from the area to get the electrodes to stick, this is more frightening to patients than having an anal plug introduced. It is recommended that perianal electrodes be used in children and that anal plugs be used in adults.

### Sensory Discrimination Training

Biofeedback training directed at increasing the patient's ability to perceive and respond to rectal distention[3,4,14] is based on sensory discrimination training. A catheter with a balloon attached to its tip is introduced into the rectum, and the balloon is distended with different volumes of air. The patient may be asked to report when he/she feels the distention or may be asked to respond to the balloon distention by contracting the pelvic floor muscles. In either case, large distentions that the patient can easily perceive are presented first, and then the volume of rectal distentions is gradually reduced until the patient has difficulty detecting when the balloon was distended. By repeatedly distending the balloon slightly above and then slightly below the patient's sensory threshold, and by providing feedback on the accuracy of detection, the patient is taught to recognize weaker and weaker distentions.

This sequence is illustrated in Figure 27.5. In many laboratories, this type of sensory training is combined with sphincter strength training by having the patient always contract in response to rectal distention and encouraging the patient to contract as strongly as possible while providing feedback on the strength of contraction and the accuracy of detection.

### Effectiveness of Biofeedback for Fecal Incontinence

Several reviews of the biofeedback literature have been published.[15–17] In the most recent and most comprehensive article,[17] 26 adult studies and 9 pediatric studies were reviewed. This represented all published studies from 1974 to 2000 that met the following criteria: a minimum of five patients studied, biofeedback technique described, and biofeedback effects not confounded with surgery. The following is a summary of this literature review.

OVERALL SUCCESS RATE. When all studies were included regardless of etiology, an average of 75% of patients showed at least a 75% reduction in fecal incontinence. However, only about 50% became completely continent.

There have been only two prospective, randomized, parallel-group experiments, and they do not allow any conclusion on the overall effectiveness of biofeedback training either because the population was too specialized[7] or because the training protocol was atypical. In the first randomized controlled trial, Whitehead and colleagues compared biofeedback plus behavioral management to behavioral management alone in children with fecal incontinence secondary to myelomeningocele.[7] Significant improvement occurred in

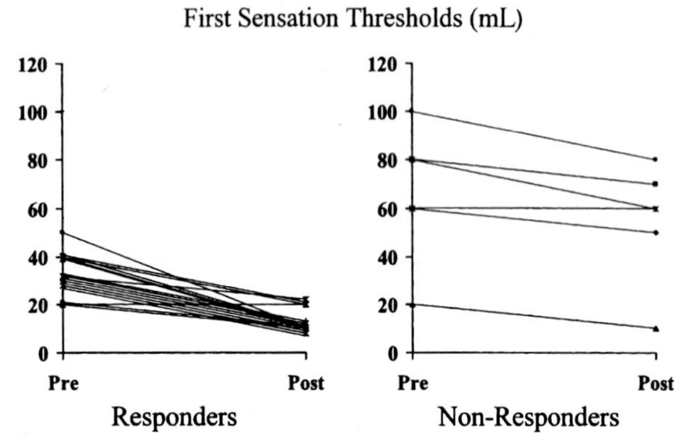

First Sensation Thresholds (mL)

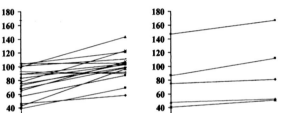

**FIGURE 27.6.** First sensation thresholds are shown before and after biofeedback training. The *left panel* shows 17 patients who had a good response to biofeedback training (continence or 75% reduction in frequency of incontinence), and the *right panel* shows 6 patients who had an inadequate response to biofeedback training. All but 1 patient with a good outcome improved sensory threshold, and all had final sensory thresholds of 20 mL or less. In contrast, 5 of 6 poor responders had final sensory thresholds in excess of 20 mL. Note also that an initial sensory threshold of 60 mL or greater was predictive of a poor response to training. Adapted from Chiarioni G, Bassotti G, Stegagnini S, et al. Sensory retraining is key to biofeedback therapy for formed stool fecal incontinence. Am J Gastroenterol. [In press].

Maximum Squeeze Pressures (mm Hg)

**FIGURE 27.7.** These data on maximum squeeze pressures before and after biofeedback training are taken from the same patients shown in Figure 27.6. Note that squeeze pressures at the end of training for successful biofeedback patients overlapped and were not significantly different from the end-of-training squeeze pressures of the patients who showed a poor response to training. Note also that initial squeeze pressures were not a significant predictor of who would respond to biofeedback training. Adapted from Chiarioni G, Bassotti G, Stegagnini S, et al. Sensory retraining is key to biofeedback therapy for formed stool fecal incontinence. Am J Gastroenterol. [In press].

both groups, suggesting that biofeedback is not superior to behavioral management for most children with myelomeningocele. However, it was already known that patients with spinal cord defects, who constitute a small subgroup of all patients with fecal incontinence, show a poorer response to biofeedback training than do patients with other etiologies for their incontinence.[9]

In the second randomized controlled trial, Miner and colleagues employed a complex crossover design that made interpretation of results difficult.[18] Their 25 adult patients were

first randomized to receive either sensory discrimination training without biofeedback on sphincter strength or equivalent distentions without feedback on the accuracy of their detection or the strength of contractions for three sessions. The sensory training group showed significant reductions in frequency of incontinence and the control group did not, but between-group differences were not statistically significant owing to small samples. Patients in the control group were subsequently given sensory training and showed improved continence. Then all 25 patients were randomized again to receive sphincter-strengthening exercises without biofeedback or were taught to squeeze in response to rectal distention with feedback. As a group, patients showed further improvements in continence with this second phase of training, but there were no significant differences between the groups, owing perhaps to the confounding effects of multiple crossovers and small sample sizes. This study suggests that sensory training is important to the elimination of incontinence, but the results are not definitive because of limited statistical power.

A third study employed a parallel-group design comparing 16 patients who received pressure biofeedback to 8 patients who received medications, but in a major design flaw, patients were not randomly assigned; they were allowed to select the treatment they preferred.[19] The biofeedback group showed significant improvements relative to baseline, but the control group did not. However, between-group comparisons were not reported and are presumed not to have been statistically significant.

Most published studies have used recordings of pressure from the anal canal rather than pelvic floor EMG activity as the basis for biofeedback. In the majority of these studies, patients were taught to squeeze in response to rectal distention with a balloon. However, comparisons between studies do not show any clear superiority for pressure versus EMG feedback,[17] and the only study to directly compare EMG to pressure feedback training showed no significant difference between the two.[20]

Several studies suggest that sensory discrimination training (ie, training directed at reducing the threshold for perception of rectal distention) is important to the success of biofeedback training.[3,4,10,14,18,21] The results of the study by Chiarioni and colleagues are shown in Figure 27.6.[14] These investigators taught 24 patients with severe, solid-stool fecal incontinence to squeeze in response to rectal distention. They evaluated these patients 3 months after the conclusion of biofeedback training and classified them as responders (greater than 75% reduction in incontinence) or nonresponders, and they compared the responders to the nonresponders with respect to changes from baseline in the threshold for perception of rectal distention and anal canal squeeze pressures. As shown in Figure 27.6, the 17 responders had significantly lower sensory thresholds following training than the nonresponders, but squeeze pressures were not significantly different in responders compared to nonresponders (Fig. 27.7). Figure 27.6 also shows that sensory thresholds measured prior to biofeedback training were also good predictors of which patients would respond to biofeedback training: patients with the most severe sensory impairments showed a poor response to biofeedback training. On the other hand, sphincter strength and severity of fecal incontinence prior to biofeedback training did not predict the response to training (see Fig. 27.7).

Although sensory discrimination training appears to be an important component of biofeedback training, it is not essential to the success of training, as is shown by the good outcomes in several studies that employed EMG biofeedback and did not include any sensory training.[17] It seems likely that sensory training is more important to patients who demonstrate loss of rectal sensation and that sensory retraining would be less important to patients with weak sphincter contractions but no loss of rectal sensation. Such direct comparisons have not been conducted.

Nonspecific components of treatment including education, attention from health care providers, and sometimes the use of laxatives or antidiarrheal agents contribute to the successful outcomes that have been reported.[6,7,18,20,21] Heymen and colleagues reported that when patients referred for a biofeedback treatment study are first placed on a systematic medical management/education program for 4 weeks, 25 to 30% of them resolve their incontinence.[22]

Reviews of the biofeedback literature report impressive outcomes: 80% improved in the 13 studies reviewed by Enck,[15] 40 to 100% improved in the 14 studies reviewed by Rao and colleagues,[23] and 75% improved in the 35 studies reviewed by Heymen and colleagues.[17] However, these impressive results should be considered cautiously because (1) there have been no uniform criteria for defining improvement or assessing outcome; (2) only two studies used parallel-group designs and random assignment of patients, and these studies lacked statistical power because of small sample sizes and did not control for placebo effects; (3) inclusion criteria differed; and (4) treatment protocols varied.

### Predictors of Outcome

Whitehead and colleagues speculated that "Demented patients, developmentally delayed patients, young children, and the severely depressed are unlikely to benefit from biofeedback training…" and that "mobility impairment is a significant risk factor for fecal incontinence in nursing home populations and will limit what can be accomplished with biofeedback…"[24] However, there are few data to support these or other guidelines for selecting patients for treatment. The available literature is summarized below:

1. *Central nervous system injury.* Cerulli and colleagues, in an early article describing the treatment of 50 patients with biofeedback, reported that patients with spinal cord injury (myelomeningocele, traumatic cord injury) were less likely to benefit than patients with damage to pelvic floor muscles.[9] Whitehead and colleagues supported this conclusion by reporting that for most children with myelomenin gocele

as a cause of fecal incontinence, biofeedback was no better than toilet skills training.[7] However, Whitehead and colleagues did identify a subgroup with less complete and lower cord lesions and frequent bowel movements, which specifically benefited from biofeedback training.

2. *Structural damage to the anal sphincters.* Reports from several laboratories indicate that severe structural damage to the anal sphincters is associated with poorer responses to biofeedback.[10,25–28]

3. *Impaired sensation.* Chiarioni and colleagues reported that severe sensory impairment was associated with poorer outcomes in biofeedback training,[14] and Norton and Kamm reported that patients with passive incontinence (loss of stool without accompanying urge), which may be associated with sensory impairment, did poorly.[25]

4. *Squeeze pressures and other manometric findings.* Most laboratories have not found that the response to biofeedback could be predicted on the basis of pretreatment manometric findings such as anal canal squeeze pressure, rectal compliance, and maximum tolerable volume for rectal distention.[26,29] However, there is an isolated report that low internal anal sphincter pressure (resting anal canal pressure) is associated with poor outcomes and is not amenable to biofeedback training.[30]

5. *Pudendal nerve terminal motor latencies.* Abnormally prolonged pudendal nerve conduction times are used in many laboratories to identify patients with pudendal nerve injuries as a cause of fecal incontinence. However, these measures are poorly correlated with the clinical response to biofeedback training.[27,31]

6. *Severity of fecal incontinence.* The severity and type of fecal incontinence do not predict the response to biofeedback training.[27,29]

7. *Depression and anxiety.* There appears to be no significant association between occurrence of fecal incontinence and anxiety or depression.[32,33] However, depression and anxiety may interfere with biofeedback treatment.[6] Depression can be associated with psychomotor retardation, a diminished ability to think or concentrate, and memory disturbance, as well as a tendency toward a lack of initiation.[34] The presence of depression could reduce the patient's capacity to learn and his/her motivation to comply with home practice.

### Innovations in the Biofeedback Treatment of Fecal Incontinence

Since the last *Atlas* was published, there have been several reports describing the combination of biofeedback with surgery to treat fecal incontinence. Positive results have been reported for high imperforate anus repair,[35] gracilis muscle transposition to create a neosphincter,[36] and anterior resection of the rectum and total colectomy with ileoanal anastomosis.[37] All of these studies were uncontrolled, and their interpretation is difficult because of small sample sizes and ascertainment bias. In the only controlled study, Hamalainen

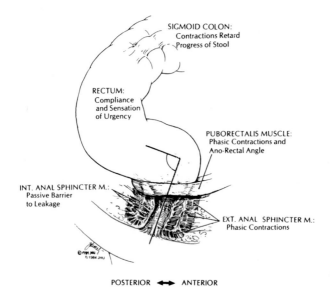

SIGMOID COLON:
Contractions Retard
Progress of Stool

RECTUM:
Compliance
and Sensation
of Urgency

PUBORECTALIS MUSCLE:
Phasic Contractions and
Ano-Rectal Angle

INT. ANAL SPHINCTER M.:
Passive Barrier
to Leakage

EXT. ANAL SPHINCTER M.:
Phasic Contractions

POSTERIOR ◄──► ANTERIOR

**FIGURE 27.8.** Anatomy of the anal canal and rectum showing the physio-logic mechanisms important to continence and defecation. The puborectalis muscle forms a sling that loops around the anal canal and is anchored ante-riorly to the symphysis pubis. Contraction of the puborectalis muscle pinches off the rectum from the anal canal by sharpening the anorectal angle. This muscle must relax to allow the rectum to funnel into the anal canal during defecation. The external anal sphincter surrounds the anal canal and is ton-ically partially contracted to maintain resting anal canal pressure above rec-tal pressure. This muscle must also relax to allow defecation to occur. Conversely, the external anal sphincter can be voluntarily contracted to increase anal canal pressure to prevent loss of stool. Reproduced with permis-sion from Whitehead WE, Schuster MM. Gastrointestinal disorders: behavioral and physiological basis for treatment. Orlando (FL): Academic Press; 1985.

and colleagues did not find that patients who received biofeedback following rectal prolapse repair did any better than patients undergoing the same surgery without biofeed-back.[30] Nevertheless, the combination of biofeedback with surgery is logical and warrants further study.

Menard and colleagues combined electrical stimulation with pelvic floor biofeedback in a mixed group of patients, including some with fecal incontinence and others with out-let dysfunction–type constipation.[38] They believed that the combination was more effective than either monotherapy, but their experimental design did not test this. It is possible that electrical stimulation augments pelvic floor biofeedback by enhancing sensations in the appropriate muscles.

Solomon and colleagues described the use of real-time ultrasonographic images of the pelvic floor muscles to teach patients with fecal incontinence to squeeze the external anal sphincter.[39] This has potential advantages because it is a direct measure of muscle contraction, but the disadvantage is that images of striated external anal sphincter muscle are poorly defined by ultrasonography and are difficult to inter-pret without special training. The investigators report that they are conducting a controlled trial of this new type of biofeedback.

Another innovation in biofeedback is the use of video arcade–type displays to motivate patients during biofeedback. To date, this has not been applied to the treatment of fecal incontinence in published reports, but encouraging results were reported in the use of biofeedback to teach relaxation to patients with irritable bowel syndrome (IBS).[40]

## PELVIC FLOOR DYSSYNERGIA

### Pathophysiology

Normally, during the act of defecation, the puborectalis sling muscle and the external anal sphincter (Fig. 27.8) relax to permit defecation, as can be demonstrated by recording EMG activity from the pelvic floor muscles or anal canal pressures during defecation (Fig. 27.9). However, some chronically constipated patients inappropriately contract[41] or fail to relax the external anal sphincter or puborectalis muscle, or both muscles, during straining and thereby obstruct defecation (Fig. 27.10). This has been called pelvic floor dyssynergia[42] or anismus.[41] A more general term, which has been incor-porated into the International Classification of Diseases 9-CM diagnostic classification system,[43] is outlet dysfunction con-stipation; this term does not specify the pathophysiologic mechanism for obstructed defecation.

Preston and Lennard-Jones first described the association of paradoxical contraction of the pelvic floor with constipa-tion,[41] and subsequent investigators confirmed their observa-tion.[44–46] This disorder of function is not attributable to a neurologic lesion since at least two-thirds of patients can learn to relax the external anal sphincter and puborectalis muscles appropriately when provided with biofeedback train-ing.[15] Paradoxical contraction of the pelvic floor during straining is believed to represent maladaptive learning.[42,47–50]

Recent reports suggest that the finding of pelvic floor dyssynergia is variable from one occasion of testing to another[51] and is less likely to be seen at home, when ambu-latory monitors are used to record the response to straining, as compared with laboratory testing. Pelvic floor dyssynergia is also observed in some asymptomatic controls and in fecally incontinent patients,[52] causing some investigators to ques-tion whether this is a distinct abnormality associated with constipation. However, most believe that although current diagnostic criteria lead to many false-positive diagnoses, there exists a subgroup of patients whose symptoms of chronic constipation and/or fecal impaction occur as a result of inability to relax the pelvic floor when straining to defe-cate. More restrictive diagnostic criteria have been recom-mended to reduce the number of false-positive diagnoses.[42]

### Types of Biofeedback Training for Fecal Incontinence

#### Sensory Training by Simulated Defecation

The earliest behavioral treatment for pelvic floor dyssynergia was simulated defecation. Bleijenberg and Kuijpers described an inpatient program in which water-filled balloons were

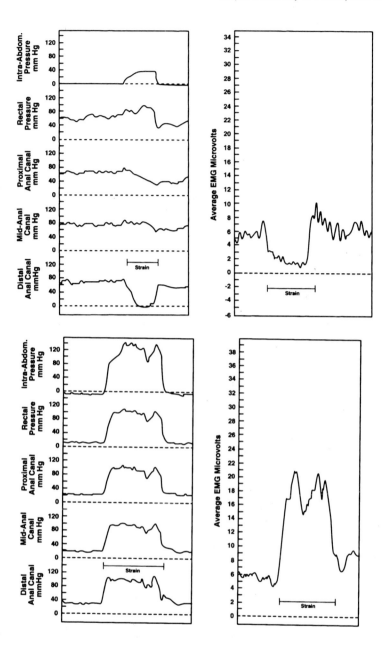

**FIGURE 27.9.** *Left panel* shows normal anal canal pressure in response to straining to defecate in a patient with colonic inertia–type constipation. Top channel shows pressure in a 10-mL air-filled rectal balloon used to detect increases in intra-abdominal pressure during straining. The next four channels show pressures in the anal canal. In the most distal channel, which is in the high-pressure zone of the anal canal, straining is associated with a decrease in anal canal pressure, which is the normal response. The *right panel*, taken from the same patient, shows the averaged electromyographic (EMG) activity recorded from an acrylic plug with metal plates on its sides and positioned in the anal canal; this patient shows normal reflex inhibition of pelvic floor EMG activity during straining. Reproduced with permission from Whitehead WE, Wald A, Diamant NE, et al. Functional disorders of the anus and rectum. In: Drossman DA, Corazziari E, Talley NJ, et al, editors. Rome II: the functional gastrointestinal disorders. McLean (VA): Degnon Associates; 2000. p. 483–532.

**FIGURE 27.10.** Left panel shows paradoxical increases in anal canal pressure in response to straining to defecate in a patient with pelvic floor dyssynergia. Top channel shows intra-abdominal pressure recorded from a 10-mL air-filled rectal balloon and reflects normal increases in pressure during straining. However, the next four channels show paradoxical increases in anal canal pressure, which would obstruct defecation, rather than decreases in anal canal pressure, which would permit defecation to occur. The *right panel*, taken from the same patient, shows that these paradoxical increases in anal canal pressure are accompanied by increases in averaged pelvic floor electromyographic activity. Compare this figure with Figure 27.9. Reproduced with permission from Whitehead WE, Wald A, Diamant NE, et al. Functional disorders of the anus and rectum. In: Drossman DA, Corazziari E, Talley NJ, et al, editors. Rome II: the functional gastrointestinal disorders. McLean (VA): Degnon Associates; 2000. p. 483–532.

introduced into the rectum and slowly pulled out while the patient was encouraged to attend to the sensations produced by the balloon and to try to facilitate balloon passage.[53] At other times, these patients had porridge introduced into the rectum to simulate stool, and they practiced defecating this. Variations on this procedure have included asking patients to attempt to defecate a balloon or simulated stool but have not employed practice in defecating porridge or other pasty substances from the rectum.[11,54]

### Electromyographic Biofeedback
A simpler form of biofeedback is to record and display the averaged EMG activity from the pelvic floor muscles and to teach patients to relax these muscles during attempts to defecate. In a typical protocol, the patient first practices decreasing EMG activity without straining. Then, as they acquire an ability to relax pelvic floor muscles to within the normal

range, they are instructed to strain very gently (increase intra-abdominal pressure minimally by contracting the abdominus rectus muscles) while keeping the EMG activity low. The amount of straining effort is gradually increased until the patient is able to produce sustained increases in intra-abdominal pressure without increases in pelvic floor EMG. Biofeedback training to relax pelvic floor EMG while straining is illustrated in Figure 27.11. Figure 27.12 shows the goal of training: relaxation of pelvic floor EMG in response to increases in abdominal pressure.

### Anal Canal Pressures
Anal canal pressures can be used to monitor pelvic floor muscles contractions and relaxations in place of EMG sensors.[49] Several technologies are available to measure anal canal pressures, including small balloons, perfusion ports, or solid-state pressure sensors. The steps in training the patient to relax the

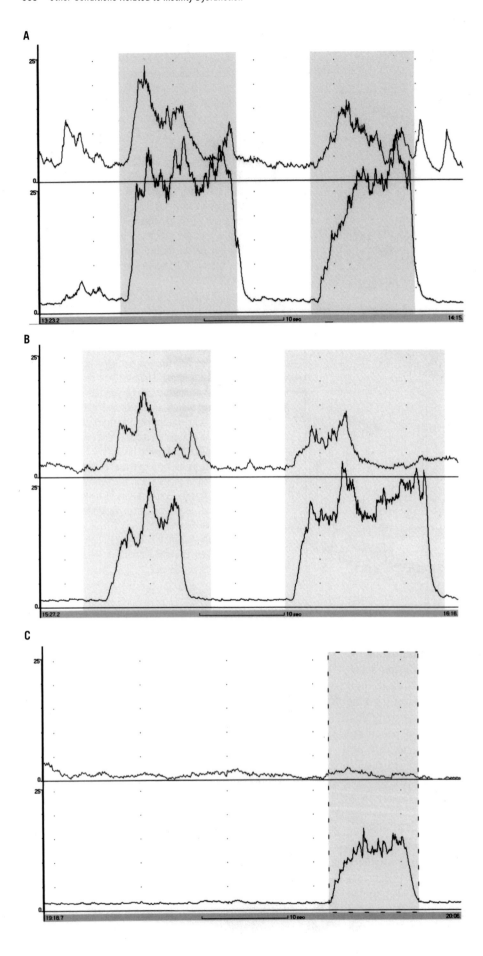

**FIGURE 27.11.** Course of biofeedback training for a patient with pelvic floor dyssynergia. In **A**, top channel is average electromyographic (EMG) activity from the pelvic floor muscles recorded from an anal plug, and the bottom channel is averaged EMG activity from the abdominus rectus muscle. The patient is being instructed to push as if defecating. In the *left panel*, pushing produces an appropriate increase in abdominal wall EMG (bottom channel; this would increase intra-abdominal pressure), but this is accompanied by an inappropriate (paradoxical) increase in pelvic floor EMG (this would increase anal canal pressure). **B** shows an intermediate stage in training: the same patient begins by contracting the pelvic floor concurrently with contracting the abdominus rectus, but halfway through the trial, the patient is able to relax the pelvic floor muscles while maintaining contraction of the abdominus rectus. **C** shows the late stage of biofeedback training in which this patient is able to push (increase abdominus rectus EMG activity) without any significant increase in pelvic floor EMG activity.

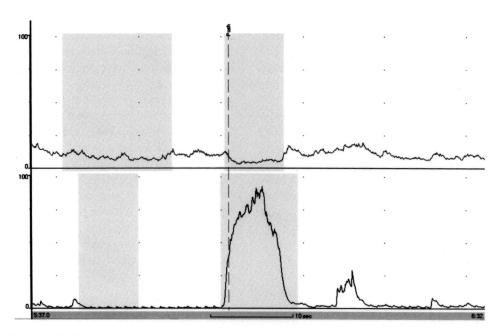

**FIGURE 27.12.** This shows the final stage of training for a patient with pelvic floor dyssynergia. Here the patient shows a reflex decrease in average pelvic floor electromyographic activity (*top tracing*) during the period of pushing to defecate.

pelvic floor are the same as for EMG biofeedback. An advantage of pressure biofeedback is that it is easy to monitor intra-abdominal pressure and provide feedback on this to the patient as well. It may also be easier to combine pelvic floor relaxation training with some sensory discrimination training by, for example, having the patient attempt to defecate a rectal balloon attached to the probe as it is gently pulled out at the end of the training session.

### *Comparison of Biofeedback Protocols*

Bleijenberg and Kuijpers systematically compared sensory training biofeedback using simulated defecation to EMG biofeedback and found that more patients benefited from EMG biofeedback.[53] Two other studies reported no difference between EMG biofeedback and simulated defecation.[55] Electromyographic biofeedback is emerging as the most commonly employed form of biofeedback for pelvic floor dyssynergia because it is at least as effective as simulated defecation, is as effective as anal canal pressure biofeedback, and is simpler to implement and better tolerated by patients than simulated defecation or pressure biofeedback.

### Efficacy of Biofeedback for Pelvic Floor Dyssynergia

Most of the studies reporting the outcome of biofeedback for constipation have been single-group, uncontrolled studies. These have been reviewed by Enck,[15] Rao and colleagues,[23] and Jones and colleagues.[56] These reviews suggest that approximately two-thirds of adult patients with pelvic floor dyssynergia benefit from biofeedback training, and, as a result, biofeedback is often regarded as the treatment of choice for this problem.[31]

Six parallel-group studies have compared biofeedback to conventional therapy, but the results have been mixed. Four of these studies involved children, and it has been suggested that the etiology of pelvic floor dyssynergia may differ for children versus adults. In the earliest controlled study, Wald and colleagues compared pressure biofeedback to mineral oil in 50 fecally incontinent children, of whom only 18 had pelvic floor dyssynergia.[49] There were no significant differences between treatments, but there was a trend for patients with pelvic floor dyssynergia to do better with biofeedback and for patients without pelvic floor dyssynergia to do better with mineral oil. Loening-Baucke compared biofeedback (pressure and EMG) to laxatives in 41 children, all of whom had pelvic floor dyssynergia, and reported that the biofeedback group did significantly better.[57] However, two recent studies comparing laxative to biofeedback found no benefit for biofeedback training.[58,59]

In adults, two controlled studies have been reported. Koutsomanis and colleagues compared EMG biofeedback training to defecate a balloon (n = 29) to guided practice of balloon defecation without visual feedback (n = 30).[60] Both groups reported subjective improvement (69% vs. 64%) associated with increased frequency of bowel movements and decreased straining. Problems with the trial were that the etiology of constipation was mixed, although approximately 75% had pelvic floor dyssynergia, and relatively few training sessions were provided (average of three). Heymen and colleagues compared four approaches to the biofeedback treatment of pelvic floor dyssynergia: EMG biofeedback training alone, EMG plus rectal balloon biofeedback training, EMG plus daily use of a home biofeedback trainer, and EMG, balloon biofeedback, and home trainer combined.[20] There were

8 to 10 subjects in each group. There was a significant increase in the frequency of unassisted bowel movements in groups 1, 2, and 4, and there was a significant decrease in the use of cathartics by groups 1, 2, and 3. There were no significant differences between groups, although the small sample sizes limited the statistical power of between-group comparisons.

Studies from St. Mark's Hospital in London, England, suggest that biofeedback may benefit constipated patients through nonspecific mechanisms rather than by modifying the pattern of paradoxical pelvic floor muscle contraction during defecation. Investigators there have reported that biofeedback benefits patients with both slow and normal colonic transit and patients without paradoxical contraction, as well as those with paradoxical contraction, of the pelvic floor.[60–63]

### Predictors of Outcome

No patient characteristics have been identified as yet that are reliable predictors of the response to biofeedback training. In particular, neither whole-gut transit time[63] nor manometric demonstration of paradoxical contraction during defecatory maneuvers[66,62,64] predicted the response to biofeedback. Gilliland and colleagues found that the success of biofeedback was related to the number of training sessions patients received,[65] and it is likely that the training and experience of the biofeedback therapist also influence success. However, the type of biofeedback training, whether EMG, pressure, or simulated defecation, does not appear to have a significant impact on clinical outcomes.

## RUMINATION SYNDROME AND AEROPHAGIA

### Indications for Biofeedback Training

Rumination syndrome[66] refers to repeated regurgitation of previously ingested food into the mouth, where it may be remasticated and either spit out or reswallowed. It is not accompanied by nausea or by propulsive vomiting. It is very common among institutionalized, developmentally disabled children and adults, in whom it may occur in up to 10%.[67] It also occurs in adults of normal intelligence, but only when they are alone. Biofeedback has been described for adult ruminators of normal intelligence, whereas various forms of operant conditioning or increased contact with nurturing adults have been described for the treatment of infant and developmentally disabled ruminators.[68,69]

Rumination appears to occur as a self-stimulatory behavior that is engaged in because it produces a pleasurable sensation. The behavioral/physiologic mechanism by which rumination occurs consists of extending the head forward to open the upper esophageal sphincter and at the same time briskly contracting the abdominus rectus muscles to force gastric contents up the esophagus.[70] Rumination is most common in the immediate postprandial period and usually disappears by 2 hours after eating. It is often mistaken for gastroesophageal reflux disease.

Aerophagia refers to excessive swallowing of air. It can be part of a self-stimulatory sequence of behaviors in developmentally disabled individuals leading to massive bloating. However, it is also a common, unrecognized cause of symptoms of bloating and belching in normal individuals. Many people unconsciously swallow more frequently when they are anxious,[71] and others swallow excessively because of excessive salivation or mucus secretion, gum chewing, or frequent snacking. Each swallow carries a few milliliters of air into the stomach, and when swallowing is frequent, it can overwhelm the body's ability to absorb the gas and clear it. The result is a large gastric air bubble, excessive belching unrelated to meals, and excessive flatus.

Both rumination syndrome and aerophagia are produced by striated muscle responses and for this reason are more likely to be amenable to biofeedback training than smooth muscle responses.

### Biofeedback for Rumination Syndrome

Shay and colleagues investigated the mechanism of rumination syndrome extensively and described a biofeedback training technique that involved providing feedback on the abdominus rectus EMG activity after meals and teaching the patient to keep these muscles relaxed during meals and in the immediate postprandial period.[71] This was reported to be successful. Soykan and colleagues offered this form of biofeedback and relaxation training to 10 adults with rumination syndrome, but 5 preferred drug treatment.[72] All 5 patients who received biofeedback reported subjective improvement, whereas 4 of 5 declining biofeedback remained symptomatic.

### Biofeedback for Aerophagia

Calloway and colleagues treated six patients with aerophagia by using an electronic stethoscope placed on the neck to amplify swallow-related sounds while patients tried to reduce the rate of swallowing.[73] A control group of six patients was treated with progressive muscle relaxation exercises not specifically targeted at swallowing. Substantial reductions in swallow frequency were achieved by four patients in the biofeedback group but only two in the relaxation group (not significantly different), and reductions in swallow frequency were correlated with reductions in symptoms. This biofeedback training protocol has not been widely used because it has proven technically difficult to reliably distinguish swallows from head movement artifact.

## GASTROESOPHAGEAL REFLUX

Gastroesophageal reflux may be associated with hiatal hernia, decreased resting pressure in the lower esophageal sphincter, or increased frequency of transient lower esophageal relaxations. Schuster first described a biofeedback procedure that enabled patients to voluntarily augment

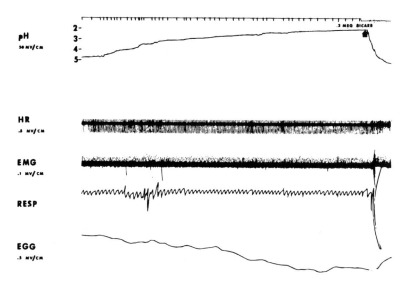

**FIGURE 27.13.** Method for training a subject to increase gastric acid secretion. A pH electrode passed transnasally was positioned in the gastric antrum and used to detect pH decreases caused by gastric acid secretion. Subjects viewed a meter that displayed the pH changes shown in the tracing. When the pH decreased by 0.1 pH unit (recorded by the event marker at the top of the figure), a points counter advanced, signaling that the subject had earned additional money. When the pH fell to approximately 2.5, sodium bicarbonate was infused into the stomach through a nasogastric tube to bring the intragastric pH back to a pH range that was more sensitive to small changes in gastric acid secretion. Adapted from Whitehead WE, Renault PF, Goldiamond I. Modification of human gastric acid secretion with operant-conditioning procedures. J Appl Behav Anal 1975;8:147–56.

lower esophageal sphincter pressure by watching a meter displaying moment-to-moment variation in sphincter pressure, but clinical results were not reported in that study.[74] Subsequently, Gordon and colleagues described a case study in which a patient with gastroesophageal reflux was treated for 10 sessions with this type of biofeedback; this patient increased lower esophageal sphincter pressure substantially, and this was associated with resolution of esophagitis and subjective improvement of heartburn.[75] Both Schuster and Gordon's group attributed these effects of biofeedback to improved smooth muscle tone, but this may not be the case: it is now known that pressures in the lower esophageal sphincter are partly attributable to the crural diaphragm, which surrounds the sphincter, and that patients can voluntarily contract this striated muscle to produce increased pressures in the lower esophageal sphincter.[76] Interest in the use of biofeedback to treat gastroesophageal reflux is minimal because proton pump inhibitors and fundoplication surgery are highly effective treatments.

## MODIFICATION OF GASTRIC ACID SECRETION

No clinical applications have been demonstrated for the operant conditioning of gastric acid secretion. It is likely that investigators will want to carry out this form of training primarily as a probe to differentiate central from peripheral mechanisms of action of investigational drugs or other agents believed to influence gastric acid secretion.

### Technique for Operant Conditioning of Gastric Acid Secretion

The essential step in providing biofeedback training for gastric acid secretion or any other secretory response is to find a way of converting the secretory response to a visual or auditory stimulus quickly. The approach used by Whitehead and coworkers was to position a pH electrode in the stomach to detect the fall in pH produced by acid secretion (Fig. 27.13).[77] These pH changes were displayed as a pen tracing on a polygraph and were also signaled by a points counter, which advanced each time the pH fell by 0.1 pH units during training to increase acid secretion and each time at least 10 seconds elapsed without a 0.1 or greater fall in pH during decrease training. A different approach was used by Welgan, who aspirated gastric secretions by continuous suction and measured pH outside the body.[78] Aspiration is relatively slow and introduces a variable and relatively long delay before a change in acid secretion can be reflected in the feedback display. Nevertheless, Welgan obtained significant changes in acid secretion as a function of training.[78]

Providing feedback that is sensitive and accurate is also difficult for gastric acid secretion. The relationship between pH and acid concentration is logarithmic rather than linear. As a consequence, acid concentration must change 10 times as much to cause a 0.1 pH change when starting at pH 2 as compared with starting at pH 3. Moreover, there are reflex mechanisms that inhibit gastric acid secretion when the pH falls to approximately 1.5. To circumvent these two difficulties, Whitehead and colleagues repeatedly titrated the contents of the stomach to pH 7 by infusing sodium bicarbonate to keep the pH of the gastric contents in a more sensitive part of the pH scale and away from the reflex brake, which would otherwise occur (see Fig. 27.13).[77] There are other sources of measurement error to contend with as well. These include a tendency for the intragastric pH electrode to become engulfed in the rugae of the stomach, where it is protected from exposure to the gastric contents, and the fact that gastric emptying can alter the relationship between acid secretion and pH change by altering the volume of the gastric residuum with which the parietal cell secretions must mix to alter pH. Displacement of the electrode by gastric contraction can provide additional problems.

Because these technical obstacles make it quite difficult for subjects to learn to alter gastric acid secretion voluntarily,

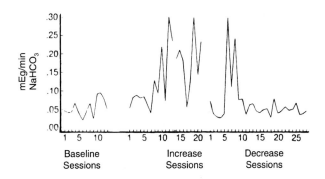

**FIGURE 27.14.** Learned control of gastric acid secretion in a healthy subject. Ordinate shows the rate of gastric acid secretion measured as the average amount of sodium bicarbonate required to repeatedly neutralize the gastric contents to pH 7.0. The baseline rate of variability was assessed during 13 90-minute sessions, after which the subject was provided with visual feedback on gastric pH and rewarded with money for increases in acid secretion (*middle panel*). After approximately 10 90-minute training sessions, the rate of secretion had increased to three times the baseline rate. Shown in the third panel is the result of rewarding the subject for decreasing acid secretion while she watched a visual display of gastric pH. Adapted from Whitehead WE, Renault PF, Goldiamond I. Modification of human gastric acid secretion with operant-conditioning procedures. J Appl Behav Anal 1975;8:147–56.

it is necessary to keep the training sessions very simple. Whitehead and colleagues found that subjects could learn to alter gastric acid secretion only if they were allowed to practice changing in one direction at a time for many hours and if they were motivated by monetary rewards (Fig. 27.14).[77] However, when subjects were asked to perform a more complex task involving alternately increasing and decreasing acid secretion, they failed to learn.

More time is required to learn to control a secretory response than a striated muscle motor response. Our best subjects required 7 to 10 90-minute training sessions before they could reliably control acid secretion. However, we trained some subjects unsuccessfully for more than 100 sessions on complex training schedules before simplifying the training schedule and then demonstrating learning effects. It is likely that the difficulty subjects had in learning to control this response was primarily attributable to the technical difficulties we had in providing accurate and immediate feedback to them on small changes in intragastric pH. With better methods of providing feedback, more rapid and more reliable learning might occur.

## GASTRIC MOTILITY

As with gastric acid secretion, no clinical indications have been identified for training patients to control gastric motility voluntarily. This training is most likely to find application by physiologists as a method of determining whether it is possible to uncouple normally correlated physiologic events such as antral motility, electrogastrographic activity, and gas-

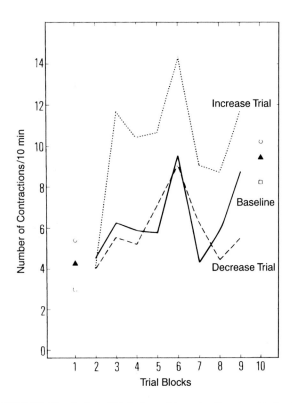

**FIGURE 27.15.** Control of 3/minute gastric contractions in subjects who received visual feedback. Data for five sessions are divided into 10 30-minute blocks. The first and last blocks are tests of voluntary control without feedback. Visual feedback was available on increase and decrease trials in blocks 2 to 9. For blocks 2 and 10, a circle indicates an increase trial, a triangle indicates a baseline period, and a square indicates a decrease trial. Reproduced with permission from Whitehead WE, Drescher VM. Perception of gastric contractions and self-control of gastric motility. Psychophysiology 1980;17:522–8.

tric emptying. It should be noted, however, that no one has investigated the effectiveness of biofeedback training for gastroparesis or gastroduodenal incoordination.

### Technique for Biofeedback Training

It is comparatively easy to obtain real-time feedback on 3 cpm antral contractions through solid-state pressure transducers or open-tipped perfused catheters or balloons positioned in the stomach and connected to external pressure transducers. Subjects learn quickly to modify this activity when provided with visual feedback and monetary incentives.[79] However, tonic contractions of the fundus may last 90 seconds or longer; it is difficult to know how to define "immediate" feedback when it may take 30 seconds to determine whether a tonic contraction has started. To date, there have been no reports of biofeedback training to modify these tonic contractions.

To improve the accuracy and sensitivity of the feedback signal, Whitehead and Drescher used an analog filter to differentiate respiratory artifact from antral contractions.[79] Digital filtering should produce better filtering and less distortion of the signal.

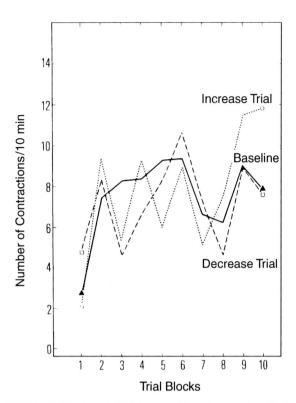

**FIGURE 27.16.** Control of 3/minute gastric contractions in subjects who practiced without feedback but with monetary incentives. Trial blocks and symbols are defined as in Figure 27.15, except that visual feedback was never available. Reproduced with permission from Whitehead WE, Drescher VM. Perception of gastric contractions and self-control of gastric motility. Psychophysiology 1980;17:522–8.

Because smooth muscle responses such as gastric motility exhibit a great deal of seemingly spontaneous variability, biofeedback experiments should incorporate differential conditioning paradigms in which subjects are asked to alternately increase and decrease contractions relative to baseline. Whitehead and Drescher used this technique and found that subjects were almost immediately able to make use of visual feedback to increase gastric contractions relative to baseline, although they were less consistent in decreasing gastric contractions relative to baseline (Fig. 27.15).[79] In the absence of visual feedback, subjects were unable to control gastric motility voluntarily as shown in Figure 27.16.

### Biofeedback Modification of the Electrogastrogram

The myoelectrical activity of the stomach, recorded as the electrogastrogram (EGG), exhibits abnormal frequencies when subjects are experiencing nausea.[80] The EGG is frequently recorded as part of the diagnostic evaluation of patients with unexplained nausea and vomiting, and in early studies, investigators reported that at least some aspects of the EGG could be modified with biofeedback training.[81,82] However, there have been no recent biofeedback studies on this topic.

## COLON MOTILITY

Early uncontrolled experiments[83,84] and a case study[85] suggested that biofeedback training might provide a useful treatment for IBS. Subsequent experience, however, suggested that biofeedback to modify colon motility is less effective than stress management training for controlling the clinical symptoms of IBS,[86] and biofeedback is no longer recommended for this disorder. Biofeedback training of colon motility seems to be useful primarily as an investigative tool.

### Techniques to Modify Colon Motility

Two different approaches to biofeedback training have been described. In one of them, pressures are recorded from the lumen of the colon, and training protocols similar to those described above for gastric motility are used. The alternative training protocol is to amplify bowel sounds with an electronic stethoscope and use this as a biofeedback signal that patients can practice increasing and decreasing. Two separate studies suggest that patients with IBS can learn to modify bowel sounds and that this is associated with modest improvements in clinical symptoms.[84,87,88] However, the relationship between bowel sounds and colon motility is complex and depends on the pitch of the sounds produced. In addition, anecdotal reports suggest that most of the sounds recorded from the abdomen by this technique are produced in the stomach or small intestine rather than in the colon.

*Acknowledgments*
Preparation of this chapter was supported in part by grant RO1 DK31369 from the National Institute of Diabetes and Digestive and Kidney Diseases.

**REFERENCES**

1. Whitehead WE, Engel BT, Schuster MM. Perception of rectal distention is necessary to prevent fecal incontinence. In: Adam G, Meszaros I, Banyai EI, editors. Advances in the physiological sciences. Vol 17. Brain and behavior. Budapest: Akademia Kiado; 1981.
2. Sun WM, Read NW, Miner PB. Relation between sensation and anal function in normal subjects and patients with faecal incontinence. Gut 1990;31:1056–61.
3. Wald A, Tunuguntla AK. Anorectal sensorimotor dysfunction in fecal incontinence and diabetes mellitus. Modification with biofeedback therapy. N Engl J Med 1984;310:1282–7.
4. Buser WD, Miner PB Jr. Delayed rectal sensation with fecal incontinence. Successful treatment using anorectal manometry. Gastroenterology 1986;91:1186–91.
5. Blanchard EB, Jurish SE, Andrasik F, Epstein LH. The relationship between muscle discrimination ability and response to relaxation training in three kinds of headaches. Biofeedback Self-Regul 1981;6:537–45.
6. Whitehead WE, Burgio K, Engel BT. Biofeedback treatment of fecal incontinence in geriatric patients. J Am Geriatr Soc 1985;33:320–4.
7. Whitehead WE, Parker L, Bosmajian L, et al. Treatment of fecal incontinence in children with spina bifida: comparison of biofeedback and behavior modification. Arch Phys Med Rehabil 1986;67:218–24.

8. Engel BT, Nikoomanesh P, Schuster MM. Operant conditioning of rectosphincteric responses in the treatment of fecal incontinence. N Engl J Med 1974;290:646–9.

9. Cerulli MA, Nikoomanesh P, Schuster MM. Progress in biofeedback conditioning for fecal incontinence. Gastroenterology 1979;76:742–6.

10. Glia A, Gylin M, Akerlund JE, et al. Biofeedback training in patients with fecal incontinence. Dis Colon Rectum 1998;41:359–64.

11. Patankar SK, Ferrara A, Larach SW, et al. Electromyographic assessment of biofeedback training for fecal incontinence and chronic constipation. Dis Colon Rectum 1997;40:907–11.

12. Cox DJ, Sutphen J, Borowitz S, et al. Simple electromyographic biofeedback treatment for chronic pediatric constipation/encopresis: preliminary report. Biofeedback Self-Regul 1994;19:41–50.

13. Eisman E, Tries J. A new probe for measuring electromyographic activity from multiple sites in the anal canal. Dis Colon Rectum 1993;36:946–52.

14. Chiarioni G, Bassotti G, Stegagnini S, et al. Sensory retraining is key to biofeedback therapy for formed stool fecal incontinence. Am J Gastroenterol 2001. [In press].

15. Enck P. Biofeedback training in disordered defecation: a critical review. Dig Dis Sci 1993;38:1953–60.

16. Rao SSC, Welcher KD, Pelsang RE. Effects of biofeedback therapy on anorectal function in obstructive defecation. Dig Dis Sci 1997;42:2197–205.

17. Heymen S, Jones KR, Ringel Y, et al. Biofeedback treatment of fecal incontinence: a critical review. Dis Colon Rectum 2001;44:728–36.

18. Miner PB, Donnelly TC, Read NW. Investigation of mode of action of biofeedback in treatment of fecal incontinence. Dig Dis Sci 1990;35:1291–8.

19. Guillemot F, Bouche B, Gower-Rosseau C, et al. Biofeedback for the treatment of fecal incontinence: long-term clinical results. Dis Colon Rectum 1995;38:393–7.

20. Heymen S, Wexner SD, Vickers D, et al. Prospective, randomized trial comparing four biofeedback techniques for patients with constipation. Dis Colon Rectum 1999;42:1388–93.

21. Latimer PR, Campbell D, Kasperski J. A component analysis of biofeedback in the treatment of fecal incontinence. Biofeedback Self-Regul 1984;9:311–24.

22. Heymen S, Jones KR, Ringel Y, et al. Biofeedback for fecal incontinence and constipation: the role of medical management and education. Gastroenterology 2001;120 Suppl 1:A397.

23. Rao SS, Enck P, Loening-Baucke V. Biofeedback therapy for defecation disorders. Dig Dis 1997;15 Suppl 1:78–92.

24. Whitehead WE, Wald A, Norton NJ. Treatment options for fecal incontinence. Dis Colon Rectum 2001;44:131–44.

25. Norton C, Kamm MA. Outcome of biofeedback for faecal incontinence. Br J Surg 1999;86:1159–63.

26. Sangwan YP, Coller JA, Barrett RC, et al. Can manometric parameters predict response to biofeedback therapy in fecal incontinence? Dis Colon Rectum 1995;38:1021–5.

27. Leroi A-M, Dorival M-P, Lecouturier M-F, et al. Pudendal neuropathy and severity of incontinence but not presence of an anal sphincter defect may determine the response to biofeedback therapy in fecal incontinence. Dis Colon Rectum 1999;42:762–9.

28. Iwai N, Nagashima M, Shimotake T, Iwata G. Biofeedback therapy for fecal incontinence after surgery for anorectal malformations: preliminary results. J Pediatr Surg 1993;28:863–6.

29. Keck JO, Staniunas RJ, Coller JA, et al. Biofeedback training is useful in fecal incontinence but disappointing in constipation. Dis Colon Rectum 1994;37:1271–6.

30. Hamalainen KJ, Raivio P, Antila S, et al. Biofeedback therapy in rectal prolapse patients. Dis Colon Rectum 1996;39:262–5.

31. Diamant NE, Kamm MA, Wald A, Whitehead WE. AGA technical review on anorectal testing techniques. Gastroenterology 1999;116:735–60.

32. Nelson R, Furner S, Jesudason V. Fecal incontinence in Wisconsin nursing homes: prevalence and associations. Dis Colon Rectum 1998;41:1226–9.

33. Heymen S, Wexner SD, Gulledge AD. MMPI assessment of patients with functional bowel disorders. Dis Colon Rectum 1993;36:593–6.

34. American Psychiatric Association. Diagnostic and statistical manual of mental disorders. 4th ed. rev. Washington (DC): American Psychiatric Association; 1999.

35. Arnbjornsson E, Breland U, Kullendorff CM, et al. Physiotherapy to improve faecal control after Stephens' rectoplasty in high imperforate anus. Z Kinderchirurgie 1986;41:101–3.

36. Sielezneff I, Bauer S, Bulgare JC, Sarles JC. Gracilis muscle transposition in the treatment of faecal incontinence. Int J Colorectal Dis 1996;11:15–8.

37. Ho Y-H, Chiang JM, Tan M, Low JY. Biofeedback therapy for excessive stool frequency and incontinence following anterior resection or total colectomy. Dis Colon Rectum 1996;39:1289–92.

38. Menard C, Trudel C, Cloutier R. Anal reeducation for postoperative fecal incontinence in congenital diseases of the rectum and anus. J Pediatr Surg 1997;32:867–9.

39. Solomon MJ, Rex J, Eyers AA, et al. Biofeedback for fecal incontinence using transanal ultrasonography. Dis Colon Rectum 2000;43:788–92.

40. Leahy A, Clayman C, Mason I, et al. Computerised biofeedback games: a new method for teaching stress management and its use in irritable bowel syndrome. J Roy Coll Physicians Lond 1998;32:552–6.

41. Preston DM, Lennard-Jones JE. Anismus in chronic constipation. Dig Dis Sci 1985;30:413–8.

42. Whitehead WE, Wald A, Diamant NE, et al. Functional disorders of the anus and rectum. In: Drossman DA, Corazziari E, Talley NJ, et al, editors. Rome II: the functional gastrointestinal disorders. McLean (VA): Degnon Associates; 2000. p. 483–529.

43. International Classificiation of Diseases. ICD-9-CM: Professional code book for physicians 2001. Washington (DC): St. Anthony Publishing; 2001.

44. Kuijpers HC, Bleijenberg G. The spastic pelvic floor syndrome. A cause of constipation. Dis Colon Rectum 1985;28:669–72.

45. Kuijpers HC, Bleijenberg G, De Moiree H. The spastic pelvic floor syndrome. Large bowel outlet obstruction caused by pelvic floor dysfunction: a radioilogical study. Int J Colorectal Dis 1986;1:44–8.

46. Roberts JP, Womack NR, Hallan RI, et al. Evidence from dynamic integrated proctography to redefine anismus. Br J Surg 1992;79:1213–5.

47. Keren S, Wagner Y, Heldenbert D, Golan M. Studies of manometric abnormalities of the rectoanal region during defecation in constipated and soiling children: modification through biofeedback therapy. Am J Gastroenterol 1988;83:827–31.

48. Loening-Baucke V. Changes in behavioural ratings with treatment of childhood encopresis. Presented at the Ambulatory Pediatric Association meeting, Washington (DC), May 1989.

49. Wald A, Chandra R, Gabel S, Chiponis D. Evaluation of biofeedback in childhood encopresis. J Pediatr Gastroenterol Nutr 1987;6:554–8.

50. Leroi AM, Berkelmans I, Denis P, et al. Anismus as a a marker of sexual abuse. Consequences of abuse on anorectal motility. Dig Dis 1995;40:141–6.

51. Duthie GS, Bartolo DCC. Anismus: the cause of constipation? Results of investigation and treatment. World J Surg 1992;16:831–5.

52. Schouten WR, Briel JW, Auwerda JJA, et al. Anismus: fact or fiction? Dis Colon Rectum 1997;40:1033–41.

53. Bleijenberg G, Kuijpers HC. Ttreatment of the spastic pelvic floor with biofeedback. Dis Colon Rectum 1987;30:108–11.

54. Kawimbe BM, Papachrysostomou M, Binnie NR, et al. Outlet obstruction constipation (anismus) managed by biofeedback. Gut 1991;35:1175–9.

55. Glia A, Gylin M, Gullberg K, Lindberg G. Biofeedback retraining in patients with functional constipation and paradoxical puborectalis contraction: comparison of anal manometry and sphincter electromyography for feedback. Dis Colon Rectum 1997;40:889–95.

56. Jones KR, Heymen S, Whitehead WE. Biofeedback for anorectal disorders. In: Drutz HP, Herschorn S, Diamant NE, editors. Urogynaecology and reconstructive pelvic surgery. London: Springer-Verlag. [In press]

57. Loening-Baucke V. Modulation of abnormal defecation dynamics by biofeedback treatment in chronically constipated children with encopresis. J Pediatr 1990;116:214–22.
58. Van der Plas RN, Benninga MA, Bueller HA, et al. Biofeedback training of childhood constipation: a randomized controlled study. Lancet 1996;348:776–80.
59. Nolan TM, Catto-Smith T, Coffey C, Wells J. Randomised controlled trial of biofeedback training in persistent encopresis with anismus. Arch Dis Child 1998;79:131–5.
60. Koutsomanis D, Lennard-Jones JE, Roy AJ, Kamm MA. Controlled randomized trial of visual biofeedback versus muscle training without a visual display for intractable constipation. Gut 1995;37:95–9.
61. Chiotakakou-Faliakou E, Kamm MA, Roy AJ, et al. Biofeedback provides long-term benefit for patients with intractable, slow and normal transit constipation. Gut 1998;42:517–21.
62. Koutsomanis D, Lennard-Jones JE, Kamm MA. Prospective study of biofeedback treatment for patients with slow and normal transit constipation. Eur J Gastroenterol Hepatol 1994;6:131–7.
63. Ho Y-H, Tan M, Goh H-S. Clinical and physiologic effects of biofeedback in outlet obstruction constipation. Dis Colon Rectum 1996;39:520–4.
64. Roy AJ, Emmanuel AV, Storrie JB, et al. Behavioural treatment (biofeedback) for constipation following hysterectomy. Br J Surg 1999;87:100–5.
65. Gilliland R, Heymen S, Altomare DF, et al. Outcome and predictors of success of biofeedback for constipation. Br J Surg 1997;84:1123–6.
66. O'Brien MD, Bruce BK, Camilleri M. The rumination syndrome: clinical features rather than manometric diagnosis. Gastroenterology 1995;108:1024–9.
67. Ball TS, Hendricksen H, Clayton JA. A special feeding technique for chronic regurgitation. Am J Ment Defic 1974;78:486–93.
68. Whitehead WE, Schuster MM. Gastrointestinal disorders: behavioral and physiological basis for treatment. New York: Academic Press; 1985.
69. Whitehead WE, Drescher VM, Morrill-Corbin E, Cataldo MF. Rumination syndrome in children treated by increased holding. Pediatr Gastroenterol Nutr 1985;4:550–6.
70. Shay SS, Johnson LF, Wong RKH, et al. Rumination, heartburn, and daytime gastroesophageal reflux. J Clin Gastroenterol 1986;8:115–26.
71. Cuevas JL, Cook EW III, Richter JE, et al. Spontaneous swallowing rate and emotional state. Possible mechanism for stress-related gastrointestinal disorders. Dig Dis Sci 1995;40:282–6.
72. Soykan I, Chen J, Kendall B, McCallum RW. The rumination syndrome: clinical and manometric profile, therapy, and long-term outcome. Dig Dis Sci 1997;42:1866–72.
73. Calloway SP, Fonagy P, Pounder RE, Morgan MJ. Behavioural techniques in the management of aerophagia in patients with hiatus hernia. J Psychosom Res 1983;27:499–502.
74. Schuster MM. Biofeedback treatment of gastrointestinal disorders. Med Clin North Am 1977;61:907–12.
75. Gordon A, Gordon E, Berelowitz M, et al. Biofeedback improvement of lower esophageal sphincter pressures and reflux symptoms. J Clin Gastroenterol 1983;5:235–7.
76. Mittal RK. The crural diaphragm, an external lower esophageal sphincter: a definitive study. Gastroenterology 1993;105:1565–67.
77. Whitehead WE, Renault PF, Goldiamond I. Modification of human gastric acid secretion with operant-conditioning procedures. J Appl Behav Anal 1975;8:147–56.
78. Welgan PR. Learned control of gastric acid secretions in peptic ulcer patients. Psychosom Med 1974;36:411–9.
79. Whitehead WE, Drescher VM. Perception of gastric contractions and self-control of gastric motility. Psychophysiology 1980;17:522–8.
80. Soykan I, Lin Z, Sarosiek I, McCallum RW. Gastric myoelectrical activity, gastric emptying, and correlations with symptoms and fasting blood glucose levels in diabetic patients. Am J Med Sci 1999;317:226–31.
81. Deckner CW, Hill JT, Bourne JR. Shaping of gastric motility in humans. In: Proceedings of the 80th Annual Convention of the American Psychological Association. Washington (DC): APA; 1972. p. 759–60.
82. Walker BB, Lawton CA, Sandman CA. Voluntary control of electrogastric activity. Psychosom Med 1978;40:610–9.
83. Bueno-Miranda F, Cerulli M, Schuster MM. Operant conditioning of colonic motility in irritable bowel syndrome (IBS) [abstract]. Gastroenterology 1976;70:A867.
84. Furman S. Intestinal biofeedback in functional diarrhea: a preliminary report. J Behav Ther Exp Psychiatry 1973;4:317–21.
85. Whitehead WE, Fedoravicius AS, Blackwell B, Wooley S. A behavioral conceptualization of psychosomatic illness: psychosomatic symptoms as learned responses. In: McNamara JR, editor. Behavioral approaches to medicine: application and analysis. New York: Plenum; 1979. p. 65–99.
86. Whitehead WE. Psychotherapy and biofeedback in the treatment of irritable bowel syndrome. In: Read NW, editor. Irritable bowel syndrome. London: Grune & Stratton; 1983. p. 245–56.
87. Radnitz CL, Blanchard EB. Bowel sound biofeedback as a treatment for irritable bowel syndrome. Biofeedback Self-Regul 1988;13:169–79.
88. Radnitz CL, Blanchard EB. A 1- and 2-year follow-up study of bowel sound biofeedback as a treatment for irritable bowel syndrome. Biofeedback Self-Regul 1989;14:333–8

# CHAPTER 28

# Motility and Pharmacologic Therapies

*James J. Galligan*

In recent years, there has been great progress in our understanding of the mechanisms controlling gastrointestinal motility. This new information has helped identify the pathophysiologic basis for many gastrointestinal motility disorders. This information has led to the development of new classes of drugs that are effective in treating gastrointestinal motility disorders that did not respond to agents available in the past. In addition, previously unknown mechanisms of drug action have been identified.

This chapter will focus on drugs used to stimulate or inhibit gastrointestinal propulsion and to treat symptoms associated with motility disorders. The first group of drugs is pro-kinetic agents, which are used to stimulate gastric accom- modation to a meal and also to stimulate gastric emptying and accelerate small and large intestinal transit. Prokinetic agents include drugs that act at least in part as 5-hydroxytryptamine (5-HT$_4$) receptor agonists (cisapride, metoclopramide), 5-HT$_1$ receptor agonists, including sumatriptan; the motilides, such as erythromycin (EM); and drugs that act as antagonists of D$_2$ dopamine receptors (domperidone). The second group of drugs is antidiarrheal agents.

Drugs in this class are opioids such as loperamide and the 5-HT$_3$ receptor antagonists, such as alosetron. Although 5-HT$_3$ receptor antagonists are used as antiemetic agents, alosetron and related agents have also been shown to be effective in treating functional diarrhea in some patients. The cellular basis for the actions of each class of drug will be discussed briefly followed by a description of the motility changes brought about by each drug.

## PROKINETIC AGENTS

### 5-HT$_4$ Receptor Agonists

#### Mechanism of Action

Drugs acting as agonists at 5-HT$_4$ receptors are effective stimulants of gastrointestinal motility and propulsion in a number of motility disorders. These receptors are localized to nerve endings of cholinergic motoneurons and interneurons in the myenteric plexus[1,2] and to some gastrointestinal smooth muscle cells.[3,4] Stimulation of 5-HT$_4$ receptors enhances acetylcholine release in ganglia and at the neuroeffector junction in the smooth muscle layers; therefore, these drugs stimulate gastrointestinal motility. These receptors are also localized to nerve endings of intrinsic primary afferent neurons, and stimulation of receptors on sensory nerve endings in the mucosal layer initiates enteric motor reflexes. 5-Hydroxytryptamine released from enterochromaffin cells in the mucosal layer is the likely source of endogenous 5-HT for the 5-HT$_4$ receptors on sensory nerve endings in the mucosal layer.[5,6]

The 5-HT$_4$ receptors belong to the superfamily of G-protein coupled receptors. These receptors couple to the stimulatory G-protein, Gs, and increase the intracellular cyclic adenosine 3′,5′-monophosphate (cAMP).[7] The increase in cAMP may stimulate mechanisms associated with acetylcholine release from enteric nerves.[8]

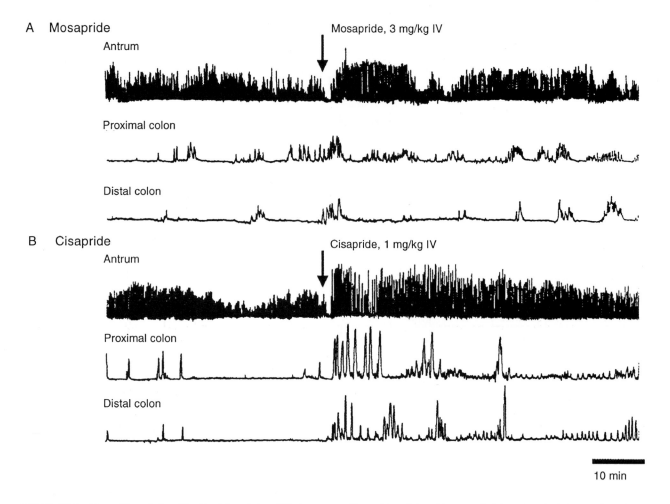

**FIGURE 28.1.** Mosapride and cisapride stimulate antral motility in conscious dogs. Motility was recorded using chronically implanted strain gauge force transducers attached to the serosal surface of the gastric antrum. Mosapride and cisapride were administered at the indicated doses (*arrows*). (Adapted from Mine et al.[13])

### *Cisapride and Mosapride*

Cisapride is effective in treating the symptoms associated with gastroesophageal reflux disease,[9] dyspepsia, and delayed gastric emptying in diabetic patients.[10] Improvement in symptoms associated with these disorders is related to cisapride-induced stimulation of gastric motility and acceleration of gastric emptying. Although cisapride stimulates upper gastrointestinal motility, it is less effective in treating symptoms associated with lower gastrointestinal motility. Cisapride has little effect on the symptoms of irritable bowel syndrome (IBS) and constipation.[11,12] These data are supported by direct studies of the actions of cisapride and mosapride, another benzamide prokinetic agent, on gastric and colonic motility in dogs.[13] In these studies, it was shown that these agents markedly enhance antral motility, whereas changes in colonic motility were less pronounced (Fig. 28.1).

The use of cisapride to treat gastric motility disorders has been restricted owing to complications caused by this agent

in patients susceptible to certain cardiac arrhythmias.[14] However, other substituted benzamide agents, such as mosapride, do not have similar cardiac actions.[15]

### Erythromycin and Related Agents

### *Mechanism of Action*

Antibiotic therapy with EM causes nausea, vomiting, and diarrhea in some patients. Initially, these effects were attributed to alterations in the normal gastrointestinal flora; however, subsequent analysis of the actions of EM on gastrointestinal tissues revealed that the antibiotic acted as an agonist at motilin receptors on gastrointestinal smooth muscle and on enteric nerves.[16,17] Erythromycin stimulates gastrointestinal motility by acting directly at motilin receptors on smooth muscle cells and at motilin receptors on enteric nerves to facilitate release of acetylcholine and other excitatory or inhibitory transmitters.[16,17] Although EM stimulates gastric, small intestinal, and colonic transit, it is particularly

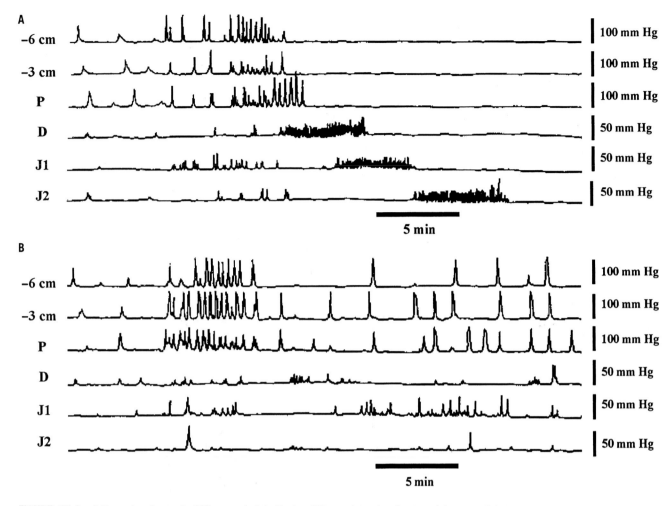

**FIGURE 28.2.** Actions of erythromycin (EM) on gastrointestinal motility recorded from healthy human volunteers. **A**, Erythromycin (40 mg, IV) induced phase 3–like contractions that began in the stomach and propagated through to the proximal jejunum. **B**, Erythromycin (200 mg) given intravenously caused phase 3–like contractions that propagated through the stomach but not into the small intestine. In both recordings, EM was admin-istered at the start of the traces. Labels to the left of the traces indicate the position of the catheter tips: D, duodenum; J1 and J2, jejunal sites 1 and 2. The position of the stomach catheters is the distance (cm) from the pylorus (P). Adapted with permission from Tack J, Janssens J, Vantrappen G, et al. Effect of erythromycin on gastric motility in controls and in diabetic gastro-paresis. Gastroenterology 1992;103:72–9.

effective in enhancing gastric motility and promoting gastric emptying in normal subjects and in patients with impaired gastric emptying as occurs in diabetics or in patients with functional dyspepsia.[18,19] The therapeutic action of EM and related agents is attributable to the ability of these drugs to enhance antroduodenal coordination and thereby facilitate gastric emptying and promote duodenal clearance. These effects are illustrated below.

### Erythromycin Stimulates Gastroduodenal Motility.

Erythromycin stimulates gastric and duodenal motility by initiating a burst of strong phasic contractions that migrate through the stomach and into the duodenum. The effects of EM have been studied in normal human volunteers in which gastrointestinal motility was recorded using perfused catheters positioned in the stomach and duodenum and proximal jejunum.[20] Erythromycin, administered intra-venously (30 or 200 mg), stimulated gastric motility by inducing strong phasic contractions that in some cases prop-agated into the small intestine (Fig. 28.2A). In other instances, these contractions did not propagate into the duo-denum, but, instead, duodenal motility was inhibited briefly (Fig. 28.2B). In the same study, the authors studied the actions of EM on gastrointestinal motility in diabetic patients with gastroparesis.[20] In some of these diabetic patients, EM produced strong phasic contractions that prop-agated from the stomach through the small intestine (Fig. (28.3A), whereas in other patients, the contractions propa-gated only through the stomach (Fig. 28.3B). In both normal subjects and diabetic patients, the properties of the migrat-ing motor complex initiated by EM were identical to those occurring spontaneously.[20]

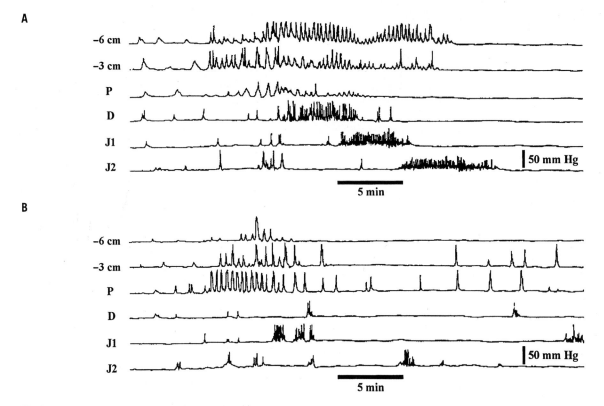

**FIGURE 28.3.** Erythromycin (EM) stimulates gastrointestinal motility in diabetic patients with gastroparesis. **A,** Erythromycin (200 mg, IV) induces phase 3–like contractions that begin in the stomach and propagate into the small intestine. **B,** In another patient, EM stimulates phase 3–like contractions that propagate through the stomach but not into the small intestine. Labels to the left of the traces indicate the position of the catheter tips: D, duodenum; J1 and J2, jejunal sites. The position of the stomach catheters is the distance (cm) from the pylorus (P). Reproduced with permission from Tack J, Janssens J, Vantrappen G, et al. Effect of erythromycin on gastric motility in controls and in diabetic gastroparesis. Gastroenterology 1992;103:72–9.

Based on the effectiveness of EM in stimulating gastrointestinal motility, there has been an effort to develop EM analogues that are devoid of antibiotic activity but that retain prokinetic properties. ABT-229 is an example of this type of compound. ABT-229 administered to healthy human volunteers stimulates both gastric emptying and antral contractions.[21] This effect is illustrated in the results from studies done in dogs instrumented with chronic serosal surface strain gauges positioned on the antrum and duodenum.[22] This study showed that ABT-229 could accelerate gastric emptying and also stimulate contractions that propagated from the antrum into the small intestine (Fig. 28.4). It is also important to note that during ABT-229-stimulated phasic contractions in the antrum, there was a simultaneous inhibition of duodenal contractions. This brief period of duodenal inhibition was followed by a propagated wave of duodenal contractions (see Fig. 28.4). These studies are important because it has been shown that EM accelerates gastric emptying in dogs[23]; therefore, the effects of EM and its motility stimulating analogues on gastric emptying and gastrointestinal motility in dogs are identical to the actions of these drugs in human subjects. However, in clinical trials, ABT-229 failed to improve symptoms in patients with gastroparesis, and this agent is no longer being pursued as a gastric prokinetic agent in humans.

It has been established that EM is an effective stimulant of gastrointestinal motility and that EM accelerates gastric emptying. The motility records shown here indicate that EM stimulates strong phasic contractions that begin in the stomach and propagate toward the pylorus. In some cases, the contractions do not propagate into the duodenum. In these instances, EM would accelerate gastric emptying without altering small intestinal transit. At other times, the contractions propagate from the stomach and along the small intestine. Under these conditions, EM would accelerate gastric emptying and decrease small intestinal transit time.

## Domperidone and Metoclopramide

### Mechanism of Action

Domperidone and metoclopramide[24,25] are two drugs that stimulate gastric motility in laboratory animals and in human subjects. Metoclopramide has multiple mechanisms of action on gastric motility (see below), including antagonism of $D_2$ dopamine receptors,[1,26] whereas domperidone is a specific $D_2$ dopamine receptor antagonist.[25] $D_2$ dopamine receptors are localized to cholinergic nerve endings in the gastric myenteric plexus, and these presynaptic $D_2$ receptors mediate inhibition of acetylcholine release. Therefore, antagonism of $D_2$

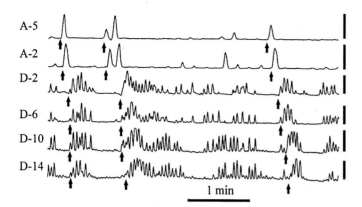

**FIGURE 28.4.** Strain gauge recordings of gastroduodenal motility in a dog treated with ABT-229. ABT-229 was administered as an intravenous infusion (2.5 or 5 μg/kg/min) prior to the start of the traces. Both doses caused similar responses. The figure shows contractions that propagate (*arrows*) from the antrum (labeled A) and into the duodenum (labeled D). Note the brief period of duodenal inhibition preceding duodenal contractions. Numbers indicate distances of the strain gauges from the pylorus. Vertical lines to the right of the traces indicate 100% of the amplitude of spontaneously occurring phase 3 contractions. Reproduced with permission from Cowles VE, Nellans IIN, Seiffert TR, et al. Effect of novel motilide ABT-229 versus erythromycin and cisapride on gastric emptying in dogs. J Pharmacol Exp Ther 2000;293:1106–11.

**FIGURE 28.5.** Electrogastrograms and running spectral analyses from a diabetic patient before and during domperidone treatment (20 mg, four times daily, oral administration). The traces illustrate that, prior to domperidone treatment, the normal 3 cycle-per-minute gastric rhythm is absent but becomes more prominent during domperidone therapy. Reproduced with permission from Koch KL, Stern RM, Stewart WR, Vasey MW. Gastric emptying and gastric myoelectrical activity in patients with diabetic gastroparesis: effect of long-term donperidone treatment. Am J Gastroenterol 1989;84:1069–75.

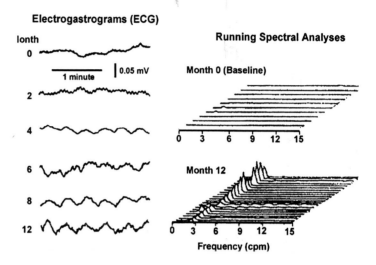

receptors results in disinhibition and an increase in acetylcholine release.[26] In addition to blocking $D_2$ receptors, metoclopramide is also an agonist at $5\text{-}HT_4$ receptors and an antagonist at $5\text{-}HT_3$ receptors. Therefore, metoclopramide can produce effects on gastrointestinal motility that are not shared by domperidone. This point is illustrated by the observations that domperidone has only proven to be effective in stimulating upper gastrointestinal motility and has little or no effect on the distal gut.[27,28] Metoclopramide stimulates both upper and lower gastrointestinal motility. These data suggest that $D_2$ receptors may be selectively localized to neurons in the upper gastrointestinal tract. Domperidone and metoclopramide are both effective antiemetic agents, although domperidone penetrates the blood-brain barrier poorly. The antiemetic effects of domperidone are likely to be mediated in the chemoreceptor trigger zone, an area of the brain that lies outside the blood-brain barrier.[25] Metoclopramide crosses the blood-brain barrier, and this may contribute to the increased number of side effects reported by patients taking metoclopramide for treatment of motility disorders.

### Effects of Domperidone and Metoclopramide on Gastric Motility

Domperidone has been used to treat effectively delayed gastric emptying and nausea and vomiting associated with diabetic gastroparesis, functional dyspepsia, and other gastric motility disorders.[29,30] For example, in diabetic patients with gastroparesis, gastric emptying was impaired compared to control subjects.[31] Electrogastrogram (EGG) recordings demonstrated that the diabetic subjects exhibited abnormal gastric electrical rhythms and tachygastria, whereas control subjects exhibited the normal three cycle per minute (cpm) electrical rhythm. After prolonged treatment with domperidone, patients reported an improvement in symptoms (reduced nausea and vomiting), and the EGG revealed the normal 3 cpm rhythm (Fig. 28.5). Interestingly, gastric emptying did not significantly improve in these patients.

Similar results were obtained in a double-blind, placebo-controlled study of the effects of domperidone in patients with idiopathic gastroparesis.[32] These patients complained of nausea, vomiting, and abdominal pain with delayed gastric emptying. Chronic motility recordings before and after domperidone treatment were similar, and there were no changes in gastric emptying of a radiolabeled solid meal after domperidone treatment. Despite the lack of effect on gastric motor function, all patients reported a marked improvement in their symptoms. However, in diabetic patients with gastroparesis, long-term (up to 6 months) treatment with domperidone caused a marked improvement in gastrointestinal symptoms (Fig. 28.6) and an increase in gastric emptying of a radiolabeled solid meal (Fig. 28.7).[33]

As discussed above, metoclopramide shares the $D_2$ recep-

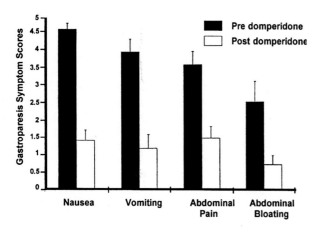

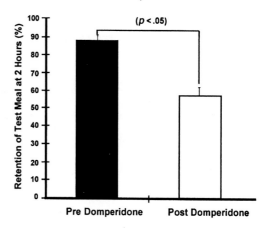

**FIGURE 28.6.** Severity of gastroparesis symptoms of nausea, vomiting, abdominal pain, and abdominal bloating at baseline (pre domperidone) and following long-term (6–48 mo) therapy with domperidone (post domperidone). The score for each of the symptoms was significantly reduced after domperidone therapy ($p < .05$; data are mean ± SEM). Adapted with permission from Soykan I, Sarosiek I, McCallum RW. The effect of chronic oral domperidone therapy on gastrointestinal symptoms, gastric emptying and quality of life in patients with gastroparesis. Am J Gastroenterol 1997;92:976–98.

**FIGURE 28.7.** The results of gastric emptying of a radionuclide solid meal (isotope labeled chicken liver and beef stew). The percent retention of the meal at baseline was 87.3 ± 3.7, abnormally slow for the test meal for which the upper limit of normal was <70% retention at 2 hours. Follow-up gastric emptying while on domperidone therapy showed a significant acceleration in gastric emptying to a mean of 57.2 ± 5.55% at 2 hours ($p < .05$; data are mean ± SEM). These data indicate that domperidone can accelerate gastric emptying in some patients with gastroparesis. Adapted with permission from Soykan I, Sarosiek I, McCallum RW. The effect of chronic oral domperidone therapy on gastrointestinal symptoms, gastric emptying and quality of life in patients with gastroparesis. Am J Gastroenterol 1997;92:976–98.

tor antagonist activity of domperidone. A study comparing the relative efficacy of domperidone versus metoclopramide in treating symptoms associated with diabetic gastroparesis found that domperidone was equally effective or somewhat better than metoclopramide in reducing symptoms such as nausea, vomiting, bloating, and early satiety, but central nervous system side effects were less prominent with domperidone.[34] This difference in side-effect profile is likely attributable to the fact that metoclopramide readily crosses the blood-brain barrier, whereas domperidone does not.[34]

## Cholecystokinin$_A$ Receptor Antagonists

### Mechanism of Action

Cholecystolkinin (CCK) is released from duodenal endocrine cells in response to the presence of lipids and/or fatty acids in the duodenum. Circulating CCK then causes an inhibition of gastric motility and a delay in gastric emptying.[35,36] Endogenously released CCK acts at CCK$_A$-type receptors in the stomach and possibly in the central nervous system to alter gastric motility. In the stomach, CCK receptors are localized to gastric smooth muscle cells[37] and to peripheral terminals of vagal afferent fibers.[38–40]

### Effects on Gastric Motility

The CCK$_A$ receptor antagonists loxiglumide and devazepide can block the inhibitory effects of a lipid meal on gastric motility and gastric emptying. For example, a magnetic resonance imaging (MRI) study of gastric emptying of a liquid lipid meal in normal subjects showed that loxiglumide administered intravenously as an infusion decreased gastric half-emptying time in all subjects (Fig. 28.8).[41] The increase in

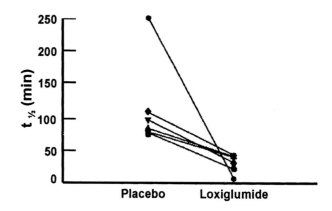

**FIGURE 28.8.** Individual gastric half-emptying times (t$_{1/2}$) of a liquid lipid meal (500 mL of 10% Intralipid) in normal subjects after treatment with placebo or with the CCK$_A$ receptor antagonist loxiglumide administered by intravenous infusion (66 μmol/kg/h for 10 minutes followed by 22 μmol/kg/h for 120 minutes to produce a steady-state plasma concentration). Loxiglumide decreased the t$_{1/2}$ in all subjects. Gastric emptying was measured using magnetic resonance imaging techniques. Reproduced with permission from Schwizer W, Borovicka J, Kunz P, et al. Role of cholecystokinin in the regulation of liquid gastric emptying and gastric motility in humans: studies with the CCK antagonist loxiglumide. Gut 1997;41:500–4.

gastric emptying was associated with an increase in antral contraction amplitude and contraction frequency (Fig. 28.9).[41] Similar data were obtained in a study using an intragastric balloon positioned in the fundus to measure gastric contractions, gastric pressures, and subject sensations following bal-

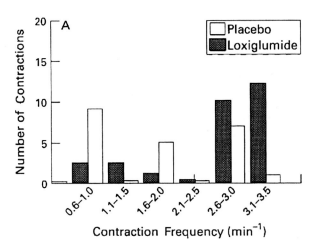

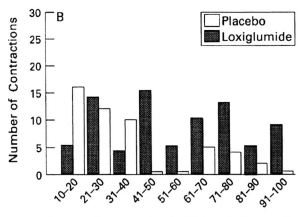

**FIGURE 28.9.** The effects of loxiglumide administered by intravenous infusion (66 µmol/kg/h for 10 minutes followed by 22 µmol/kg/hr for 120 minutes to produce a steady-state plasma concentration) on the frequency (**A**) and amplitude (**B**) of distal gastric contractions in normal subjects. Loxiglumide increased the average frequency of contractions (2.9 ± 0.2/min versus 1.5 ± 0.7/min after placebo) and the average amplitude of contractions (56 ± 22% of basal diameter versus 27 ± 16% after placebo). Reproduced with permission from Schwizer W, Borovicka J, Kunz P, et al. Role of cholecystokinin in the regulation of liquid gastric emptying and gastric motility in humans: studies with the CCK antagonist loxiglumide. Gut 1997;41:500–4.

**TABLE 28.1.** Fundic Tonic and Phasic Pressure Activity during Gastric Distention Following Intraduodenal Saline or Intraduodenal Lipid Infusion in Normal Human Subjects

|  | Saline-Placebo | Saline-Loxiglumide | Lipid-Placebo | Lipid-Loxiglumide |
|---|---|---|---|---|
| Tonic activity (cm H$_2$O) | 9 ± 1 | 9 ± 1 | 3 ± 0* | 6 ± 0† |
| Pressure oscillations |  |  |  |  |
| Amplitude (cm H$_2$O) | 6 ± 1 | 7 ± 1 | 1 ± 0* | 3 ± 1† |
| Rate (contractions/min) | 1 ± 0 | 1 ± 0 | 0 ± 0* | 1 ± 0† |

Lipid or saline was administered via a nasogastric tube, the tip of which was positioned in the duodenum. Fundic pressures were measured using an intragastric balloon connected to a flexible double-lumen gastric tube that was swallowed by the patients. The bag was positioned in the fundus and inflated with air, and pressures (tonic and phasic) in response to the various experimental conditions were recorded. These data indicate that loxiglumide has no effect on basal pressures or contractile activity. However, loxiglumide partly reverses the lipid-induced reduction in basal pressure and contractile activity. Reproduced with permission from Feinle C, D'Amato, Read NW. Cholecystokinin-A receptors modulate gastric sensory and motor responses to gastric distention and duodenal lipid. Gastroenterology 1996;110:1379–85.

Data are mean ± SEM of all subjects.
* Significantly different from saline-placebo and lipid-loxiglumide ($p < .001$).
† Significantly different from saline-loxiglumide ($p < .001$).

did not affect the volume/pressure relationship after intraduodenal saline. These data indicate that endogenous CCK released in response to the lipid stimulus was responsible for the change in gastric distensibility.[42] Intraduodenal lipid reduced the pressures at which subjects felt a sensation of fullness and discomfort following intragastric balloon inflation. This effect of intraduodenal lipid was also blocked by loxiglumide treatment. Loxiglumide did not change the fullness or discomfort pressures in subjects receiving intraduodenal lipid (see Fig. 28.10).[42] These data indicate that CCK$_A$ receptor antagonists might be used to treat gastric motility disorders exacerbated by lipid-containing meals. Cholecystokinin$_A$ receptor antagonists might also be useful in treating early satiety.

## GASTRIC ACCOMMODATION AGENTS

### Sumatriptan

***Mechanism of Action and Therapeutic Use***
Sumatriptan is a 5-HT$_1$ receptor agonist that is used to treat migraine headaches. One of the actions of sumatriptan is to alleviate the nausea and vomiting often associated with migraine attacks. Early studies found that sumatriptan caused a delay in liquid gastric emptying, and these authors concluded that reduction in nausea and vomiting caused by sumatriptan was likely to be centrally mediated.[43] Subsequently, it was shown that sumatriptan delayed gastric emptying of both solids and liquids, and the delay in liquid emptying was caused by a drug-induced lag phase.[44] Studies in cats using a gastric barostat to measure gastric fundus tone showed that sumatriptan caused a dose-dependent relaxation of the fundus and that this effect was

loon inflation before and after intraduodenal infusions of lipids.[42] These authors showed that the CCK$_A$ receptor antagonist loxiglumide did not change tonic or phasic gastric contractile activity following intraduodenal saline infusion (Table 28.1). However, intraduodenal infusion of lipid (20% Intralipid®) reduced tonic pressure and the rate and amplitude of phasic gastric contractions. The inhibitory effect of intraduodenal lipid was blocked by intravenous loxiglumide treatment (see Table 28.1). Intraduodenal lipid also altered the gastric volume/pressure relationship, and this was shown to be due to activation of CCK$_A$ receptors (Fig. 28.10). In these studies, it was shown that intraduodenal lipid shifted the volume/pressure relationship downward and to the right, and loxiglumide treatment partly reversed this effect. Loxiglumide

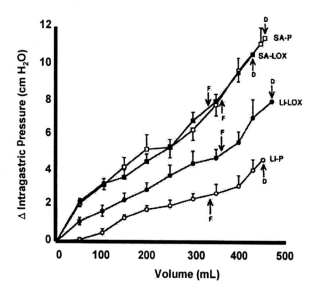

**FIGURE 28.10.** Intragastric pressure-volume relationship during four experimental conditions: duodenal saline infusion-placebo (SA-PP), duodenal saline infusion-intravenous loxiglumide (SA-LOX), intraduodenal lipid infusion-intravenous loxiglumide (LI-LOX), and intraduodenal lipid-placebo (LI-P). Loxiglumide was administered as an infusion at an initial rate of 30 mg/kg/h for 10 minutes and then at 10 mg/kg/h for the remainder of the study. *Arrows* indicate threshold volumes for feelings of fullness (F) and discomfort (D). Lipid or saline was administered via a nasogastric tube, the tip of which was positioned in the duodenum. Intragastric pressures were measured using an intragastric balloon connected to a flexible double-lumen gastric tube that was swallowed by the patients. The bag was positioned in the fundus and inflated with indicated volumes of air, and the resulting pressures were recorded. Reproduced with permission from Feinle C, D'Amato, Read NW. Cholecystokinin-A receptors modulate gastric sensory and motor responses to gastric distention and duodenal lipid. Gastroenterology 1996;110:1379–85.

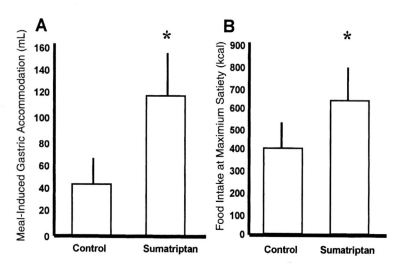

**FIGURE 28.11.** Sumatriptan increases gastric accommodation in response to a meal and also increases the amount of food intake required to reach satiety in patients with functional dyspepsia. **A,** Gastric accommodation in response to a meal under control conditions and after treatment with 6 mg (SQ) of the 5-HT$_1$ receptor agonist sumatriptan. Sumatriptan increased meal-induced gastric relaxation. Gastric relaxation was measured using a barostat. **B,** Food intake required to reach satiety in patients treated with placebo or sumatriptan (6 mg). Sumatriptan increased the amount of calories needed to reach satiety. Asterisks indicate significantly different ($p < .05$) from placebo treatment (control). Reproduced with permission from Tack J, Piessevaux H, Coulie B, et al. Role of impaired gastric accommodation to a meal in functional dyspepsia. Gastroenterology 1998;115:1346–52.

blocked following pretreatment of the cats with an inhibitor of nitric oxide synthase.[45] These data suggest that 5-HT$_1$ receptors may be localized to inhibitory neurons in the stomach and that stimulation of the 5-HT$_1$ receptors caused release of nitric oxide and subsequent relaxation of fundic smooth muscle.[45]

Functional dyspepsia is associated with a variety of symptoms that may be caused by alterations in gastric motor function. One change in gastric motor function in dyspeptic patients is an impairment of receptive relaxation of the proximal stomach in response to ingestion of a meal.[46] Failure of the proximal stomach to relax may contribute to early satiety. The 5-HT$_1$ receptor agonist sumatriptan reduces early satiety in some patients with functional dyspepsia. This therapeutic effect is associated with enhancement of vagally mediated receptive relaxation in dyspeptic patients. This conclusion is based on studies measuring gastric accommodation using a barostat balloon.[46] It was found that sumatriptan increased meal-induced gastric relaxation and the amount of food intake required to reach

satiety in dyspeptic patients (Fig. 28.11).

## ANTIDIARRHEAL AGENTS

### Opiates and Opioid Compounds

Morphine and related opiates are powerful antidiarrheal drugs. In humans, opiates and opioid compounds delay gastrointestinal propulsion but stimulate gastrointestinal motility.[47] Opiates and opioids act to inhibit the release of acetylcholine and nonadrenergic noncholinergic inhibitory neurotransmitters from enteric nerves in the human gastrointestinal tract.[48–50] These effects are likely mediated by $\mu$ and $\delta$ opioid receptors.[48–53]

### Loperamide

Although opiates and opioids are powerful antidiarrheal drugs, their abuse potential and addiction liability limit their usefulness for the routine treatment of diarrhea. However,

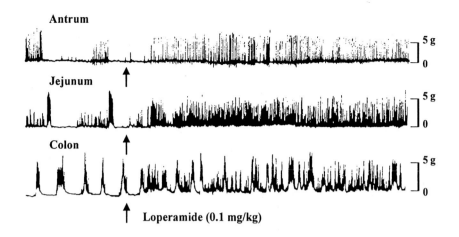

**FIGURE 28.12.** The effects of oral administration of loperamide (0.1 mg/kg) on gastrointestinal motility in conscious dogs. Loperamide disrupted the normal cyclic pattern of gastrointestinal contractions and induced continuous contractile activity through the length of the gut. Gastrointestinal contractions were recorded using chronically implanted serosal surface strain gauges oriented to record circular muscle contractions. Reproduced from Fioramonti J, Fargeus MJ, Bueno L. Stimulation of gastrointestinal motility by loperamide in dogs. Dig Dis Sci 1987;32:64–6, with permission from Kluwer Academic/Plenum Publishers.

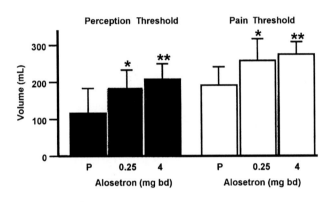

**FIGURE 28.13.** Mean barostat bag volumes at the first sensation threshold and at the threshold for abdominal pain during isobaric distention of the left colon with a barostat in patients with irritable bowel syndrome. Comparisons between placebo and alosetron 0.25 mg bd and 4 mg bd given orally for 7 days before the distention challenge. Error bars are the standard deviation of the mean. $*p < .02$; $**p < .001$ versus placebo-treated subjects. Reproduced with permission from Delvaux D, Mamét J-P, Campos-Oriola R, Frexinos J. Effect of alosetron on responses to colonic distention in patients with irritable bowel syndrome. Aliment Pharmacol Ther 1998;12:849–55.

agents are available with limited blood-brain barrier permeability and sites of action that are restricted to the periphery. Loperamide is an agent in this class.[51] It acts at opioid receptors in the enteric nervous system to alter gastrointestinal motility.[48,52] The overall effect of loperamide is to delay gastrointestinal transit time by stimulating gastrointestinal motility. Although contractile activity is increased, there is a disruption in the normal propulsive patterns of motility, leading to a delay in transit time. This disruption is illustrated in Figure 28.12, which shows that loperamide administered orally to conscious dogs disrupted the normal cyclic pattern of fasting motility.[53]

### 5-Hydroxytryptamine (5-HT₃) Receptor Antagonists

Colonic motility is altered in some patients with IBS who also exhibit visceral hypersensitivity. Visceral hypersensitivity is a prominent symptom in many patients with IBS, and hypersensitivity appears to be attributable in part to activation of 5-HT$_3$ receptors on visceral afferents and in the central nervous system.[54,55] For example, colorectal distentions that did not elicit painful sensations in normal subjects did so in patients with IBS. Furthermore, the 5-HT$_3$ receptor antagonist granisetron raised the sensation and pain thresholds in the subjects with IBS.[56] 5-Hydroxytryptamine released from enterochromaffin cells located in the gastroin-

testinal mucosal layer is an important mediator of a number of intestinal stimuli, including mechanical stimulation of the mucosa. 5-HT$_3$ released from enterochromaffin cells then acts at 5-HT$_3$ receptors localized to intrinsic intestinal sensory neurons and extrinsic primary afferent neurons to elicit gastrointestinal reflexes and sensations.[55,57] 5-HT$_3$ receptors are a family of multimeric ligand gated cation channels that are similar in overall structure to nicotinic acetylcholine receptors.[58,59]

### Alosetron

Alosetron is the first 5-HT$_3$ receptor antagonist that has been used to treat symptoms associated with diarrhea-predominant IBS and was shown to be effective only in female patients.[60,61] Alosetron increases sensation and pain thresholds in patients with IBS (male and female) measured as barostat volumes eliciting the first sensation and abdominal pain (Fig. 28.13). This effect was associated with an increase in the slope of the pressure/volume relationship, suggesting that alosetron decreases colonic wall tension (Table 28.2).[62] In addition, alosetron delays colonic transit by an apparent selective action on the left colon of patients with IBS.[63] In the same subjects, small bowel transit, right colonic transit, and rectosigmoid transit were unaffected when transit was measured as the progression of radiopaque

**TABLE 28.2.** Pressure/Volume Relationship during Isobaric Distention of the Left Colon with a Barostat in Patients with Irritable Bowel Syndrome

|  | Slope of the P/V Curve (mL/mm Hg) Mean ± SD | Difference vs Placebo* |
|---|---|---|
| Placebo | 5.93 ± 1.28 | — |
| Alosetron 0.25 mg bd | 7.62 ± 1.17 | NS |
| Alosetron 4 mg bd | 9.78 ± 1.17 | .034 |

Comparison of the slope of the pressure (P)/volume (V) curve on placebo and alosetron. Data show that there is an increase in the steepness of the pressure P/V curve after alosetron (4 mg) treatment, indicating an increase in colonic compliance. Reproduced with permission from Delvaux D, Mamet J-P, Campos-Oriola R, Frexinos J. Effect of alosetron on responses to colonic distention in patients with irritable bowel syndrome. Aliment Pharmacol Ther 1998;12:849–55.

*Data analyzed by analysis of variance. NS, not significant.

**TABLE 28.3.** Effect of Alosetron on Transit Parameters in Patients with Irritable Bowel Syndrome

|  | Placebo | Alosetron | p |
|---|---|---|---|
| Mean whole-gut transit (h) | 58.9 (17.8, 113.8) | 72.2 (20, 140.9) | .128 |
| Small bowel transit (min) | 335.0 (190, 490.0) | 330.0 (200, 510.0) | .513 |
| Colonic transit | 53.2 (13.0, 107.6) | 64.2 (15.5, 135.6) | .036 |
| Left colonic transit | 11.5 (0, 23.0) | 22.5 (0, 52.0) | .006 |
| Right colonic transit | 7.0 (1.0, 23.0) | 6.5 (0, 31.0) | .571 |
| Rectosigmoid transit | 8.0 (0, 24.0) | 4.5 (0, 23.0) | .378 |

Mean whole-gut transit was measured as the time from ingestion to defecation of orally administered radiopaque markers. Radiography was used to detect the markers in the stool. Colonic transit was measured as the difference between mean whole-gut transit and mouth to cecum transit. Mouth to cecum transit was measured using the hydrogen breath test after the subjects consumed a meal containing nonabsorbable carbohydrates (baked beans). Segmental colonic transit was measured as the progression of radiopaque markers through each colonic segment as seen on a plain abdominal radiography. Alosetron slowed colonic transit in patients with IBS. The effect on whole colonic transit was principally attributable to a delay in left colonic transit. Reproduced with permission from Houghton LA, Foster JM, Whorwell PJ. Alosetron, a 5-HT₃ receptor antagonist delays colonic transit in patients with irritable bowel syndrome and healthy volunteers. Aliment Pharmacol Ther 2000;14:77–782.

Results are expressed as the median with the range in parentheses.

markers through the gastrointestinal tract (Table 28.3).[63] The effects of alosetron on colonic transit and rectal sensation are consistent with the reported decrease in the frequency of bowel movements and reports of diarrhea as well as an increase in the number of pain-free days reported by patients with IBS.[60] A delay in colonic transit may also contribute to constipation as a side effect of alosetron therapy.[61]

Alosetron has been withdrawn from the American market following reports of severe constipation and ischemic colitis in female patients receiving alosetron for treatment of IBS symptoms. However, other 5-HT₃ receptor antagonists are somewhat effective in the treatment of IBS.[64] 5-HT₃ receptors may still prove to be a useful target for drugs used to treat the symptoms of diarrhea-predominant IBS if it can be shown that ischemic colitis is not a consequence of 5-HT₃ receptor antagonism.

## REFERENCES

1. Briejer MR, Akkermans LMA, Schuurkes JAJ. Gastrointestinal prokinetic benzamides: the pharmacology underlying stimulation of motility. Pharmacol Rev 1995;47:631–51.
2. Prins NH, Akkermans LM, Lefebvre RA, Schuurkes JA. 5-HT₄ receptors on cholinergic nerves involved in contractility of canine and human large intestine longitudinal muscle. Br J Pharmacol 2000;131:927–32.
3. Baxter GS, Craig DA, Clarke DE. 5-Hydroxytryptamine₄ receptors mediate relaxation of the rat oesophageal tunica muscularis mucosae. Naunyn Schmiedebergs Arch Pharmacol 1991;343:439–46.
4. Prins NH, Van Haselen JFWR, Lefebvre RA, et al. Pharmacological characterization of 5-HT₄ receptors mediating relaxation of canine isolated rectum circular smooth muscle. Br J Pharmacol 1999;127:1431–7.
5. Grider JR, Kuemmerle JF, Jin J-G. 5-HT released by mucosal stimuli initiates peristalsis by activating 5-HT₄/₅-HT₁ₚ receptors on sensory CGRP neurons. Am J Physiol 1996;270:G778–82.
6. Grider JR, Foxx-Orenstein AE, Jin J-G. 5-Hydroxytryptamine₄ receptor agonists initiate the peristaltic reflex in human, rat and guinea pig intestine. Gastroenterology 1998;115:370–80.
7. Dumuis A, Sebben M, Bockaert J. The gastrointestinal prokinetic benzamide derivatives are agonists at the non-classical 5-HT₄ receptor positively coupled to adenylate cyclase in neurons. Naunyn Schmiedebergs Arch Pharmacol 1989;340:403–10.
8. Kilbinger H, Wolf D. Effects of 5-HT₄ receptor stimulation on basal and electrically evoked release of acetylcholine from guinea-pig myenteric plexus. Naunyn Schmiedebergs Arch Pharmacol 1992; 345:270–5.
9. Castell D, Silvers D, Littlejohn T, et al. Cisapride 20 mg b.d. for preventing symptoms of GERD induced by a provocative meal. The CIS-USA-89 study group. Aliment Pharmacol Ther 1999;13:787–94.
10. Pandolfino JE, Howden CW, Kahrilas P. Motility-modifying agents and management of disorders of gastrointestinal motility. Gastroenterology 2000;118:S32–47.
11. Farup PG, Hovdenak N, Wetterus S, et al. The symptomatic effect of cisapride in patients with irritable bowel syndrome and constipation. Scand J Gastroenterol 1998;33:128–31.
12. Schutze K, Brandstatter G, Dragosics B, et al. Double blind study of the effect of cisapride on constipation and abdominal discomfort as components of the irritable bowel syndrome. Aliment Pharmacol Ther 1997;11:387–94.
13. Mine Y, Yoshikawa T, Oku S, et al. Comparison of effect of mosapride citrate and existing 5-HT₄ receptor agonists on gastrointestinal motility in vivo and in vitro. J Pharmacol Exp Ther 1997;283:1000–8.
14. Tonini M, De Ponti F, Di Nucci A, Crema F. Review article: cardiac adverse effects of gastrointestinal prokinetics. Aliment Pharmacol Ther 1999;13:1585–91.
15. Carlsson L, Amos GJ, Andersson B, et al. Electrophysiological characterization of the prokinetic agents cisapride and mosapride in vivo and in vitro: implications for proarrhythmic potential? J Pharmacol Exp Ther 1997;282:220–7.
16. Peeters TL. Erythromycin and other macrolides as prokinetic agents. Gastroenterology 1993;105:1886–99.
17. Sarna SK, Gonzalez A, Ryan RP. Enteric locus of action of prokinetics: ABT-229, motilin and erythromycin. Am J Physiol 2000;G744–52.
18. Sturm A, Holtmann G, Goebell H, Gerken G. Prokinetics with gastroparesis: a systematic analysis. Digestion 1999;60:422–7.
19. Koch KL. Diabetic gastropathy: gastric neuromuscular dysfunction in diabetes mellitus: a review of symptoms, pathophysiology, and treatment. Dig Dis Sci 1999;44:1061–75.
20. Tack J, Janssens, J, Vantrappen G, et al. Effect of erythromycin on gastric motility in controls and in diabetic gastroparesis. Gastroenterology 1992;103:72–9.
21. Verhagen MA, Samsom M, Maes B, et al. Effects of a new motilide, ABT-229, on gastric emptying and postprandial antroduodenal motility in healthy volunteers. Aliment Pharmacol Ther 1997;11:1077–86.
22. Cowles VE, Nellans HN, Seiffert TR, et al. Effect of novel motilide ABT-229 versus erythromycin and cisapride on gastric emptying in dogs. J Pharmacol Exp Ther 2000;293:1106–11.

23. Chiba T, Thomforde GM, Kost LJ, et al. Motilides accelerate regional gastrointestinal transit in the dog. Aliment Pharmacol Ther 2000;14:955–60.

24. Schulze-Delrieu K. Metoclopramide. Gastroenterology 1979;77:768–79.

25. Barone JA. Domperidone: a peripherally acting dopamine₂ receptor antagonist. Ann Pharmacother 1999;33:429–40.

26. Takahashi T, Kurosawa S, Wiley J, Owyang C. Mechanism for the gastrokinetic action of domperidone. In vitro studies in guinea pigs. Gastroenterology 1991;101:703–10.

27. Lanfranchi GA, Bazzocchi G, Fois F, et al. Effect of domperidone and dopamine on colonic motor activity in patients with the irritable bowel syndrome. Eur J Clin Pharmacol 1985;29:307–10.

28. Cann PA, Read NW, Holdsworth CD. Oral domperidone: double-blind comparison with placebo in the irritable bowel syndrome. Gut 1983;24:1135–40.

29. Prakash A, Wagstaff AJ. Domperidone. A review of its use in diabetic gastropathy. Drugs 1998;56:429–45.

30. McCallum RW, Brown RL. Diabetic and nondiabetic gastroparesis. Curr Treat Options Gastroenterol 1998;1:1–7.

31. Koch KL, Stern RM, Stewart WR, Vasey MW. Gastric emptying and gastric myoelectrical activity in patients with diabetic gastroparesis: effect of long-term domperidone treatment. Am J Gastroenterol 1989;84:1069–75.

32. Davis RH, Clench MH, Mathias JR. Effects of domperidone in patients with chronic unexplained upper gastrointestinal symptoms: a double-blind, placebo-controlled study. Dig Dis Sci 1988;33:1505–11.

33. Soykan I, Sarosiek I, McCallum RW. The effect of chronic oral domperidone therapy on gastrointestinal symptoms, gastric emptying and quality of life in patients with gastroparesis. Am J Gastroenterol 1997;92:976–80.

34. Patterson D, Abell T, Rothstein R, et al. A double blind multicenter comparison of domperidone and metoclopramide in the treatment of diabetic patients with symptoms of gastroparesis. Am J Gastroenterol 1999;94:1230–4.

35. Borovicka J, Kreiss C, Asal K, et al. Role of cholecystokinin as a regulator of solid and liquid gastric emptying in humans. Am J Physiol 1996;271:G448–53.

36. McLaughlin J, Grazia-Lucà M, Jones MN, et al. Fatty acid chain length determines cholecystokinin secretion and effect on human gastric motility. Gastroenterology 1999;116:46–53.

37. Grider JR, Makhlouf GM. Distinct receptors for cholecystokinin and gastrin on muscle cells of stomach and gallbladder. Am J Physiol 1990;259:G184–90.

38. Raybould HE, Roberts ME, Dockray GJ. Reflex decreases in intragastric pressure in response to cholecystokinin in rats. Am J Physiol 1987;253:G165–70.

39. Hölzer P, Turkelson CM, Solomon TE, Raybould HE. Intestinal lipid inhibits gastric emptying via CCK and a vagal capsaicin-sensitive afferent pathway in rats. Am J Physiol 1994;267:G625–9.

40. Blackshaw LA, Grundy D. Effects of cholecystokinin (CCK-8) on two classes of gastroduodenal vagal afferent fibre. J Auton Nerv Syst 1990;31:191–201.

41. Schwizer W, Borovicka J, Kunz P, et al. Role of cholecystokinin in the regulation of liquid gastric emptying and gastric motility in humans: studies with the CCK antagonist loxiglumide. Gut 1997;41:500–4.

42. Feinle C, D'Amato M, Read NW. Cholecystokinin-A receptors modulate gastric sensory and motor responses to gastric distention and duodenal lipid. Gastroenterology 1996;110:1379–85.

43. Houghton LA, Fowler P, Keene ON, Read NW. Effect of sumatriptan, a new selective 5-HT₁-like agonist, on liquid emptying in man. Aliment Pharmacol Ther 1992;6:685–91.

44. Coulie B, Tack J, Maes B, et al. Sumatriptan, a selective 5-HT₁ receptor agonist, induces a lag phase for gastric emptying of liquids in humans. Am J Physiol 1997;272:G902–8.

45. Coulie B, Tack J, Sifrim D, et al. Role of nitric oxide in fasting gastric fundus tone and in 5-HT₁ receptor mediated relaxation of gastric fundus. Am J Physiol 1999;276:G373–7.

46. Tack J, Piessevaux H, Coulie B, et al. Role of impaired gastric accommodation to a meal in functional dyspepsia. Gastroenterology 1998;115:1346–52.

47. Manara L, Bianchetti A. The central and peripheral influences of opioids on gastrointestinal propulsion. Annu Rev Pharmacol Toxicol 1985;25:249–73.

48. Burleigh DH. Opioid and non-opioid actions of loperamide on cholinergic nerve function in human isolated colon. Eur J Pharmacol 1988;152:39–46.

49. Hoyle CH, Burnstock G, Jass J, Lennard-Jones J. Enkephalins inhibit non-adrenergic, non-cholinergic neuromuscular transmission in the human colon. Eur J Pharmacol 1986;131:159–60.

50. Bauer AJ, Sarr MG, Szurszewski JH. Opioids inhibit neuromuscular transmission in circular smooth muscle of human and baboon jejunum. Gastroenterology 1991;101:970–6.

51. Heel RC, Brogden RN, Speight TM, Avery GS. Loperamide: a review of its pharmacological properties, and therapeutic efficacy in diarrhea. Drugs 1978;15:33–52.

52. Anton AAHP, Canters LLJ, Awouters FHL, Niemegeers CJE. Normalization of small intestinal propulsion with loperamide-like antidiarrheals in rats. Eur J Pharmacol 1990;17:357–64.

53. Fioramonti J, Fargeas MJ, Bueno L. Stimulation of gastrointestinal motility by loperamide in dogs. Dig Dis Sci 1987;32:641–6.

54. Sanger GJ. Hypersensitivity and hyperreactivity in the irritable bowel syndrome: an opportunity for drug discovery. Dig Dis 1999;17:90–9.

55. Humphrey PPA, Bountra C, Clayton N, Kozlowski K. Review article: the therapeutic potential of 5-HT₃ receptor antagonists in the treatment of irritable bowel syndrome. Aliment Pharmacol Ther 1999;13 Suppl 2:31–8.

56. Prior A, Read NW. Reduction of rectal sensitivity and post-prandial motility by granisetron, a 5-HT₃ receptor antagonist, in patients with the irritable bowel syndrome. Aliment Pharmacol Ther 1993;7:175–80.

57. Bertrand PP, Kunze WA, Furness JB, Bornstein JC. The terminals of myenteric intrinsic primary afferent neurons of the guinea-pig ileum are excited by 5-hydroxytryptamine acting at 5-hydroxytryptamine-3 receptors. Neuroscience 2000;101:459–69.

58. Derkach V, Surprenant A, North RA. 5-HT₃ receptors are membrane ion channels. Nature 1989;339:706–9.

59. Maricq AV, Peterson AS, Brake AJ, et al. Primary structure and functional expression of the 5-HT₃ receptor, a serotonin-gated ion channel. Science 1991;254:432–7.

60. Bardhan KD, Bodemar G, Geldof H, et al. A double-blind, randomized placebo-controlled dose ranging study to evaluate the efficacy of alosetron in the treatment of irritable bowel syndrome. Aliment Pharmacol Ther 2000;14:23–34.

61. Camilleri M, Northcutt AR, Kong S, et al. Efficacy and safety of alosetron in women with irritable bowel syndrome: a randomised, placebo-controlled trial. Lancet 2000;355:1035–40.

62. Delvaux D, Mamet J-P, Campos-Oriola R, Frexinos J. Effect of alosetron on responses to colonic distention in patients with irritable bowel syndrome. Aliment Pharmacol Ther 1998;12:849–55.

63. Houghton LA, Foster JM, Whorwell PJ. Alosetron, a 5-HT₃ receptor antagonist, delays colonic transit in patients with irritable bowel syndrome and healthy volunteers. Aliment Pharmacol Ther 2000;14:77–782.

64. Maxton DG, Morris J, Whorwell PJ. Selective 5-hydroxytryptamine antagonism: a role in irritable bowel syndrome and functional dyspepsia? Aliment Pharmacol Ther 1996;10:595–9.

# CHAPTER 29

# Pediatric Gastrointestinal Motility

*Carlo Di Lorenzo and Paola Ciamarra*

## APPROACH TO THE PEDIATRIC PATIENT

Motility disorders are very common in children. They include conditions also found in adult subjects, such as intestinal pseudo-obstruction, rumination syndrome, and gastro-esophageal reflux, and other disorders more specific to pediatric subjects, such as infantile regurgitation, toddlers' diarrhea, and functional fecal retention. A variety of diagnostic techniques have been used to diagnose and investigate such disorders, including radiologic, scintigraphic, and transit studies using breath analyzers. Because of its perceived invasive nature and the difficulty encountered in establishing control values in normal subjects, for many years, manometry was considered a "research" technique rather than an established diagnostic test in pediatrics. This is not the case anymore, and, currently, there are several well-established pediatric motility centers in the United States, with the demand for evaluations often outnumbering the ability to perform timely testing. Basic training in the evaluation and treatment of motility disorders is now part of the curriculum for training in pediatric gastroenterology.[1] It is essential to emphasize that although manometry tests are now used with increasing frequency in children of all ages, they will produce completely worthless results if not tailored to the specific characteristics and needs of pediatric patients. Rather than being a comprehensive description of the motility events throughout the entire gastrointestinal tract, this chapter will focus on the main differences between motility patterns and disorders in children and adults.

The physician performing the test must be familiar with the patterns of gastrointestinal motility (Fig. 29.1) and the developmental and behavioral aspects of pediatrics (Table 29.1). Infants and toddlers rarely cooperate with medical testing. Sedation is often needed to place the catheter with full recovery from sedation needed before starting the study. An exception is the performance of anorectal manometry in a newborn or infant to rule out Hirschsprung's disease. Anesthesia does not affect the presence of the rectoanal inhibitory reflex, and the test may be performed in a sedated child when the only goal is to evaluate whether such a reflex is present. Although strain-gauge catheters small enough to be used in toddlers are now available, most studies in children continue to use water-perfused catheters. The size of the catheters and the water infusion rate differ in children from adult standards and need to be adjusted to the different age and size of the patient. As an example, the catheter with recording sites spaced 5 cm apart, routinely used in adults to evaluate esophageal motility, will not be appropriate in a newborn whose esophagus is less than 10 cm long. Prolonged motility studies with multilumen-perfused catheters may place infants and toddlers at risk for serious water intoxication.

**TABLE 29.1.** Pediatric Patient: What to Consider in the Evaluation

Poor cooperation
Artifacts
Effect of sedation
Size of catheters
Numbers of recording sites
Age-related normal values
Infusion rates
Interaction with parents and medical personnel

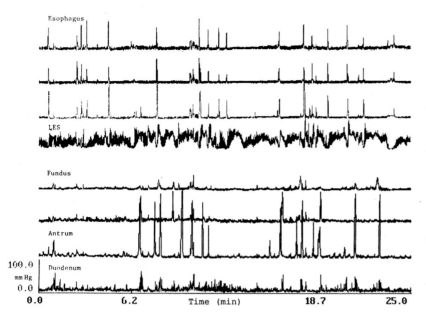

**FIGURE 29.1.** Motor events in the upper gastrointestinal tract. The figure depicts the type of contractions found in the different areas of the upper gastrointestinal tract. In this child, there are eight recording sites spaced 5 cm apart measuring pressure changes in the esophageal body, lower esophageal sphincter (LES), gastric fundus, gastric antrum, and duodenum. As in healthy adults, the highest-amplitude contractions (>150 mm Hg) in the foregut of children are found in the distal portion of the stomach. Phasic propagated contractions are also found in the esophagus and duodenum. The gastric fundus produces slow tonic changes that are not reliably measured by side-hole motility catheters. Little is known in pediatrics about the motor activity of the pylorus, fundus, and small bowel distal to the duodenum because of the relative inaccessibility of these areas to measuring devices. New instruments, such as miniaturized manometric sleeves and the electronic barostat, are beginning to shed some light on the function of these areas in children of different sizes and ages.

Motility studies need to be interpreted based on the patient's age and developmental status. For example, a lack of high-amplitude propagated contractions (HAPCs) after a meal is an abnormal finding in a young toddler but may be normal in an adolescent.[2] Migrating motor complexes (MMCs) cycle more frequently in younger children.[3] Manometric patterns are impossible to interpret when crying or movement artifacts are superimposed onto intraluminal pressure changes. A nonthreatening environment and entertainment appropriate to the patient's developmental stage (tapes, toys, reading material) are often necessary to calm the patient and successfully complete the test. Well-trained nursing personnel are essential to create a relaxing, collaborative ambiance for patients and parents. Allowing parents to attend the examination and making them leave if the child does not feel comfortable with them can be useful for a good outcome. Observation of the child–caregiver's interaction in a stressful environment, such as during performance of motility testing, may provide important clues on the presence of a behavioral disorder as the cause of the patient's symptoms. The presence of a disturbed caregiver–child interaction in conjunction with normal motility studies can shift the attention to social and mental health issues. It is important that the physician is present or immediately available throughout most of the motility testing, in view of the fact that study protocols often need to be modified based on the child's age, behavior, and indications for the testing.

Indications for motility testing in children differ from those in adults, reflecting the different medical conditions found in pediatrics (Table 29.2). Some of the motility tests, such as esophageal manometry, are more commonly used in adults, whereas others, such as colonic manometry, seem to be more useful in children. There is no role for motility testing in the evaluation of most childhood functional bowel disorders.

**TABLE 29.2.** Indications for Motility Testing in Children as Proposed by a Working Group of the American Motility Society

**Esophageal manometry**

1. To diagnose achalasia and other primary motility disorders
2. To evaluate dysphagia and chest pain of noncardiac origin in children and adolescents
3. To place pH electrodes for esophageal pH-metry when there are anatomic malformations (ie, hiatal hernia) or to place it without radiographs
4. To aid in the diagnosis of diseases that may have esophageal dysmotility, like connective tissue disease or chronic intestinal pseudo-obstruction

**Antroduodenal manometry**

1. To confirm the pathophysiology underlying intestinal failure in children with chronic intestinal pseudo-obstruction
2. To assess upper gastrointestinal motility when colectomy is considered for intractable constipation
3. When necessary to distinguish between rumination and vomiting

**Colonic manometry**

1. To evaluate persistent constipation unresponsive to conventional treatment and of uncertain cause
2. To characterize the physiology responsible for symptoms of chronic intestinal pseudo-obstruction and to assess the presence or absence of colonic involvement
3. To determine the physiology associated with persistent symptoms following successful surgery for Hirschsprung's disease
4. In patients with unexplained symptoms, which might be related to motility problems
5. Prior to intestinal transplantation, to decide whether to retain the colon at the time of transplantation

**Anorectal manometry**

1. To diagnose a nonrelaxing internal anal sphincter
2. To evaluate postoperative patients with Hirschsprung's disease who have obstructive symptoms or fecal incontinence
3. To evaluate postoperative patients after imperforate anus repair
4. To decide if the patient is a candidate for biofeedback therapy

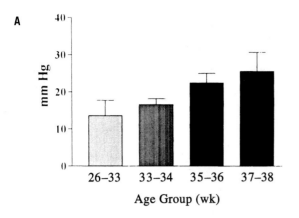

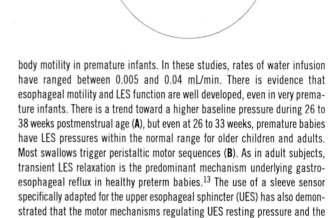

**FIGURE 29.2.** Esophageal manometry in preterm newborns. **A**, Lower esophageal sphincter (LES) pressure in preterm children between 26 and 38 weeks postconceptional age. The LES pressure of children between 33 and 38 weeks relates to preprandial values. Data from Omari et al.[12] **B**, Esophageal motor patterns in response to swallows in healthy preterm children between 26 and 33 weeks postmenstrual age. Data from Omari et al.[13] Swallow-unrelated pressure waves are usually nonperistaltic, with the majority of sequences being synchronous, incomplete, or retrograde. The use of manometry assembly with side-hole recording ports in the 1970s suggested that the LES pressure in newborns and premature babies was lower than in older children and that the esophageal peristalsis was uncoordinated. Data from Boix-Ochoa and Canals.[14] Newly developed miniaturized feeding catheters, with sleeve sensors, have allowed a more accurate evaluation of LES and esophageal body motility in premature infants. In these studies, rates of water infusion have ranged between 0.005 and 0.04 mL/min. There is evidence that esophageal motility and LES function are well developed, even in very premature infants. There is a trend toward a higher baseline pressure during 26 to 38 weeks postmenstrual age (**A**), but even at 26 to 33 weeks, premature babies have LES pressures within the normal range for older children and adults. Most swallows trigger peristaltic motor sequences (**B**). As in adult subjects, transient LES relaxation is the predominant mechanism underlying gastroesophageal reflux in healthy preterm babies.[13] The use of a sleeve sensor specifically adapted for the upper esophageal sphincter (UES) has also demonstrated that the motor mechanisms regulating UES resting pressure and the onset of UES relaxation are well developed in premature infants as young as 33 weeks postmenstrual age. Data from Omari et al.[15]

## ESOPHAGUS

The motor function of the esophagus has been thoroughly studied in children and preterm infants (Fig. 29.2). The esophagus includes three functional regions: the upper esophageal sphincter, the esophageal body, and the lower esophageal sphincter. Each of these regions may display motility abnormalities (Figs. 29.3 to 29.10), leading to symptoms such as dysphagia, chest pain, vomiting, and decreased oral intake. Although manometry remains the gold standard for the diagnosis of esophageal motility disorders, other tests, such as radiographic or scintigraphic studies, may often provide relevant, complementary information.

## STOMACH AND SMALL BOWEL

Most catheters used to study antroduodenal manometry in adults are suitable for use in toddlers and older children. Fluoroscopy or endoscopy is used to facilitate catheter placement in the antrum and duodenum. When using fluoroscopy, it may be advantageous to infuse erythromycin 1 mg/kg intravenously over 30 minutes during the passage of the catheter. Erythromycin induces clusters of powerful propagated contractions in the antrum within 10 minutes of infusion, allowing an easier progression of the catheter through the pylorus. Most investigators study gastrointestinal motility in children for at least 4 hours during fasting and 1 hour after feeding. Children have a shorter MMC cycle compared to adults, and 4 hours are sufficient in most children with normal motility to observe at least one MMC.[3] The meal is individualized based on the patient age and clinical condition, with an attempt being made to administer a meal with at least 10 kcal/kg or 400 kcal, with >30% kcal deriving from lipids. Drugs such as erythromycin and/or octreotide are often administered during a motility study to test their potential as therapeutic agents.

The analysis of antroduodenal manometry includes an evaluation of fasting and postprandial motility (Figs. 29.11 to 29.14). During fasting, the presence of phase 3 of the MMCs, its site of origin, direction of propagation, duration and frequency of contractions, and presence of a tonic component are evaluated. After the meal, conversion to a "fed" state is determined by the absence of MMCs and the presence of an increase in the number and strength of antral and duodenal contractions. Computer analysis may be used to quantitate the amount of motility generating the "motility index," a value that takes into account the frequency and amplitude of contractions. Caution should be exercised in interpreting manometry studies performed in dilated bowels because the ability to increase intraluminal pressure is inversely proportional to the gut diameter (Laplace's law). Features of normal gastric and small bowel motility in children of different ages have been described.[3,4]

### Gastric Motility Disorders

Disorders in gastric motility are associated with abnormal storage, trituration, and emptying of food. Gastroparesis is a syndrome characterized by symptoms resulting from impaired

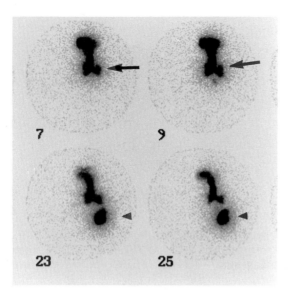

**FIGURE 29.3.** Upper esophageal sphincter (UES) dysfunction: radionuclide salivagram demonstrating salivary aspiration in the trachea and main bronchi (*arrows*). Late images show radioactivity in the stomach (*arrowheads*). Chronic aspiration is one of the factors responsible for highest morbidity and mortality in children with neurologic deficits. Although manometry has been used to investigate pharyngeal and UES function in children with a variety of central nervous system abnormalities,[16] its use in pediatrics is fraught with problems. Manometry is not well tolerated in young children with cognitive and developmental delay, and sedation cannot be used when repeated swallow sequences are needed. Perfused catheters dripping water in the pharynx cause frequent gagging and choking episodes. Swallowing causes sudden movements of the larynx and UES discordant with the movement of the motility catheter. Information of UES pressure values in normal children is scanty. In view of all of these factors, the clinical utility of manometry in the evaluation of UES function is limited, and less invasive ways to evaluate its function have been sought. The radionuclide salivagram is being increasingly used to identify patients who have abnormal swallowing dynamics.[17] This test is currently considered the most sensitive technique to detect aspiration.[18] The salivagram consists in the sublingual administration of technetium-99m sulfur colloid in a drop of water. Serial images are then obtained for 60 minutes and evaluated for entrance of the tracer into the airways. It is felt that the salivagram is an effective tool for demonstrating aspiration of oral contents caused by abnormal UES function. Additionally, it provides information on the clearance of aspirated material, allowing evaluation of the airways protective mechanisms.

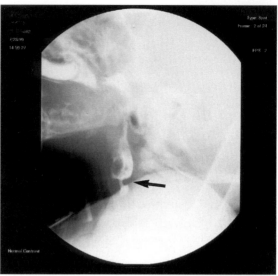

**FIGURE 29.4.** Cricopharyngeal achalasia. The radiologic study demonstrates a horizontal "bar" during swallowing (*arrow*). Cricopharyngeal achalasia has been described in newborns and older children. It occurs when the upper esophageal sphincter fails to open completely or to open in synchrony with pharyngeal contractions. Symptoms include choking and gagging, cough while swallowing, food refusal, drooling, and recurrent pneumonia caused by aspiration. Symptoms are usually more severe when swallowing liquids rather than solids, a differentiating feature from patients with a fixed, lumen-occluding lesion. Upper esophageal sphincter dysfunction may occur as a consequence of a variety of neuromuscular diseases (muscular dystrophy, mitochondrial deletions, minimal change myopathy, cerebral palsy) and abnormalities of the central nervous system that alter cranial nerve function (ie, Arnold-Chiari malformation). A modified barium swallow with different consistency boluses, the so-called "cookie swallow," is the most useful test to detect this dysfunction. Cricopharyngeal achalasia is demonstrated radiologically as a persistent horizontal "bar" during swallowing often accompanied by aspiration of radiopaque material. Esophageal manometry provides information complementary to the radiologic study but is often difficult to perform in neonates and infants. Brainstem magnetic resonance imaging should be performed to rule out Arnold-Chiari malformation in every child with cricopharyngeal achalasia. Therapy includes dietary modifications in younger children such as thickening of food and beverages or gastrostomy tube feeding. In older children, resolution of symptoms can be achieved with either bougienage, surgical and laser myotomy, or botulinum toxin injection.

emptying of intraluminal contents from the stomach into the duodenum, in the absence of a mechanical obstruction. It is a condition seldom found in children except in the neonatal period. In older children, it may be found in association with systemic disease (often during the acute phase of a viral illness) or after surgery. Symptoms of gastroparesis include postprandial fullness, anorexia, early satiety, bloating, emesis several hours after meal, halitosis, and epigastric pain. The most accurate and sensitive measure of gastric emptying is the emptying scan. A solid meal, usually containing technetium[99m]-labeled eggs, is used in older children, whereas milk or formula is used in infants. Scintigraphic studies in pediatrics are fraught with shortcomings. Infants and uncooperative toddlers may not be able to lie motionless under the gamma camera for extended periods of time. Standard test meals cannot be given to infants with dietary protein allergies or be refused by children who do not like that specific meal. There are no normal values obtained from healthy children. Manometry may be used to evaluate the contractile response of the gastric antrum to the ingestion of food and to differentiate rumination from other causes of vomiting (Figs. 29.15 to 29.17).

Rapid gastric emptying associated with dumping syndrome is even less common in children. Accelerated emptying may be attributable to either decreased gastric compliance and accommodation, most commonly caused by vagal denervation, or loss of pyloric function as a result of surgical bypass or performance of gastric drainage procedures (pyloroplasty, pyloromyotomy).

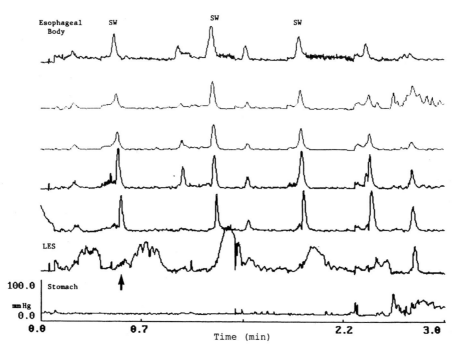

**FIGURE 29.5.** Example of normal esophageal peristalsis. The recording sites are spaced 3 cm apart, with five sensors positioned in the esophageal body, one at the level of the lower esophageal sphincter (LES) and the bottom one in the stomach. The figure shows normal peristalsis in the esophageal body and normal pressure and relaxation (*arrow*) of the LES. Protocols to perform and evaluate esophageal manometry in children are similar to those used in adults. Esophageal manometry catheters are usually placed nasally in infants and children and orally in newborns, who are obligate nose breathers. Ideal spacing between recording sites varies with the age of the child, with most laboratories using at least four sensors spaced 3 cm apart. The length of the esophagus varies depending on the age of the child, ranging from 10 cm or less in the preterm infant to 40 cm in the adolescent. The catheter is initially introduced into the stomach and slowly pulled through the LES. The measurement of LES pressure is performed relative to intragastric pressure. Ideally, one recording site is then placed at the level of the LES, with the more proximal recording sites spanning the esophagus and one more distal recording site in the stomach. Several swallows are obtained so that esophageal peristalsis and LES relaxation can be assessed. Blowing air in the child's face (the Santmyer reflex) is a technique useful to induce swallowing in infants younger than 11 months and neurologically disabled children.[19] In older and more cooperative children, it is preferable to obtain at least 10 "wet" swallows, gently inserting in the child's mouth approximately 1 to 5 mL of water at room temperature. Normal values obtained from asymptomatic, healthy children are not available. In general, contractions in the distal esophagus with an amplitude <40 mm Hg are considered hypotensive, whereas contractions > 180 mm Hg are considered hypertensive. SW, swallow.

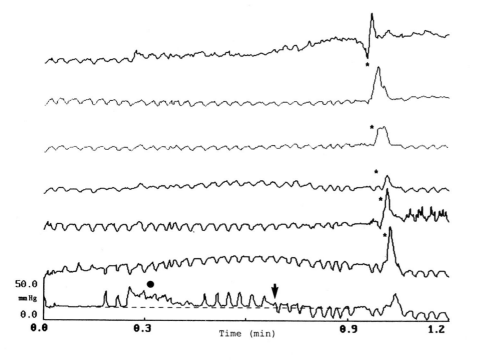

**FIGURE 29.6.** Lower esophageal sphincter (LES) pull-through. The recording sites are spaced 3 cm apart, with the top six in the esophagus and the most distal recording site being slowly pulled through the LES. It is possible to identify a hypotensive (baseline pressure ~10 mm Hg) LES (●) and the pressure inversion point (*arrow*) when the recording sensor moves from the abdomen into the chest. The dotted line indicates baseline gastric pressure. The *asterisk* indicates a peristaltic wave. Inspiration causes negative deflections within the chest and positive deflection (increases in pressure) within the abdomen. Asking the patient to take a deep breath during a pull-through helps to determine whether the catheter is still in the stomach or has already reached the esophagus. In this example, the LES is found distal to the diaphragm, ruling out a hiatal hernia.

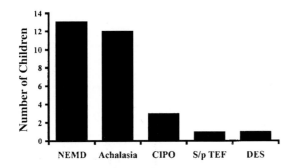

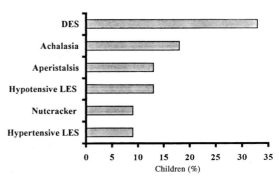

**FIGURE 29.7.** Esophageal motility disorders in children (data from Rosario et al[20]). Esophageal manometry has been used to evaluate dysphagia and chest pain of noncardiac origin in children and adolescents. Criteria for the diagnosis of different esophageal motility disorders (achalasia, diffuse esophageal spasm, nutcracker esophagus, and nonspecific esophageal motor disorders) are identical in children and adults. The figure summarizes the results of the largest published pediatric series evaluating esophageal motility in 154 children presenting with swallowing-related upper gastrointestinal symptoms (dysphagia, chest pain, food impaction, vomiting).[20] Abnormal motility was found in the esophagus of 30 among the 45 children without gastroesophageal reflex. The most common abnormality was the presence of a nonspecific esophageal motor disorder, a condition that was associated with food impaction and characterized mainly by simultaneous, retrograde, or low-amplitude contractions. NEMD, nonspecific esophageal motor disorder; CIPO, chronic intestinal pseudo-obstruction; S/p TEF, status post tracheoesophageal fistula repair; DES, diffuse esophageal spasm.

**FIGURE 29.8.** Type of esophageal motor dysfunction in children with chest pain (data from Glassman et al[21]). Another large series has evaluated the manometric abnormalities in children with chest pain.[21] It was found that diffuse esophageal spasm (DES) and achalasia were the most common motility disorders identified. In DES, the esophagus retains its ability to propagate primary peristaltic contractions most of the time. Radiographically, it may appear as a "corkscrew" esophagus. Manometry reveals contractions of greater than normal amplitude and prolonged duration, with approximately 30% occurring simultaneously at different levels of the esophagus. In a typical case, these nonperistaltic, high-amplitude, prolonged contractions are associated with chest pain or dysphagia. At times, there are multipeaked, repetitive contractions following a single swallow indicative of a dysfunction of the autonomic nervous system. Diffuse esophageal spasm is likely to be an underdiagnosed entity in pediatrics. Treatment for this entity has included the use of calcium channel blockers, nitrates, or acid suppressant with variable results. Surgical myotomy is an option reserved for patients whose medical treatment fails. LES, lower esophageal sphincter.

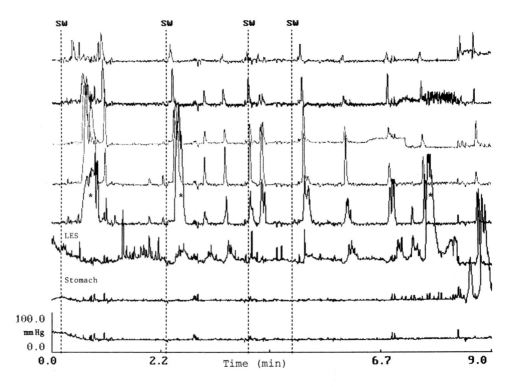

**FIGURE 29.9.** Example of nutcracker esophagus. High-amplitude, prolonged peristaltic contractions, with pressure in excess of 250 mm Hg, indicated by an asterisk. Nutcracker esophagus has been reported in children with chest pain or dysphagia. It may represent a consequence of abnormal inhibitory neuronal innervation and may be secondary to diabetic neuropathy.[22] Manometry represents the most sensitive technique to diagnose spastic disorders of the esophagus. LES, lower esophageal sphincter; SW, swallow.

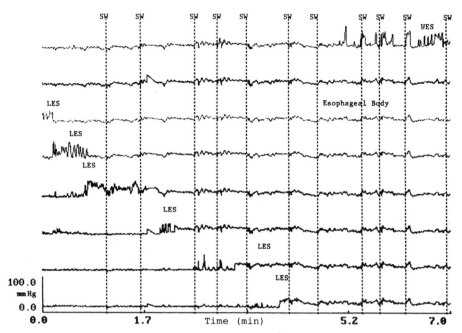

**FIGURE 29.10.** Esophageal achalasia. Typical manometric tracing of a child with achalasia during an esophageal pull-through. There is no peristalsis in the body of the esophagus and evidence of incomplete lower esophageal sphincter (LES) relaxation. Swallows trigger identical pressure changes throughout the esophagus, a pattern named "mirror images." The intraesophageal baseline pressure is higher than the intragastric baseline pressure. Manometric features found in achalasia include loss of esophageal peristalsis, absent or incomplete LES relaxation in response to a swallow, increased or normal LES pressure, and elevated intraesophageal pressure. The resting LES pressure tends to be elevated but is the least consistent of the manometric changes, with one in three patients with achalasia having baseline sphincter pressure within the normal range. The term "vigorous" achalasia is used when there are nonperistaltic spasm-like contractions. Esophageal achalasia is the most common primary esophageal motor disorder in children. Achalasia is thought to result from postganglionic denervation of the esophageal smooth muscle. This condition should be suspected in children presenting with progressive dysphagia, recurrent emesis, weight loss, chest pain, and aspiration pneumonia. The mean age at the time of diagnosis in pediatric patients is 8.8 years, with some cases being diagnosed even in infancy. It starts as an obstruction at the level of the gastroesophageal junction with subsequent dilation of the lower esophagus due to the absence of esophageal peristalsis. Esophageal manometry represents a very sensitive and specific diagnostic technique in achalasia. The two most successful modalities for a definitive cure are pneumatic dilation and esophageal myotomy, even though botulinum toxin injection has been found to provide short-term benefit in children who are poor surgical candidates. SW, swallow, UES, upper esophageal sphincter.

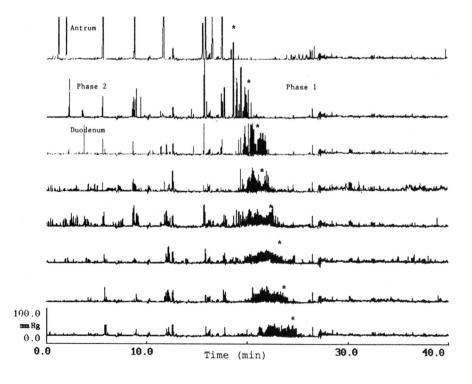

**FIGURE 29.11.** Normal antroduodenal fasting motility. The three phases of the migrating motor complex (MMC) are identified. The MMC consists of three distinctive phases that occur in sequence and slowly migrate along the length of the small bowel. In phase 1, there is motor quiescence, followed by a period of apparently random contractions of variable amplitude, called phase 2. Phase 3 (*) is characterized by a 4- to 10-minute period with a distinctive pattern of uninterrupted, propagating contractions occurring at a frequency of 3/min in the stomach, 11 to 12/min in the duodenum, and 7 to 9/min in the distal ileum. Most phase 3 contractions originate in the antrum (~70%) or in the duodenum (~30%).[23] Each cycle lasts 100 to 200 minutes, and once a phase 3 contraction reaches the distal ileum, a new phase 3 contraction is generated in the proximal gut. The onset and migration of MMCs in the small bowel are under the control of the enteric nervous system and are independent of extrinsic innervation.

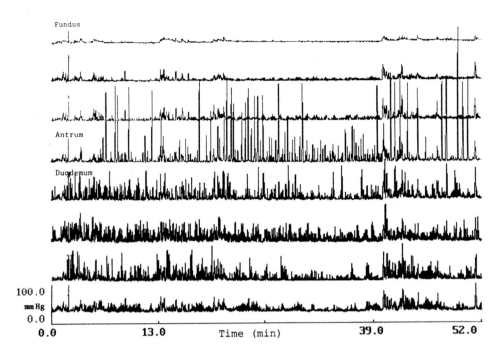

**FIG 29.12.** Normal postprandial motility. Feeding abolishes the cyclic migrating motor complex (MMC) pattern and replaces it with a postprandial pattern characterized by random, phasic contractions (similar to phase 2 activity) that may last several hours, after which the fasting pattern resumes if no food is ingested. The ability to switch to a postprandial motility pattern is controlled by extrinsic nerves and is missing in patients with vagotomy or bowel denervation. It has been suggested that manometric evidence of normal MMCs and the presence of an intact postprandial motor activity excludes an enteric neuromuscular disorder and suggests a reassessment of the diagnostic work-up in children presenting with a diagnosis of pseudo-obstruction.[9]

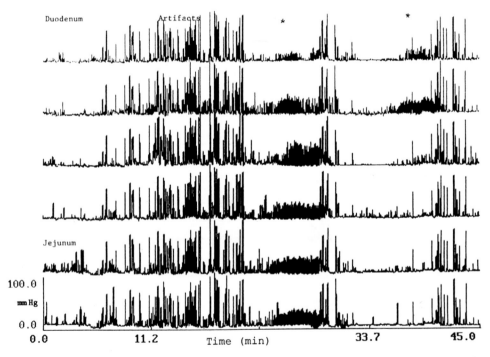

**FIGURE 29.13.** Example of artifacts in a child with prolonged periods of crying. The asterisks indicate phase 3 contractions of the migrating motor complex. In children, artifacts are very common (*left side of the tracing*). If contractions with almost the same amplitude and shape are recorded simultaneously at all recording sites, it is likely that they are caused by motion, crying, coughing, or talking. The presence of frequent artifacts makes the use of software analysis of motility studies in children very challenging. The software may misinterpret any change in pressure as a real contractile event, overestimating the motility index and the number of simultaneous contractions. This is one of the reasons why interpretation of manometry studies in children is performed mainly by visual analysis of the tracing.

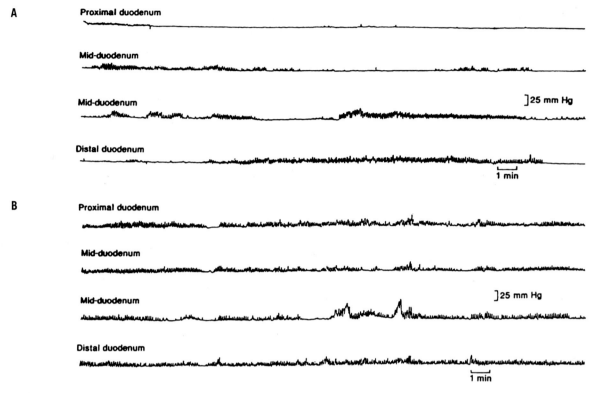

**A**

Proximal duodenum

Mid-duodenum

Mid-duodenum

]25 mm Hg

Distal duodenum

1 min

**B**

Proximal duodenum

Mid-duodenum

Mid-duodenum

]25 mm Hg

Distal duodenum

1 min

**FIGURE 29.14.** Examples of duodenal motor activity during fasting in preterm infants able to tolerate enteral feedings (**A**) and not able to tolerate enteral feedings (**B**). In the proximal leads, there are longer periods of quiescence in **A**, whereas in **B**, small-amplitude contractions occupy most of the recording. Much is known about the ontogeny of intestinal motility in premature babies. There is a striking increase in the number and amplitude of small bowel contractions between 29 and 32 weeks postconception. The migrating motor complex (MMC) appears between 32 and 35 weeks gestational age.[24] With increasing age, there is also an increase in the average duration of the MMC and the rate of phase 3 propagation. Initiation of enteral feedings within 2 weeks of age induces a more rapid maturation of motor patterns, with more phase 3 and fewer nonpropagating clusters than age-matched unfed infants.[25]

There is no difference in the ability of gastric or transpyloric formula feedings to induce a postprandial intestinal motor response. Preterm intestinal motility responses are affected by changes in the caloric density of formula, with very diluted formula not being able to stimulate a fed response in the preterm infant.[26] It has also been suggested that manometry may be used to predict feeding readiness in preterm infants.[27] Infants who were initially feeding intolerant were able to tolerate feedings when they developed more periods of motor quiescence and less clustered activity. Periods of intestinal motor quiescence significantly increase with postnatal age and are associated with an elevation in gastrin and peptide YY plasma concentration.[28] Reproduced with permission from Berseth CL, Nordyke CK. Manometry can predict feeding readiness in preterm infants. Gastroenterology 1992;103:1523–8.

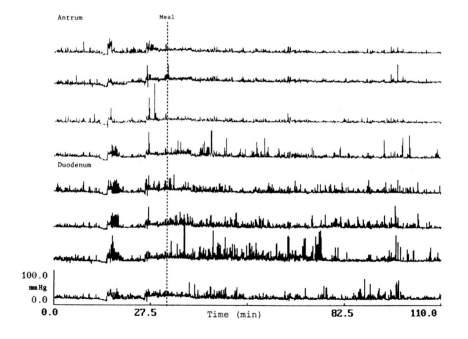

Antrum

Meal

Duodenum

100.0
mm Hg
0.0

0.0          27.5          Time (min)          82.5          110.0

**FIGURE 29.15.** Example of postprandial antral hypomotility. After ingestion of a solid meal, this child with postviral gastroparesis has a normal motor response in the duodenum, with an increase in the number and strength of contractions and no detectable antral contractions. Postviral gastroparesis is an entity recently described in children after a short viral illness, often a rotavirus gastroenteritis.[29] It is associated with postprandial antral hypomotility and normal contraction amplitude during fasting, suggesting a disturbance of the enteric nervous system rather than the smooth muscle. In most cases, symptoms resolve spontaneously within 6 to 24 months. When evaluating postprandial gastric motility, it is important to administer a solid meal because liquids may not stimulate antral contractions.

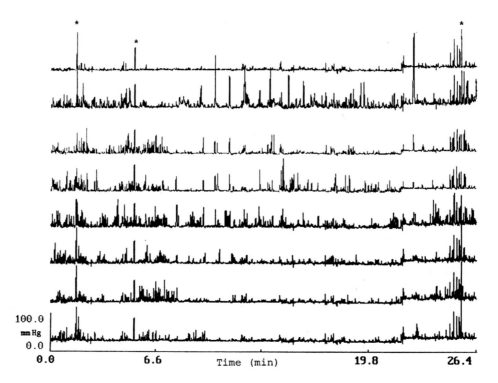

**FIGURE 29.16.** Antroduodenal manometry in a child with rumination. The asterisks indicate brief, simultaneous, postprandial pressure increases (called "R" waves) at all recording sites, associated with regurgitation. These pressure changes are likely to represent unconscious acts (eg, contractions of abdominal muscles) aimed at increasing the intra-abdominal pressure and induce regurgitation. Rumination is a behavioral disorder characterized by effortless regurgitation of partially digested food. The regurgitation occurs during or imme-diately after the meal, differentiating this condition from gastroparesis, in which the patient may vomit material ingested several hours before. The presence of esophagitis is unusual. Rumination is believed to be caused by the coexistence of functional and psychiatric abnormalities and is recognized with increased frequency, especially in adolescent females. The presence of normal fasting motility and the characteristic postprandial motility pattern allows differentiation of children with rumination from others with intrinsic motility disorders.[30]

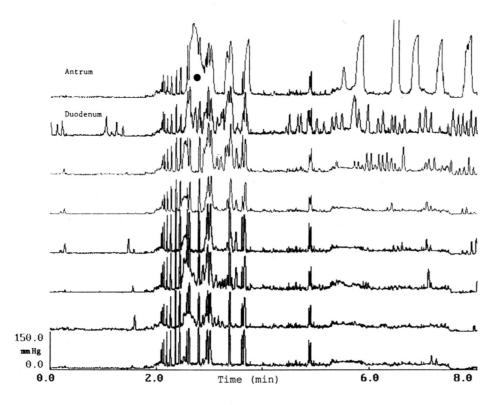

**FIGURE 29.17.** Vomiting in a child with a motility disorder. There is an episode of vomiting associated with a prolonged, high-amplitude antral contraction. In this example, the emesis is associated with a gastric motor event, and it is possible to identify the abnormal antral contraction (•), partially masked by the artifacts caused by the act of retching.

## Small Bowel Motility Disorders

Abnormalities in small bowel motility have been described in many childhood gastrointestinal disorders. It has been suggested that abnormal small bowel motility may play a pathogenic role in some children with severe abdominal pain or nonulcer dyspepsia.[5,6] It is now believed that rather than having a baseline abnormal motor function, some children with functional bowel disorders may have an exaggerated motor response to a heterogeneous group of physical or psychosocial stimuli.

The most severe form of intestinal dysmotility in children is chronic intestinal pseudo-obstruction (CIP), a term that refers to a heterogeneous group of gastrointestinal nerve and muscle disorders with similar phenotypic presentation.[7] Based on a strict definition of the syndrome, CIP should be diagnosed only when a mechanical obstruction has been entertained in the differential diagnosis and has been ruled out.[8] In reality, there are many other severe forms of motility disorders involving the small bowel that do not necessarily present with obstructive signs and symptoms. These are often referred to as "mild" forms of CIP. Because pseudo-obstruction is caused by a failure of the "intestinal pump," the most revealing diagnostic tests in CIP are those involving the evaluation of gastrointestinal motility. Differently from adults, children with CIP rarely have esophageal dysmotility, and a normal esophageal manometry should not rule out CIP. The measurement of upper gastrointestinal motility is critical in the evaluation of the child with CIP. Small bowel motility is always abnormal in children with CIP involving the upper gastrointestinal tract.[9] Other diagnoses, including factitious disorders or behavioral problems in the child or the family, should be ruled out when the manometry study is normal. In subjects with neuropathy, there are normal-amplitude, uncoordinated contractions (Figs. 29.18 to 29.21).

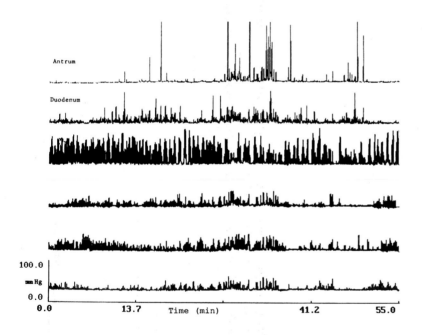

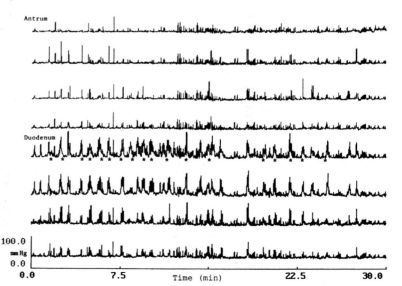

**FIGURE 29.18.** Antroduodenal manometry: neuropathic motor disorder. There is a prolonged cluster of high-amplitude duodenal contractions in the mid-duodenum (*). Some of the contractions exceed 100 mm Hg. Prolonged clusters of stationary, nonpropagating contractions have been reported in children with enteric neuropathy caused by in utero exposure to alcohol.[31]

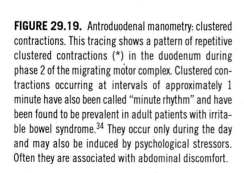

**FIGURE 29.19.** Antroduodenal manometry: clustered contractions. This tracing shows a pattern of repetitive clustered contractions (*) in the duodenum during phase 2 of the migrating motor complex. Clustered contractions occurring at intervals of approximately 1 minute have also been called "minute rhythm" and have been found to be prevalent in adult patients with irritable bowel syndrome.[34] They occur only during the day and may also be induced by psychological stressors. Often they are associated with abdominal discomfort.

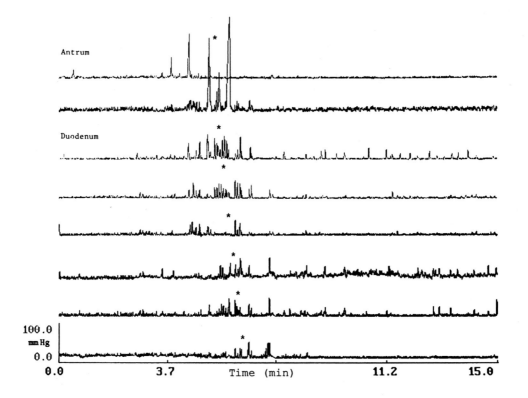

**FIGURE 29.20.** Antroduodenal manometry: abnormal phase 3. The tracing shows a short (~2 minutes) phase 3 contraction of the migrating motor complexes, followed by phase 1 activity. Short, poorly formed, or abnormally propagating phase 3 contractions have been described in children with pseudo-obstruction.[32] Other authors have noted that these abnormalities do not discriminate children with motility disorders from controls.[4]

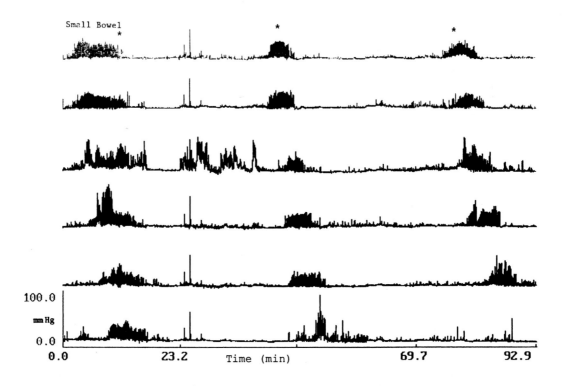

**FIGURE 29.21.** Antroduodenal manometry in a child after small bowel transplantation. There are three phase 3 (*) of the migrating motor complexes in 90 minutes, with very minimal phase 2 activity. The alternation of phase 1 and phase 3, with little phase 2, is a typical feature of the bowel devoid of extrinsic innervation[35] and is also found during sleep.

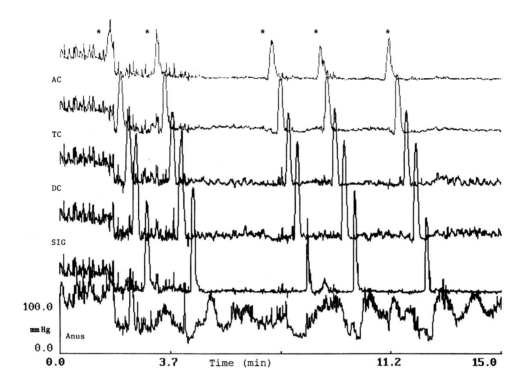

**FIGURE 29.26.** Example of a cluster of high-amplitude propagated contractions (HAPCs) (*) associated with relaxation of the internal anal sphincter. Once the HAPCs carry the stool to the distal colon, the rectal wall is distended, and there is a reflex contraction of the rectum with relaxation of the internal anal sphincter, pushing fecal material into the anal canal. Bisacodyl-induced HAPCs are quantitatively and qualitatively similar to naturally occurring HAPCs. In selected cases, such as in children receiving total parenteral nutrition or restricted fluid intake, it may be possible to shorten diagnostic colonic manometry using bisacodyl rather than waiting for spontaneous HAPCs.[38] AC, ascending colon; TC, transverse colon; DC, descending colon; SIG, sigmoid colon.

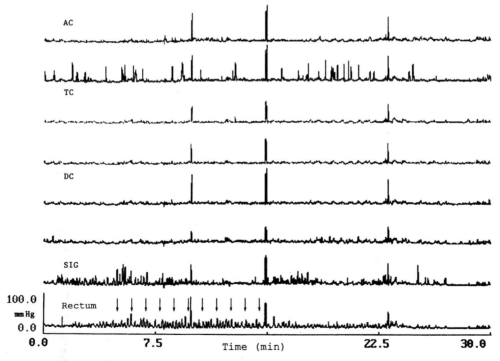

**FIGURE 29.27.** Example of a rectal motor complex (RMC), indicated by the *arrows*. The RMC is a cluster of phasic contractions, occurring every 1 to 2 hours, sustained for than 3 minutes, followed by motor quiescence.[39,40] The RMC is not synchronous with the small intestine MMC and has uncertain physiologic significance. It has been hypothesized that it may keep the rectum devoid of stools at night. AC, ascending colon; TC, transverse colon; DC, descending colon; SIG, sigmoid colon.

may be no improvement after appropriate behavioral and medical treatment. These children may suffer from a neuromuscular colonic disorder. The diagnosis of such disorders relies either on pathologic studies of bioptic specimens or on evaluation of colonic motility. Histopathologic studies are helpful mainly in the diagnosis of Hirschsprung's disease, the most common neuropathy in children. The pathologic diagnosis of other neuromuscular colonic diseases is much more challenging because of the lack of age- and location-matched control specimens. Thus, colonic manometry and anorectal manometry are being increasingly used to differentiate different causes of intractable constipation (Figs. 29.28 to 29.30).[11]

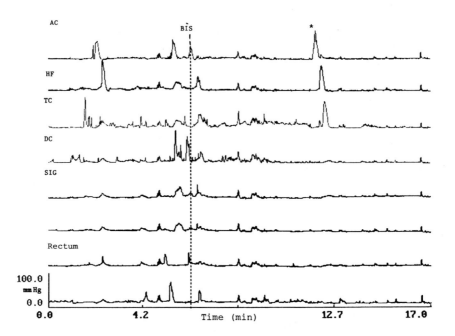

**FIGURE 29.28.**   Example of abnormal colonic motility. The figure shows a high-amplitude propagated contraction (HAPC) (*) migrating only to the transverse colon (TC). There are no propagated contractions in the distal colon either before or after stimulation with bisacodyl (BIS) (*dotted line*). The lack of propagation of HAPCs into the distal colon is indicative of colonic neuropathy. This pattern is often found in the ganglionated colon of children who remain constipated after surgery for Hirschsprung's disease.[41] AC, ascending colon; HF, hepatic flexure; SIG, sigmoid colon.

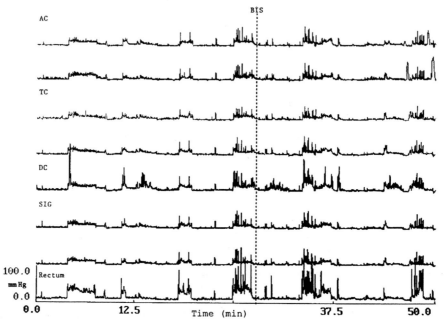

**FIGURE 29.29.**   Example of abnormal colonic motility. The figure shows the absence of propagated contractions both before and after stimulation with bisacodyl (BIS) (*dotted line*). In the absence of severe colonic dilation, the presence of only low-amplitude contractions and the total absence of contractions are features suggestive of a colonic myopathy.[42] AC, ascending colon; TC, transcending colon; DC, descending colon; SIG, sigmoid colon.

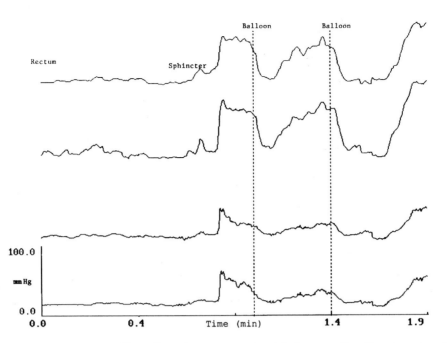

**FIGURE 29.30.** Example of normal anorectal motility. The motility catheter with four radially oriented recording sites, spaced 1 cm apart, is pulled from the rectum into the anal sphincter (*left side of the tracing*). The recording sites are then positioned at the level of the anal sphincter (*right side of the tracing*), and the rectal balloon is inflated. There is a complete relaxation of the anal sphincter on rectal distention. The presence of the rectoanal inhibitory reflex rules out Hirschsprung's disease. Contrary to earlier reports, there is now evidence that the rectoanal inhibitory reflex is present even in premature infants younger than 34 weeks postmenstrual age.[43] Abnormal rectoanal inhibitory reflex has also been reported in children with neuronal intestinal dysplasia.[44] When performing anorectal manometry in newborns, only the anal resting pressure and the rectoanal reflex are evaluated. In infants and toddlers, the examiner also evaluates the effect of rectal distention on the urge to defecate and the presence of withholding behaviors. The protocol to perform anorectal manometry in older children is very similar to the protocol used in adults.

## REFERENCES

1. Rudolph CD, Winter HS. NASPGN guidelines for training in pediatric gastroenterology. NASPGN Executive Council, NASPGN Training and Education Committee. J Pediatr Gastroenterol Nutr 1999;29 Suppl:S1–26.
2. Di Lorenzo C, Flores AF, Hyman PE. Age-related changes in colon motility. J Pediatr 1995;127:593–6.
3. Uc A, Hoon A, Di Lorenzo C, Hyman PE. Antroduodenal manometry in children with no upper gastrointestinal symptoms. Scand J Gastroenterol 1997;32:681–5.
4. Tomomasa T, Di Lorenzo C, Morikawa A, et al. Analysis of fasting antroduodenal manometry in children. Dig Dis Sci 1996;41:2195–203.
5. Di Lorenzo C, Hyman PE, Flores AF, et al. Antroduodenal manometry in children and adults with severe non-ulcer dyspepsia. Scand J Gastroenterol 1994;29:799–806.
6. Cucchiara S, Bortolotti M, Colombo C, et al. Abnormalities of gastrointestinal motility in children with nonulcer dyspepsia and in children with gastroesophageal reflux disease. Dig Dis Sci 1991;36:1066–73.
7. Di Lorenzo C. Pseudo-obstruction: current approaches. Gastroenterology 1999;116:980–7.
8. Rudolph CD, Hyman PE, Altschuler SM, et al. Diagnosis and treatment of chronic intestinal pseudo-obstruction in children: report of consensus workshop. J Pediatr Gastroenterol Nutr 1997;24:102–12.
9. Cucchiara S, Borrelli O, Salvia G, et al. A normal gastrointestinal motility excludes chronic intestinal pseudoobstruction in children. Dig Dis Sci 2000;45:258–64.
10. Hyman PE, Di Lorenzo C, McAdams L, et al. Predicting the clinical response to cisapride in children with chronic intestinal pseudo-obstruction. Am J Gastroenterol 1993;88:832–6.
11. Di Lorenzo C, Flores AF, Reddy SN, Hyman PE. Use of colonic manometry to differentiate causes of intractable constipation in children. J Pediatr 1992;120:690–5.
12. Omari TI, Miki K, Fraser R, et al. Esophageal body and lower esophageal sphincter function in healthy premature infants. Gastroenterology 1995;109:1757–64.
13. Omari TI, Benninga MA, Barnett CP, et al. Characterization of esophageal body and lower esophageal sphincter motor function in the very premature neonate. J Pediatr 1999;135:517–21.
14. Boix-Ochoa J, Canals J. Maturation of the lower esophagus. J Pediatr Surg 1976;11:749–56.
15. Omari TI, Snel A, Barnett C, et al. Measurement of upper esophageal tone and relaxation during swallowing in premature infants. Am J Physiol 1999;277:G862–6.
16. Putnam PE, Orenstein SR, Pang D, et al. Cricopharyngeal dysfunction associated with Chiari malformation. Pediatrics 1992;89:871–6.
17. Heyman S, Respondek M. Detection of pulmonary aspiration in children by radionuclide "salivagram." J Nucl Med 1989;30:697–9.
18. Finder JD, Yellon R, Charron M. Successful management of tracheotomized patients with chronic saliva aspiration by use of constant positive airway pressure. Pediatrics 2001;107:1343–5.
19. Orenstein SR, Giarrusso VS, Proujansky R, Kocoshis SA. The Santmyer swallow: a new and useful infant reflex. Lancet 1988;13:345–6.
20. Rosario JA, Medow MS, Halata MS, et al. Nonspecific esophageal motility disorders in children without gastroesophageal reflux. J Pediatr Gastroenterol Nutr 1999;28:480–5.
21. Glassman MS, Medow MS, Berezin S, Newman LJ. Spectrum of esophageal disorders in children with chest pain. Dig Dis Sci 1992;37:663–6.
22. Solzi GF, Di Lorenzo C. Nutcracker esophagus in a child with insulin-dependent diabetes mellitus. J Pediatr Gastroenterol Nutr 1999;29:482–4.

23. Dooley CP, Di Lorenzo C, Valenzuela JE. Variability of migrating motor complex in humans. Dig Dis Sci 1992;37:723–8.

24. Ittmann PI, Amarnath R, Berseth CL. Maturation of antroduodenal motor activity in preterm and term infants. Dig Dis Sci 1992;37:14–9.

25. Berseth CL, Nordyke CK. Enteral nutrients promote postnatal maturation of intestinal motor activity in preterm infants. Am J Physiol 1993;264:G1046–51.

26. Koenig WJ, Amarnath RP, Hench V, Berseth CL. Manometrics for preterm and term infants: a new tool for old questions. Pediatrics 1995;95:207–9.

27. Berseth CL, Nordyke CK. Manometry can predict feeding readiness in preterm infants. Gastroenterology 1992;103:1523–8.

28. Baker J, Berseth CL. Postnatal change in inhibitory regulation of intestinal motor activity in human and canine neonates. Pediatr Res 1995;38:133–9.

29. Sigurdsson L, Flores A, Putnam PE, et al. Postviral gastroparesis: presentation, treatment, and outcome. J Pediatr 1997;131:751–4.

30. Khan S, Hyman PE, Cocjin J, Di Lorenzo C. Rumination syndrome in adolescents. J Pediatr 2000;136:528–31.

31. Uc A, Vasiliauskas E, Piccoli DA, et al. Chronic intestinal pseudo-obstruction associated with fetal alcohol syndrome. Dig Dis Sci 1997;42:1163–7.

32. Fell JM, Smith VV, Milla P. Infantile chronic idiopathic pseudo-obstruction: the role of small intestinal manometry as a diagnostic tool and prognostic indicator. Gut 1996;39:306–11.

33. Guze CD, Hyman PE, Payne VJ. Family studies of infantile visceral myopathy: a congenital myopathic pseudo-obstruction syndrome. Am J Med Genet 1999;85:114–22.

34. Kellow JE, Gill RC, Wingate DL. Prolonged ambulant recordings of small bowel motility demonstrate abnormalities in the irritable bowel syndrome. Gastroenterology 1990;98:1208–18.

35. Mousa H, Bueno J, Griffiths J, et al. Intestinal motility after small bowel transplantation. Transplant Proc 1998;30:2535–6.

36. Di Lorenzo C, Flores AF, Tomomasa T, Hyman PE. Effect of erythromycin on antroduodenal motility in children with chronic functional gastrointestinal symptoms. Dig Dis Sci 1994;39:1399–404.

37. Bassotti G, Crowell MD, Whitehead WE. Contractile activity of the human colon: lessons from 24 hour studies. Gut 1993;34:129–33.

38. Hamid SA, Di Lorenzo C, Reddy SN, et al. Bisacodyl and high-amplitude-propagating colonic contractions in children. J Pediatr Gastroenterol Nutr 1998;27:398–402.

39. Kumar D, Williams NS, Waldron D, Wingate DL. Prolonged manometric recording of anorectal motor activity in ambulant subjects: evidence of periodic activity. Gut 1989;30:1007–11.

40. Prior A, Fearn UJ, Read NW. Intermittent rectal motor activity: a rectal motor complex? Gut 1991;32:1360–3.

41. Di Lorenzo C, Solzi GF, Flores AF, et al. Colonic motility after surgery for Hirschsprung's disease. Am J Gastroenterol 2000;95:1759–64.

42. Di Lorenzo C, Flores AF, Reddy SN, et al. Colonic manometry in children with chronic intestinal pseudo-obstruction. Gut 1993;34:803–7.

43. Benninga MA, Omari TI, Haslam RR, et al. Characterization of anorectal pressure and the anorectal inhibitory reflex in healthy preterm and term infants. J Pediatr 2001;139:233–7.

44. Koletzko S, Ballauff A, Hadziselimovic F, Enck P. Is histological diagnosis of neuronal intestinal dysplasia related to clinical and manometric findings in constipated children? J Pediatr Gastroenterol Nutr 1993;17:59–65.

C H A P T E R  3 0

# Gastroesophageal Surgery

*Nagammapudur S. Balaji and Jeffrey H. Peters*

The majority of the surgery for benign esophageal disorders includes interventions for gastroesophageal reflux disease and motility disorders of the esophagus and pharyngoesophageal segment.

Accurate preoperative assessment is imperative for optimal outcomes. Preoperative assessment enables the identification of the correct pathologic disorder, grading the severity of disease, and subsequent planning of appropriate interventions. Esophageal manometry plays a key role in the preoperative assessment of esophageal disorders. Subsequently, objective assessment of surgical outcomes is equally important to quantify success or failure. Manometric evaluation of the esophagus is an integral part of evaluation of persistent symptoms or new symptoms following surgery.

## TECHNIQUE

Esophageal manometry can be done using the water-perfused or the solid-state catheter systems. Irrespective of the type of system used, the lower esophageal high-pressure zone (LEHPZ), esophageal body, and upper esophageal sphincter (UES) are assessed in states of rest and during the act of swallowing a standard liquid bolus.

At our institution, we use an eight-channel water-perfused catheter system for the procedure. In addition to the standard methods of assessment of the LEHPZ, we perform the slow motorized pull-through for a dynamic evaluation of the same (Fig. 30.1).[1] This method enables us to obtain a circumferential and dynamic evaluation of the LEHPZ, that is, a limitation of the water-perfused systems because of the unidirectional pressure sensors. The UES is evaluated as a routine in every patient. However, patients with potential cervical dysphagia undergo a detailed UES evaluation using an eight-channel (spaced 1 cm apart) water-perfused catheter that is custom made and permits detailed evaluation of the pharyngoesophageal segment both pre- and postoperatively.[2]

## MANOMETRIC ASSESSMENT OF THE ESOPHAGUS BEFORE AND AFTER ANTIREFLUX SURGERY

The rationales for manometry preoperatively in gastroesophageal reflux disease in order of importance are as follows:
1. *Exclusion of primary motility disorders and evaluation of esophageal body function.* The most important parameter of interest with concern to surgical therapy and outcome is the capacity of the esophageal body to propel bolus in an aboral direction in a peristaltic fashion, which is measured by the contraction amplitudes and wave progression. Contraction amplitudes of >30 mm Hg have been conventionally chosen to indicate adequate esophageal function. However, recent evidence from the literature disputes the same. Studies have shown that the outcomes after Nissen fundoplication in patients with esophageal contraction amplitudes <30 mm Hg are no different from the rest.[3,4] However the possibility of surgical failure should be anticipated, and this may influence the surgeon to prefer a partial fundoplication to a Nissen fundoplication.

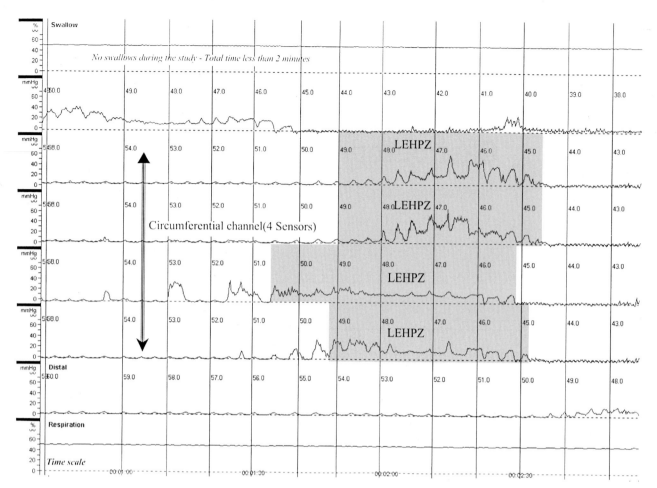

**FIGURE 30.1.** Normal lower esophageal high-pressure zone (LEHPZ). Tracings of the LEHPZ as noticed on the motorized pull-through. The motorized puller withdraws the catheter at a controlled rate of 1 mm/s. The pull-through is commenced with the circumferential channels (*highlighted* and with four pressure sensors), which are all at the same level positioned 5 cm distal to the LEHPZ (determined by the station pull) and hence in the stomach. It can be noted that the four circumferential channels traverse the LEHPZ (*highlighted portion*) from the stomach (*left of the highlighted area*) to enter into the esophageal body (*right of the highlighted portion*). The recording channels above and below the highlighted area lie 5 cm proximal and 5 cm distal to the circumferential channel, respectively. The asymmetry of the LEHPZ is well demonstrated in the pressure tracings of the four different sensors oriented at 90 degrees to each other. This is owing to the configuration of the crural sling attachment to the esophagus in a variable fashion. The vertical lines and adjoining numbers indicate the distance from the nares.

2. *Characterization of the LEHPZ.* The LEHPZ is composed of the diaphragmatic crura and the lower esophageal sphincter (LES) and constitutes the "mechanical barrier to reflux."[5,6] The parameters that have been shown to influence the probability of reflux are predominantly the resting pressure and the abdominal length of the same.[7] Patients with a defective resting pressure and a short abdominal length have an 88% chance of objective reflux owing to the mechanical incompetence of the barrier.[7] The separation of the two components of the LEHPZ (crura and LES), as manifested by a double hump, signifies a hiatal hernia, and the pressure in the hiatal sac measured as the plateau pressure may influence the patterns of reflux.[8]

3. *Placement of the probe for the 24-hour ambulatory pH study (identification of the upper border of the LEHPZ).*

In contrast, manometric evaluation of the postoperative patient after antireflux surgery is done to (1) assess new-onset/recurrent symptoms of reflux or dysphagia, (2) exclude secondary motility disorders (pseudoachalasia), and (3) assess the physiologic outcomes after surgery and relate them to symptomatic surgical outcomes.

Figure 30.2 depicts a defective LEHPZ prior to an antireflux procedure (Laparoscopic Nissen), and Figure 30.3 represents the configuration of a symmetric and competent wrap.

Manometry is also of diagnostic help in the evaluation of postoperative symptoms following surgery and in the detection of physiologic abnormalities contributing to the patients' symptoms.

The illustration in Figure 30.4 depicts the consequence of a tight fundoplication exhibiting a high resting pressure and partial relaxation and a secondary motility disturbance in the body exhibiting simultaneous contractions (pseudoachalasia).

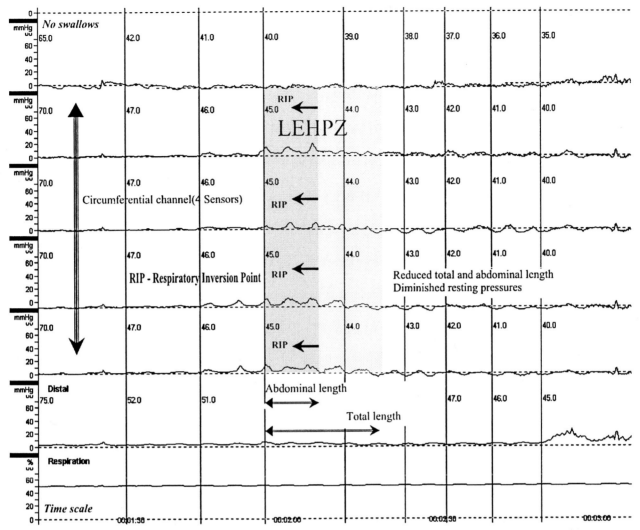

**FIGURE 30.2.** Defective lower esophageal high-pressure zone (LEHPZ) (preoperative). Motorized pull-through study of the LEHPZ. The LEHPZ is highlighted and the pressures are measured in the four sensors positioned at the same level in the catheter. It is fairly symmetric; however, the short overall length, abdominal length, and virtually absent high-pressure zone are distinct and denote overt incompetence. This sphincter is typical of a patient with advanced gastroesophageal reflux disease (GERD), and the above patient's pH score was 174.0. This patient was also noted to have Barrett's esophagus and underwent antireflux surgery.

In addition, esophageal manometry provides information on the topographic location of the LEHPZ and stomach in preoperative patients and the wrap in postoperative patients. Manometry serves only as a useful adjunct in the above scenario as the videoesophagogram would be the best investigation for anatomic mapping of the viscera.

Figure 30.5 reveals the tracing of an intrathoracic stomach as evidenced from the deflection patterns in pressure noted with the respiratory cycle.

## MANOMETRIC ASSESSMENT OF THE ESOPHAGUS BEFORE AND AFTER SURGERY FOR ACHALASIA (MYOTOMY AND A PARTIAL WRAP)

Preoperative diagnosis of achalasia rests on the finding of an aperistaltic esophagus, a hypertensive sphincter that is nonrelaxing, and frequently a pressurized esophagus.

Figure 30.6 is a classic example of the usefulness of manometry and the motorized pull-through study in particular. A basal pressure corresponding to the gastric baseline merging into a hypertensive LEHPZ that then transitions into a pressurized esophageal body is seen. This is typical in addition to esophageal aperistalsis.

Postoperative manometry in the evaluation of the effectiveness of surgery is not a routine practice; however, manometry done for persistent symptoms provides details about the altered physiology of the LEHPZ after surgery.

Figure 30.7 is a representation of a successful physiologic outcome after a myotomy and partial fundoplication for achalasia (see Fig. 30.6). The symmetry of the LEHPZ is a consistent feature after a wrap, and the resting pressure has dropped to ranges within the normal range. The disappearance of the pressurization in the esophagus is yet another feature noted indicating the absence of outflow obstruction.

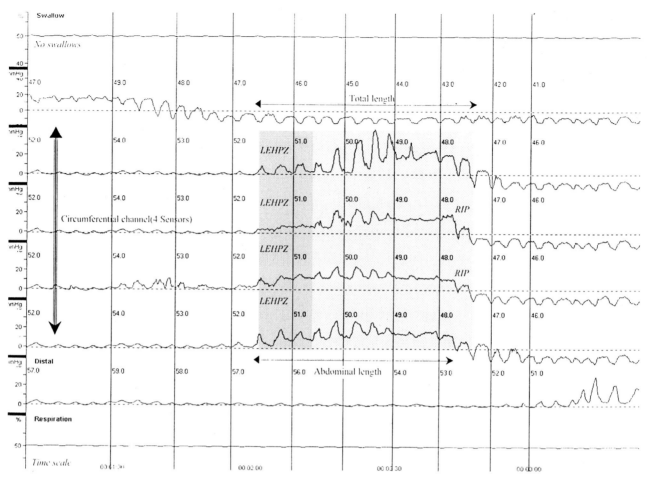

**FIGURE 30.3.** Lower esophageal high-pressure zone (LEHPZ) after antireflux surgery. The tracings depict what is achieved after a Nissen fundoplication aimed at reconstituting the LEHPZ. As noted, there is a competent sphincter with normal overall, abdominal length, and resting pressures (mea-sured in mm Hg). A characteristic appearance seen after antireflux surgery is the symmetry of the LEHPZ, which is a consequence of the complete wrap around the lower esophagus encompassing the LEHPZ.

## MANOMETRIC EVALUATION OF THE UPPER ESOPHAGEAL SPHINCTER BEFORE AND AFTER CRICOPHARYNGEAL MYOTOMY

Patients with suspected UES dysfunction as a cause of dysphagia will benefit from a detailed manometric study of the UES. The use of the custom-made eight-channel catheter with channels placed 1 cm apart enables accurate circumferential characterization of the UES and the pharynx. The variables that are known to predict surgical outcomes after cricopharyngeal myotomy are the residual pressure at relaxation and the bolus pressures attained during the passage of 5-mL liquid bolus.[9] Normalization of the above variables are physiologic markers of a successful outcome.

Cricopharyngeal bars that are radiologically defined indentations of the posterior pharyngeal wall seen on lateral swallows of a barium swallow are not uncommonly seen as incidental findings on routine videoesophagograms.[10,11] The significance of these in contributing to oropharyngeal dysphagia is controversial. The manomet-ric characteristics of the UES are largely unaffected.[12] However, they can contribute to dysphagia in the presence of associated pharyngeal dysfunction, resulting in an inability to overcome the elevated intrabolus pressure in the region above the UES.[13]

Figure 30.8 reveals inadequate relaxation on dry swallows to atmospheric pressure and an abnormally elevated bolus pressure in a patient who presented with dysphagia.

Figure 30.9 exhibits a return of variables seen as abnormal in Figure 30.7 (preoperatively) to within normal levels and is a physiologic measure of the outcome of cricopharyngeal myotomy for the relief of dysphagia.

The results of surgery are not always as expected, as in the following situation. An inappropriately long myotomy without precise manometric localization of the UES can be a disaster. The tracings in Figure 30.10 were those in a patient post–cricopharyngeal myotomy. The myotomy was extended into the proximal esophagus, resulting in the failure of the proximal esophageal body. The above may be secondary to inaccurate preoperative manometric localization of the UES.

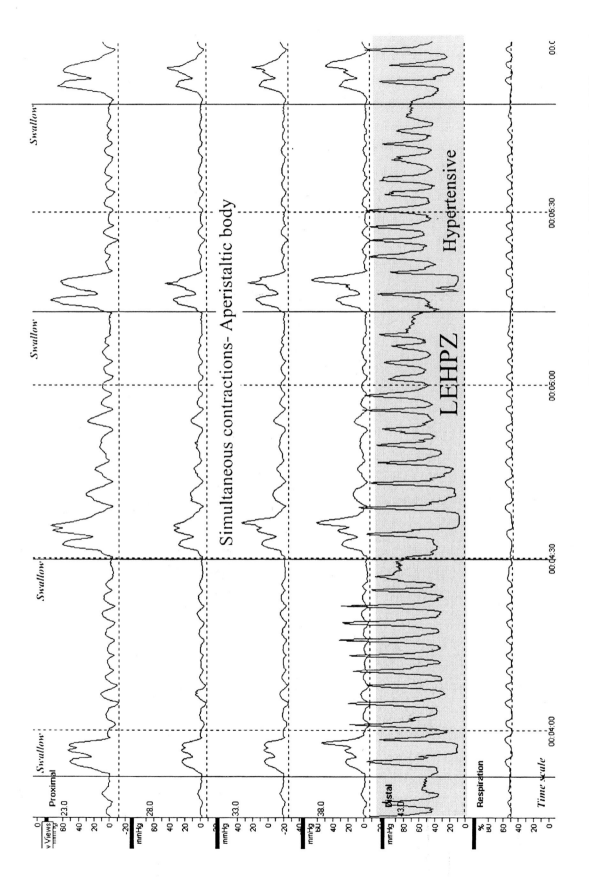

**FIGURE 30.4.** Pseudoachalasia. The tracings above are seen as part of the esophageal body study with the most proximal channel at 1 cm below the lower border of the upper esophageal sphincter. The proximal four channels in this patient were lying in the esophageal body and the fifth channel from above in the LEHPZ. This patient was referred with continuing dysphagia after antireflux surgery, and her body study revealed a hypertensive LEHPZ. This is the feature of a tight wrap and as a consequence has developed esophageal body dysfunction as seen by the nonperistaltic but simultaneous wave progression. Note the elevated bolus pressures (initial hump) averaging to >20 mm Hg and partial relaxation (residual pressures >8), which signify outlet resistance.

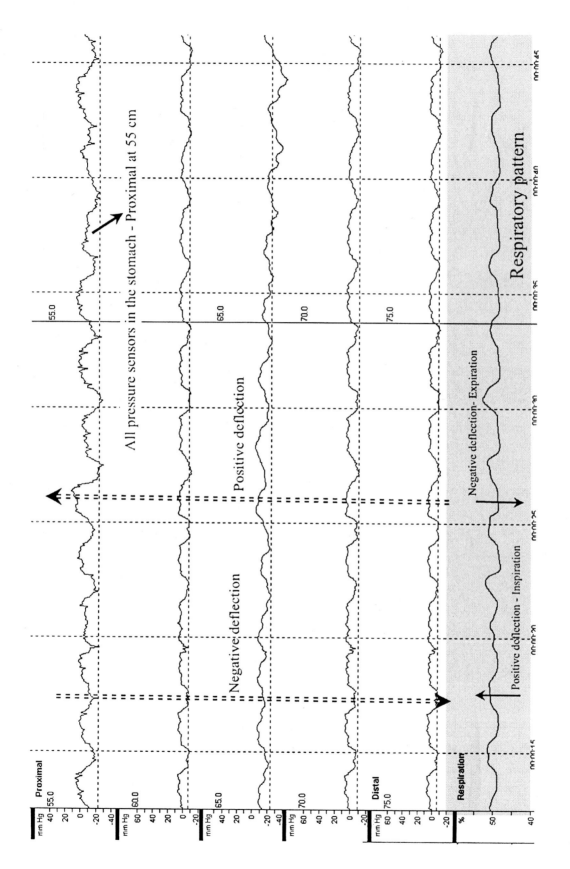

**FIGURE 30.5.** Intrathoracic stomach. The above figure reveals the patterns noticed with all of the pressure sensors in the stomach (distal at 75 cm and proximal at 55 cm from the nares). Note that the deflection patterns in all five channels are in reverse direction to the respiratory pattern. This would imply that the sensors are in an environment with a thoracic pattern of influence on the pressure sensors. This patient was found to have an intrathoracic stomach secondary to traumatic disruption of the diaphragmatic hiatus. This pattern is to be recognized at the start of the procedure as it could lead to misinterpretation if missed. There would be no respiratory inversion point to represent the transition from the abdominal to the thoracic segment of the LEHPZ as the whole segment is within the thorax.

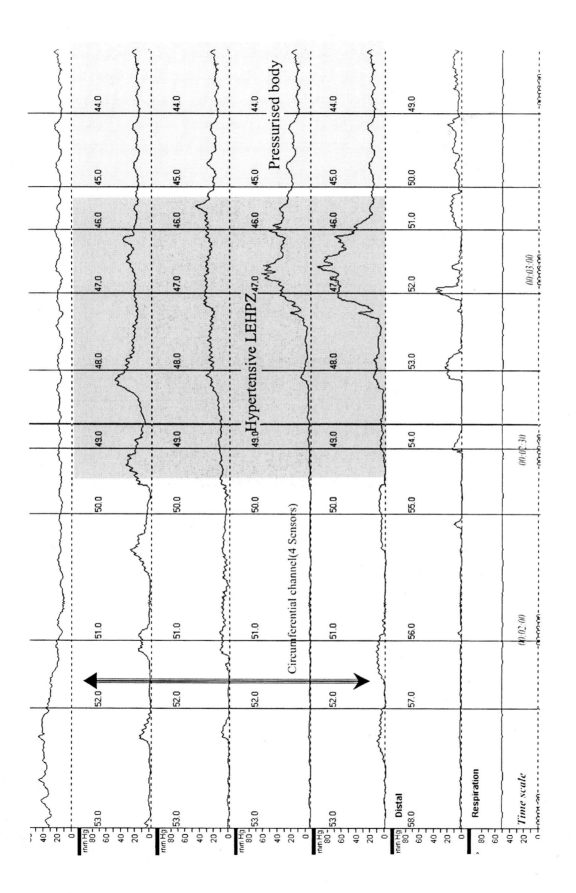

**FIGURE 30.6.** Achalasia—LEHPZ motorized pull-through. The characteristics shown here are typical of achalasia. As the circumferential sensor passes from the stomach (*left*) into the LEHPZ (*highlighted*), it is noted that the LEHPZ is of a hypertensive nature. Although a hypertensive LEHPZ can occur as an isolated feature, the pressurized body that is seen after the sensors pass into the esophageal body (*right*) is characteristic of achalasia.

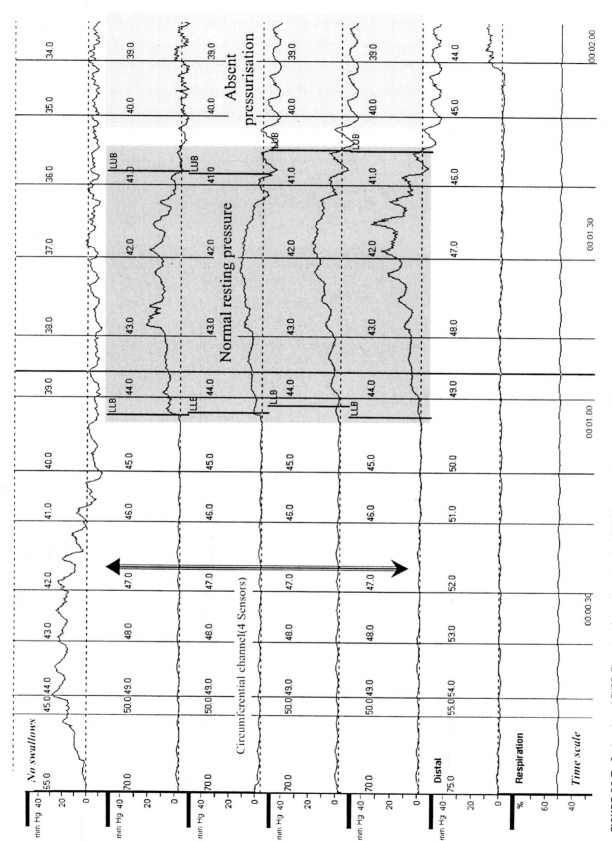

**FIGURE 30.7.** Postmyotomy LEHPZ. The return from a hypertensive LEHPZ to a normotensive state after myotomy for achalasia is well shown. Note that the symmetric nature of the LEHPZ is attributable to the partial wrap of the distal 3 cm of the esophagus, which is usually coupled with myotomy to protect against potential reflux. The disappearance of esophageal pressurization is attributable to the absence of outflow resistance after surgery.

**FIGURE 30.8.** Defective UES—premyotomy. The detailed UES study above is done using an eight-channel water-perfused catheter, with each channel 1 cm apart. When appropriately positioned, a minimum of two channels lie in the pharynx and two channels in the UES. In the study above, channels 1 to 3 are in the pharynx and channels 4 to 7 are in the UES. As can be seen, there is no relaxation of the UES to the baseline (0 mm Hg) during a 5-mL swallow (average pressure noted to be >10 mm Hg), and the intrabolus pressure is elevated. The pharyngeal bolus pressures are also elevated (>16 mm Hg), signifying resistance to flow at the region of the UES. The failure of the UES pressures to attain a subatmospheric pressure drop and an elevated bolus pressure are the best prognostic indicators for good functional outcome after surgery.

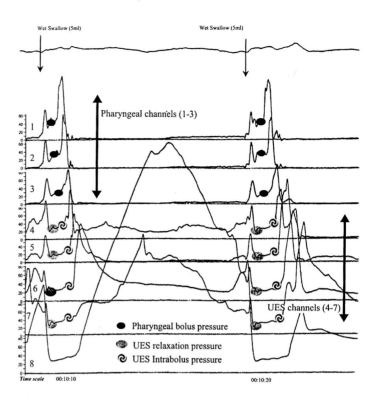

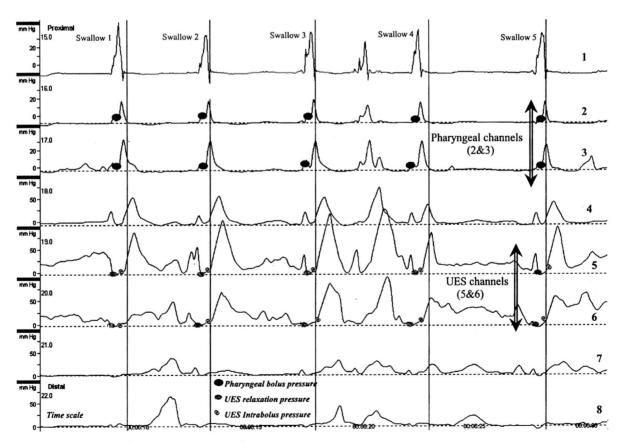

**FIGURE 30.9.** Post–cricopharyngeal myotomy—detailed UES study. The detailed UES study above is done using an eight-channel water-perfused catheter, with each channel 1 cm apart. When appropriately positioned, a minimum of two channels lie in the pharynx and two channels in the UES. In the study above, channels 1 to 3 are in the pharynx and channels 5 and 6 are in the UES. The changes seen after cricopharyngeal myotomy are the subatmospheric pressure drop at relaxation and the return of elevated bolus pressures to normal values.

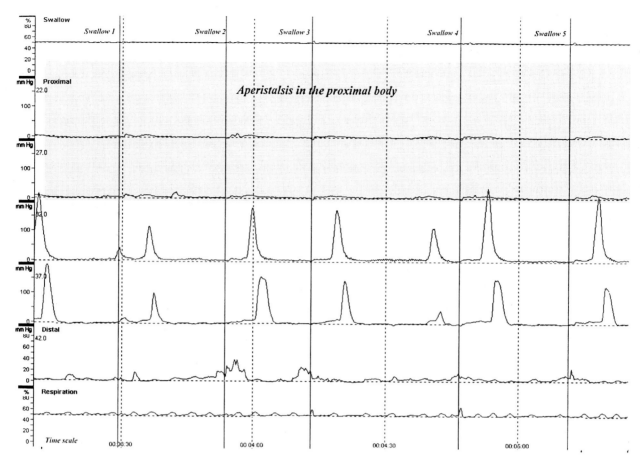

**FIGURE 30.10.** Dysfunctional proximal esophageal segment after cricopharyngeal myotomy. Accurate manometric localization of the UES is necessary for purposes of myotomy during surgery. The UES is not a well-defined anatomic sphincter and is difficult to localize at surgery. The proximal limit of myotomy is made easier in the presence of a Zenker's diverticulum. However, inadvertent extended myotomy in the distal direction onto the esophageal body can result in proximal esophageal dysfunction. In the figure, proximal body dysfunction was noted in a patient who complained of persistent dysphagia after cricopharyngeal myotomy. No peristalsis or any form of contractile activity is observed in the proximal segment in contrast to a normal distal body.

## REFERENCES

1. Costantini M, Bremner RM, Crookes P, DeMeester TR. The slow motorized pull-through: an improved technique to evaluate the lower esophageal sphincter. Gastroenterology 1992;102:A53.
2. Mason RJ, Bremmer CG, DeMeester TR, et al. Pharyngeal swallowing disorders: selection for and outcome after myotomy. Ann Surg 1998;228:598–608.
3. Bremner RM, Bremmer CG, DeMeester TR, et al. The effect of symptoms and nonspecific motility abnormalities on outcomes of surgical therapy for gastroesophageal reflux disease. J Thorac Cardiovasc Surg 1994;107:1244–9.
4. Beckingham IJ, Cariem AK, Bornman PC, et al. Oesophageal dysmotility is not associated with poor outcome after laparoscopic Nissen fundoplication. Br J Surg 1998;85:1290–3.
5. Kahrilas PJ. Anatomy and physiology of the gastroesophageal junction. Gastroenterol Clin North Am 1997;26:467–86.
6. Kahrilas PJ, Lin S, Chen J, Manka M. The effect of hiatus hernia on gastrooesophageal junction pressure. Gut 1999;44:476–82.
7. Zaninotto G, DeMeester TR, Schwizer W, et al. The lower esophageal sphincter in health and disease. Am J Surg 1988;155:104–11.
8. Balaji NS, Wajed SJ, Bremner CD, DeMeester TR. The significance of the plateau pressure in a hiatal hernia noted on esophageal manometry. Gastroenterology 2001;120:A429.
9. Mason RJ, Bremner CG. Myotomy for pharyngeal swallowing disorders. Adv Surg 1999;33:375–411.
10. Olsson R, Ekberg O. Videomanometry of the pharynx in dysphagic patients with a posterior cricopharyngeal indentation. Acad Radiol 1995;2:597–601.
11. Ekberg O, Nylander G. Dysfunction of the cricopharyngeal muscle. A cineradiographic study of patients with dysphagia. Radiology 1982;143:481–6.
12. Dantas RO, Cook IJ, Dodds WJ, et al. Biomechanics of cricopharyngeal bars. Gastroenterology 1990;99:1269–74.
13. Olsson R, Nilsson H, Ekberg O. An experimental manometric study simulating upper esophageal sphincter narrowing. Invest Radiol 1994;29:630–5.

# CHAPTER 31

# Gastric and Small Bowel Surgery

*Gordon L. Kauffman Jr*

In the experience of most gastrointestinal (GI) surgeons, surgical intervention for the complications of peptic ulcer disease (PUD) is significantly lower than in years past. The next generation of GI surgeons will have less experience with both the primary operations and the surgical treatment of patients with the untoward effects of these procedures. Indications for surgery in patients with PUD have traditionally been intractability, bleeding, perforation, obstruction, and, in the case of gastric ulcer, concern about the risk of an underlying carcinoma. Surgical options include proximal gastric vagotomy (PGV), truncal vagotomy and antrectomy (V&A), truncal vagotomy and pyloroplasty (V&P), and subtotal gastrectomy. Two to five decades ago, surgical treatment for the complications of PUD was common. Today, patients who exhibit the complications of any of these procedures are older and have comorbid conditions that place them at high risk for further surgical intervention.

## POSTGASTRECTOMY SYNDROMES

The term "postgastrectomy syndromes" encompasses several conditions that can be defined, such as early and late dumping syndrome, postvagotomy diarrhea, postoperative delayed gastric emptying, chronic gastroparesis, alkaline reflux gastritis, afferent loop syndrome, and anastomotic strictures. Unfortunately, there is a great deal of overlap between the symptoms of these conditions, making a truly definitive diagnosis difficult. If an inappropriate remedial operation is undertaken, the results can be less than optimal. On average, 25 to 35% of patients who have surgery for PUD have symptoms that fall under the rubric of a postgastrectomy syndrome.

The causes of these physiologic abnormalities are thought to be related to removal of the antrum, destruction of the pylorus by resection, or pyloroplasty and/or vagal denervation of the GI tract below the gastroesophageal junction. With the introduction of PGV, the frequency of these postgastrectomy syndromes has dropped dramatically. Remedial surgery should be reserved only for those patients who have failed, after sufficient time, to develop spontaneous adaptive mechanisms with or without the use of medications.[1,2]

## REMEDIAL SURGERY FOR EARLY DUMPING SYNDROME

Early dumping syndrome is thought to be a vasomotor response to food, perhaps hypertonic solutions entering the duodenum following V&A or V&P. Postprandial weakness, dizziness, palpitations, diaphoresis, nausea, and crampy abdominal pain followed by explosive diarrhea may be fre-

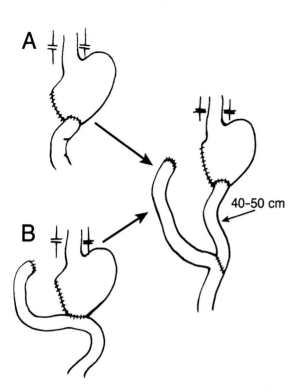

**FIGURE 31.1.** Conversion of gastroduodenostomy (**A**) or gastrojejunostomy (**B**) to Roux-en-Y reconstruction with the Roux limb that must be at least 40 to 50 cm in length. Following a gastroduodenostomy, the surgery requires that the anastomosis be dismantled and a Roux-en-Y reconstruction be formed. In some cases, following gastrojejunostomy, the afferent limb can be transected and an enteroenterostomy between the afferent and efferent limb, 40 to 50 cm distal to the anastomosis, can be formed.

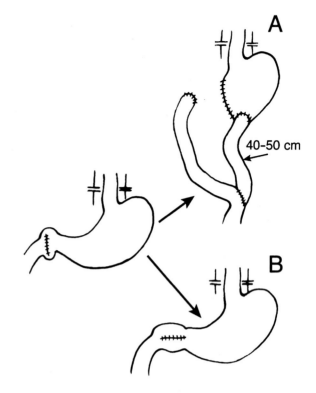

**FIGURE 31.2.** Conversion of a vagotomy and pyloroplasty to either distal gastrectomy with Roux-en-Y reconstruction (**A**) or reversal of the pyloroplasty (**B**). The former is the procedure of choice as the efficacy of the latter is not well established.

quently observed in patients with early dumping syndrome. The vasoactive substance or substances that mediate this symptom complex include serotonin, kinins, neurotensin, and vasoactive intestinal polypeptide in addition to other, as yet unidentified mediators. Medical therapy involves separating the solid and liquid phases of a meal, eating meals of low carbohydrate content, and perhaps adding pectin to the diet to delay gastric emptying.[3,4] Somatostatin administration has some beneficial effect in certain patients by inhibiting the release of these putative peptide mediators.[5]

Remedial surgery for early dumping syndrome involves procedures that are designed to delay gastric emptying. Following V&A with either a gastroduodenal or gastrojejunal anastomosis, conversion to a Roux-en-Y gastrojejunostomy with jejunojejunostomy is considered to be the remedial procedure of choice (Fig. 31.1).[6] Following V&P, a distal gastrectomy with Roux-en-Y gastrointestinal reconstruction (Fig. 31.2A) is the best surgical option. Reversing the pyloroplasty (Fig. 31.2B) is another option; however, there is little experience with this approach. Although advocated by some surgeons, positioning an 8- to 10-cm antiperistaltic jejunal loop between the gastric remnant and isoperistaltic jejunum (Fig. 31.3) has been associated with delayed gastric emptying, the

formation of bezoars, and weight loss such that the loop often had to be removed.[7,8]

## REMEDIAL SURGERY FOR LATE DUMPING SYNDROME

Late dumping syndrome symptoms occur 1 to 2 hours after a meal and are similar to those of early dumping. They are primarily related to hypoglycemia. It is thought that the release of enteroglucagon sensitizes the pancreatic beta cells to release excessive amounts of insulin, resulting in hypoglycemia. Adjusting the diet to separate the solid and liquid phases of a meal alters the release of enteroglucagon from the small bowel. Somatostatin administration may also be of some benefit by inhibiting the release of insulin. Rarely is remedial surgery indicated for this syndrome.

## REMEDIAL SURGERY FOR POSTVAGOTOMY DIARRHEA

Postvagotomy diarrhea occurs in nearly 20% of patients who have had a truncal vagotomy. In general, it is self-limited and responds to antidiarrheal medications. Approximately 1 to 2% of patients complain of incapacitating diarrhea follow-

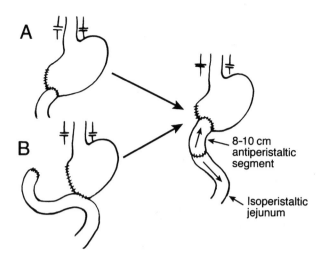

**FIGURE 31.3.** Conversion of postdistal gastrectomy reconstitution of gastro-duodenostomy (**A**) or gastrojejunostomy (**B**) to include an 8- to 10-cm segment of antiperistaltic jejunum between the duodenum and isoperistaltic jejunum. Antiperistaltic segments larger than 8 to 10 cm are associated with significant delays in gastric emptying. Care must be taken to avoid mesenteric twisting of the antiperistaltic segment, which would lead to ischemia and necrosis.

ing truncal vagotomy. Frequent watery and explosive bowel movements, unrelated to meals, characterize this syndrome. Medical therapy, in addition to antidiarrheal medications, includes ingesting meals with low fluid content, the intake of frequent smaller meals, and the use of increased dietary fiber. Studies suggest that many of these patients have a rapid transit time from stomach to colon. Again, the use of somatostatin has been beneficial in some patients.

Two surgical procedures have been suggested to treat those patients who are incapacitated by the diarrhea and have failed dietary and medical therapy. The first is to reverse an 8- to 10-cm segment of jejunum, 100 cm distal to the ligament of Treitz in an antiperistaltic orientation (Fig. 31.4A).[7] This procedure has had reasonable success in the hands of those who designed the procedure yet has not been exploited by many other GI surgeons because the results have not been uniformly positive. An alternative surgical approach consists of reversing 180 degrees of antiperistaltic ileum, allowing the other 180 degrees of ileum to be isoperistaltic (Fig. 31.4B).

Again, because of the relative infrequency of this problem, no large studies are available to evaluate the efficacy of the procedure. In the hands of those who designed this approach, however, the results have been gratifying.[9]

## REMEDIAL SURGERY FOR ACUTE AND LONG-TERM GASTROPARESIS

Acute and more long-term postoperative gastroparesis may occur in 10 to 15% of patients who have had a truncal vagotomy, in particular when combined with distal gastrectomy

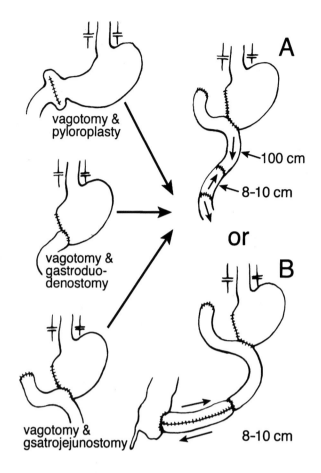

**FIGURE 31.4.** Following either vagotomy and pyloroplasty, vagotomy and gastroduodenostomy, or vagotomy and antrectomy, interposition of an 8- to 10-cm segment of antiperistaltic jejunum can be positioned either 100 cm distal to gastrojejunostomy in continuity (**A**) or 180 degrees of the circumference just proximal to the ileocecal valve (**B**).

to include resection of the gastric pacemaker, irrespective of whether reconstitution of the GI tract is by gastroduodenostomy or gastrojejunostomy. Preoperative duodenal obstruction may predispose to postoperative acute gastroparesis. The symptoms include epigastric fullness, abdominal discomfort, postprandial nausea, and vomiting of undigested food and are similar to those seen in gastric outlet obstruction. Other causes of gastric dysmotility must be ruled out: diabetic gastropathy, autonomic neuromuscular disease, hypothyroidism, electrolyte imbalance, and the use of anticholinergic drugs. Postvagotomy and gastric resection gastric atony seem to be related to parasympathetic denervation as the result of truncal vagotomy and resection of the gastric pacemaker, located on the greater curvature of the gastric wall. Radionuclide gastric emptying studies using both liquid- and solid-phase meals, upper gastrointestinal barium studies, and esophagogastroduodenoscopy (EGD) should confirm the presence of delayed gastric emptying and allow the physician to determine whether there is a mechanical gastric outlet obstruction. This, coupled with electrogas-

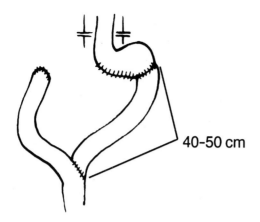

**FIGURE 31.5.** Near-total gastrectomy with Roux-en-Y reconstruction for postgastrectomy gastric atony requires that the Roux-en-Y limb also be 40 to 50 cm in length.

trography, discussed elsewhere in this volume, may also give a clue as to the potential role of endogenous pacemaker abnormalities or high resistance to gastric outflow as the cause of delayed gastric emptying.

Medical therapy for postoperative gastric atony includes nasogastric suction, enteral tube feedings directly into the duodenum, an attempt at ingestion of frequent small meals, and the use of metoclopramide or erythromycin to promote gastric motility.

Since this problem is relatively infrequent, a number of surgical options have emerged as potentially efficacious. The most aggressive surgical approach is to do a near-total gastrectomy with a Roux-en-Y gastrojejunal reconstruction (Fig. 31.5). This procedure has been reported to benefit two-thirds of patients.[2]

A less aggressive approach is to resect the gastrojejunostomy that may be dysfunctional because of position or stenosis. This procedure should allow the patient to retain about 25% of the proximal stomach. It should be combined with a posterior gastrojejunostomy (Fig. 31.6A) and may be combined with a distal Braun enteroenterostomy (Fig. 31.6B).[10] This enteroenterostomy will allow pancreaticobiliary secretions to bypass the gastrojejunostomy and as such may offer an advantage by reducing the risk of developing alkaline reflux gastritis. On the other hand, it may predispose to marginal ulceration as the protons secreted from the stomach are not readily neutralized by pancreatic bicarbonate. If acute gastric atony occurs following truncal V&P, the recommended surgical approach is a hemigastrectomy and posterior gastrojejunostomy with or without a Braun enteroenterostomy. Finally, there may be situations in which the gastrojejunostomy can be identified, but because of extensive scarring to the liver and/or pancreas, the surgeon deems that the resection will place the patient at great risk for complications or death. In such a situation, a "plasty" can be performed in which vertical incision is made through the gastrojejunostomy that is closed horizontally (Fig. 31.7). This will reduce the resistance to the outflow gastric luminal contents and may provide some degree of symptomatic relief.

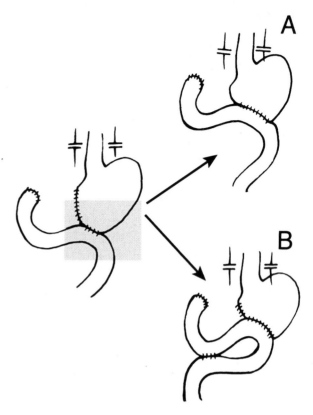

**FIGURE 31.6. A**, Resection of gastrojejunostomy with greater gastric resection (*shaded area*) and formation of a posterior gastrojejunostomy (**A**) or posterior gastrojejunostomy with a Braun jejunojejunostomy between the afferent and efferent limbs (**B**) are both legitimate options for reconstruction.

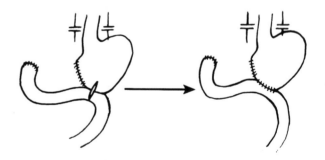

**FIGURE 31.7.** A "plasty" of stenotic gastrojejunostomy can be performed when resection is considered to be technically prohibitive, thus reducing the gastric outflow resistance and enhancing gastric emptying. A vertical incision is made through the gastrojejunostomy, which is then closed horizontally.

## REMEDIAL SURGERY FOR ALKALINE REFLUX GASTRITIS

Alkaline reflux gastritis occurs in nearly 2% of patients who have had gastric surgery, primarily in those who have had a gastrojejunal anastomosis without a Braun jejunojejunostomy. Chronic abdominal discomfort in the epigastrium that is burning in nature and nausea brought on by the ingestion of a meal suggest the diagnosis. It seems to take months to years for the symptom complex to occur postoperatively. Since symptoms are brought on by eating, patients tend to eat less frequently, lose weight, and become anemic. It is not clear what single enzyme or combination of enzymes in hepatobiliary secretions refluxing into the stomach and bathing the mucosa is the primary cause of the condition. Proton pump inhibitors are rarely of any benefit. It has been considered a diagnosis of exclusion, but, endoscopically, the entire gastric mucosa is erythematous, friable, and covered by bile. When the gastroenterologist and surgeon are convinced that alkaline reflux gastritis is the correct diagnosis, consideration can be given to surgical conversion from a V&A or V&P to a distal gastrectomy with a Roux-en-Y biliary diversion (Fig. 31.8). The Roux limb should be at least 40 to 50 cm in length to preclude reflux of hepatobiliary secretions up the limb and into the gastric lumen. The clinical results suggest that, provided that the diagnosis is correct, nearly 90% of patients will experience endoscopic and symptomatic improvement.[11–14]

## REMEDIAL SURGERY FOR AFFERENT LOOP SYNDROME

The afferent loop syndrome is a real entity following gastrojejunal reconstruction following a distal or hemigastrectomy, with or without truncal vagotomy. When the afferent limb is too long because of technical error, there can be a mechanical obstruction at the afferent limb—gastric anastomosis, causing the hepatobiliary secretions to accumulate in the limb, resulting in distention and colicky pain, and the pain is completely relieved when the pressure in the limb overcomes the obstruction and allows the accumulated hepatobiliary contents to rush into the gastric lumen. This is often associated with nausea and bilious vomiting that produces symptomatic relief. Thus, it is incumbent on the surgeon to create the shortest afferent limb possible to prevent this complication.

If the afferent loop syndrome persists unrecognized, bacterial overgrowth in the afferent limb may occur, leading to the signs and symptoms associated with the blind loop syndrome. Revision to shorten the afferent limb (Fig. 31.9)[14,15] or decompression of the obstructed afferent limb with an enteroenterostomy (Fig. 31.10) usually is associated with symptomatic improvement.[10]

## REMEDIAL SURGERY FOR ANASTOMOTIC STRUCTURES

Anastomotic strictures may occur as a result of a technical error, an error in positioning or the jejunum, or anastomotic ulceration with edema, scarring, and fibrosis. Anastomotic ulceration can be caused by an incomplete vagotomy, retained

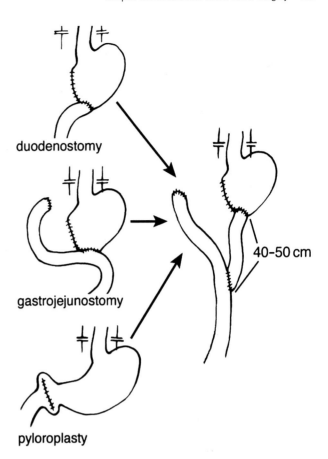

**FIGURE 31.8.** Conversion of gastroduodenostomy, gastrojejunostomy, or pyloroplasty to a Roux-en-Y biliary diversion for alkaline reflux gastritis requires that the afferent limb be 40 to 50 cm in length. Following vagotomy and pyloroplasty, a formal gastric resection is required.

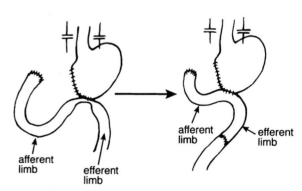

**FIGURE 31.9.** Patients who have had a gastrojejunostomy with a long afferent limb are prone to develop "kinking" at the gastrojejunostomy of the afferent limb. This causes afferent limb syndrome, which can be handled surgically by resecting the gastrojejunostomy and bringing the afferent limb as close to the ligament of Treitz as possible.

antrum following distal gastrectomy, a long afferent limb, or inadequate gastrectomy. Marginal ulcers may present with epigastric pain or GI bleeding. If they are not diagnosed and treated, the result can be gastric outlet obstruction caused by edema, initially, followed by healing with fibrosis. A contrast study from above may show a tapered narrowing at the anas-

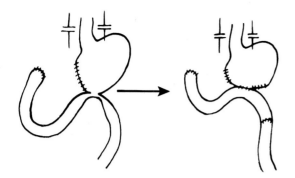

**FIGURE 31.11.** Resection of a nonfunctional gastrojejunostomy with a larger gastric resection (*shaded area*) and new posterior gastrojejunostomy is appropriate.

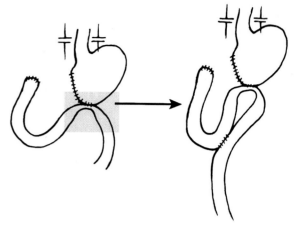

**FIGURE 31.10.** In situations in which it is difficult to resect the gastrojejunostomy and shorten the afferent limb, a Braun enteroenterostomy between the afferent and efferent limbs is a legitimate alternative to treating afferent limb syndrome.

tomosis. An EGD may reveal a narrowed gastrojejunostomy, which, in conjunction with compromised gastric neuromuscular activity, may cause a functional gastric outlet obstruction. An EGD will also reveal retained gastric secretions and/or a bezoar. Both solid- and liquid-phase radionuclide gastric emptying studies will confirm abnormal gastric emptying. Dietary manipulation may provide some symptomatic improvement, but, in most cases, remedial surgery offers the best opportunity for success. The recommended procedure is to resect the anastomosis, thereby reducing the gastric reservoir and creating a new, posterior gastrojejunostomy with or without a Braun jejunojejunostomy (Fig. 31.11).[16]

## SUMMARY

Postgastrectomy syndromes, by and large, are reflective of some type of gastric neuromuscular disorder, whether a result of truncal vagotomy that interferes with pyloric function, resection, or pyloroplasty or inadvertent resection of the gastric pacemaker. The gastroenterologist and GI surgeon should allow a significant amount of time to elapse between the initial surgery and consideration to remedial surgical intervention as most symptoms will dissipate with time. Medical forms of therapy, including dietary considerations, are all legitimate. Unfortunately, little is known about the role of *Helicobacter pylori* antral colonization in the causation of many of these postgastric surgery dysmotility syndromes. Remedial surgery is the last resort and should be considered only when all other courses of action fail. Everyone caring for these patients should do so with a positive attitude to be conveyed to the patient regarding the final outcome.

### REFERENCES

1. Delcore R, Cheung LY. Surgical options in postgastrectomy syndromes. Surg Clin North Am 1991;212:57–75.
2. Egon JC, Miedema BW, Kelly KA. Postgastrectomy syndromes. Surg Clin North Am 1992;72:445–65.
3. Jenkins DJA, Gassull MA, Leeds AR. Effect of dietary fiber on complications of gastric surgery: prevention of postprandial hypoglycemia by pectin. Gastroenterology 1977;73:215–7.
4. Speth PAJ, Jansen JBMJ, Lamers CBHW. Effect of acarbose, pectin, a combination of acarbose with pectin, and placebo on postprandial reactive hypoglycemia after gastric surgery. Gut 1983;24:798–802.
5. Geer R, Richards WO, D'Dorisio TM, et al. Efficacy of octreotide acetate in treatment of severe postgastrectomy dumping syndrome. Ann Surg 1990;212:678–87.
6. Miedema BW, Kell KA. The Roux operation for postgastrectomy syndromes. Am J Surg 1990;161:256–61.
7. Sawyers JL, Herrington JL Jr. Antiperistaltic jejunal segments for control of the dumping syndrome and postvagotomy diarrhea. Surgery 1971;69:263–7.
8. Sawyers JL, Herrington HL Jr. Superiority of antiperistaltic jejunal segments in management of severe dumping syndrome. Ann Surg 1973;178:311–21.
9. Cuschieri A. Longterm evaluation of a reservoir jejunal interposition with an isoperistaltic conduit in the management of patients with the small stomach syndrome. Br J Surg 1982;69:386–8.
10. Vogel SB, Drane WE, Woodward ER. Clinical and radionuclide evaluation of bile diversion by Braun enteroenterostomy: prevention and treatment of alkaline reflux gastritis. Ann Surg 1994;219:458–65.
11. Sawyers JL, Herrington JL Jr, Buckspan GS. Remedial operation for alkaline reflux gastritis and associated postgastrectomy syndromes. Arch Surg 1980;115:519–23.
12. Ritchie WF Jr. Alkaline reflux gastritis: an objective assessment of its diagnosis and treatment. Ann Surg 1980;192:288–96.
13. Madura JA, Grosfeld JL. Biliary diversion: a new method to prevent enterogastric reflux and reverse the Roux stasis syndrome. Arch Surg 1997;132:245–9.
14. Lygidakis NJ. The value of revisional surgery for the treatment of postoperative alkaline reflux gastritis. World J Surg 1982;6:226–9.
15. Herrington JL Jr. Experience with the surgical management of the afferent loop syndrome. Ann Surg 1966;164:797–809.
16. Kelly KA, Becker JM, Van Heerden JA. Reconstructive gastric surgery. Br J Surg 1981;68:687–91.

# CHAPTER 32

# Colonic and Anorectal Surgery

*Howard S. Kaufman*

Motility disorders of the distal gastrointestinal tract range from intractable constipation and obstructed defecation to total fecal incontinence. Proper radiographic and physiologic evaluations as outlined in the previous chapter should be guided by findings elicited on a comprehensive history and physical examination. Iatrogenic causes such as medications that result in constipation or diarrhea must be ruled out and eliminated if possible. With the possible exception of rectal prolapse, medical management for these disorders should be exhausted prior to consideration of surgical therapy. Modification of dietary habits, appropriate use of bulking agents, and behavioral modification may result in acceptable improvements to quality of life. Patients should be counseled that surgical intervention may restore function to an acceptable level; however, perfect bowel habits or continence is often an unrealistic expectation. In addition, many procedures may fail with time. Finally, as the "end-organ" of the process of defecation, the various components of the pelvic floor may be primarily or secondarily involved. Multidisciplinary approaches to these clinical disorders are often warranted, and cross-referral to a variety of pelvic floor specialists, including behavioral therapists, is frequently indicated.

## CONSTIPATION

Constipation is a widely encompassing term that has been applied to a variety of types of defecatory dysfunction. Confusion in diagnosis can result as this symptom may have markedly different definitions for patients and physicians. Numerous factors may contribute to the slowing of or obstruction to normal patterns of defecation and include extracolonic (Table 32.1),[1] intestinal (small and large), and outlet (pelvic floor) disorders.

### Evaluation

In the evaluation of the constipated patient, a useful operational definition for constipation includes ≤ two stools per week and/or straining at stool ≤20% of the time.[2] A detailed history and physical examination are essential. Bowel habits should be carefully elucidated with detail paid to the duration of symptoms, frequency and consistency of stool, and association with abdominal and/or pelvic pain. A diary of bowel habits can be helpful. The use of adjuncts necessary to achieve successful fecal evacuation should also be discussed, including fiber and water intake, laxative and/or enema use, and the need for transanal or transvaginal digital manipulation. The extracolonic causes of constipation may be uncovered in the past medical and surgical histories. Since numerous drugs can slow intestinal transit, all medications (prescription, nonprescription, and herbal supplements) should be carefully reviewed. A history of physical and/or sexual abuse is often associated with obstructed

**TABLE 32.1.** Extracolonic Causes of Constipation

| | |
|---|---|
| Endocrine and metabolic | Carcinomatosis |
| | Diabetes mellitus |
| | Glucagonoma |
| | Hypercalcemia |
| | Hyperparathyroidism |
| | Hypokalemia |
| | Hypopituirism |
| | Hypothyroidism |
| | Milk-alkali syndrome |
| | Pheochromocytoma |
| | Porphyria |
| | Pregnancy |
| | Uremia |
| Neurologic cerebral | Parkinson's disease |
| | Stroke |
| | Tumors |
| Spinal | Cauda equina tumor |
| | Ischemia |
| | Iatrogenic |
| | Meningocele |
| | Multiple sclerosis |
| | Paraplegia |
| | Shy-Drager syndrome |
| | Tabes dorsalis |
| | Trauma |
| Peripheral | Autonomic neuropathy |
| | Chagas' disease |
| | Multiple endocrine neoplasia, type 2B |
| | von Recklinghausen's disease |
| Drugs | Anesthetic |
| | Analgesic |
| | Antacids (calcium and aluminum compounds) |
| | Anticholingeric |
| | Anticonvulsant |
| | Antidepressant |
| | Antiparkinsonian |
| | Barium sulfate |
| | Calcium channel blockers |
| | Diuretics |
| | Ganglion blockers |
| | Hematinics (iron) |
| | Hypotensives |
| | Laxative abuse |
| | Monoamine oxidase inhibitor |
| | Metals (arsenic, lead, mercury, phosphorus) |
| | Opiates |
| | Paralytic agents |
| | Psychotherapeutics |
| Myopathic | Amyloidosis |
| | Dermatomyositis |
| | Myotonic dystrophy |
| | Scleroderma |

Reproduced with permission from Pfeifer J, Agachon F, Wexner SD. Surgery for constipation: a review. Dis Colon Rectum 1996;39:444–60.

defecation secondary to anismus, and appropriate referrals should be made prior to pursuing surgical therapy. A review of systems including a past gynecologic and obstetric history should query other associated symptoms that may unveil alternative diagnoses and additional sequelae of pelvic floor dysfunction.

Physical examination may uncover an extraintestinal cause of constipation. The abdomen can appear normal or be distended and tympanitic. Massive protuberance may be apparent in extreme cases of megarectum and megacolon. Rectal and pelvic examinations are essential components of the examination and should be performed in the presence of a chaperone. The patient should be examined at rest, during straining, and while trying to expel an examining finger. Rectal prolapse, pelvic organ prolapse (especially rectocele), and failure of the puborectalis to relax may be easily diagnosed on physical examination. The levator ani muscles should be palpated to delineate occult defects such as posterolateral hernias (Fig. 32.1) or spasm with associated pain. Anal stricture from previous anorectal surgery will often preclude an adequate digital examination, and examination and/or biopsy of a stricture may be necessary under sedation or anesthesia to rule out malignancy.

Following history and physical examination, specific investigations of the colon and pelvic floor are obtained as described in detail above. Endoscopic or contrast enema evaluation of the colon and rectum should be obtained to rule out an obstructing lesion. In the absence of an otherwise defined cause, tests of colonic transit with radiopaque markers or scintigraphic techniques should be ordered. Negative results may be repeated if the patient still complains of constipation. Pelvic floor evaluation should be initiated if prolapse or perineal descent is seen on physical examination. Evacuation proctography with the addition of vesical,

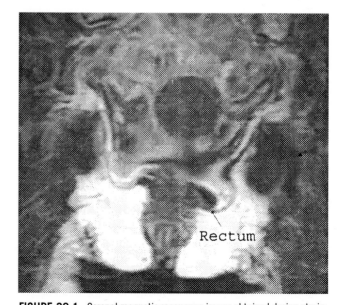

**FIGURE 32.1.** Coronal magnetic resonance image obtained during straining from a patient with obstructed defecation. Note bilateral levator hernias with rectum protruding through the left levator hernia.

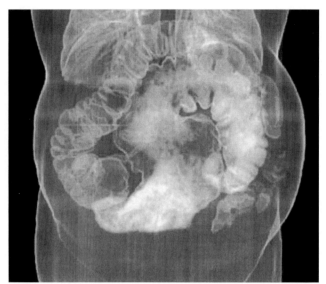

**FIGURE 32.2.** Adult Hirschsprung's disease. Multidetector computed tomographic image with three-dimensional reconstruction showing the outline of protuberant abdomen with a massively dilated and stool-filled sigmoid colon.

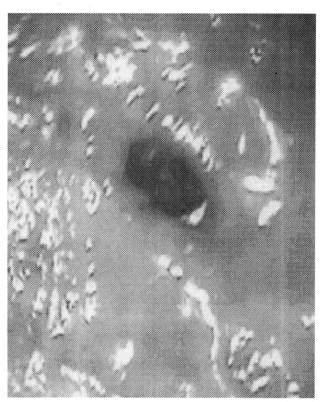

**FIGURE 32.3.** Colorectal anastomotic stricture following sigmoid colectomy for malignancy.

vaginal, and enteral contrast as indicated is useful to demonstrate the anatomic causes of obstructed defecation secondary to pelvic floor disease. Finally, patients with documented slow transit constipation (STC) should have additional tests of gastric and small intestinal motility if symptoms suggest a generalized gastrointestinal motility disorder.

### Surgery for Constipation

Slow transit constipation is uncommon and should be diagnosed on the basis of an abnormal radiopaque marker or scintigraphic studies. Mechanical and functional causes such as Hirschsprung's disease (Fig. 32.2), volvulus, rectal prolapse, tumors, anastomotic strictures (Fig. 32.3), and pseudo-obstruction must be excluded prior to considering colectomy for STC.

The most common procedure for STC is subtotal colectomy with ileorectal (or ileo- to distal sigmoid) anastomosis (Fig. 32.4). In most surgical series, only 5 to 10% of patients who are referred for refractory constipation are candidates for surgical management.[3–5] Success rates of >88% have been reported following careful patient selection. Two special categories of patients with STC deserve mention. Patients with pelvic floor disorders and STC should be treated with pelvic floor retraining prior to IRA. Outcomes are similar to patients with STC alone following retraining. In addition, patients with a history suggestive of upper gastrointestinal motility disorders warrant additional evaluation prior to consideration of colectomy with IRA. Redmond and colleagues further categorized patients into those with colonic inertia alone or those with a more generalized intestinal dysmotility problem.[6] In 37 consecutive patients operated on for colonic inertia, 19 of 21 (90%) patients with colonic inertia had successful outcomes at a mean of 7.5

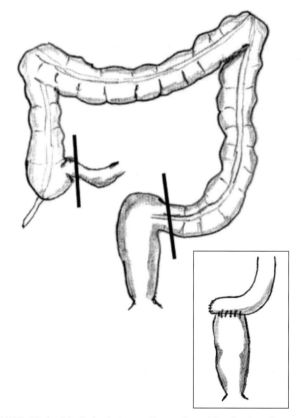

**FIGURE 32.4.** Extent of colonic resection performed for slow transit constipation with reconstruction by side-to-end ileorectostomy (*inset*).

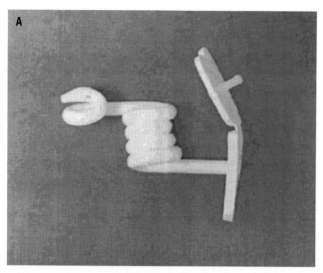

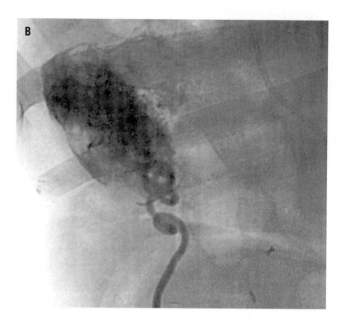

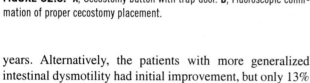

**FIGURE 32.5. A,** Cecostomy button with trap door. **B,** Fluoroscopic confirmation of proper cecostomy placement.

years. Alternatively, the patients with more generalized intestinal dysmotility had initial improvement, but only 13% had prolonged relief.

A variety of other surgical procedures have been used less commonly and reported for the treatment of constipation including restorative proctocolectomy (ileal pouch-anal anastomosis) and anorectal myectomy.[7,8] However, despite its role in the treatment of short segment Hirschsprung's disease,[9] long-term results for anorectal myectomy in the treament of STC have been poor.[8,10] Finally, encouraging results with the Malone antegrade continence enema (ACE) in the pediatric population have prompted some investigators to apply this option to adults with constipation and incontinence. This procedure leaves the colon in situ and relies on antegrade lavage of stool via a catheter placed into a surgically raised appendicostomy or cecostomy. Patients usually irrigate every 1 to 3 days to evacuate the colon. Most published data include only pediatric patients. In a small series, 75% of 16 adult patients who had severe fecal incontinence (n = 10) or constipation (n = 6) in whom the ACE procedure was performed reported overall satisfaction.[11] The mean time for defecation was reduced from 175 to 40 minutes in the constipated group. This procedure can now be safely performed percutaneously under fluoroscopic[12] (Fig. 32.5) or colonoscopic[13] (Fig. 32.6) guidance with a button cecostomy replacing the surgical appendicostomy.

## RECTAL PROLAPSE

Rectal prolapse (procidentia) results when the full thickness of the rectum intussuscepts through the anal canal (Fig. 32.7). Although this disorder can affect infants and young children, it is unusual in adults before the fifth decade and more commonly affects the elderly. The female-to-male ratio is 5:1. Rectal prolapse may result from lower rectal herniation through the anorectal ring or from higher rectorectal intussusception progressing to full-thickness rectal prolapse. Many congenital and acquired defects have been implicated in the etiology of procidentia and include neurologic disorders (congenital anomaly, cauda equina lesion, spinal cord tumors and injury, and dementia), chronic straining to stool, perineal descent and other pelvic organ prolapse syndromes, and postoperative conditions following hemorrhoidectomy, fistulectomy, and low pelvic anastomosis. Anatomic findings associated with rectal prolapse include a redundant rectosigmoid, deep pouch of Douglas, lack of posterior mesorectal fixation, levator ani diastasis, and weak anal sphincters. A colorectal neoplasm may also serve as a lead point for the intussusception.

### Evaluation

Patients usually present with a chief complaint of protrusion of the rectum. Constipation has been reported in 25 to 50% of patients with prolapse.[14] Soiling, mucus drainage, or gross fecal incontinence accompanies full-thickness rectal prolapse in up to 75% of patients.[15] Most patients will have some resolution of these symptoms following repair. At least 100 surgical procedures have been described to treat rectal prolapse. For simplicity, these procedures are broadly characterized into those performed via the abdominal route and those performed through a perineal approach. The latter set of procedures is usually reserved for more debilitated patients as results from abdominal procedures have been associated with lower long-term recurrence rates.

The most popular abdominal operation for prolapse in the United States has been the Ripstein procedure (Fig. 32.8). Ripstein described the modern anterior sling rectopexy in 1965.[16] Although Ripstein anecdotally reported a very low recurrence rate, his personal series of over 1,500 patients was

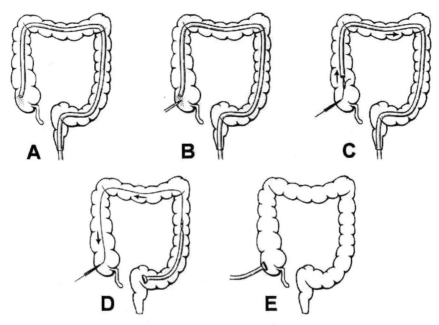

**FIGURE 32.6.** Schematic diagram of colonoscopic cecostomy procedure. **A**, Colonoscopy is performed to the cecum, and the anterior abdominal wall is transilluminated. **B**, After prepping and draping the anterior abdominal wall, a 0.5-cm incision is made, and a trocar is passed into the cecum. **C**, A guidewire is passed through the trocar and grasped with a snare passed through the accessory channel of the colonoscope, and the colonoscope is removed. **D**, The guidewire is tied to a 20F pull-type percutaneous endoscopic gastrostomy tube and pulled retrograde through the colon and out the anterior abdominal wall. **E**, Properly placed percutaneous cecostomy. Reproduced with permission from Rivera MT, Kugathasan S, Berger W, Werlin SL. Percutaneous colonoscopic cecostomy for management of chronic constipation in children. Gastrointest Endosc 2001;53:225–8. Copyright © 2001 American Society for Gastrointestinal Endoscopy.

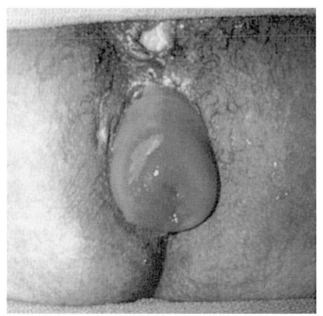

**FIGURE 32.7.** Circumferential full-thickness rectal prolapse.

never published in detail. Despite initially encouraging results, constipation was frequently experienced by patients in longer-term follow-up and was attributed to the anterior sling causing obstruction to defecation. Modifications employing an incomplete anterior wrap have been designed to avoid this problem. Recurrence rates of complete prolapse range from 5 to 10%.[16–18]

Other related suspensions/fixation procedures include the Wells procedure, direct suture rectopexy, posterior Ivalon sponge rectopexy, and resection rectopexy (Frykman-Goldberg procedure) (Fig. 32.9).[15,19] There have been no prospective randomized trials to compare these techniques. Moreover, there are no data to suggest that the addition of a foreign sling provides any advantage to simple suture fixation alone in large retrospective series. Debate continues as to the value and extent of resection when combined with rectopexy.[20]

Perineal operations for rectal prolapse have usually been reserved for more infirm and unfit patients who cannot tolerate an abdominal approach. Although easily tolerated, perianal encirclement procedures such as the Thiersch wire have largely been abandoned because of poor success rates and high rates of recurrence and fecal impaction. Full-thickness rectosigmoidectomy (Altemeier procedure) with or without levatoroplasty or rectomucosectomy with plication of the distal rectal wall (Delorme procedure) can be performed with minimal morbidity in this less fit patient population.

The Altemeier procedure can be performed under general or regional anesthesia after a full mechanical bowel preparation. Pre- and perioperative parenteral antibiotics should be given. The distal rectum is divided >1 cm above the dentate line. The mesorectal blood supply is divided and ligated, allowing for continued prolapse of the nonfixed (and often redundant) rectosigmoid after entering the peritoneal cavity anteriorly. Sigmoid mesentery is then similarly controlled and divided. After (optional) levatoroplasties have been performed, a handsewn or stapled end-to-end coloanal

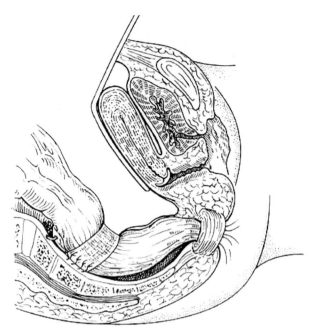

**FIGURE 32.8.** Anterior sling rectopexy (Ripstein procedure). Reproduced with permission from Nicholls RJ, Banerjee A. Rectal prolapse and solitary rectal ulcer syndrome. In: Nicholls RJ, Dozois RR, editors. Surgery of the colon and rectum. London: Churchill Livingston; 1997. p. 722.

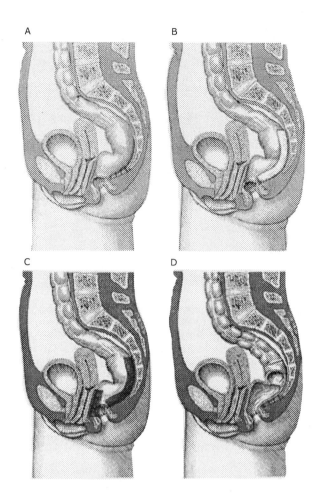

**FIGURE 32.9. A**, Simple suture rectopexy. Four sutures fix the rectum to the presacral facia. **B**, Posterior Ivalon sponge rectopexy. **C**, Anterior and posterior Marlex rectopexy. **D**, Sigmoid resection and suture rectopexy. Reproduced with permission from Duthie GS, Bartolo DCC. Abdominal rectopexy for rectal prolapse: a comparison of techniques. Br J Surg 1992;79:107–13.

anastomosis is completed. Although Altemeier and colleagues reported a recurrence rate of only 3% following perineal rectosigmoidectomy,[21] other authors have reported failures in up to 60% of patients.[22]

Delorme, a French army surgeon, first described mucosal stripping of the prolapsed rectum of three young men in 1900.[23] Following circumferential mucosectomy, plication of the circular smooth muscle of the distal rectum and anal canal is performed in at least four quadrants to accordian the distal rectum (Fig. 32.10). Finally, an end-to-end mucosa-to-mucosa anastomosis is performed. There was little interest in Delorme's procedure until the 1970s, when several small series were reported.[24,25] Recurrence rates are higher (12 to 22%) than for most abdominal procedures; however, constipation and incontinence usually improve.

In conclusion, rectal prolapse is a multifactorial disease mostly affecting the elderly. For younger and fit patients, abdominal approaches offer low recurrence rates. Recently, laparoscopic approaches to suture rectopexy, sling rectopexy, and resection rectopexy have been described with satisfactory results.[26] Regardless of the abdominal technique, continence is usually improved following repair. Elderly and debilitated patients, as well as younger patients with multiple medical problems, are best served by a perineal procedure.

## RECTOCELE

Rectoceles (Fig. 32.11) are thought to result from tears in the rectovaginal fascia or disruption of the distal rectovaginal fascia from the perineal body occurring during vaginal childbirth. Long-term straining to stool is another mechanism of potential fascial disruption. Since up to 80% of asymptomatic female volunteers have fluoroscopic evidence of a rectocele, selection of appropriate surgical candidates is difficult. Attempts to correlate bowel symptoms with the degree of posterior prolapse have been difficult. In a prospective evaluation of 143 women with uterovaginal prolapse, there was only a weak statistical correlation between the severity of bowel symptoms and the degree of posterior vaginal wall prolapse (Fig. 32.12).[27] Furthermore, a specific stage of posterior prolapse that was reliably associated with defecatory dysfunction could not be identified.

In the absence of strict anatomic criteria, surgical candidates may include women who complain of protrusion or bulging of the rectum into the posterior vaginal wall, difficult defecation, constipation (defined by straining), the need for assisted defecation by splinting the posterior vaginal wall, and dyspareunia. Physical examination should include a pelvic examination in the presence of a chaperone, and the

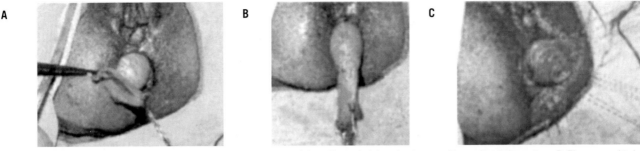

**FIGURE 32.10.** Delorme procedure. **A**, The rectal mucosa is stripped from the underlying circular smooth muscle of the rectum. **B**, The mucosal tube is developed until the full extent of the prolapse is reached. **C**, The circular smooth muscle is plicated prior to completing the mucosa-to-mucosa anastomosis above the dentate line.

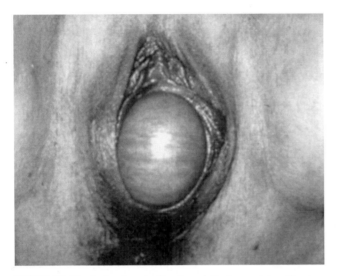

**FIGURE 32.11.** Rectocele protruding through the hymenal ring. (Courtesy of Geoffrey W. Cundiff, MD.)

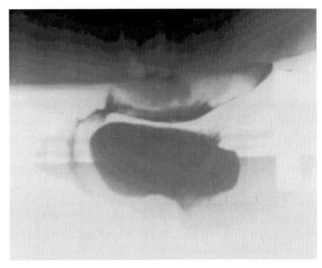

**FIGURE 32.13.** Nonemptying rectocele seen during quadruple-contrast videoproctography.

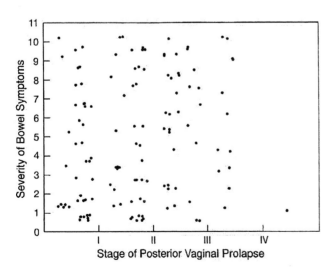

**FIGURE 32.12.** Scattergram of severity of bowel symptoms and stage of posterior vaginal prolapse according to the measurement at point Bp. There is a weakly positive correlation ($r = 0.23$, $p = .006$); women with more advanced posterior vaginal prolapse were more bothered by their bowel function than were women with less advanced posterior vaginal prolapse. Reproduced with permission from Weber AM, Waters MD, Ballard LA, et al. Posterior vaginal prolapse and bowel function. Am J Obstet Gynecol 1998;179:1446–9.

stage of prolapse should be recorded according to the standards of the International Continence Society.[28] Confirmation of a nonemptying rectocele on video proctography is helpful (Fig. 32.13). Parodoxic contraction of the puborectalis should be ruled out by examination, physiologic testing, or proctography and treated by pelvic floor physical therapy prior to performing operative repair of rectocele. Other sequelae of pelvic relaxation commonly coexist, and symptoms and/or physical findings suggestive of anterior and apical (vault) prolapse (Fig. 32.14) warrant further investigation and specialist referral.

### Surgical Management

The surgical approach to rectocele repair has differed according to surgeon specialty, with gynecologic and colorectal surgeons using transvaginal and transanal techniques, respectively. The most common gynecologic repair, posterior colporrhaphy, involves midline plication of the endopelvic fascia with or without levatoroplasty (Fig. 32.15). Fascial defects are not precisely identified and repaired but oversewn. The resulting vaginal narrowing and transverse submucosal ridge have been associated with dys-

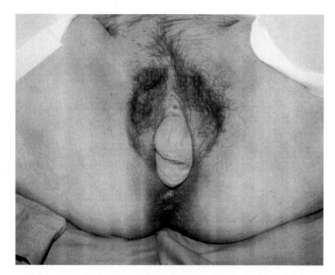

**FIGURE 32.14.** Vaginal vault prolapse associated with rectocele and obstructed defecation.

pareunia or apareunia in up to 50% of patients.[29] Moreover, bowel function does not necessarily improve postoperatively. In a retrospective review of 231 women following posterior colporrhaphy, the vaginal anatomic defect remained corrected in 76% of patients.[30] However, whereas prolapse symptoms decreased from 62 to 31%, symptoms of constipation (22% versus 33%), incomplete evacuation (27% versus 38%), fecal incontinence (4% versus 11%), and sexual dysfunction (18% versus 27%) worsened (pre- versus postoperative values, respectively).

Transanal rectocele repair, performed in the prone-jackknife position, involves plication of the rectal muscularis propria with subsequent attachment of the plicated anterior rectal wall to the levator ani muscles. The results have also been variable, with 75 to 95% of women reporting improvement in bowel function in surgical series with stringent patient selection.[31–33] The presence of anismus on preoperative evaluation has been associated with less satisfactory outcomes.[33]

Based on cadaveric dissections and intraoperative observations, numerous authors have employed a modified transvaginal approach to rectocele repair.[34–37] Richardson identified five common locations of rectovaginal fascial disruption (Fig. 32.16), and the discrete defect approach to rectocele repair is aimed at specific repair of these fascial breaks (Fig. 32.17).[34] Early results have been encouraging, with significant anatomic improvement in the amount of posterior vaginal wall excursion and genital hiatus lengthening with strain at 12 months.[36] Kenton and colleagues also reported improved symptoms in 46 patients evaluated 1 year following discrete defect rectocele repair.[37] Symptomatic improvement has also been reported with respect to protrusion (90%), difficult defecation (54 to 63%), and dyspareunia (33 to 92%).[35–37] Although the need for vaginal splinting was eliminated in 63% of patients who preoperatively required assistance with defecation in one series, 64% resumed manual assistance in another report.[36,37] Longer follow-up will support the concepts behind this repair, and randomized trials comparing these techniques are needed.

## ANAL FISSURE

The differential diagnosis for acute anal pain includes anal fissure, thrombosed external hemorrhoid, and undrained sepsis. Patients with anal fissure complain of severe pain following defecation. There may be associated bright red blood that is passed at the end of defecation or noted on the toilet tissue. The majority of acute anal fissures will heal with medical therapy, which is directed at elimination of hard stools and decreasing internal anal sphincter (IAS) spasm. (Fig. 32.18). Fiber and fluid intake are titrated to result in soft, formed stools. Sitz baths may decrease IAS spasm and provide symptomatic relief. Topical nitroglycerine 0.2% applied three times per day as a direct nitric oxide donor will also relax the IAS.

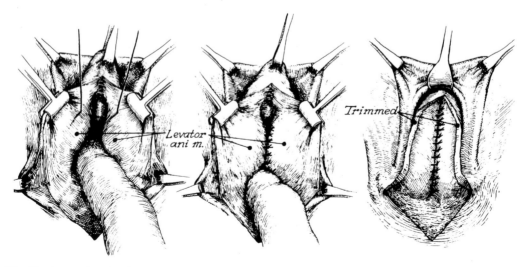

**FIGURE 32.15.** Classic posterior colporrhaphy with midline levator plication. Reproduced with permission from Wheeless CR. Atlas of pelvic surgery. Baltimore: Williams and Wilkins; 1997. p.47.

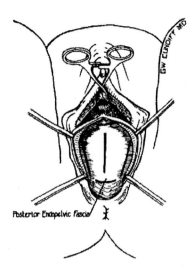

**FIGURE 32.16.** Potential locations for rents in the rectovaginal fascia, as seen through posterior colporrhaphy incision with cervix retracted anteriorly Adapted with permission from Richardson AC. The rectovaginal septum revisited: its relationship to rectocele and its importance in rectocele repair. Clin Obstet Gynecol 1993;36:976–83.

A fissure may be seen by gently parting the buttocks of a patient placed in the lateral decubitus position. The fissure will be seen as a linear tear most often in the posterior midline, although 10% of fissures occur anteriorly in women. Lateral fissures suggest alternative pathology such as Crohn's disease, malignancy, acquired immune deficiency syndrome, and tuberculosis and warrant further investigation. If a fissure cannot be seen easily on inspection of the perianal area, digital rectal examination and/or endoscopy is warranted to rule out other causes of pain. However, these maneuvers should not be performed if a fissure can easily be documented and sepsis is not suspected.

With time, an unhealed acute anal fissure will progress to a chronic anal fissure with progressive thinning of the anoderm and exposure of underlying fibers of the IAS. Pain becomes less severe, and the patient should tolerate digital rectal examination and/or anoscopy. However, the main force of insertion of either an examining finger or scope should be directed away from the fissure to decrease discomfort. Topical lidocaine is often helpful to eliminate postexamination discomfort. Additional morphologic changes may occur within the anal canal such as a hypertrophied anal papilla and sentinel tag at the distal-most aspect of the fissure (Fig. 32.19). Therapy for chronic anal fissure is again directed at avoidance of hard stools and straining; however, <10% of chronic fissures will heal without intervention.

Several lines of indirect evidence support the hypothesis that anal fissure may be secondary in anodermal ischemia. The posterior and most commonly anterior commissures of the anal canal have been shown to have less complete anastomotic blood flow by both postmortem angiography[38] and laser Doppler flowmetry.[39] High resting pressures within the anal canal occur commonly in patients with fissure,[40] and this phenomenon may further reduce blood flow to the posterior and/or anterior regions of the anal canal. Therapy is therefore directed at chemical or mechanical relaxation of the IAS and subsequent restoration of perfusion to the ischemic areas, resulting in re-epithelialization of the ulcerated fissure.

### Chemical Sphincterotomy

Although the treatment of chronic anal fissure had traditionally required random disruption of the IAS by stretch or controlled surgical division of the distal IAS by lateral internal anal sphincterotomy (see below), chemical sphincterotomy has now become the first line of therapy. Nitric oxide is a mediator of IAS relaxation. Topical nitroglycerine acts as a

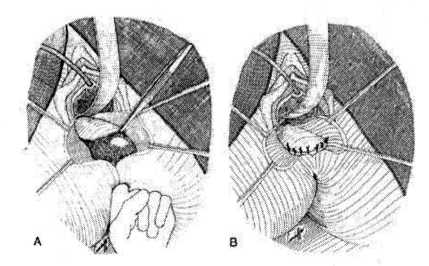

**FIGURE 32.17.** Discrete defect rectocele repair. **A**, The inferior separation of the rectovaginal fascia as defined by the forceps elevating the rectovaginal fascia and the herniation of rectal muscularis determined by the rectal finger. **B**, The break is closed using simple interrupted stitches. Reproduced with permission from Cundiff GW, Addison WA. Management of pelvic organ prolapse. Obstet Gynecol Clin North Am 1998;25:907–21.

**FIGURE 32.18.** Anorectal manometric tracing from a patient with a chronic anal fissure refractory to medical therapy. Note the high internal sphincter resting pressures and spasm.

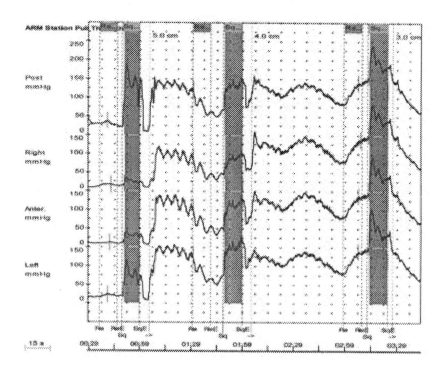

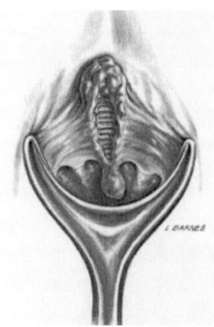

**FIGURE 32.19.** Chronic anal fissure showing hypertrophied anal papilla, sentinel tag, and underlying internal anal sphincter muscle fibers. Reproduced with permission from Corman ML. Colon and rectal surgery. 4th ed. Philadelphia: Lippincott-Raven; 1998. p. 208.

direct nitric oxide donor and mediates relaxation of the IAS by increasing cyclic guanosine monophosphate levels within the smooth muscle cells. Nitroglycerine 0.2% ointment must be diluted from the commercially available 2% concentration prescribed for cardiac disorders. A small amount of 0.2% ointment is applied to the skin at the anal verge overlying the internal sphincter two to three times per day for 8 weeks.

Healing occurs in up to three-quarters of patients with chronic fissures.[41,42] Younger patients are more susceptible to the most common side effect, headache, and this treatment should be avoided in a patient with a history of vascular headaches. Premedication with acetaminophen is suggested during the first several doses as headaches become less severe with duration of therapy.

Botulinum toxin A (Botox) has been evaluated in the treatment of chronic anal fissure. As a potent neurotoxin, it binds to presynaptic colonergic nerve terminals and inhibits the release of acetylcholine at the neuromuscular junction. The mode of botulinum toxin on the IAS is unclear as there are no acetylcholine receptors in the smooth muscle of the IAS. The precise location for injection of botulinum toxin is debatable and possibly imprecise. Various authors advocate injection into the internal sphincter, intersphincteric groove, and, less commonly, the external sphincter. Injection into the internal sphincter on either side of the fissure has been associated with healing in 96% of fissures.[43] As an invasive therapy, complications of perianal hematoma, sepsis, and pain during injection have been reported.[44,45] Temporary fecal incontinence has been reported in 7% of patients.[45] A randomized trial has been published comparing botulinum toxin with 0.2% nitroglycerine cream, reporting healing rates of 96% and 60%, respectively.[43] There were no relapses at a mean follow-up of 15 months. None of the patients in the botulinum toxin group reported adverse events.

### Lateral Internal Anal Sphincterotomy

This procedure may be performed either by a closed or an open technique. Open lateral interal sphincterotomy (Fig. 32.20) requires an operating room setting and may be done

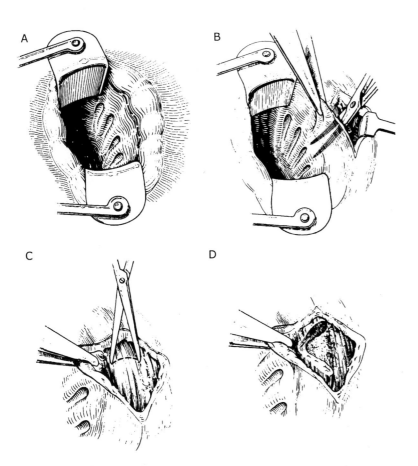

**FIGURE 32.20.** Open internal sphincterotomy. **A,** An intra-anal incision is placed just inside the cutaneous margin of the anal canal at the site of the inter-sphincteric groove. **B,** The mucosa of the anal canal is dissected from the internal anal sphincter. The inter-sphincteric space is then exposed. **C,** Once the internal sphincter has been carefully dissected from the mucosa and the external sphincter, it is divided. **D,** It is usual to divide only the lower half of the internal anal sphincter. Reproduced with permission from Keighly MRB, Williams NS. Surgery of the anus, rectum and colon. London: WB Saunders; 1993. p. 378.

in either the prone jackknife or lithotomy position and under general or regional anesthesia. A 2-cm curvilinear incision is made overlying the intersphincteric groove, and the internal sphincter is dissected laterally from the external sphincter and medially from the anal submucosa. The distal half of the sphincter is elevated within a clamp and divided using the scissors or electrocautery. The incision is closed with absorbable sutures.

A less invasive technique of closed lateral internal sphincterotomy was introduced by Notaras in 1971.[46] The advantages to this procedure include the ability to perform in the office setting under local anesthesia and improved long-term continence versus the open procedure demonstrated in one retrospective large series from the University of Minnesota.[47] This procedure (Fig. 32.21) is performed again in the lateral aspect of the anal canal by placing a #11 blade or cataract Beaver blade into the interal sphincteric groove with the knife parallel to the interal sphincter fibers. The blade is slowly rotated 90 degrees toward the anoderm. A finger may be placed on top of the anoderm to gauge the depth of penetration of the knife through the internal sphincter fibers. The knife is turned back and removed. A finger is used to deliver hemostasis and disrupt any remaining fibers of the distal half to third of the anal canal.

Acute postoperative morbidity has been reported in up to 36% of patients and includes urinary retention, hematoma, and incontinence. Although there have been no prospective randomized trials comparing open versus closed sphinctero-

tomy, a large retrospective series of 864 patients treated with open (n = 512) or closed (n = 343) lateral internal sphincterotomy has been published.[47] Recurrence rates were less than 12% in both groups, and less than 4% of patients required reoperation. Evaluated in a retrospective survey, differences were reported in long-term function including difficulty controlling flatus (30.3% versus 23.6%), seepage (26.7% versus 16.1%), and the occurrence of accidental bowel movements (11.8% versus 3.1%) in the open versus closed sphincterotomy groups, respectively.

## Recurrent Anal Fissure

Despite the effectiveness of chemical and surgical sphincterotomies, up to 10% of patients will go on to develop recurrent fissures. Moreover, women who have sustained sphincter injuries during vaginal delivery may have occult sphincter defects and not be suitable candidates for lateral internal sphincterotomy. In this population and in patients who have failed lateral internal anal sphincterotomy, more extensive evaluation of the anal canal is indicated. Manometry and anal ultrasonography should be obtained in patients with refractory fissure. In the absence of persistent IAS hypertonia, a variety of local advancement flaps have been suggested.[48,49] Both the V-Y and houseflap (Fig. 32.22) anoplasties resurface the area of the fissure, bringing in new blood supply and repairing the ulcerated defect without further detriment to the IAS. Uniform healing of 15 patients

**FIGURE 32.21.** Lateral subcutaneous sphincterotomy. **A,** The intersphincteric groove is identified. **B,** This shows the intersphincteric groove in a coronal section 90 degrees from the chronic anal fissure. **C,** A fine cataract knife is inserted in the intersphincteric plane with the knife going parallel to the fibers of the internal anal sphincter. The blade is then rotated through 90 degrees. **D,** The lower fibers of the internal anal sphincter are divided. A finger is placed in the anal canal to ensure that the mucosa is breeched. **E,** At the completion of the procedure, a defect will be palpable in the internal anal sphincter. Reproduced with permission from Keighly MRB, Williams NS. Surgery of the anus, rectum and colon. London: WB Saunders; 1993. p. 381.

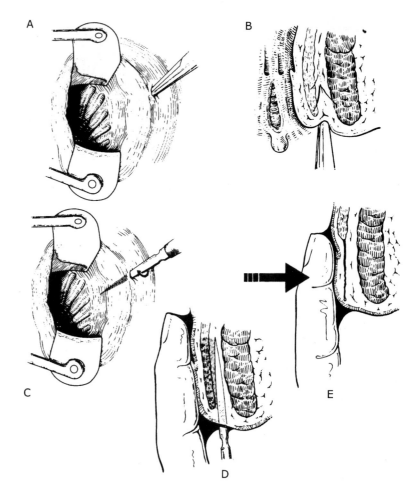

treated with island advancement flap anoplasty (Fig. 32.23) has been reported at 18 months.[48]

## FECAL INCONTINENCE

Incontinence represents an inability to store solid or liquid feces or flatus and expel it at a proper place at a proper time. The maintenance of continence to stool is a complex process that depends on multiple events and systems working in concert. Any one or more of the components of this mechanism from the formation and delivery of formed stool to defects in the muscle or neural control of the anal sphincter complex may impair the continence mechanism. The prevalence of this condition is probably understated because of its associated social stigmata. In a telephone survey of nearly 7,000 individuals from 2,570 households, the incidence of fecal incontinence was determined to be 2.2%.[50] Thirty percent of affected individuals were >65 years of age, and approximately two-thirds were female. Thirty-six percent reported incontinence to solid stool, 54% to liquid stool, and 60% to flatus. Fecal incontinence is the second leading cause of institutionalization in the elderly, and the annual cost of adult diapers in chronic care facilities was estimated at $500,000,000 in 1993.[51]

Most surgically treatable causes of fecal incontinence result from traumatic injury to the sphincter(s) from obstetric injury, previous anorectal surgery, or social trauma. Congenital abnormalities such as spina bifida, meningomyelocele, and imperforate anus, as well as acquired central and peripheral neurologic disorders, may cause fecal incontinence. Anatomic anorectal and colorectal disorders such as rectal prolapse, inflammatory bowel disease, and low rectal cancers, as well as functional disorders such as fecal impaction with overflow, can produce fecal incontinence.

### Evaluation of the Incontinent Patient

A careful history is essential in determining the etiology of fecal incontinence and must include a comprehensive survey of bowel and bladder habits. A history of trauma (surgical, obstetric, or accidental) is encouraging as patients with well-defined anatomic sphincter defects have the highest success rates following surgical repair. Numerous scoring systems for incontinence have been proposed; however, unlike urinary incontinence, attempts at standardization have not been successful across institutions. Recent progress toward this goal has been made with the Fecal Incontinence Severity Index.[52] This type frequency matrix (Fig. 32.24) was validated by Rockwood and col-

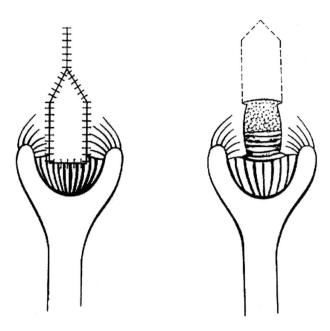

**FIGURE 32.22.** Houseflap anoplasty for recurrent anal fissure. Reproduced with permission from DeMarta DA, Nogueras JJ. An approach to the recurrent or persistent anal fissure. Semin Colon Rectal Surg 1997;8:29–35.

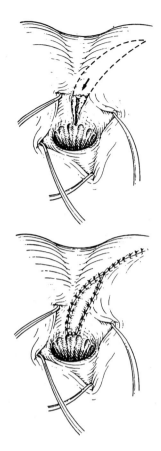

**FIGURE 32.23.** Island advancement flap anoplasty for recurrent anal fissure. Reproduced with permission from Nyam DCNK, Wilson RG, Stewart KJ, et al. Island advancement flaps in the management of anal fissures. Br J Surg 1995;2:326–8.)

leagues with respect to patient and surgeon ranking of the severity of symptoms associated with fecal incontinence.[52] A Fecal Incontinence Quality of Life (FIQL) instrument has also been validated.[53] Surgeons and patients had similar correlations using this instrument.

A comprehensive physical evaluation may occasionally confirm a history of some underlying medical condition; however, it is usually unrevealing with respect to the etiology of incontinence. Alternatively, a careful anorectal and perineal evaluation is essential in determining the etiology and will often suggest the best line of therapy. Patients are examined both in the left lateral decubitus position and in lithotomy (women). Inspection of the perineum may reveal scar tissue suggestive of previous trauma or the presence of other associated anorectal pathology such as fistula in ano (Fig. 32.25). A scarred and narrowed perineal body suggests previous obstetric injury (Fig. 32.26). A widened perineal

body may suggest an associated pelvic floor disorder including perineal descent. Patients are asked to strain in order to identify other associated pelvic floor disorders such as rectal prolapse, pelvic organ prolapse, rectocele, and/or perineal descent. Digital examination is always informative and can identify a gaping anus and anatomic defects in both the internal and external anal sphincters.

Further evaluation of the incontinent patient may include endoscopic, manometric, neourophysiologic, and imaging tests. Surgical repair is most often guided by findings on

|  | 2 or More Times a Day | Once a Day | 2 or More Times a Week | Once a Week | 1 to 3 Times A Month | Never |
|---|---|---|---|---|---|---|
| a. Gas | ☐ | ☐ | ☐ | ☐ | ☐ | ☐ |
| b. Mucus | ☐ | ☐ | ☐ | ☐ | ☐ | ☐ |
| c. Liquid Stool | ☐ | ☐ | ☐ | ☐ | ☐ | ☐ |
| d. Solid Stool | ☐ | ☐ | ☐ | ☐ | ☐ | ☐ |

**FIGURE 32.24.** Fecal Incontinence Severity Index type by frequency, symptom matrix. Reproduced with permission from Rockwood TH, Church JM, Fleshman JW, et al. Patient and surgeon ranking of the severity of symptoms associated with fecal incontinence. Dis Colon Rectum 1999;42:1525–32.

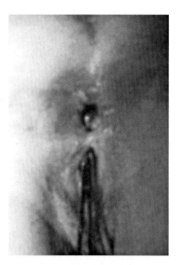

**FIGURE 32.25.** Patient in prone-jackknife position with fecal incontinence secondary to obstetric injury with persistent rectovaginal fistula and associated Crohn's disease. The surgical clamp is placed through the fistula.

transanal ultrasonography (Fig. 32.27), whereas pudendal nerve evaluation may be of prognostic significance for success following sphincteroplasty.

### Treatment Options

For patients with mild symptoms, dietary modification and loperamide or codeine phosphate are safe and often effective. Biofeedback is often attempted, especially in the absence of a structural sphincter defect. Surgical therapy for incontinence is most effective for well-defined external sphincter defects resulting from obstetric, surgical, or accidental trauma. Overlapping sphincteroplasty (Fig. 32.28) is the preferred method of repair for these injuries, and overall success rates of 50 to 80% have been reported in short-term follow-up.[54,55] Postoperative continence is usually dependent on the degree of incontinence preoperatively. Patients who are incontinent to solids and liquids have a less favorable result following sphincteroplasty. Gilliland and colleagues reported that patients with either unilateral or bilateral pudendal nerve terminal motor latency (PNTML) abnormalities have significantly less satisfactory results after sphincteroplasty.[56] Of 100 patients who underwent overlapping sphincteroplasty, 62% of patients with normal PNTML studies had a satisfactory result versus 17% of 12 patients with pudendal neuropathy at a median of 24 months follow-up. However, others have reported symptomatic and manometric improvement in patients after sphincteroplasty, despite preoperative evidence of pudendal neuropathy.[57] Age has also been suggested to correlate with outcomes in women undergoing sphincteroplasty for obstetric-related trauma.[58] Of 38 patients with normal PNTML values, 24 patients <40 years of age had a 40% difference in functional outcome when compared with 14 patients >40 years old.

Recent reports suggest that the long-term results for overlapping sphincteroplasty may not be durable. Malouf and col-

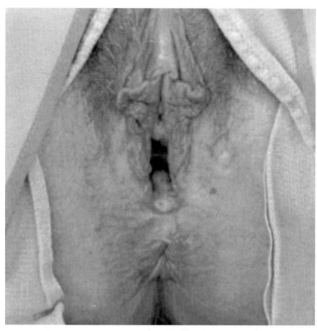

**FIGURE 32.26.** Narrowed and scarred perineal body from previous failed repair of obstetric injury.

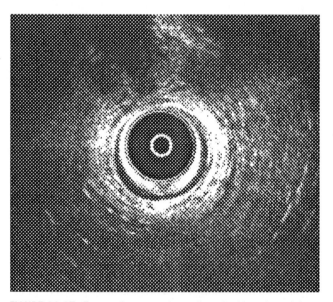

**FIGURE 32.27.** Transanal sonogram image through mid-anal canal showing internal and external anal sphincter defects.

leagues interviewed 47 of 55 patients who had undergone overlapping sphincteroplasty for obstetric injuries with a median follow-up of 77 months.[59] Earlier evaluation (15 months) of the entire group had found that 76% of 55 patients were continent to liquid and solid stool. Of 38 evaluable patients at later follow-up, 53% were using pads, and 66% reported restricting daily activities because of incontinence. New evacuation disorders developed in 37% of patients. These observations have recently been supported by discouraging data from the Cleveland Clinic, with only 14% of 63 patients reporting total continence at a median follow-up of

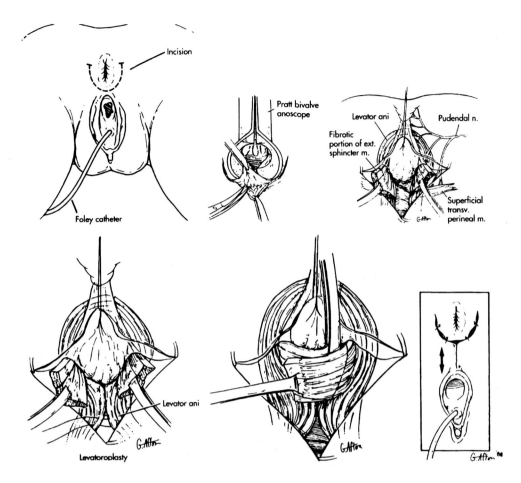

**FIGURE 32.28.** Overlapping sphincteroplasty. The patient is in the prone-jack-knife position. A curvilinear incision is made over the area of the internal anal sphincter and flaps are raised. The sphincter is dissected out, and the anterior scar is identified and maintained. Care is taken not to extend the dissection to the posterolateral positions bilaterally in order to avoid pudendal nerve injury. The midline scar is divided, and the scar and muscles are overlapped and secured with interrupted sutures (slowly absorbable or nonabsorbable). The perineal skin may require a Y- type closure to lengthen the perineal body. Reproduced with permission from Bernstein M. Rectovaginal fistula. In: Cameron JL, editor. Current surgical therapy. 6th ed. St. Louis: Mosby; 1998. p. 296.

69 months.[60] However, 15 of 63 patients (36%) reported the best possible FIQL score of 16.

Numerous procedures have been described for patients with neuropathic or idiopathic fecal incontinence and include pelvic floor repair, lengthening of the anal canal, and muscular adjuncts to the damaged sphincter muscle.[61] Sir Alan Parks described the post anal repair in 1975 as a procedure to restore the angle of the anorectal junction and increase the length of the anal canal.[62] The technical aspects of this procedure involve exposure and plication of the pubococcygeus, puborectalis, and ischiococcygeus muscles through the intersphincteric plane. Although early results of post anal repair were encouraging, with 74% of 140 patients reporting complete continence of liquid and semisolid stool, long-term results have been less favorable.[64,65] Only 28% of patients reported marked improvement after 2 years. In a series of 124 patients operated on during a 10-year period, 71% of patients followed for > 3 years reported an improvement in the degree of incontinence.[65] However, numerous physiologic parameters failed to reveal improvement of continence. Furthermore,

63% of patients continued to have some degree of soiling, with 50% continuing to use pads. Only 34% of patients were completely continent of liquids, solids, and gas.

Total pelvic floor repair as described by Keighley combines an anterior levatoroplasty and external sphincter plication with a standard post anal repair. Preliminary data from 20 patients included 10 patients who developed complete continence, 8 patients reported moderate benefit, and 2 patients had no improvement of symptoms.[65] Eleven additional patients who remained incontinent after post anal repair were treated with a staged total pelvic floor repair. Only 1 patient regained full control, 7 had some improvement, and 3 had no clinical benefit.

Muscle transposition is a surgical option when the sphincter muscle mass is significantly diminished or after multiple other attempts at less aggressive surgery have failed. The nonstimulated graciloplasty was first described by Pickrell and colleagues in 1952.[66] Although this muscular bulking procedure has had some success in children, the transposed gracilis cannot maintain the tonic high-pressure

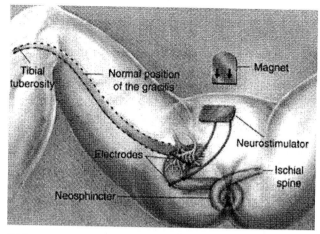

**FIGURE 32.29.** Configuration of the anal dynamic graciloplasty, showing the transposed gracilis muscle, electrodes, neurostimulator, and external magnet. After Baeten CGMI, Geerdes BP, Adang EMM, et al. Anal dynamic treatment of intractable fecal incontinency. N Engl J Med 1995;332:1600–5.

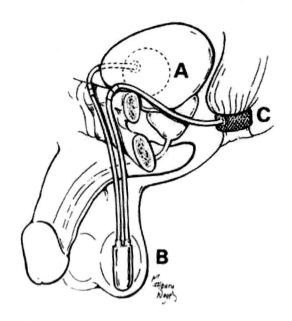

**FIGURE 32.30.** Artificial anal sphincter implanted in a male. The reservoir sits in the space of Retzius and is attached to a cuff surrounding the anal canal. Reproduced with permission from Wong WD, Jensen LL, Bartolo DCC, Rothenberger DA. Artificial anal sphincter. Dis Colon Rectum 1996;39:1345–51.

zone necessary to maintain continence in adults. However, chronic low-frequency stimulation of the native type 2 fast-twitch gracilis skeletal muscle fibers results in conversion to type 1 slow-twitch fibers, which are capable of prolonged contraction. Baeten and colleagues performed the first stimulated graciloplasty in 1986 in Maastricht (Fig. 32.29).[67] The results from his unit have been published on 52 patients.[68] At a median follow-up of 2.1 years, 73% of patients were continent. Median frequency of defecation decreased from 5 per 24 hours to 2 per 24 hours through week 156. Median time to defecation was significantly increased, as well as enema retention time.

A multicenter evaluation of dynamic graciloplasty (and gluteoplasty) has been published that includes the data from Maastricht.[69] One hundred thirty-nine patients were enrolled in 12 centers. Overall, 66% of patients who underwent graciloplasty achieved a successful outcome. Major wound complications occurred in 32% and included 13 cases of tissue necrosis of the anus, neoanus, or transposed muscle. Fourteen patients developed abscesses. A total of 102 reoperations were performed. Success and complication rates were significantly correlated with center experience. However, because of the high complication rate with frequent need for reoperation, the approval of the U.S. Food and Drug Administration was not sought for this application.

Gluteus maximus transposition has recently been revisited for treatment of refractory incontinence. Several small series have been reported with early success rates of 40 to 60%.[70,71] The variable anatomy of the inferior gluteal neurovascular supply adds to the technical problems associated with this procedure. In addition, stimulation of the gluteal muscles requires higher voltages, and the results for the stimulated gluteal transposition have not been as encouraging as for the graciloplasty.[69]

An artificial anal sphincter is under investigation, and several centers have reported success in a limited number of patients.[72–74] The artificial sphincter is a modification of the AMS 800 urinary sphincter made by American Medical Systems (Minneapolis, Minnesota). An inflatable cuff is positioned around the anus, and a pressure-regulated balloon reservoir is implanted in the space of Retzius (Fig. 32.30). A control pump is connected to the balloon and to the cuff and is implanted in the labia of a woman or the scrotum of a man. When the patient experiences the urge to defecate, the control pump is compressed, forcing water out of the cuff and into the reservoir. The cuff then refills gradually over 7 to 10 minutes, and continence is re-established. Data from a pilot study including 12 patients have been published.[74] There was no operative mortality, and overall morbidity was 33%. Nine patients (75%) reported improvement in continence and quality of life. A multicenter prospective trial has recently been completed but not published.

Success with sacral nerve stimulation in patients with urinary incontinence has led several investigators to pursue this therapy for fecal incontinence. Implantation of a permanent stimulator into five women for incontinence of solid or liquid stool resulted in improvements in continence scores (scale 0–20) from a median of 16 to 2.[75] Although one patient required lead replacement at 12 months, there were no early complications or side effects. Short-term physiologic results have been published from an additional 17 patients. Seventy-four percent of this group was completely continent of stool. Mean resting pressure, volume of voluntary contraction, volume of first sensation, pressure for urge to defecate, and volume for urge sensation were all significantly improved. These measures were maintained in 5 patients who went on to permanent stimulator implantation.

In contrast, Malouf and colleagues showed that there were no consistent alterations in physiologic measures that paralleled symptomatic improvements in patients implanted with a permanent stimulator.[75]

Finally, fecal diversion remains an option for those who have failed multiple attempts at sphincter repair or augmentation. Colostomy is also advocated for patients with severe neurologic dysfunction. End-colostomy is preferred by most surgeons for total fecal diversion. However, some patients with severe colonic dysmotility may benefit from ileostomy. As discussed for constipation, the ACE procedure is gaining popularity in the adult population and can be placed via minimally invasive techniques.[11–13]

## SUMMARY

Surgical management of colorectal and anorectal motility disorders requires careful assessment and planning as well as a substantial time investment for counseling. Although some mechanical problems such as rectal prolapse are easily treated with satisfactory long-term results, formidable challenges still exist in developing satisfactory and durable remedies to disorders of colonic motility and fecal storage and evacuation.

## REFERENCES

1. Pfeifer J, Agachan F, Wexner SD. Surgery for constipation: a review. Dis Colon Rectum 1996;39:444–60.
2. Drossman DA, Sandler RS, McKee DC, Loritz AJ. Bowel patterns among patients not seeking health care. Gastroenterology 1982;83:529–34.
3. Nyam DCNK, Pemberton JH, Ilstrup DM, Rath DM. Long-term results of surgery for chronic constipation. Dis Colon Rectum 1997;40:273–9.
4. Wexner SD, Daniel N, Jagelman DG. Colectomy for constipation: physiologic investigation is the key to success. Dis Colon Rectum 1991;34:851–6.
5. Sunderland GT, Poor FW, Lauder J, Finlay IG. Video-proctography in selecting patients with constipation for colectomy. Dis Colon Rectum 1992;35:235–7.
6. Redmond JM, Smith GW, Barofsky I, et al. Physiological tests to predict long-term outcome of total abdominal colectomy for intractable constipation. Am J Gastroenterol 1995;90:748–53.
7. Hosie KB, Kmiot WA, Keighley MR. Constipation: another indication for restorative proctocolectomy. Br J Surg 1990;77:801–2.
8. Martelli H, Devroede G, Arhan P, Duguay C. Mechanisms of idiopathic constipation: outlet obstruction. Gastroenterology 1978;75:623–31.
9. Fishbein RH, Handelsman JC, Schuster MM. Surgical treatment of Hirschsprung's disease in adults. Surg Gynecol Obstet 1986;163:458–64.
10. Pinho M, Yoshioka K, Keighley MRB. Long term results of anorectal myectomy for chronic constipation. Br J Surg 1989;76:1163–4.
11. Krogh K, Laurberg S. Malone antegrade continence enema for faecal incontinence and constipation in adults. Br J Surg 1998;85:974–7.
12. Shandling B, Chait PG, Richards BY. Percutaneous cecostomy: a new technique in the management of fecal incontinence. J Pediatr Surg 1996;31:534–7.
13. Rivera MT, Kugathasan S, Berger W, Werlin SL. Percutaneous colonoscopic cecostomy for management of chronic constipation in children. Gastrointest Endosc 2001;53:225–8.
14. Jurgeleit HC, Corman ML, Coller JA, et al. Procidentia of the rectum: Teflon sling repair of rectal prolapse, Lahey Clinic experience. Dis Colon Rectum 1975;18:464–7.
15. Duthie GS, Bartolo DCC. Abdominal rectopexy for rectal prolapse: a comparison of techniques. Br J Surg 1992;79:107–13.
16. Ripstein CB. Surgical care of muscle rectal prolapse. Dis Colon Rectum 1965;8:34–8.
17. Tjandra JJ, Fazio VW, Church JM, et al. Ripstein procedure is an effective treatment for rectal prolapse without constipation. Dis Colon Rectum 1993;36:501–7.
18. Gordon PH, Hoexter B. Complications of the Ripstein procedure. Dis Colon Rectum 1978;21:277–80.
19. Frykman HM, Goldberg SM. The surgical treatment of rectal procidentia. Surg Gynecol Obstet 1969;129:1225–30.
20. Kuijpers HC. Treatment of complete rectal prolapse: to narrow, to wrap, to suspend, to fix, to encircle, to placate or to resect? World J Surg 1992;16:826–30.
21. Altemeier WA, Culbertson WR, Schowengerdt CJ, et al. Nineteen years experience with the one stage perineal repair of rectal prolapse. Ann Surg 1971;173:993–1006.
22. Wassef R, Rothenberger D, Goldberg S. Rectal prolapse. Curr Probl Surg 1986;23:397–451.
23. Delorme R. Sue le traitement des prolapses du rectum toteaux pour l'excision de la mucueuse rectele ou rectocolique. Bull Mem Soc Chir Paris 1900;26:498.
24. Senapati A, Nicholls RJ, Thomson JPS, Phillips RKS. Results of Delorme's procedure for rectal prolapse. Dis Colon Rectum 1994;37:456–60.
25. Oliver GC, Vachon D, Eisenstat TE, et al. Delorme's procedure for complete rectal prolapse in severely debilitated patients. Dis Colon Rectum 1994;37:461–7.
26. Graf W, Stefansson T, Arvidssom D, Pahlman L. Laparoscopic suture rectopexy. Dis Colon Rectum 1995;38:211–2.
27. Weber AM, Walters MD, Ballard LA, et al. Posterior vaginal prolapse and bowel function. Am J Obstet Gynecol 1998;179:1446–9.
28. Bump RC, Mattiasson A, Bo K, et al. The standardization of terminology of female pelvic organ prolapse and pelvic floor dysfunction. Am J Obstet Gynecol 1996;175:10–7.
29. Francis WJ, Jeffcoate TN. Dyspareunia following vaginal operations. J Obstet Gynaecol Br Emp 1961;68:1–10.
30. Kahn MA, Stanton SL. Posterior colporrhaphy: its effects on bowel and sexual function. Br J Obstet Gynaecol 1997;104:882–6.
31. Sullivan ES, Leaverton GH, Hardwick CE. Transrectal perineal repair: an adjunct to improved function after anorectal surgery. Dis Colon Rectum 1968;11:196–214.
32. Murthy VK, Orkin BA, Smith LE, Glassman LM. Excellent outcome using selective criteria for rectocele repair. Dis Colon Rectum 1996;39:374–8.
33. Tjandra JJ, Ooi BS, Tang CL, et al. Transanal repair of rectocele corrects obstructed defecation if it is not associated with anismus. Dis Colon Rectum 1999;42:1544–50.
34. Richardson AC. The rectovaginal septum revisited: its relationship to rectocele and its importance in rectocele repair. Clin Obstet Gynecol 1993;36:976–83.
35. Cundiff GW, Addison WA. Management of pelvic organ prolapse. Obstet Gynecol Clin North Am 1998;25:907–21.
36. Cundiff GW, Weidner AC, Visco AG, et al. An anatomic and functional assessment of the discrete defect rectocele repair. Am J Obstet Gynecol 1998;179:1451–6.
37. Kenton K, Shott S, Brubaker L. Outcome after rectovaginal fascia reattachment for rectocele repair. Am J Obstet Gynecol 1999;181:1360–4.
38. Klosterhalfen B, Vogel P, Rixen H, et al. Topography of the inferior rectal artery: a possible cause of chronic, primary anal fissure. Dis Colon Rectum 1989;32:43–52.
39. Schouten WR, Briel JW, Auwerda JJ. Relationship between anal pressure and anodermal blood flow: the vascular pathogenesis of anal fissures. Dis Colon Rectum 1994;37:664–9.
40. Nothmann BJ, Schuster MM. Internal anal sphincter derangement with anal fissures. Gastroenterology 1974;67:216–20.

41. Carapeti EA, Kamm MA, McDonald PJ, et al. Randomised controlled trial shows that glyceryl trinitrate heals anal fissures, higher doses are not more effective, and there is a high recurrence rate. Gut 1999;44:727–30.

42. Lund JN, Scholefield JH. Follow-up of patients with chronic anal fissure treated with topical glyceryl trinitrate [letter]. Lancet 1998;352:1681.

43. Brisinda G, Maria G, Bentivoglio AR, et al. A comparison of injections of botulinum toxin and topical nitroglycerin ointment for the treatment of chronic anal fissure. N Engl J Med 1999;341:65–9.

44. Jost WH. One hundred cases of anal fissure treated with botulin toxin: early and long-term results. Dis Colon Rectum 1997;40:1029–32.

45. Jost WH, Schanne S, Mlitz H, et al. Perianal thrombosis following injection therapy into the external anal sphincter using botulinum toxin [letter]. Dis Colon Rectum 1995;38:781.

46. Notaras MJ. The treatment of anal fissure by lateral subcutaneous sphincterotomy—a technique and results. Br J Surg 1971;58:96–100.

47. Garcia-Aguilar J, Belmonte C, Wong WD, et al. Open vs. closed sphincterotomy for chronic anal fissure: long term results. Dis Colon Rectum 1996;39:441–3.

48. Nyam DCNK, Wilson RG, Stewart KJ, et al. Island advancement flaps in the management of anal fissures. Br J Surg 1995;2:326–8.

49. DeMarta DA. An approach to the recurrent or persistent anal fissure. Semin Colon Rectal Surg 1997;8:29–35.

50. Nelson R, Norton N, Cautley E, Furner S. Community based prevalence of anal incontinence. JAMA 1995;274:559–61.

51. Jorge JMN, Wexner SD. Etiology and management of fecal incontinence. Dis Colon Rectum 1993;36:77–97.

52. Rockwood TH, Church JM, Fleshman JW, et al. Patient and surgeon ranking of the severity of symptoms associated with fecal incontinence. Dis Colon Rectum 1999;42:1525–32.

53. Rockwood TH, Church JM, Fleshman JW, et al. Fecal Incontinence Quality of Life Scale: quality of life instrument for patients with fecal incontinence. Dis Colon Rectum 2000;43:9–16.

54. Certeceko GC, Fazio VW, Jagelman DG, et al. Anal sphincter repair: a report of 60 cases and a review of the literature. Aust N Z J Surg 1988;58:703–10.

55. Fleshman JW, Dreznick Z, Fry RD, Kodner IJ. Anal sphincter repair for obstetric injury: manometric evaluation of functional results. Dis Colon Rectum 1991;34:1061–7.

56. Gilliland R, Altomare DF, Moreira H Jr, et al. Pudendal neuropathy is predictive of failure following anterior overlapping sphincteroplasty. Dis Colon Rectum 1998;41:1516–22.

57. Simmang C, Birnbaum EH, Kodner IJ, et al. Anal sphincter reconstruction in the elderly: does advancing age affect outcome? Dis Colon Rectum 1994;37:1065–9.

58. Rasmussen O, Puggaard L, Christiensen J. Anal sphincter repair ipatients with obstetric trauma: age affects outcome. Dis Colon Rectum 1999;42:193–5.

59. Malouf AJ, Norton CS, Engel AF, et al Long-term results of overlapping anterior anal-sphincter repair for obstetric trauma Lancet 2000;355:260–5.

60. Halverson A, Hull T. Long-term repair of overlapping sphincteroplasty [abstract]. Dis Colon Rectum 2001;44:A10.

61. Pinho M, Keighley MRB. Results of surgery in idiopathic faecal incontinence. Ann Med 1990;22:425–33.

62. Parks AG. Anorectal incontinence. Proc R Soc Med 1975;68:681–9.

63. Browning GGP, Parks AG. Post-anal repair for neuropathic faecal incontinence; correlation of clinical results and anal canal pressures. Br J Surg 1983;70:101–4.

64. Jameson JS. Audit of postanal repair in the treatment of fecal incontinence. Dis Colon Rectum 1994;37:369–72.

65. Pinho M, Ortiz J, Oya M, et al. Total pelvic floor repair for the treatment of neuropathic fecal incontinence. Am J Surg 1992;163: 340–3.

66. Pickrell K, Georgiade N, Maguire C, Crawford H. Gracilis muscle transplant for rectal incontinence. Surgery 1956;40:34–63.

67. Baeten C, Spaans F, Fluks A. An implanted neuromuscular stimulator for fecal continence following previously implanted gracilis muscle: report of a case. Dis Colon Rectum 1988;31:134–7.

68. Baeten CG, Geerdes BP, Adang EM, et al. Anal dynamic treatment of intractable fecal incontinence. N Engl J Med 1995;332:1600–5.

69. Madoff RD, Rosen HR, Baeten CG, et al. Safety and efficacy of dynamic muscle plasty for anal incontinence: lessons from a prospective multicenter trial. Gastroenterology 1999;116:549–56.

70. Christiansen J, Ronholt Hansen C, Rasmussen O. Bilateral gluteus maximus transposition for anal incontinence. Br J Surg 1995;83:903–5.

71. Pearl RK, Prasad ML, Nelson RL, et al. Bilateral gluteus maximus transposition for anal incontinence. Dis Colon Rectum 1991; 34:478–81.

72. Christiansen J, Sparso B. Treatment of anal incontinence by an implantable prosthetic anal sphincter. Ann Surg 1992;215:383–6.

73. Wong WD, Jensen LL, Bartolo DCC, Rothenberger DA. Artificial anal sphincter. Dis Colon Rectum 1996;39:1345–51.

74. Lehur PA, Michot F, Denis P, et al. Results of artificial sphincter in severe anal incontinence: report of 14 consecutive implantations. Dis Colon Rectum 1996;39:1352–55.

75. Malouf AJ, Vaizey CJ, Nicholls RJ, Kamm MA. Permanent sacral nerve stimulation for fecal incontinence. Ann Surg 2000;232:143–8.

76. Ganio E, Luc AR, Clerico G, Trompetto M. Sacral nerve stimulation for treatment of fecal incontinence: a novel approach for intractable fecal incontinence. Dis Colon Rectum 2001;44:619–29.

CHAPTER 33

# Future Directions in Gastrointestinal Motility

*Kenneth L. Koch, Michael D. Crowell, and Marvin M. Schuster*

## INTRODUCTORY COMMENTS

This *Atlas* underscores the fact that the field of gastrointestinal (GI) motility is multidisciplinary and requires the integration of molecular and cell biology, organ physiology, and symptomatology. Thus, smooth muscle cells, neural circuits, interstitial cells of Cajal, hormones, gut–brain interactions, and emotions are all within the field of neuromuscular function and dysfunction of the gut.

It is well appreciated by clinicians that most patients with heartburn do not have esophageal ulcers, most patients with dyspepsia do not have a peptic ulcer, and most patients with constipation do not have mechanical obstruction of the colon. To diagnose GI motility disorders, clinicians must think beyond structural alterations of the gut.

The ongoing interaction of multiple disciplines is defining a new specialty—neurogastroenterology—with a focus on the study of the neuroenteric and hormonal functions of the gut and on the diagnosis and treatment of neuromuscular disorders. The neurogastroenterologist of the future will assess the normal and disturbed neuromuscular function of the GI and biliary tracts in relation to many poorly explained GI symptoms such as dysphagia, abdominal pain, nausea, bloating, and constipation.

Thus, the future of GI motility encompasses cells to systems. Future studies of individual cells such as the interstitial cells of Cajal will reveal new mechanisms that will uncover the origin of rhythmicity itself. Receptors that affect the function of the interstitial cells, as well as their rhythmic

and dysrhythmic activity, will be an exciting area for future studies in physiology and new therapeutics. The interaction of GI neuromuscular activity and the perception of symptoms is another area that is open for clinical investigation and new discoveries in physiology and pathophysiology. Studies that correlate GI neuromuscular dysfunction and GI symptoms will lead to new diagnostic tests and new drug and nondrug therapies. In the future, the relationships between treatment of neuromuscular dysfunction and improvement in symptoms will become clearer.

From the esophagus to the anal canal, each area of the GI tract has distinct and unique neuromuscular properties and whole organ functions. Thus, the smooth muscle cells of the esophagus need to be studied and compared with the smooth muscle cells of other GI organs. Likewise, the cells of the enteric nervous system throughout the GI tract have different roles in integrating neural and interstitial cell inputs to achieve normal neuromuscular function of the GI tract. The role of the intrinsic nervous system and the extrinsic parasympathetic and sympathetic nervous system inputs to the gut is still poorly understood, and further research is required. Whole animal research has been in decline in the past 20 years, and more efforts are needed in the future to integrate basic science studies, intact organ physiology, and animal and human studies of physiology of the digestive system. Neuromuscular function of the gut has an underappreciated role in hunger and satiety and should be investigated as it affects nutrition, obesity, and eating disorders.

## ESOPHAGUS

When neuromuscular abnormalities of the GI tract are present, symptoms may be severe, but the dysfunction of the particular organ is often subtle. Thus, for example, esophageal symptoms, such as dysphagia, atypical chest pain, and heartburn, are very common, but the barium swallow, upper GI series, and upper endoscopy are entirely normal in many patients. Findings such as transient lower esophageal sphincter relaxations are subtle neuromuscular abnormalities that have key roles in allowing the reflux of acid from the stomach into the esophagus. Another example of such subtlety of neuromuscular dysfunction is the sustained contractions of esophageal longitudinal muscle that is recorded in patients who have chest pain of esophageal origin. The longitudinal muscle contractions are detected by ultrasonographic methods, however, and not by typical intraluminal pressure catheters. Thus, refinements in measuring devices will also continue to reveal new and subtle neuromuscular dysfunctions that correlate with symptoms. In the future, new patterns of normal and abnormal neuromuscular activity of the esophagus will be described. These new technologies will lead to the appreciation of new pathophysiology patterns and new treatments.

## STOMACH

It is appreciated now that gastric intraluminal pressure transducers record only lumen-occluding contractions. Ultrasonography, scintigraphy, and magnetic resonance imaging reveal the more subtle non–lumen-occluding corpus and antral contractions, which are most prominent after ingestion of meals. Abnormalities of gastric myoelectrical rhythm are subtle electrical events that correlate with increased or decreased contractions and are associated with symptoms of nausea. Gastric dysrhythmias are not detected by radiography, endoscopy, or gastric emptying studies, but bradygastrias and tachygastrias affect gastric emptying patterns and are recorded in patients with dyspepsia symptoms. Failure of the gastric fundic muscle to relax is important in the generation of epigastric fullness and pain. Failure of the antrum and pylorus to relax normally also impedes proper gastric emptying. NOS-deficient mice develop gastroparesis and increased pyloric contractions, abnormalities that are reversed with sildenaphil or insulin therapy. On the basis of new pathophysiologic findings, new classes of drugs will be discovered to treat gastric electrical dysrhythmias, relax contracted gastric smooth muscle, and increase contraction of weak antral smooth muscle. Therapies in the future will range from antiarrhythmics to prokinetic and muscle relaxation agents to electrical stimulation and pacemaker therapies.

## BILIARY SYSTEM

The gallbladder and biliary tree continue to present many mysteries in neuromuscular function. Endoscopic retrograde cholangiopancreatography and biliary manometry have advanced our understanding in this area. Magnetic resonance cholangiopancreatography may also uncover functional aspects of this very complex area. Combined manometric and scintigraphic techniques will continue to advance diagnostic and therapeutic approaches in this very difficult area.

## SMALL BOWEL

The small bowel remains a very difficult area to study, and the mainstay method of motility investigation is solid-state or perfused catheters. Further information concerning the integration, coupling, and entrainment of the multiple electrical pacemakers of the small intestine may point the way toward successful electrical stimulation of the small intestine. The patterns of small bowel motility are difficult to interpret, but myopathies and neuropathies can be differentiated. Scintigraphy and breath hydrogen tests are used to determine oral-cecal transit times, but these measures have not been associated with particular GI symptoms. Video capsules may be modified to record pressure or myoelectrical events. Future developments may require new methodologic approaches such as the swallowed capsule to study the small intestine in health and disease.

## COLON

Interest in colonic neuromuscular function will continue in the future because irritable bowel syndrome and constipation symptoms are common and frequently debilitating. The descending and more proximal colon are difficult to study clinically in the intact human. The basic science knowledge of neuromuscular function of the right colon, transverse colon, or descending colon will be integrated further with colonic motility studies in health and disease in humans. New investigative tests are needed to study neuromuscular function of the colon, but it will be important to associate specific lower GI symptoms with abnormal neuromuscular function to make these tests clinically relevant.

## SPHINCTERS

We need new methodology and studies applied to the coordination of sphincters and adjacent nonsphincter muscle. Further developments in biofeedback therapy are needed to improve the technique and expand its border to other areas of the alimentary tract (as has been done with pelvic musculature).

## SUMMARY

In summary, over the past 9 years since the first *Atlas of Gastrointestinal Motility* was published, much has been accomplished in basic research and clinical areas of GI motility. Comparison of the two books emphasizes both the technological advances that have been made in measuring various aspects of motility and the more sophisticated understanding of neuromuscular activities of the gut that has been achieved. New technologies have uncovered new pathophysiologies, and all of these efforts will ultimately help to improve clinical diagnosis and to design new drug and nondrug therapies, such as biofeedback and electrical pacing. These therapies of the future will be used to correct many of the neuromuscular abnormalities of the GI tract and thus improve the associated symptoms.

Hopefully, this atlas will help the clinician and the researcher confront future challenges in the rapidly evolving field of GI motility and neurogastroenterology.

# INDEX